Clinical Progress in Sports Medicine

Clinical Progress in Sports Medicine

Edited by Ellis Baker

SYRAWOOD
PUBLISHING HOUSE
New York

Published by Syrawood Publishing House,
750 Third Avenue, 9th Floor,
New York, NY 10017, USA
www.syrawoodpublishinghouse.com

Clinical Progress in Sports Medicine
Edited by Ellis Baker

International Standard Book Number: 978-1-68286-623-8 (Hardback)

Cataloging-in-Publication Data

Clinical progress in sports medicine / edited by Ellis Baker.
p. cm.
Includes bibliographical references and index.
ISBN 978-1-68286-623-8
1. Sports medicine. 2. Clinical medicine. 3. Sports sciences. I. Baker, Ellis.
RC1210 .C55 2018
617.102 7--dc23

Printed in China.

TABLE OF CONTENTS

Preface IX

Chapter 1 **Experiences of Injuries and Injury Reporting among Swedish Skydivers** 1
Mats Jong, Anton Westman and Britt-Inger Saveman

Chapter 2 **The Effect of Acute *Rhodiola rosea* Ingestion on Exercise Heart Rate, Substrate Utilisation, Mood State, and Perceptions of Exertion, Arousal, and Pleasure/Displeasure in Active Men** 11
Michael J. Duncan and Neil D. Clarke

Chapter 3 **A Review of Treatments for Iliotibial Band Syndrome in the Athletic Population** 19
Corey Beals and David Flanigan

Chapter 4 **Validation of the Continuum of Care Conceptual Model for Athletic Therapy** 25
Mark R. Lafave, Dale Butterwick and Breda Eubank

Chapter 5 **Effects of Cooling on Ankle Muscle Strength, Electromyography, and Gait Ground Reaction Forces** 31
Amitava Halder, Chuansi Gao and Michael Miller

Chapter 6 **Immediate Effects of Neurodynamic Sliding versus Muscle Stretching on Hamstring Flexibility in Subjects with Short Hamstring Syndrome** 39
Yolanda Castellote-Caballero, Maríe C. Valenza, Emilio J. Puentedura, César Fernández-de-las-Peñas and Francisco Alburquerque-Sendín

Chapter 7 **Strength Gains as a Result of Brief, Infrequent Resistance Exercise in Older Adults** 47
James Fisher, James Steele, Pat McKinnon and Stephen McKinnon

Chapter 8 **A Structured and Flexible Language for Physical Activity Assessment and Characterization** 54
Pedro Silva, Maria Teresa Andrade, Pedro Carvalho and Jorge Mota

Chapter 9 **Nutritional Considerations for Performance in Young Athletes** 63
JohnEric W. Smith, Megan E. Holmes and Matthew J. McAllister

Chapter 10 **A Meta-Analysis of Soccer Injuries on Artificial Turf and Natural Grass** 76
Jay H. Williams, Emmanuel Akogyrem and Jeremy R. Williams

Chapter 11 **Functional Popliteal Artery Entrapment Syndrome: Poorly Understood and Frequently Missed? A Review of Clinical Features, Appropriate Investigations, and Treatment Options** 82
Matthew Hislop, Dominic Kennedy, Brendan Cramp and Sanjay Dhupelia

Chapter 12 **Validity and Reliability of Farsi Version of Youth Sport Environment Questionnaire**........90
Mohammad Ali Eshghi, Ramin Kordi, Amir Hossein Memari, Ahmad Ghaziasgar, Mohammad-Ali Mansournia and Seyed Hojjat Zamani Sani

Chapter 13 **Physiological and Psychophysical Responses to Listening to Music during Warm-Up and Circuit-Type Resistance Exercise in Strength Trained Men**........95
Hamid Arazi, Abbas Asadi and Morteza Purabed

Chapter 14 **Incidence and Time to Return to Training for Stress Fractures during Military Basic Training**........101
Alexander M. Wood, Richard Hales, Andre Keenan, Alexandra Moss, Michael Chapman, Trish Davey and Andrew Nelstrop

Chapter 15 **The Injury/Illness Performance Project (IIPP): A Novel Epidemiological Approach for Recording the Consequences of Sports Injuries and Illnesses**........106
Debbie Palmer-Green, Colin Fuller, Rod Jaques and Glenn Hunter

Chapter 16 **The Incidence of Concussion in a Professional Australian Rugby League Team, 1998–2012**........115
Jason Savage, Chloe Hooke, John Orchard and Richard Parkinson

Chapter 17 **Quantifying the "Slosh Stomach": A Novel Tool for Assessment of Exercise-Associated Gastroparesis Symptoms in Endurance Athletes**........122
Amy Sue Biondich and Jeremy D. Joslin

Chapter 18 **Examining Measures of Weight as Risk Factors for Sport-Related Injury in Adolescents**........127
Sarah A. Richmond, Alberto Nettel-Aguirre, Patricia K. Doyle-Baker, Alison Macpherson and Carolyn A. Emery

Chapter 19 **Graded Exercise Testing Protocols for the Determination of VO_2max: Historical Perspectives, Progress, and Future Considerations**........132
Nicholas M. Beltz, Ann L. Gibson, Jeffrey M. Janot, Len Kravitz, Christine M. Mermier and Lance C. Dalleck

Chapter 20 **Efficiency of an Active Rehabilitation Intervention in a Slow-to-Recover Paediatric Population following Mild Traumatic Brain Injury**........144
Sarah Imhoff, Philippe Fait, Frédérike Carrier-Toutant and Geneviève Boulard

Chapter 21 **A Scoping Review of the Associations of Golf with Eye Injuries in Adults and Children**........155
Evan Jenkins, Roger Hawkes and Andrew Murray

Chapter 22 **Muscle Activation Differs between Three Different Knee Joint-Angle Positions during a Maximal Isometric Back Squat Exercise**........161
Paulo Henrique Marchetti, Josinaldo Jarbas da Silva, Brad Jon Schoenfeld, Priscyla Silva Monteiro Nardi, Silvio Luis Pecoraro, Julia Maria D'Andréa Greve and Erin Hartigan

Chapter 23 **Validity of a Smartphone-Based Application for Determining Sprinting Performance**........167
Robert Stanton, Melanie Hayman, Nyree Humphris, Hanna Borgelt, Jordan Fox, Luke Del Vecchio and Brendan Humphries

Chapter 24 **Plasma Cytokine Profiles in Long-Term Strenuous Exercise**....172
Hilde G. Nielsen, Olav Øktedalen, Per-Kristian Opstad and Torstein Lyberg

Chapter 25 **The Influence of Methylsulfonylmethane on Inflammation-Associated Cytokine Release before and following Strenuous Exercise**....179
Mariè van der Merwe and Richard J. Bloomer

Chapter 26 **Comparison of Muscle Onset Activation Sequences between a Golf or Tennis Swing and Common Training Exercises using Surface Electromyography**....188
John M. Vasudevan, Andrew Logan, Rebecca Shultz, Jeffrey J. Koval, Eugene Y. Roh and Michael Fredericson

Chapter 27 **Cervical Spine Involvement in Mild Traumatic Brain Injury**....197
Michael Morin, Pierre Langevin and Philippe Fait

Chapter 28 **Trajectories of Physical Activity Predict the Onset of Depressive Symptoms but not their Progression**....217
Kaisa Kaseva, Tom Rosenström, Taina Hintsa, Laura Pulkki-Råback, Tuija Tammelin, Jari Lipsanen, Xiaolin Yang, Mirka Hintsanen, Christian Hakulinen, Katja Pahkala, Mirja Hirvensalo, Nina Hutri-Kähönen, Olli T. Raitakari and Liisa Keltikangas-Järvinen

Permissions

List of Contributors

Index

PREFACE

Sports medicine is a field of study that deals with the prevention and treatment of injuries occurring due to sports and exercise. It also studies and evaluates the overall physical fitness of athletes. Musculoskeletal injuries, underperformance syndrome, sports cardiology are some of the primary concerns of this field. This book explores all the important aspects of sports medicine in the present day scenario. It is compiled in such a manner, that it will provide in-depth knowledge about the theory and practice of sports medicine. The readers would gain knowledge that would broaden their perspective about the field.

All of the data presented henceforth, was collaborated in the wake of recent advancements in the field. The aim of this book is to present the diversified developments from across the globe in a comprehensible manner. The opinions expressed in each chapter belong solely to the contributing authors. Their interpretations of the topics are the integral part of this book, which I have carefully compiled for a better understanding of the readers.

At the end, I would like to thank all those who dedicated their time and efforts for the successful completion of this book. I also wish to convey my gratitude towards my friends and family who supported me at every step.

Editor

1

Experiences of Injuries and Injury Reporting among Swedish Skydivers

Mats Jong,[1,2] Anton Westman,[3] and Britt-Inger Saveman[4]

[1] *Department of Nursing, Mid Sweden University, Sundsvall, Sweden*
[2] *Mid Sweden Research & Development Centre, Västernorrland County Council, 851 70 Sundsvall, Sweden*
[3] *Department of Physiology and Pharmacology, Karolinska Institutet, 171 77 Stockholm, Sweden*
[4] *Department of Nursing, Umeå University, 901 87 Umeå, Sweden*

Correspondence should be addressed to Mats Jong; mats.jong@miun.se

Academic Editor: S. John Sullivan

The objective was to illuminate the experience of injuries and the process of injury reporting within the Swedish skydiving culture. Data contained narrative interviews that were subsequently analyzed with content analysis. Seventeen respondents (22–44 years) were recruited at three skydiving drop zones in Sweden. In the results injury events related to the full phase of a skydive were described. Risk of injury is individually viewed as an integrated element of the recreational activity counterbalanced by its recreational value. The human factor of inadequate judgment such as miscalculation and distraction dominates the descriptions as causes of injuries. Organization and leadership act as facilitators or constrainers for reporting incidents and injuries. On the basis of this study it is interpreted that safety work and incident reporting in Swedish skydiving may be influenced more by local drop zone culture than the national association regulations. Formal and informal hierarchical structures among skydivers seem to decide how skydiving is practiced, rules are enforced, and injuries are reported. We suggest that initial training and continuing education need to be changed from the current top-down to a bottom-up perspective, where the individual skydiver learns to see the positive implications of safety work and injury reporting.

1. Introduction

Skydiving, sport parachuting from aircraft, engages more than 800,000 participants in over one hundred countries who make more than 6 million jumps per year. It is a competitive sport with national and international championships in several disciplines [1].

Skydiving can be viewed as an "extreme sport," by being associated with a risk of death or serious injury [2]. Skydiving activities are dependent on rules and regulations issued by authorities, but it is also suggested that the policing role of more experienced skydivers sets limits of risk behavior to an even higher degree than formal regulations [3].

The risks associated with modern skydiving have not been satisfactorily described in the scientific literature. Because of lack of unified reporting systems and differences in definitions of injury, the reporting and comparisons of incidents and injuries are hard to make. Injury rates of 170 per 100,000 jumps with an accompanying hospital admission rate of 18 per 100,000 jumps have been reported from the United States [4] and similar rates have been reported from European countries [5–7]. In Sweden, an injury rate of 48 per 100,000 jumps has been reported [8].

Most countries in the world do not have reliable figures on the epidemiology of incidents and injuries. The International Parachuting Commission (IPC) has identified four member countries (France, Finland, Norway, and Sweden) which collect reliable and valid data as the countries have compulsory national routines for reporting of injury events. The IPC has a reporting system for injuries and fatal incidents, but severe problems in acquiring reliable data have made it necessary to identify elements that may influence the reporting culture in the different member states [1]; that is, what makes the individual skydiver choose to abide to formal rules connected to reporting of incidents and injuries.

Studies of Swedish skydiving have used epidemiological designs to describe fatal and nonfatal injury events [8, 9]. A report is compulsory for an incident/injury that leads to a health care visit [10]. The validity of the nonfatal data may be questioned since the performance of the compulsory Swedish system has been reported as having a sensitivity of 0.37 and a specificity of 0.91 [11]. Reasons for this grave underreporting of injuries, several of which were serious or even life threatening, are not known. Social or cultural factors that may play a role are difficult to assess through epidemiological quantitative designs.

A qualitative interview study may provide grounds for understanding and clarifying why individuals, despite the compulsory reporting obligations, choose not to report adverse events [11]. A study from Wales found "culture," or more specifically, "reporting culture" among surgeons to be one explanatory variable for a discrepancy between surgeons and theatre nurses. Approximately 55% of surgeons and 91.5% of theatre nurses report all or more than 50% of mucocutaneous and percutaneous injuries occurring in operating theatres. The cumbersome administrative procedure, the attitude, personal characteristics of the surgeon, and lack of feedback were given as important reasons for not reporting incidents [12]. According to Roberts and Rousseau [13], can management attitudes and institutional climate greatly influence the success or failure of reporting efforts in high reliability organizations. In high-reliability theory, incident reporting/response systems are important instruments to effectively synthesize and share information with the relevant people across an organization so that appropriate action can be made to prevent or reduce the risk of accidents and disasters [14]. This is also the basic idea for reporting incident and injury events within the sport of skydiving. For instance, a reported incident related to technical failure of a specific piece of the parachute equipment may lead to modification or market withdrawal.

Although most skydivers are pursuing their air sport as a leisure time activity and not as a job, individual, organizational, subcultural (e.g., "reporting culture"), and social aspects may influence the motivation and other incentives to report incidents and injuries. To date, no studies have given voice or studied how skydivers describe events leading to incidents and injury, or how this relates to injury risks and injury reporting.

The objective of the present study was to illuminate the experience of injuries and the process of injury reporting within the Swedish skydiving culture.

2. Method

This study is based on a qualitative approach, where data was collected in narrative interviews that were subsequently analyzed with content analysis [15]. A qualitative study can provide a scientific ground to interpret phenomena on the basis of the meanings the studied group of people assign them [16].

2.1. Respondents. Inclusion of respondents was made through a convenience sampling procedure; that is, respondents readily at hand and willing to participate in the study were interviewed. Respondents were recruited through a personal contact on three different skydiving drop zones in Sweden. Efforts were made to include respondents from a broad spectrum of skydivers regarding age, sex, and experience of skydiving.

Twenty people were invited to the study; three chose not to participate because of time constraints. The total sample of 17 respondents consisted of six women and 11 men between the ages of 22 and 44 (median = 29). They had been skydiving between one and 25 years (median = 6) and had made between 14 and 3400 jumps (median = 750).

2.2. Interviews. Each interview began with a short presentation of the study, followed by a broad question "Could you please tell me about events where you have been injured or have nearly injured yourself while skydiving?" Follow-up questions, if necessary, were asked in accordance with an interview guide (Table 1). Interviews were digitally recorded and lasted between half an hour and two hours and were later transcribed verbatim. The interviews were conducted in places chosen by the respondents, either at drop zones, at respondents' home, in cafés, or at their work.

2.3. Data Analysis. The text data underwent a qualitative content analysis where an attempt was made to determine and interpret both the manifest (what is said) and the latent content (what it means) of the text, referred to as categories and/or themes [15, 17]. The description of the analytic procedure is simplified as the three steps that were intertwined and overlapping.

The First Step. To achieve an overall understanding of the text, each transcript was read several times. Along with the reading, meaning units were identified and given a temporary code in the body of the text. The coding was used to more easily link and sort text passages connected to each other.

The Second Step. During the process of coding and sorting the meaning units, three categories, were identified. In the first category named *descriptions of incidents and injury events,* a coding scheme was used. The scheme that aimed to describe mechanisms in skydiving injuries (phase of jump, mechanism of incident, and mechanism of injury) was developed by Ellitsgaard [6] and further developed by Westman and Björnstig [8]. We used one part of the scheme as a phase of deduction to gain better comprehensive understanding (c.f. Ricoeur [18], page 71–88). The categories *human factor as a contributor to incidents and injuries* and *organization and leadership as facilitators or constrainers for reporting* emerged inductively; that is, no premade coding scheme was used and they were formulated from the manifest

Table 1: The interview guide.

Yourself as a skydiver	What constitutes skydiving culture for you	Injuries during skydiving?
(i) Favorite way to skydive (ii) Positive and negative aspects as a skydiver (iii) Deliberately putting yourself in potentially dangerous situations (iv) Affected by others to stretch limits	(i) Skydiving culture versus other sport cultures (ii) In your own club, other clubs, internationally (iii) Experiences while skydiving or being on other drop zones	(i) Descriptions of events leading to injury, the injury itself (ii) Emergency procedures (iii) Incidents/near injury events (iv) Thoughts and feelings before and after incidents and injury (v) Injury reported to SFF (vi) If injured, why continue
Risk behavior—yours and others	**Differences between male and female skydivers**	**Safety issues**
(i) Reporting, grounding (ii) Discussions on club or national level (iii) Talking to risk takers, what do you say and how do they react	(i) The way to skydive (ii) Risk taking (iii) Attitudes (iv) Injuries (v) Skill and expertise	(i) Strategies for your own safety (ii) Strategies to identify others' safety issues (iii) Suggestions or ideas for improvement of safety issues (iv) Educative efforts (v) Rules and regulations

content of the text passages relating to incidents and injury events and the reporting of incidents.

The Third Step. this step aimed to compare prior steps, codes, and categories with the entire text to obtain a sense of what it is about, to seek and identify a common theme, and to more comprehensively understand and interpret the findings. The identified theme named *skydiving culture—A place for joy, playfulness, and safety awareness* provides a description and an understanding of the cultural context present throughout the prior identified categories.

2.4. Ethical and Methodological Considerations. The research performed in this study is not regulated by the Swedish legislation of research on humans [19]. The authors took into account ethical issues that may have appeared through pursuing the study.

Prior to each interview, the interviewer informed the respondent of the study's aim, how long the interview would take, that participation was voluntary, and that the respondent could terminate study participation at any time. The interviewer also informed the respondent that no individual would be named and that respondent integrity and confidentiality would be respected in the presentation of the findings.

In order to enhance trustworthiness and transferability [15], the structuring and analytic procedure was regularly discussed among the three authors. When necessary, codes, categories, and theme were revised, reorganized, added, or omitted to account for the interrelations of the parts and the whole. A second way trustworthiness and transferability [15] was enhanced was through presenting and discussing findings in a group comprised by an expert panel of ten skydiving instructors associated with various skydiving clubs in Sweden. The discussion confirmed the general content of categories and theme and no additional changes were made. In the presentation of quotes, the numbers within parentheses represents the consecutive number of the interviewee; *m* refers to male and *f* to female.

The first two authors (Mats Jong and Anton Westman) are experienced skydivers with approximately 25 years each in the sport. Their preunderstanding was a necessary requisite to conduct interviews with skydivers on their own terms, that is, by sharing the same language and culture. Mats Jong and Anton Westman had no personal connections to the respondents prior to the interview. During the interviews, all respondents were perceived by the interviewers as being able to speak easily and freely even though the subjects related to experiences of incidents, injury, and death. During the analysis, the two interviewers strived to put their preunderstanding in the background to stay open for what came out from the text. The third author (Britt-Inger Saveman) had no previous knowledge or experience in the sport but had extensive knowledge in the methodology used and the topic of injury and injury prevention; thereby, the author has been able to approach the topic without preunderstanding.

In this study, the term "skydiving culture" refers to each respondent's self-defined notion and what it means to them from an individual perspective, including how they experience its relation to injury risks and injury reporting.

3. Results

To present an overall understanding of the topic and the context of the skydiving culture, the theme is presented first, followed by the three categories.

3.1. Skydiving Culture—A Place for Joy, Playfulness, and Safety Awareness. Skydivers express a constant awareness of imminent injury or death balanced by the positive experiences of being able to pursue the sport. Participating in skydiving activities is interpreted as including a form of risk negotiation where the risk of potential injury is balanced against individual benefits in the form of pleasure, progression, and learning in skydiving. In the narratives, it is possible to identify attitudes of risk behavior differing between males and females; caution is referred to as a feminine characteristic, and the will to develop and progress by pushing limits is referred to as a masculine characteristic. Regardless of the gender of the skydiver, these attitudes toward risk behavior remained the same.

> *"It's about the same as anywhere else, girls are not that eager to show off or show how tough they are; girls care more about safety, and at the same time a bit timid and do not dare to test their limits. In that sense, it's a kind of danger too because they need to learn too. In the end, I believe guys turn out as more skillful skydivers, but girls probably think more about how they do things. (1, f, 150 jumps)"*

Skydiving is viewed as a sport where males and females can participate and compete on equal terms, but in relation to risk exposure and behavior a recurrent attitude is that it differs between males and females.

Joy, playfulness, and safety awareness are expressed by both experienced skydivers and those new in the sport. These aspects are associated with several dimensions of interaction relating not only to a sense of belonging to a special group, but also to the direct experience of in-air activities. The aspects of social life and community are also described as important by the respondents:

> *"Skydiving contains elements of joy in a higher degree than other sports. Many sports tend to focus on the elite athlete, but even though we have systems of supporting the elite competitors, there is so much that's just playing—just for fun! Many skydivers jump for several years without competing, or even practicing for competition—they do it just for the fun of doing it. I believe that is unusual in other sport activities. (13, f, 300 jumps)"*

Both the degree of playfulness and the degree of safety awareness are interpreted as dependent on the subculture of the local drop zone. Respondents that have skydived abroad express the view that there is a higher degree of safety awareness among Swedish skydivers compared with skydivers in other countries. Safety awareness and playfulness are interwoven in the culture of the sport where fellow skydivers, for example, check each other's equipment prior to boarding the aircraft. A skydiving novice expressed it as:

> *"Safety awareness does not make you less cool, it's quite fantastic that people push for safety (7, f, 90 jumps)."*

Skydiving can be dangerous but the experiences of joy and delight outweighs the thoughts of giving up the sport. A view is that "every" skydiver knows that each skydive is a potential injury event or could even lead to death. Risk and injury are considered a constant ingredient in skydiving and the respondents think about it differently. Some want to make the sport as safe as possible, even if it means more regulations are needed while others express "pushing the limits" individually as part of learning what skydiving is or can be. Crossing the limit can lead to injury, but pushing the limit may also lead to learning. An expressed attitude is that the sport and its pursuers are individualists and hence responsible for their own risk-taking acts leading to incidents. Incidents and critical events lead to reflections of one's own and others' risk in the sport. Such incidents can serve as eye openers and affect the attitude toward skydiving. An experienced skydiver puts this into words:

> *"Once again, you have an eye-opener and think about the risks in skydiving. I think more of an attitude to life when I think, for example, of an accident like this (a friend's death); you are reminded how fragile life is and how fast it may end. Back again to this respect, an awareness that is so important to hold on to. I am definitely guilty of losing it from time to time, when I just push through, and everything works fine. At the same time, I am so grateful to be here and do what we do, and if that has affected my attitude to skydiving, I'm unsure. Still, it is a reminder to respect what we are doing and not to forget that. (4, m, 2300 jumps)"*

When asked what constitutes "skydiving culture" the respondents often reflect around evening parties and drinking beer. As expressed in the narratives, the safety control system that aimed to prevent incidents with skydivers under the influence of alcohol seems to work properly; often because of self-regulation where individuals stay on the ground when they have drunk too much the previous day. A breath alcohol tester is used to confirm that the skydiver is not intoxicated and ready to jump. Even if the control system works well, the respondents claim that it fails from time to time and some jump despite the control system. Reflecting on skydiving culture, a respondent says:

> *"Well I think about case, for example, and it's nice. That's what really constitutes skydiving culture; drinking beer. Unfortunately it is so. I say unfortunately, it is not so serious to tell new students, "ah well, when you're done with your student training, you're supposed to buy beer and case with it." Some students had a cake instead, really much nicer and more fun. Case is simple, just buy beer, it happens all the time, so it constitutes skydiving culture. (10, m, 800 jumps)"*

Authors note: case is a tradition of buying fellow skydivers "a case of beer" when passing through different check points or levels in the skydiving sport, for example, after completing student training, first 8-way formation, and first jump from hot air balloon.

3.2. Descriptions of Incidents and Injury Events. All respondents in this study had experienced incidents or injury incidents associated with skydiving that occurred at different phases of a jump: from aircraft exit, free fall, parachute opening, parachute flight, and landing. During aircraft exit, bruising and minor lacerations are mentioned as well as strained arms when exiting late while the other group members jump off the plane. Several incidents were described as caused by inadequate separation from other skydivers in free fall resulting in or nearly resulting in impact with other skydivers, evoking fear and anger. A respondent describes an incident.

> *"Well, there was this scary thing which happened; a kind of close call, some guy opened his parachute below me during a big-way jump (authors' remark; in a formation skydiving jump with 20 other skydivers), which scared me a lot. I was terrified and landed with tears in my eyes. (8, f, 350 jumps)"*

Several incidents happened during parachute opening, for example, when total or partial malfunctions of the main parachute necessitated reserve parachute activation. Examples of malfunctions were twisted lines resulting in violently spinning main parachutes or inability to release steering toggles. In conjunction to malfunctions, injury events have occurred because of reduced plan time for a normal parachute landing, or an increased sink rate because of malfunction or a smaller reserve parachute. Free fall instability during deployment of the parachute has resulted in events described as "horse shoe malfunctions" causing, for example, a sprained ankle while landing under two parachutes.

Incidents associated with wing parachute flight include, for example, downwind landing (high speed—more difficult to come to a stop) resulting in a fractured wrist and several near miss mid-air collision incidents at low altitude. Other examples of incidents include experienced skydivers describing incidents when they miscalculate hook turns, resulting in bruises and fractures. A respondent who fractured an ankle says,

> *"Well, once I injured my ankle. I made a turn, kind of low, honestly speaking. I flared too low and hit the grass. It was a hook turn where I waited too long to flare, I landed on my feet but it hurt a lot in one foot. In a way I was lucky, it could have turned out a lot worse if I had been a couple of decimetres lower. (15, m, 1300 jumps)"*

Basically, all respondents gave descriptions of incidents or injury events associated with landing, some resulting in bruises, scratches, sprains, and strains but also more severe injuries including sprained crucial ligaments and fractures of legs and spines. Events occurred both during unintentional and intentional high-speed landings but also in normal low-speed landings. The quote below from a respondent shows an example of the complexity in an injury event while landing outside the drop zone:

> *"Well, everything looked just fine. I was planning to land at the nicest spot on the area of clear-cut forest, right in between two tree stumps. It was hard to plan the exact position, but I thought that I could land there. But as I came lower I saw that there was an uprooted tree pointing straight up making the landing area less optimal, at that time I had no choice. I had to land there. My idea was to land in front of one stump and jump over it. It looked just fine, but wasn't under the grass. I stumbled when my feet reached the ground. My feet stuck and my body continued, hands down in full flare (Authors remark; braking), with no chance to catch myself. My head went straight into the tree stump and everything turned black, and I could hear my neck and back crunch. (2, m, 150 jumps)"*

3.3. Human Factor as a Contributor to Incidents and Injuries. Inadequate judgment such as miscalculations and failing to pay attention dominates these descriptions as causes to incidents. Additionally, a number of events are described as possibly attributing to female skydivers having less muscular strength than male skydivers.

Miscalculation of exit point from aircraft is described as a factor causing landings outside (forest areas, roads, and in pasture-land) the drop zones (the designated landing area). Another described miscalculation relates to landings at drop zones but where the respondents nearly hit ground obstacles.

A lack of insight into one's own competence and neglecting to undergo proper training about flight characteristics of new equipment was described that as resulting in injuries, for example, using a new wing parachute and realizing that it flew faster at landing than anticipated. Failing in attention and judgment was described as affecting reasons for deviating from set plans, leading to incidents and at times injuries, especially in connection with high speed landings. Parachute traffic, inadequate preparation, and lack of concentration were other reasons mentioned. An experienced respondent gives an example of how different distractions compounded while performing a high speed landing led to an incident:

> *"What really happened during that jump was that I deviated from my original plan and began improvising, simultaneously other things happened. I had some kind of attention overload, approaching in a different angle than I was used to, the wind had changed, and additionally there were other parachutes drawing attention. I judged that I would be able to turn around and approach in the direction I was aiming to, which added some extra degrees to my turn, and since I had to pay attention to some other chutes I probably had lost some altitude before I initiated my turn. (4, m, 2300 jumps)"*

A recurrent statement from the respondents is that females and males perform skydiving in different ways. Mentioned by both sexes is the view that females by flying their parachutes too passively do not learn the flying characteristics of their parachute, which may lead to increased risk of injury when encountering situations requiring flexibility and fast unreflective response. An experienced respondent puts this in words by saying,

> *"I believe guys hurt themselves for other reason than girls. I can imagine guys hurt themselves more because they are pushing themselves a little*

bit harder, exceeding their limits. I imagine girls hurt themselves more, not necessarily because they push themselves, but rather because they cannot handle the situation. I believe that if you would expose guys and girls to—it may sound prejudiced, but I believe that if you put guys and girls in exactly the same situations, then girls would suffer more injuries. (6, m, 1400 jumps)"

Respondents give examples of when they have been unable to deploy their parachute because of not being able to locate the main parachute activation handle or not having the strength to pull it out—resulting in a need to activate the reserve parachute.

3.4. Organization and Leadership as Facilitators or Constrainers for Reporting. Whether or not an incident or an injury event is reported to the Swedish Parachuting Association (Svenska Fallskärmsförbundet, SFF) is expressed as depending on a number of distinct reasons. Important emerging issues relate to an individuals' knowledge and definition of what injuries are supposed to be reported, the safety and reporting culture at the local drop zone, organizational structure, and the administration of reports. Additionally, the hierarchical structure in the skydiving culture serves either as a facilitator or a constrainer for reporting. The respondents describe comparable injuries that may be reported in some circumstances but not in others. A recurring view among respondents is that injury severity influences injury reporting propensity. Minor bruises and distortions are described as commonly occurring but rarely reported, whereas major injuries (e.g., fractures) are described as being reported to a higher degree. An important incentive to send in a report is whether the injured person expects long-term consequences, for instance, if the injury may lead to impaired mobility. Respondents report that the regulations are complex and wish for more clarity in some aspects:

"Today we have all these forms and what is written in the regulations for skydiving, and then it's not, per definition, really an injury (describing a frostbite), more plain stupidity. I consider the regulations good in many ways, but some issues are dense and stupid. And the form for reporting, maybe we could have incidents on three levels: incidents, injuries, and injuries defined as physical injury; that may include frostbite by definition, but I believe it is not done. (3, m, 1300 jumps)"

An expressed desire is to see the positive implications from reporting and to be given feedback from the skydiving association and the local club on how the administration of reporting benefits the skydiving community. The respondents also express a need to update and modernize the reporting system. Additionally more experienced skydivers need to take more responsibility in teaching newcomers about reporting and safety issues and to a higher degree enforce the formal routines on the drop zones. A novice female respondent expresses it as follows:

"I think it is laziness which decides if you report or not. You need to fill out all these papers, and that's strenuous. I think you would do it if there's a routine—if I sprain my ankle, someone should come and put that paper in my hand and say that I must do it. If not for that, I would actually not have a thought of reporting. For people like me, you know, I have no routine on how to do it. Other people on the drop zone must show me how to. (7, f, 90 jumps)"

Although report submission is part of the jump leader's duties, respondents point out that during jump days, the jump leader is quite busy which may constrain reporting of incidents and injuries

Authors note: on a Swedish skydiving drop zone on a given jump day, ultimate responsibility for safety issues is bestowed an assigned instructor, the jump leader. This person is also responsible to make sure that all incidents related to equipment malfunctions, and injuries leading to health care contacts are reported [10].

The role of the jump leader is, according to the respondents, quite unclear among many skydivers, which may contribute to a chaotic situation when incidents occur. Another task of the jump leader, which is highlighted in most interviews, is the commission of restraints as a consequence from unsafe actions or rule violation behavior. What decides if the jump leader acts or not is described as depending on who is reporting and who made the violation. When an experienced skydiver violates regulations resulting in incidents, jump leaders are described as having different incentives not to confront them; sometimes it may be due to an anticipated negative reaction, or they may hesitate because the skydiver is more experienced than themselves. An experienced respondent says,

"If they would tell me that I am grounded because of unsafe behavior, then I would take the discussion at the end of the day. But, at the same time, if I am aware that what I was doing was wrong, then I would accept the decision. I think it's necessary to enforce the authority and formal assignment, but my opinion is that not many jump leaders do so. The experience level should not be so influential because the rules are clear, you can be experienced or inexperienced and as long as there are rules and regulations you should stick to them. (6, m, 1400 jumps)"

An expressed view in the narratives is that skydiving clubs in Sweden tend to interpret the national regulations in various ways, which also affects incident reporting. Some clubs are believed to conform to the regulations very strictly and even enforce higher demands than the national regulations on their members by, for example, totally prohibiting high-speed landings. On the other side of the spectrum are clubs, which are considered less conforming to the regulations, informally, allowing people to use equipment not suitable to their experience level.

Depending on the openness of the local drop zone, it is described that skydivers occasionally avoid showing other skydivers that they hurt themselves. Thereby injuries are not reported for fear of exposing themselves as having made a bad judgment or being embarrassed for having poor skills.

4. Discussion

The Swedish national rules and regulations regarding safety aspects seem to suggest conformity in the country as a whole regarding skydiving activities, but present results imply the opposite. The respondents express variability between the Swedish clubs (drop zones) regarding safety issues and abidance to national rules and regulations. This is in line with a previous finding of variability between the Swedish clubs regarding reported nonfatal injury rates 1999–2003 [8] and also with findings of Laurendeau and van Brunschot [3], suggesting that the individual skydiver listens more to fellow skydivers than to rules and regulations about safety measures and skill level required to, for example, jump with a specific parachute or start performing high speed landings.

On the individual level, the interpretation is that the risk of injury is viewed as an integrated element of the recreational activity, counterbalanced by its recreational value. The balancing act between risk of injury, death, and recreational value has several implications. In our study respondents claim that they have awareness when their limit is reached and back off when they come too close to the line of danger. However, they simultaneously expressed that challenging the limits is a means of progression and learning. Challenging the limits is described by Lyng [20] as an act of "edgework," where the person explores the limits of his/her ability and/or the technology used while maintaining enough control to successfully negotiate the edge. Laurendeau and van Brunschot [3] develop this further in the skydiving context, saying that edge workers sustain an illusion of control when they are "crowding the edge." In high-risk skydiving activities, if injuries do occur, edgework can represent an attempt to push the responsibility away from them, to someone else or some other factor outside themselves. Several experienced respondents in our study who have had incidents and injuries express a high degree of self-responsibility, taking into account that incidents happen to them because of their own poor judgment (human error) or lack of skill. Noticeably, they acknowledge their own deficiencies but might be influenced by interview directions, where they were encouraged to speak from their own self-experienced perspective and not so much from how they perceive the skill of others. The results are similar to Laurendeau and van Brunschot [3], where it also was expressed that skydivers acknowledged occurred incidents as situations for learning and progressing. Our finding is also to some extent contrasting to the study of Laurendeau and van Brunschot [3], where participants expressed a distance between themselves and those who suffered from injury or died, stating that the "other person" was doing things that they would never do. They took a stance of "blaming the victim," possibly with a subconscious objective to preserve their own sense of control over risks in the sport.

Landing errors due to poorly executed high speed landings have, worldwide, become an important cause of skydiving-related injuries and deaths [1, 21]. Parachute associations and parachute manufacturers' recommend that only highly skilled skydivers perform these maneuvers, but only a limited number of countries or drop zones use regulations to prevent inexperienced skydivers from performing high speed landings [10, 22]. Nevertheless, drop zones, parachute associations, regulatory authorities, and the skydiving community itself have acknowledged the need for skydivers to be better educated about canopy control and are, hence, arranging canopy piloting courses on basic and advanced levels all over the world (http://www.dropzone.com/).

One of the jump leaders' policing duties includes alcohol use, because in Sweden, as in most countries, it is prohibited to skydive under the influence of alcohol and drugs [10]. From our findings, it appears that alcohol consumption and partying are integrated elements in Swedish skydiving culture, as in the North American and Australian skydiving cultures [23–26]. Control systems exist to prevent skydivers from jumping under the influence of alcohol (jump leader, breath testers), but a previous study [9] found that two out of the 37 fatalities in Swedish skydiving 1964–2003 had a blood alcohol level elevated to the point of impairing cognitive functions [27]. Problems and potential risks in skydiving associated with alcohol and illicit drug use need to be more clearly addressed in the safety work within the skydiving community. In line with the discussion above, it may be most important at the local drop zone level.

Worth noting is that respondents have described some incidents relating to the free fall sequence. In Sweden, a hard helmet is compulsory until you have a B-license (>100 jumps after student status) [10], but as a voluntary action most skydivers in Sweden, regardless of rating, use hard helmets to prevent injury [3]. This may be described as a self-policing act. In surfing the reverse is seen, where experienced surfers make the choice not to use head protection, referring to impaired hearing and feeling restrained [28].

From the findings, we can see that inadequate judgment is described as a major cause and contributing factor to incidents. There are other contributors, which conjointly result in an unwanted event. Stressors affecting judgment can emerge during the full sequence of a jump, from prejump activities to landing. When several stressors emerge simultaneously, the person is at risk of making a hasty/bad decision. This is similar to the concept of "sensory overload," where input of several "never-ending" cognitive stimuli results in mood changes and irrational psychological behavior [29].

The incidents or injury events described in this study chiefly appear to be perceived by the respondents as attributable to human error (i.e., inadequate decision). Reasons for this operator-oriented view among respondents might be connected to their levels of knowledge, insights of the risk associated with the sport, and their innate motivation for pursuing the sport. The complexity of the chain of events leading to an incident can, at times, be connected to the equipment used; for example, the placing of handles for deploying the reserve parachute may be different depending on bodily position. Problems with the technical equipment (airplane, parachute, altimeters, helmets, etc.) are, in general, rare and not explicitly mentioned by the respondents in this study. Technical equipment is controlled for quality and accuracy in order to adhere to industrial standards. Nevertheless, there are equipment-related incidents mentioned by the respondents that possibly occurred due to insufficient muscular strength. Skydivers need to test the deployment systems on the ground from time to time to ensure that they have sufficient muscle strength to activate their parachute, and additionally the parachute industry must continue to monitor their standards to prevent gear-related incidents.

Our results suggest that the skydiving community and subculture have an influence on safety awareness and on reporting of incidents and injuries among Swedish skydivers. It is, in line with high-reliability theory [14], necessary to raise this issue further to understand how subculture can facilitate reporting so that appropriate action can be taken to prevent or reduce the risk of incidents and injuries. Healthcare researchers [12] and other high reliability organizations [13] have similarly put forth issues of subculture and workplace climate factors, such as burdensome administration and lack of feedback, as obstacles for reporting. Barach and Small [30] have, in other types of aviation, noted similar results where fear of reprisal, lack of trust, code of silence, and skepticism are mentioned as reporting barriers.

It may not only be necessary to identify errors for reporting, the people involved in the "culture" need to see the results and how it is used in order to see the meaning of from reporting. In a study by Waring [31], the participating physicians see reporting as pointless, since the "errors are an inevitable and potentially unmanageable feature of medical work." Another article from the healthcare setting puts forth that incident reporting does have a role in safety work and care processes, by indirectly affecting the attitudes and knowledge of those working there [32]. Barach and Small [30] conclude that confidential incident reporting systems have a decisive role in identifying errors on the system level and that it is necessary to shift from a punitive to a collaborative mindset that seeks to identify and understand the underlying system failures. In that sense, reporting circumvents the culture of blame [31].

In this study, "skydiving culture" as a concept was understood from the participants self-defined understanding. A more comprehensive and complex concept of skydiving culture, including issues of gender, injury risks, risk behavior, and subculture has been scrutinized from a sociological perspective by several authors in the North American and Australian contexts [3, 23, 26, 33], Wade [24], and Brymer [25] in the North American and Australian contexts.

Organization and leadership aspects within the skydiving community can serve both as facilitators as well as constrainers to reporting. Following this line, perhaps a way of addressing safety issues and improving incident and injury reporting would be to work bottom up instead of top down, to initiate/promote discussions at local drop zones, educate jump leaders more thoroughly, and influence all categories of skydivers to reflect on how they pursue skydiving, the related risk taking, and incidents. This has similarities to the conclusions from a review on the safety systems topic within healthcare settings where it was stressed that in order to learn the lesson and take adequate actions inside and across organizations, local and national systems must work together closely giving constant feedback to those involved in reporting incidents [34]. Our proposition to national parachuting associations is to promote a system, preferably web-based, where skydivers can report incidents anonymously and injuries related to all aspects of skydiving, including while aboard aircraft. This is in line with a proposition made by Nilsson et al. [35]. Starting in 2013, the Swedish Parachuting Association (SFF) launched such a system in part because of the contributions from our research group.

The present findings suggest that jump leaders and other instructors act inconsistently when critical situations/incidents occur, for instance, depending on who is reporting and who had a violation. It also appears that respondents (with knowledge of the content) view the regulations as adequate and even express that jump leaders should be more stringent in enforcing them. Power structures might become relevant when the "formal" power of the jump leader is overridden by a skydiver with more experience or higher instructor ratings, thereby holding more "informal power" on the hierarchical ladder. In line with the writings of Laurendeau et al. [3, 23, 26, 33] the hierarchical structures play a substantial role in the Swedish skydiving setting; again they pinpoint variations among the Swedish clubs regarding safety issues and abidance to national rules and regulations.

Because of the qualitative approach and the limited sample size of this study, it is impossible to generalize the findings to the larger population of skydivers on a national or international level in quantitative terms. By presenting quotes as well as validating the analysis in a group of expert skydiving instructors, we have tried to enhance trustworthiness and transferability [15]. Although an effort was made to include a broad range of skydivers with respect to age and gender, the sample has a relatively high level of experience (years of skydiving and number of jumps). This may have affected the data in different ways but probably by enhancing data quality in that experienced respondents have acquired knowledge of the subject matter and have extensive personal experience of incidents and injuries; thereby, they provide reliable accounts of their experiences.

5. Conclusion

On the basis of the results presented above, it is interpreted that safety work and incident reporting in Swedish skydiving may be influenced more by local drop zone culture than by the national association policy. Formal and informal hierarchical structures among skydivers seem to dictate how skydiving is practiced, how rules are enforced, and if incidents or injuries are reported. These findings suggest that a change of safety work doctrine may be of value, from a present top-down to a bottom-up perspective, further empowering the individual skydiver. In practical terms, this could mean ensuring a fast, comprehensive bidirectional flow of information between the skydiver and reporting agency after having submitted an incident or injury incident report, thereby giving meaning to both the adverse event and the act of reporting.

Conflict of Interests

The authors declare that there is no conflict of interests regarding the publication of this paper.

Acknowledgments

The authors wish to thank Petter Alfsson-Thor, National Safety Officer of the Swedish Parachute Association (SFF), for sharing thoughts and discussing the meaning of the results. Also the authors thank the Department of Surgical and Perioperative Sciences, Division of Surgery, Umeå University, for support during the course of the study. The study was funded by grants from the Västernorrland County Council, Mid Sweden University and Umeå University.

References

[1] IPC Technical and Safety Committee, IPC Safety Survey Report—2011: International Parchuting Commission (IPC), Fedération Aéronautique Internationale (FAI), 2012.

[2] J. C. Hunt, "Divers' accounts of normal risk," *Symbolic Interaction*, vol. 18, no. 4, pp. 439–462, 1995.

[3] J. Laurendeau and E. G. van Brunschot, "Policing the edge: risk and social control in skydiving," *Deviant Behavior*, vol. 27, no. 2, pp. 173–201, 2006.

[4] T. H. Barrows, T. J. Mills, and S. D. Kassing, "The epidemiology of skydiving injuries: world freefall convention, 2000-2001," *The Journal of Emergency Medicine*, vol. 28, no. 1, pp. 63–68, 2005.

[5] D. S. R. Baiju and L. A. James, "Parachuting: a sport of chance and expense," *Injury*, vol. 34, no. 3, pp. 215–217, 2003.

[6] N. Ellitsgaard, "Parachuting injuries: a study of 110,000 sports jumps," *British Journal of Sports Medicine*, vol. 21, no. 1, pp. 13–17, 1987.

[7] P. J. Steinberg, "Injuries to Dutch sport parachutists," *British Journal of Sports Medicine*, vol. 22, no. 1, pp. 25–30, 1988.

[8] A. Westman and U. Björnstig, "Injuries in Swedish skydiving," *British Journal of Sports Medicine*, vol. 41, no. 6, pp. 356–364, 2007.

[9] A. Westman and U. Björnstig, "Fatalities in Swedish skydiving," *Accident Analysis and Prevention*, vol. 37, no. 6, pp. 1040–1048, 2005.

[10] Riksinstruktören, *Swedish Regulations for Sport Parachuting*, Swedish Parachute Association (SFF), Västerås, Sweden, 2013.

[11] A. Westman, M. Sjöling, A. Lindberg, and U. Björnstig, "The SKYNET data: demography and injury reporting in Swedish skydiving," *Accident Analysis and Prevention*, vol. 42, no. 2, pp. 778–783, 2010.

[12] J. Cutter and S. Jordan, "The systems approach to error reduction: factors influencing inoculation injury reporting in the operating theatre," *Journal of Nursing Management*, vol. 21, no. 8, pp. 989–1000, 2012.

[13] K. H. Roberts and D. M. Rousseau, "Research in nearly failure-free, high-reliability organizations: having the bubble," *IEEE Transactions on Engineering Management*, vol. 36, no. 2, pp. 132–139, 1992.

[14] D. L. Cooke and T. R. Rohleder, "Learning from incidents: from normal accidents to high reliability," *System Dynamics Review*, vol. 22, no. 3, pp. 213–239, 2006.

[15] U. H. Graneheim and B. Lundman, "Qualitative content analysis in nursing research: concepts, procedures and measures to achieve trustworthiness," *Nurse Education Today*, vol. 24, no. 2, pp. 105–112, 2004.

[16] N. K. Denzin and Y. S. Lincoln, *Handbook of Qualitative Research*, Sage, Thousand Oaks, Calif, USA, 2nd edition, 2000.

[17] L. Baxter, "Content analysis," in *Studying Interpersonal Interaction*, B. M. Montgomery and S. Duck, Eds., The Guilford communication, pp. 554–582, Guilford, New York, NY, USA, 1991.

[18] P. Ricoeur, *Interpretation Theory: Discourse and the Surplus of Meaning*, Texas Christian U.P, Fort Worth, Tex, USA, 2 edition, 1976.

[19] *Legislation (2003:460) on Ethical Approval for Research on Humans*, SFS, 2004.

[20] S. Lyng, *Edgework: The Sociology of Risk Taking*, Routledge, New York, NY, USA, 2005.

[21] M. Vidovic and N. Rugai, "Are hook turns a major obstacle to safe skydiving? A study of skydiving fatalities in the United States from 1992 to 2005," *Perceptual and Motor Skills*, vol. 105, no. 3, part 1, pp. 795–802, 2007.

[22] USPA and United States Parachute Association, *USPA Safety & Training, Advisor Handbook*, USPA—United States Parachute Association, Fredericksburg, 2012, http://www.uspa.org.

[23] J. Laurendeau, *Blue skies, Black death: risk Subculture issues, and gender in the contemporary skydiving community [Masters thesis]*, University of Calgary, Calgary, Canada, 2000.

[24] S. Wade, *The culture of skydiving [Masters thesis]*, Western Kentucky University, Bowling Green, Ky, USA, 2011.

[25] G. E. Brymer, *Extreme Dude! A Phenomenological Perspective on the Extreme Sport Experience [Monography]*, University of Wollongong, Wollongong, Australia, 2005.

[26] J. Laurendeau, ""He didn't go in doing a skydive": sustaining the illusion of control in an edgework activity," *Sociological Perspectives*, vol. 49, no. 4, pp. 583–606, 2006.

[27] D. Breitmeier, I. Seeland-Schulze, H. Hecker, and U. Schneider, "The influence of blood alcohol concentrations of around 0.03% on neuropsychological functions—a double-blind, placebo-controlled investigation," *Addiction Biology*, vol. 12, no. 2, pp. 183–189, 2007.

[28] D. M. Taylor, D. Bennett, M. Carter, D. Garewal, and C. Finch, "Perceptions of surfboard riders regarding the need for protective headgear," *Wilderness and Environmental Medicine*, vol. 16, no. 2, pp. 75–80, 2005.

[29] S. Marshall, "Stress-seekers in everyday life," in *Why Man Takes Chances*, S. Klausner, Ed., pp. 59–72, Doubleday, New York, NY, USA, 1968.

[30] P. Barach and S. D. Small, "Reporting and preventing medical mishaps: lessons from non-medical near miss reporting systems," *British Medical Journal*, vol. 320, no. 7237, pp. 759–763, 2000.

[31] J. J. Waring, "Beyond blame: cultural barriers to medical incident reporting," *Social Science and Medicine*, vol. 60, no. 9, pp. 1927–1935, 2005.

[32] J. E. Anderson, N. Kodate, R. Walters, and A. Dodds, "Can incident reporting improve safety? Healthcare practitioners'

views of the effectiveness of incident reporting," *International Journal for Quality in Health Care*, vol. 25, no. 2, pp. 141–150, 2013.

[33] J. Laurendeau, "The "crack choir" and the "cock chorus": the intersection of gender and sexuality in skydiving texts," *Sociology of Sport Journal*, vol. 21, no. 4, pp. 397–417, 2004.

[34] R. P. Mahajan, "Critical incident reporting and learning," *British Journal of Anaesthesia*, vol. 105, no. 1, pp. 69–75, 2010.

[35] J. Nilsson, C. Fridén, V. Burén, and B. O. Äng, "Development and validation of a web-based questionnaire for surveying skydivers," *Aviation Space and Environmental Medicine*, vol. 82, no. 6, pp. 610–614, 2011.

2

The Effect of Acute *Rhodiola rosea* Ingestion on Exercise Heart Rate, Substrate Utilisation, Mood State, and Perceptions of Exertion, Arousal, and Pleasure/Displeasure in Active Men

Michael J. Duncan[1,2] and Neil D. Clarke[1]

[1] *Department of Biomolecular and Sports Sciences, Coventry University, Coventry CV1 5HB, UK*
[2] *Human Performance Laboratory, Department of Biomolecular and Sports Sciences, Coventry University, James Starley Building, Priory Street, Coventry CV 5HB, UK*

Correspondence should be addressed to Michael J. Duncan; michael.duncan@coventry.ac.uk

Academic Editor: Laura Guidetti

The aim of this study was to examine the effect of acute *Rhodiola rosea* (*R. rosea*) ingestion on substrate utilisation, mood state, RPE, and exercise affect. Ten males (mean age ± S.D. = 26 ± 6 years) completed two 30-minute cycling trials at an intensity of 70% of $\dot{V}O_{2\,max}$ following ingestion of either 3 mg·kg^{-1} body mass of *R. rosea* or placebo using a double-blind, crossover design. During exercise, heart rate and RPE were recorded. Participants completed measures of mood state and exercise affect before and after exercise. Expired air samples were taken during exercise to determine substrate utilisation. Repeated measures analysis of variance indicated that RPE was significantly lower at 30 minutes into exercise versus placebo ($P = 0.003$). Perceptions of arousal ($P = 0.05$) and pleasure were significantly higher after exercise with *R. rosea* compared to placebo ($P = 0.003$). Mood state scores for vigor were also higher in *R. rosea* condition compared to placebo ($P = 0.008$). There were no significant differences in energy expenditure, carbohydrate, or fat oxidation between conditions ($P > 0.05$). Ingestion of *R. rosea* favourably influenced RPE and exercise affect without changes in energy expenditure or substrate utilization during 30-minute submaximal cycling performance.

1. Introduction

Rhodiola rosea (*R. rosea*) is an herb that grows in mountainous regions of North America, Europe, and Asia. It has been used in traditional folk medicine for centuries as a treatment for fatigue and mood disorders [1]. *R. rosea* has been extensively studied by scientists in the former Soviet Union and has predominantly been found to result in favourable effects on exercise performance [2]. However, this prior work has been lacking in experimental control [3]. Some recent studies have supported the results of earlier work by identifying antioxidant and anti-inflammatory properties of *R. rosea* [3, 4]. Another work has suggested ingestion of *R. rosea* appears to be effective, either acutely [5] or with daily supplementation [6], for reducing perceived fatigue and improving cognition [5, 7], as well as reducing markers of physiological and psychological stress [7, 8].

Although *R. rosea* ingestion has been identified as a means to reduce physical fatigue, its efficacy during exercise is unclear. Animal based research has shown increased swim time to exhaustion in rats [3, 9] but the impact of *R. rosea* ingestion on exercise performance in humans is equivocal. Some studies have shown no effect of *R. rosea* ingestion on exercise performance [4, 10–12] whilst others have supported its use [13, 14]. The array of protocols and supplementation doses used in prior studies has also limited comparisons between studies and provides one potential explanation for the discrepancy in their findings. For example, de Bock et al. [13] reported that an acute dose of *R. rosea* increased time to exhaustion during an incremental cycle ergometer protocol. Conversely, in the same study, 4 weeks of *R. rosea* supplementation did not significantly improve cycling performance. This was the first study to show an acute impact of *R. rosea* ingestion on human exercise performance. More recent research by Noreen et al. [14] examined the efficacy of a 3 $mg{\cdot}kg^{-1}$ body mass dose of *R. rosea* on 6-mile cycle time trial performance in 18 active women. They reported that *R. rosea* significantly decreased submaximal exercise heart rate, reduced RPE, and improved time trial performance time. Noreen et al. [14] subsequently suggested that acute *R. rosea* ingestion might be employed by active individuals while exercising to complete a set distance in the shortest time.

Such data are interesting; as if *R. rosea* does positively impact on exercise, it may be safe and legal way to enhance exercise performance in athletes and the exercise experience in recreational gym users. The mechanism by which *R. rosea* might improve performance is also unclear. Abidov et al. [15] demonstrated that an extract of *R. rosea* significantly prolonged the duration of exhaustive swimming in rats and stimulated ATP synthesis in muscle during exercise. These findings led Perfumi and Mattioli [16] to speculate that, in addition to enhancing the catecholaminergic system, the ability of *R. rosea* to increase performance involves an improvement in cellular energy metabolism. However, some studies have suggested that *R. rosea* acts to acutely increase endogenous opioid production or receptor sensitivity [2, 13] which subsequently impacts on brain dopamine and serotonin and cardiac activity and attenuates the perception of effort at a given workload [14]. However, as only two studies have examined acute *R. rosea* ingestion on exercise performance to date, further data is needed on this topic. Moreover, both de Bock et al. [13] and Noreen et al. [14] employed performance based protocols to examine the effect of *R. rosea* ingestion. While these are valuable in understanding the effect of a nutritional supplement on performance responses, different protocols may be better placed to evidence any effect of *R. rosea* on exercise performance. For example, using steady state submaximal exercise in the presence of *R. rosea* and placebo would allow for power output to remain constant across a given period. This then allows for better like-for-like comparison of data between the active supplement and placebo trials. Moreover, when employing protocols where intensity is modified throughout (as is the case with both time trials and time to exhaustion) understanding any impact of the exercise protocol of substance ingested becomes more difficult because even small increases in exercise intensity have been shown to markedly change feelings of pleasure during exercise [17].

Furthermore, given the postulation that *R. rosea* acts through increased opioid production, it is perhaps surprising that few studies have examined its impact on affect. Noreen et al. [14] reported no effect of *R. rosea* ingestion on mood state, as assessed using the POMS questionnaire. However, changes in mood state with exercise have been reported following ingestion of a range of substances including caffeine [18, 19] and carbohydrate [20]. Hedonic theory [21] postulates that hedonic responses (i.e., pleasure versus displeasure) following a behaviour influence decisions regarding whether or not to repeat that behaviour. As a consequence if nutritional manipulation enhances the pleasure response to exercise, according to hedonic theory, it may mean individuals are more likely to exercise [21]. This is important as different exercise intensities and individual fitness will create variability in the affective response to exercise [22–24] and the effect of nutritional manipulation on these responses is not well known. Changes in mood and feelings of pleasure may be one reason why individuals do not participate in regular exercise and physical activity [19] and favourable affective states benefit exercise performance [25]. Research by DaSilva et al. [26] has also identified that affective and perceptual responses to exercise differ depending on adiposity status. Assuming that the affective response to exercise is the same in recreational exercises compared to high level performers may therefore lead to erroneous conclusions regarding the exercise-affect relationship. Thus, while the extant literature examining the effect of *R. rosea* ingestion has focused on performance measures, the current study seeks to develop this work by employing a model that can be applied to recreational exercisers and is more applicable to the exercising public in general.

The aim of this study was to examine the effect of acute *R. rosea* ingestion on substrate utilisation, mood state, RPE, perceptions of arousal, and pleasure/displeasure in a population of recreationally active men. It was hypothesized that ingestion of *R. rosea* would positively influence perceived exertion during exercise as well as enhancing mood and perceptions of arousal and pleasure/displeasure before and after cycling exercise. Testing these hypotheses will address gaps in knowledge on the effect of *R. rosea* by examining their effects on an active but not performance oriented group, more typical of regularly active individuals in the general population. The study will also combine physiological and psychological measures to address gaps in the literature base by assessing substrate utilisation, heart rate, RPE, mood state, and perceptions of arousal and pleasure/displeasure to provide a multidisciplinary investigation of the effect of *R. rosea* during exercise.

2. Method

2.1. Design. This study employed a within-participants double-blind cross-over design whereby participants visited the laboratory on 3 occasions at the same time of day in a well-rested and well-hydrated state. Ten male, recreational exercisers (mean age ± S.D. = 26 ± 6 years) participated in this study. All participants were asked to refrain from vigorous exercise and maintain normal dietary patterns in the 48 hours prior to testing and were asked not to consume caffeine for 24 hours before testing. During the first visit participants completed a familiarization session with the measures to be used in the subsequent experimental trials and completed an incremental exercise test to assess $\dot{V}O_{2\,max}$. Inclusion criteria included being male and habitually engaged in recreational physical activity of more than 3 but less than 10 hours per week and not including formal competitive sports performance. Participants were excluded if they had a musculoskeletal or cardiovascular contraindication to exercise, were taking any medication that could impact mood/affect, engaged in less than 3 or more than 10 hours physical activity per week, or were engaged in competitive sports activity as part of their habitual physical activity.

TABLE 1: Descriptive information (mean ± S.D.) of participants' height, body mass, resting heart rate, and maximal oxygen uptake.

Height (m)		Mass (kg)		Resting heart rate (bpm)		$\dot{V}O_{2\,max}$ (mL·kg^{-1}·min^{-1})	
M	S.D.	M	S.D.	M	S.D.	M	S.D.
1.72	0.03	67.7	6.3	79.8	17.3	50.5	6.6

The incremental exercise test was performed on a mechanically braked cycle ergometer (Monark Exercise AB, Sweden) to assess $\dot{V}O_{2\,max}$ following previously published guidelines [27]. Initially, participants were fitted to the ergometer and performed a 5 min warm-up at 25 Watts. The initial work rate for the test was 80 Watts with the work rate increasing by 40 Watts every 3 minutes. This protocol, using 3-minute stages rather than a ramp protocol, was employed based on prior research suggesting that this form of protocol provides more reliable physiological measures, particular for the population characteristics examined in this study (i.e., active but not cycling trained specifically) [27]. Participants were asked to maintain their pedal cadence at 70 rpm and were given visual feedback from the Monark control box in order to do this. Expired air was collected via the Douglas bag technique during the final minute of each incremental exercise stage. Samples were analyzed for oxygen and carbon dioxide content (Servomex, Crowborough, England) and expired air volume (Harvard dry gas meter, Harvard Apparatus, Kent, England) with values for oxygen consumption ($\dot{V}O_2$) and carbon dioxide production ($\dot{V}CO_2$) subsequently calculated. Heart rate (Polar Electro, Kempele, Finland) and rating of perceived exertion (RPE), using the Borg 6–20 RPE scale [28], were recorded during the final 15 seconds of each workload. Exercise was continued to exhaustion in order for measurement of $\dot{V}O_{2\,max}$ to be made. Participants were judged to have reached $\dot{V}O_{2\,max}$ if they presented at least 3 of the following: (a) a respiratory exchange ratio of greater than 1.1, (b) a heart rate during the last stage of testing that was ±10 beats of age predicted maximum heart rate, (c) an RPE of 18 or greater, (d) a plateau in VO_2 with an increase in workload, and (e) volitional fatigue. These criteria were employed based on those commonly used for maximal oxygen uptake [29]. All participants met these criteria during their incremental exercise test. Mean ± S.D. of participants' baseline $\dot{V}O_{2\,max}$ values was 50.5 ± 6.6 mL·kg^{-1}·min^{-1} (range: 38.8–58.4 mL·kg^{-1}·min^{-1}). Descriptive information for the participants is presented in Table 1.

2.2. Experimental Protocol. On completion of the $\dot{V}O_{2\,max}$ testing and following a period of at least 72 hours participants completed two 30-minute submaximal cycling trials at a workload of 70% $\dot{V}O_{2\,max}$ in a fasted state. Self-report of dietary intake was employed to assess and control dietary intake in the 24 hours prior to exercise trials. This was used to ensure that the same/similar per testing meals were consumed prior to experimental trials and that caffeine and alcohol had not been consumed in the 24 hours prior to testing. The duration and intensity of exercise were chosen as it sits within the American College of Sports Medicine guidelines for the prescription of exercise for health benefit [30]. On a molecular basis, the main active ingredients of *R. rosea* appear to be Tyrosol and its glucoside known as salidroside and following oral ingestion of 100 mg·kg^{-1} salidroside, the half-life of salidroside appears to be 1.32 ± 0.22 h [31]. Therefore, conditions were randomised, separated by 48–72 hours, and consisted of a *R. rosea* condition where 3 mg·kg^{-1} body mass of *R. rosea* (Indigo Herbs, Glastonbury, UK) placed in a coloured, opaque gelatin capsule or a placebo (3 mg·kg^{-1} body mass of maltodextrin, (MyProtein, Northwich, UK)) was ingested with 250 mL water. The capsules were indistinguishable between *R. rosea* and placebo conditions and were ingested 60 min before exercise on an empty stomach. The amount of total maltodextrin ingested was approximately 170 mg and thus highly unlikely to have had any impact on exercise performance or metabolism [14]. The dose of *R. rosea* used was based on the previous work of de Bock et al. [13] and Noreen et al. [14] who observed improvements in endurance performance following acute ingestion of *R. rosea*.

During each of the cycling trials, heart rate was monitored (Polar RS400, Polar Electro Oy, Kempele, Finland) continuously and assessed every 10 minutes. Participants were also asked to provide ratings of perceived exertion (RPE) using the Borg 6–20 scale [28]. Prior to commencing the experimental trials the memory-anchoring approach [32] was employed whereby participants were asked to remember a time when they were at rest (attributed to RPE of 6) and a time when they had reached a level of exertion that was maximal attributed to RPE of 20. The RPE scale was presented to students for 1 minute prior to their rating of perceived exertion at each time point and was not visible other than this. Prior to any substance ingestion, 60 min after ingestion (at the onset of each exercise bout) and immediately on completion of each exercise bout, participants also completed the feeling scale (FS) as a measure of pleasure and displeasure [33]. This is an 11-item single-item scale ranging from +5 (very good) to −5 (very bad) that is used to quantify pleasure/displeasure. The Felt Arousal Scale (FAS) was also used as a measure of arousal [34]. This is a six-item scale ranging from 1 (low arousal) to 6 (high arousal). Mood state was also assessed using the fatigue and vigour subscales of the Brunel Mood State Inventory (BRUMS) [35]. This is a well-established, reliable, and valid measure of mood state that has been previously employed to assess the mood state response to various exercise modes [18, 35, 36]. The fatigue and vigor subscales were chosen in particular as prior research [1, 7] has suggested *R. rosea* may particularly influence feelings of fatigue and/or vigor.

Participants were introduced to these scales during their first visit to the laboratory (prior to establishment of $\dot{V}O_{2\,max}$). Standardised instructions for completing the FS and FAS were read to participants at the beginning of each trial.

3. Substrate Oxidation

Prior to cycling (but whilst seated on the exercise bike) at 14 min and 29 min during each exercise bout expired air samples were collected using the Douglas bag technique to estimate fat and carbohydrate (CHO) oxidation rates. The collection time was 60 s and samples were analysed for oxygen and carbon dioxide content (Servomex, Crowborough, England) that was calibrated at two points before each assessment using gases of known concentrations (15.12% O_2, 5.1% CO_2) in accordance with manufacturers guidelines and expired air volume (Harvard dry gas meter, Harvard Apparatus, Kent, England) with values for oxygen consumption ($\dot{V}O_2$) and carbon dioxide production ($\dot{V}CO_2$) subsequently calculated. Energy expenditure (Kcal·min^{-1}) and the oxidation rates for carbohydrate and fat (g·min^{-1}) were then calculated according to the Weir [37] and Frayn [38] equations, respectively.

3.1. Statistical Analysis. Data were analysed in a number of ways. A series of 2 (substance ingested) × 4 (time point) ways repeated measures analysis of variance was used to examine any differences in heart rate and RPE. A series of 2 (substance ingested) X 3 (time point, before ingestion, after ingestion but before exercise, and after exercise) ways repeated measures analysis of variance was used to examine any differences in mood state and perceptions of arousal and pleasure/displeasure and substrate utilisation. Where any significant differences were discovered, Bonferroni pairwise multiple comparisons were used to determine where the differences lay. Partial η^2 was used as a measure of effect size, statistical significance was set at $P = 0.05$ a priori, and the Statistical Package for Social Sciences (Version 20) was used for all analysis (SPSS Inc., IL, USA).

4. Results

In respect to heart rate, results indicated no significant interactions or main effect due to the substances ingested. There was however a significant main effect for time (F 3, 27 = 266.7, $P = 0.0001$, $P\eta^2 = 0.967$) where heart rate was significantly increased throughout the exercise bout irrespective of substance ingested. Mean ± SE of heart rate (bpm) was 77 ± 4 at rest compared to 151 ± 4, 158 ± 4, and 162 ± 4 at 10, 20, and 30 minutes into the exercise bout, respectively. Bonferroni comparisons indicated that heart rate was significantly different at all time points ($P = 0.001$ in all cases).

In the case of RPE, results indicated a significant substance × time interaction (F 3, 27 = 6.12, $P = 0.003$, $P\eta^2 = 0.405$, see Figure 1). RPE data were not significantly different at rest and at 10 and 20 minutes into the exercise bout between the two conditions. However, RPE in the placebo condition was significantly higher than that in the *R. rosea* condition 30 minutes into the exercise bout ($P = 0.003$).

Scores from the fatigue subscale of the BRUMS indicated a significant main effect across time (F 2, 18 = 12.879, $P = 0.0001$, $P\eta^2 = 0.589$) where scores were significantly higher

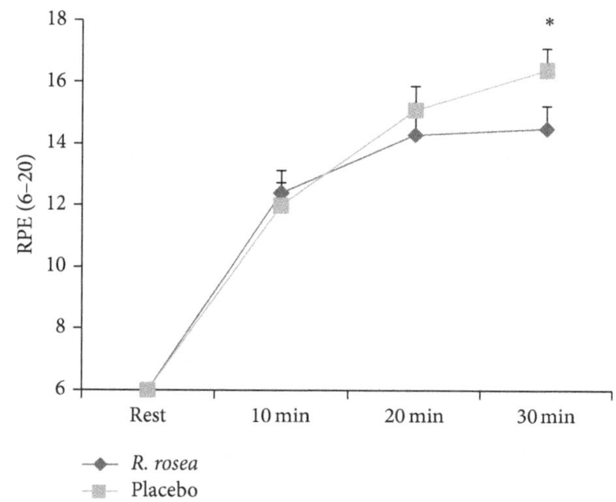

Figure 1: Mean ± SE of RPE (6–20) at rest and during 30 min submaximal cycling between *R. rosea* and placebo conditions ($^*P = 0.003$).

after exercise compared to before exercise ($P = 0.028$) and compared to before exercise but after ingestion ($P = 0.008$). There were no other significant main effects of interactions for fatigue subscale data. In regard to the vigor subscale of the BRUMS, there was no significant substance × time interaction. There were however significant main effects for time (F 2, 18 = 4.435, $P = 0.027$, $P\eta^2 = 0.350$) and for the substance ingested (F 2, 9 = 11.692, $P = 0.008$, $P\eta^2 = 0.565$). Scores for vigor were significantly lower at after exercise compared to after ingestion but before exercise ($P = 0.04$). Mean ± SE for vigor scores was 6.9 ± 0.56 before ingestion, 7.4 ± 0.44 after ingestion but before exercise, and 5.6 ± 0.74 after exercise. For the substance ingested, scores for vigor were significantly higher in the *R. rosea* condition ($P = 0.008$) compared to the placebo. Mean ± SE for vigor was 7.6 ± 0.52 in the *R. rosea* condition compared to 5.7±0.57 in the placebo condition.

Perceptions of arousal were also significantly different in the presence of *R. rosea* compared to placebo (F 1, 9 = 5.0, $P = 0.05$, $P\eta^2 = 0.357$) with scores for arousal being higher (3.1 ± 0.19) in the presence of *R. rosea* compared to placebo (2.8 ± 0.11). When data for feeling of pleasure/displeasure were assessed, there was however a significant condition × time effect (F 2, 18 = 12.795, $P = 0.0001$, $P\eta^2 = 0.587$, see Figure 2). This followed a similar pattern to RPE with no significant difference evident before ingestion ($P = 0.591$) or after ingestion but before exercise ($P = 0.08$). There was however significantly lower scores for pleasure after exercise in the placebo condition compared to the *R. rosea* condition ($P = 0.003$).

Energy expenditure was significantly higher during exercise (F 2, 18 = 130.921, $P < 0.001$, $P\eta^2 = 0.936$) (see Figure 3), irrespective of the trial (F 1, 9 = 1.198, $P = 0.302$, $P\eta^2 = 0.117$). The rate of total carbohydrate oxidation (Figure 4) was not significantly different between trials (F 1, 9 = 0.317, $P = 0.587$, $P\eta^2 = 0.034$). Carbohydrate oxidation remained relatively

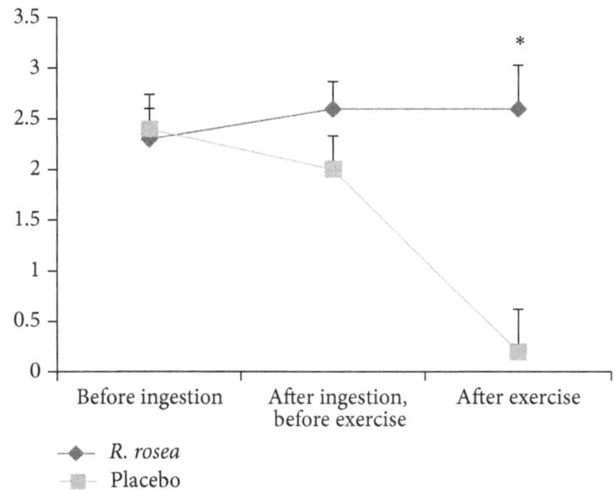

FIGURE 2: Mean ± SE of perception of pleasure/displeasure before ingestion, after ingestion but before exercise, and after exercise between *R. rosea* and placebo conditions ($^*P = 0.003$).

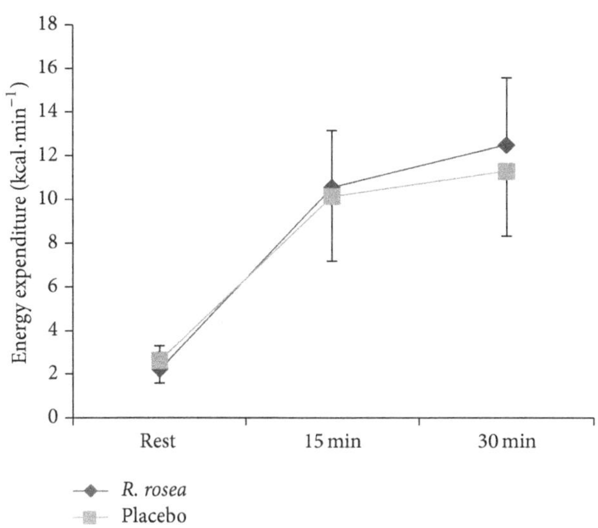

FIGURE 3: Mean ± S.D. energy expenditure (Kcal·min^{-1}) during 30 min submaximal cycling between *R. rosea* and placebo conditions.

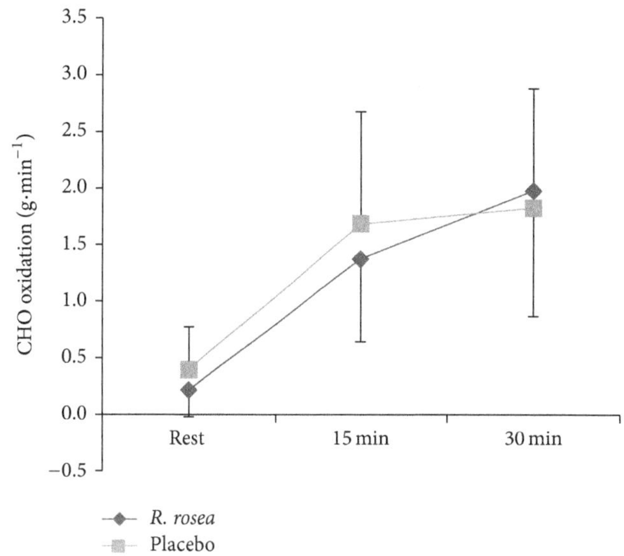

FIGURE 4: Mean ± S.D. total CHO oxidation rate (g·min^{-1}) during 30 min submaximal cycling between *R. rosea* and placebo conditions.

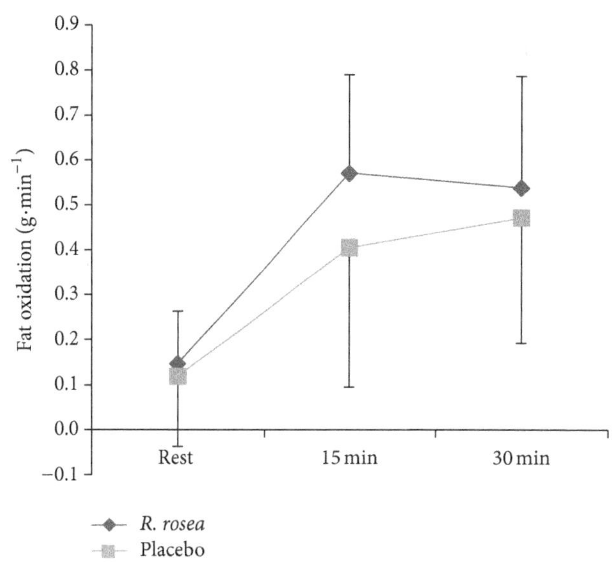

FIGURE 5: Mean ± S.D. fat oxidation rate (g·min^{-1}) during 30 min submaximal cycling between *R. rosea* and placebo conditions.

constant throughout exercise but was higher compared with the rest (F 2, 18 = 13.902, $P < 0.001$, $P\eta^2 = 0.770$). The rate of fat oxidation (Figure 5) was higher than that at rest during exercise (F 1, 11 = 25.131, $P < 0.001$, $P\eta^2 = 0.736$) but there was no significant main effect due to the substances ingested (F 1, 9 = 0.950, $P = 0.355$, $P\eta^2 = 0.095$).

5. Discussion

Acute *R. rosea* ingestion has been reported to improve exercise performance [13, 14] in performance based tasks. Authors have suggested that this performance enhancement may result from *R. rosea's* action as an opioid producer [2, 13]. However, use of performance based exercise tasks (e.g., time trial) in prior studies makes it difficult to assess the effect of the substance ingested apart from the exercise intensity in tasks where intensity will fluctuate. Arguably, the sue of a constant load exercise protocol for 30 minutes is a more externally valid form of exercise for most individuals as it mirrors the minimum exercise recommendations for healthy adults [30]. No study to date has assessed the effects of *R. rosea* ingestion on mood, perceptions of exertion, arousal, and feelings of pleasure/displeasure during steady state exercise. In the current study, RPE and affect were measured prior to, during, and after 30-minute submaximal cycling at a moderate exercise intensity after ingestion of 3 mg·kg^{-1} *R. rosea* of placebo. This study is novel in that results demonstrated dampened RPE, greater vigor, perception of arousal, and pleasure in the presence of *R. rosea* compared to placebo. In the case of RPE and feelings of pleasure, these changes were seen at the end of the 30 min exercise bout. Thus, this data indicate that acute *R. rosea* ingestion positively modifies affect during relatively brief, steady state exercise at moderate intensity.

Previous studies have speculated that the ingestion of *R. rosea* can improve exercise performance via altered energy metabolism [16], activated by the synthesis or resynthesis of ATP in mitochondria and stimulated restorative energy processes after intense exercise [15]. However, the results of the present study suggest that altered substrate utilization is not responsible for the improved performance. The discrepancy between the findings of the present study in this respect and those of prior work [15, 16] may be due to varying preexercise fed state across studies. In the present study the Frayn [38] equation was employed to assess fat oxidation as this is the most widely applied equation for fat oxidation available. However, we acknowledge that other equations are also available [39] and may be preferable in future work. It is also important to note that there is no gold standard to validate whole body substrate oxidation but that assessment of substrate oxidation using indirect calorimetry may be prone to large errors [40]. Therefore, the acute increase in endogenous opioid production may play a role in enhancing exercise performance in the presence of *R. rosea* and is evidenced through changes in perceived exertion and exercise affect rather than changes in physiological markers.

The present study does have some limitations. The task used employed a bout of steady state exercise at a moderate intensity. Prior research has tended to employ protocols involving time trial performance [14] or time to exhaustion [13], neither of which is applicable to the typical exercising public. While the protocol employed in the present study may be valid when examining steady state exercise at a moderate intensity, it also might not fully address the typical training session undertaken by many recreational exercisers and athletes. However, given the lack of studies examining the effect of *R. rosea* on exercise performance such steady state protocols are useful in developing the extant literature in this area. We do acknowledge that by controlling exercise intensity based on a percentage of $\dot{V}O_{2\,max}$ we are unable to determine if participants were exercising below, at, or above their lactate threshold. Exercise across these different intensities may however change affective responses [22]. This should be considered in future studies. Future research might subsequently benefit from using a standardised protocol to mimic the type of exercise session commonly undertaken in gyms (e.g., combined aerobic and resistance exercise) in order to determine if *R. rosea* ingestion is practically useful in a more ecologically valid exercise task. The current study also examined participants who were recreationally active but were not specifically cycling trained. It has been suggested that less fit individuals may experience greater fatigue and discomfort during exercise which may reduce feelings of pleasure compared to more highly trained individuals. It may therefore be useful to compare the responses of participants of different training status in order to make more conclusive statements regarding the effect of *R. rosea* on variables such as perception of exertion, arousal, and pleasure. Furthermore, a posteriori power calculations indicated a sample size of 28 would have been required to detect a difference of $P = 0.05$ at 95% power. However, due to the paucity of data on effects of *R. rosea* on exercise performance this study was exploratory in nature and subsequently used a relatively small number of participants. The current study may therefore be underpowered. Finally, the assessment of affect immediately on completion of the cycling bout might have resulted in elevated scores for feeling states due to the cessation of exercise as has been suggested previously [17]. It may be that the trajectory of pleasure and displeasure during and after exercise exhibits two distinct phases [22]. The first phase involves a decline or increase of affective responses during exercise, whereas the second phase involves an improvement or rebound of affective responses after exercise. As measures of affect were only taken on completion of the exercise bouts, the data presented here are only representative of the rebound phase of exercise in the presence of *R. rosea* and placebo. Future research should therefore attempt to assess affect during exercise in addition to immediately on cessation in order to more effectively capture the time course of affective responses to exercise following ingestion of different substances.

6. Conclusions

Ingestion of *R. rosea* favourably influenced RPE and exercise affect without changes in energy expenditure or substrate utilization during 30 minutes of submaximal cycling performance at moderate intensity in regularly active adults. These changes support the efficacy of acute *R. rosea* ingestion in positively enhancing psychophysiological responses to submaximal exercise performance.

Conflict of Interests

The authors declare that there is no conflict of interests regarding the publication of this paper.

References

[1] T. B. Walker and R. A. Robergs, "Does Rhodiola rosea possess ergogenic properties?" *International Journal of Sport Nutrition and Exercise Metabolism*, vol. 16, no. 3, pp. 305–315, 2006.

[2] R. P. Brown, P. L. Gerbarg, and Z. Ramazanov, "Rhodiola rosea: a phytomedicinal overview," *HerbalGram*, vol. 56, pp. 40–52, 2002.

[3] M. Abidov, S. Grachev, R. D. Seifulla, and T. N. Ziegenfuss, "Extract of Rhodiola rosea radix reduces the level of C-reactive protein and creatinine kinase in the blood," *Bulletin of Experimental Biology and Medicine*, vol. 138, no. 1, pp. 63–64, 2004.

[4] A. Skarpanska-Stejnborn, L. Pilaczynska-Szczesniak, P. Basta, and E. Deskur-Smielecka, "The influence of supplementation with Rhodiola rosea L. extract on Selected redox parameters in professional rowers," *International Journal of Sport Nutrition and Exercise Metabolism*, vol. 19, no. 2, pp. 186–199, 2009.

[5] V. A. Shevtsov, B. I. Zholus, V. I. Shervarly et al., "A randomized trial of two different doses of a SHR-5 Rhodiola rosea extract versus placebo and control of capacity for mental work," *Phytomedicine*, vol. 10, no. 2-3, pp. 95–105, 2003.

[6] A. A. Spasov, G. K. Wikman, V. B. Mandrikov, I. A. Mironova, and V. V. Neumoin, "A double-blind, placebo-controlled pilot study of the stimulating and adaptogenic effect of Rhodiola rosea SHR-5 extract on the fatigue of students caused by stress during an examination period with a repeated low-dose regimen," *Phytomedicine*, vol. 7, no. 2, pp. 85–89, 2000.

[7] V. Darbinyan, A. Kteyan, A. Panossian, E. Gabrielian, G. Wikman, and H. Wagner, "Rhodiola rosea in stress induced fatigue—a double blind cross-over study of a standardized extract SHR-5 with a repeated low-dose regimen on the mental performance of healthy physicians during night duty," *Phytomedicine*, vol. 7, no. 5, pp. 365–371, 2000.

[8] L. Mattioli, C. Funari, and M. Perfumi, "Effects of Rhodiola rosea L. extract on behavioural and physiological alterations induced by chronic mild stress in female rats," *Journal of Psychopharmacology*, vol. 23, no. 2, pp. 130–142, 2009.

[9] F. T. Lee, T. Y. Kuo, S. Y. Liou, and C. T. Chien, "Chronic Rhodiola rosea extract supplementation enforces exhaustive swimming tolerance," *The American Journal of Chinese Medicine*, vol. 37, no. 3, pp. 557–572, 2009.

[10] T. B. Walker, S. A. Altobelli, A. Caprihan, and R. A. Robergs, "Failure of Rhodiola rosea to alter skeletal muscle phosphate kinetics in trained men," *Metabolism: Clinical and Experimental*, vol. 56, no. 8, pp. 1111–1117, 2007.

[11] S. N. Colson, F. B. Wyatt, D. L. Johnston, L. D. Autrey, Y. L. FitzGerald, and C. P. Earnest, "Cordyceps sinensis- and Rhodiola rosea-based supplementation in male cyclists and its effect on muscle tissue oxygen saturation," *Journal of Strength and Conditioning Research*, vol. 19, no. 2, pp. 358–363, 2005.

[12] C. P. Earnest, G. M. Morss, F. Wyatt et al., "Effects of a commercial herbal-based formula on exercise performance in cyclists," *Medicine and Science in Sports and Exercise*, vol. 36, no. 3, pp. 504–509, 2004.

[13] K. de Bock, B. O. Eijnde, M. Ramaekers, and P. Hespel, "Acute Rhodiola rosea intake can improve endurance exercise performance," *International Journal of Sport Nutrition and Exercise Metabolism*, vol. 14, no. 3, pp. 298–307, 2004.

[14] E. E. Noreen, J. G. Buckley, S. L. Lewis, J. Brandauer, and K. J. Stuempfle, "The effects of an acute does of Rhodiola rosea on endurance exercise performance," *Journal of Strength and Conditioning Research*, vol. 27, no. 3, pp. 839–847, 2013.

[15] M. Abidov, F. Crendal, S. Grachev, R. Seifulla, and T. Ziegenfuss, "Effect of extracts from Rhodiola rosea and Rhodiola crenulata (Crassulaceae) roots on ATP content in mitochondria of skeletal muscles," *Bulletin of Experimental Biology and Medicine*, vol. 136, no. 6, pp. 585–587, 2003.

[16] M. Perfumi and L. Mattioli, "Adaptogenic and central nervous system effects of single doses of 3% rosavin and 1% salidroside Rhodiola rosea L. extract in mice," *Phytotherapy Research*, vol. 21, no. 1, pp. 37–43, 2007.

[17] P. Ekkekakis, G. Parfitt, and S. J. Petruzzello, "The pleasure and displeasure people feel when they exercise at different intensities: decennial update and progress towards a tripartite rationale for exercise intensity prescription," *Sports Medicine*, vol. 41, no. 8, pp. 641–671, 2011.

[18] M. J. Duncan and S. W. Oxford, "The effect of caffeine ingestion on mood state and bench press performance to failure," *Journal of Strength and Conditioning Research*, vol. 25, no. 1, pp. 178–185, 2011.

[19] T. A. Astorino, T. Cottrell, A. T. Lozano, K. Aburto-Pratt, and J. Duhon, "Effect of caffeine on RPE and perceptions of pain, arousal, and pleasure/displeasure during a cycling time trial in endurance trained and active men," *Physiology and Behavior*, vol. 106, no. 2, pp. 211–217, 2012.

[20] S. H. Backhouse, N. C. Bishop, S. J. H. Biddle, and C. Williams, "Effect of carbohydrate and prolonged exercise on affect and perceived exertion," *Medicine and Science in Sports and Exercise*, vol. 37, no. 10, pp. 1768–1773, 2005.

[21] D. Kahneman, B. L. Fredrickson, C. A. Schreiber, and D. A. Redelmeier, "When more pain is preferred to less: adding a better end," *Psychological Science*, vol. 4, no. 6, pp. 401–405, 1993.

[22] P. Ekkekakis, E. E. Hall, and S. J. Petruzzello, "Variation and homogeneity in affective responses to physical activity of varying intensities: an alternative perspective on dose-response based on evolutionary considerations," *Journal of Sports Sciences*, vol. 23, no. 5, pp. 477–500, 2005.

[23] K. A. Barbour, T. M. Edenfield, and J. A. Blumenthal, "Exercise as a treatment for depression and other psychiatric disorders: a review," *Journal of Cardiopulmonary Rehabilitation and Prevention*, vol. 27, no. 6, pp. 359–367, 2007.

[24] M. D. Hoffman and D. R. Hoffman, "Exercisers achieve greater acute exercise-induced mood enhancement than nonexercisers," *Archives of Physical Medicine and Rehabilitation*, vol. 89, no. 2, pp. 358–363, 2008.

[25] E. O. Acevedo, D. L. Gill, A. H. Goldfarb, and B. T. Boyer, "Affect and perceived exertion during a two-hour run," *International Journal of Sport Psychology*, vol. 27, no. 3, pp. 286–292, 1996.

[26] S. G. DaSilva, L. Guidetti, C. F. Buzzachera et al., "The influence of adiposity on physiological, perceptual, and affective responses during walking at a self-selected pace," *Perceptual and Motor Skills*, vol. 109, no. 1, pp. 41–60, 2009.

[27] L. Moseley and A. E. Jeukendrup, "The reliability of cycling efficiency," *Medicine and Science in Sports and Exercise*, vol. 33, no. 4, pp. 621–627, 2001.

[28] G. Borg, "Perceived exertion as an indicator of somatic stress," *Scandinavian Journal of Rehabilitation Medicine*, vol. 2, no. 2, pp. 92–98, 1970.

[29] A. W. Midgley, L. R. McNaughton, R. Polman, and D. Marchant, "Criteria for determination of maximal oxygen uptake: a brief critique and recommendations for future research," *Sports Medicine*, vol. 37, no. 12, pp. 1019–1028, 2007.

[30] American College of Sports Medicine, *ACSM's Guidelines for Exercise Testing and Prescription*, Lippincott Williams & Wilkins, Baltimore, Md, USA, 2013.

[31] N. Guo, Z. Hu, X. Fan et al., "Simultaneous determination of Salidroside and its aglycone metabolite p-tyrosol in rat plasma by liquid chromatography-tandem mass spectrometry," *Molecules*, vol. 17, no. 4, pp. 4733–4754, 2012.

[32] R. J. Robertson, *Perceived Exertion for Practitioners*, Human Kinetics, Champaign, Ill, USA, 2004.

[33] C. J. Hardy and W. J. Rejeski, "Not what, but how one feels: the measurement of affect during exercise," *Journal of Sport and Exercise Psychology*, vol. 11, pp. 304–317, 1989.

[34] S. Svebak and S. Murgatroyd, "Metamotivational dominance. A multimethod validation of reversal theory constructs," *Journal of Personality and Social Psychology*, vol. 48, no. 1, pp. 107–116, 1985.

[35] P. Terry and A. Lane, *User Guide for the Brunel Mood State Inventory (BRUMS)*, University of Southern Australia, Queensland, Australia, 2003.

[36] P. C. Terry and A. M. Lane, "Normative values for the profile of mood states for use with athletic samples," *Journal of Applied Sport Psychology*, vol. 12, no. 1, pp. 69–85, 2000.

[37] J. B. Weir, "New methods for calculating metabolic rate with special reference to protein metabolism," *Journal of Physiology*, vol. 109, no. 1-2, pp. 1–9, 1949.

[38] K. N. Frayn, "Calculation of substrate oxidation rates in vivo from gaseous exchange," *Journal of Applied Physiology Respiratory Environmental and Exercise Physiology*, vol. 55, no. 2, pp. 628–634, 1983.

[39] A. E. Jeukendrup and G. A. Wallis, "Measurement of substrate oxidation during exercise by means of gas exchange measurements," *International Journal of Sports Medicine*, vol. 26, supplement 1, pp. S28–S37, 2005.

[40] Y. Schutz, "On problems of calculating energy expenditure and substrate utilization from respiratory exchange data," *European Journal of Nutrition*, vol. 36, no. 4, pp. 255–262, 1997.

3

A Review of Treatments for Iliotibial Band Syndrome in the Athletic Population

Corey Beals[1] and David Flanigan[2]

[1] *Department of Surgery, Wexner Medical Center, 395 W. 12th Avenue Columbus, OH 43210, USA*
[2] *Department of Sports Medicine, Wexner Medical Center, 2050 Kenny Road, Suite 3100 Columbus, OH 43221, USA*

Correspondence should be addressed to David Flanigan; david.flanigan@osumc.edu

Academic Editor: Adrian W. Midgley

Iliotibial band syndrome (ITBS) is a common injury in runners and other long distance athletes with the best management options not clearly established. This review outlines both the conservative and surgical options for the treatment of iliotibial band syndrome in the athletic population. Ten studies met the inclusion criteria by focusing on the athletic population in their discussion of the treatment for iliotibial band syndrome, both conservative and surgical. Conservative management consisting of a combination of rest (2–6 weeks), stretching, pain management, and modification of running habits produced a 44% complete cure rate, with return to sport at 8 weeks and a 91.7% cure rate with return to sport at 6 months after injury. Surgical therapy, often only used for refractory cases, consisted of excision or release of the pathologic distal portion of the iliotibial band or bursectomy. Those studies focusing on the excision or release of the pathologic distal portion of the iliotibial band showed a 100% return to sport rate at both 7 weeks and 3 months after injury. Despite many options for both surgical and conservative treatment, there has yet to be consensus on one standard of care. Certain treatments, both conservative and surgical, in our review are shown to be more effective than others; however, further research is needed to delineate the true pathophysiology of iliotibial band syndrome in athletes, as well as the optimal treatment regimen.

1. Introduction

Iliotibial band syndrome is a common knee injury caused by inflammation of the distal portion of the iliotibial band (ITB), which results in lateral knee pain. The distal iliotibial band slides over the lateral femoral epicondyle, and during repetitive flexion and extension activities of the knee excessive friction and potential irritation results in pain. Potential risk factors for the development of iliotibial band syndrome include preexisting iliotibial band tightness, high weekly mileage, time spent walking or running on a track, interval training, and muscular weakness of knee extensors, flexors, and hip abductors [1, 2]. Populations who expose their knees to a greater amount of flexion and extension activities, such as athletes, particularly long distance athletes, put themselves at a higher risk for iliotibial band syndrome. Due to the pathophysiology of IT band syndrome, runners have been a group often looked at for prevalence and management of this syndrome. ITB syndrome has been documented to have as high as a 22.2% incidence of all lower extremity injuries in runners [3]. Despite a clear pathophysiology, it is unclear why this syndrome affects some athletes greater than others. Few studies have shown any direct relationship between biomechanical factors and the development of iliotibial bad syndrome [1, 2, 4–6].

Athletes with ITB syndrome typically complain of a sharp or burning pain roughly 2 cm superior to the lateral joint line [3]. The pain may radiate proximally or distally, and in less severe cases, the pain may quickly subside upon cessation of activities. Often pain will occur as activities proceed. It is not uncommon that the athlete will experience popping on the lateral aspect of the knee with activities.

ITB syndrome is a clinical diagnosis and most often additional diagnostic studies are not necessary. It should be suspected in overuse and nontraumatic cases of knee pain where rest has not been helpful. Ober's test is one

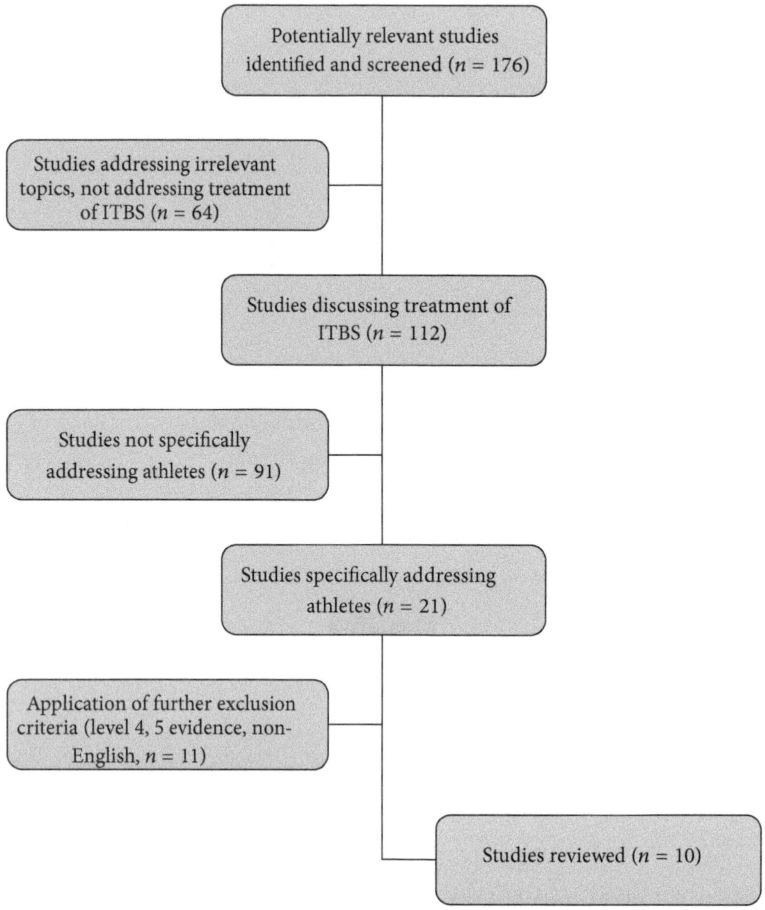

FIGURE 1: Flow chart displaying search process for review.

of numerous physical exam tests often used to assess the tightness of the ITB. If the leg can be passively stretched to a position horizontal but not completely adducted to a table, this constitutes minimal tightness. If the leg can be passively adducted to horizontal at best, this constitutes moderate tightness, and if it cannot be passively adducted to horizontal, this is maximal tightness [7]. Popping of the ITB over the lateral femoral condyle can also occur in this position as the knee is brought through range of motion. Palpation over the ITB during this maneuver typically will reproduce pain. History, however, is much more important than physical exam in diagnosis and short-term resolution of symptoms following corticosteroid injection and be both diagnostic and therapeutic.

MRI may be of use if there is doubt about the diagnosis as well as to exclude an intra-articular problem such as a lateral meniscal tear; however, isolated ITBFS often does not lead to MRI abnormalities and can be misdiagnosed if a minor but different lesion is present. Two studies revealed that in patients with iliotibial band syndrome, MRI studies have shown that the distal portion of the ITB may thicken, and a bursa deep to the iliotibial band over the lateral epicondyle becomes inflamed and filled with fluid [8, 9]. When the athletic population was isolated, normal, or cystic, poorly defined signal intensities at the distal portion of the ITB predominated. Only in chronic cases was a thickening of the distal ITB at the level of the lateral femoral epicondyle seen [8].

While the majority of patients respond to a nonsurgical, conservative approach, this does not occur for all, and escalation of treatment is necessary. This is especially true in athletes that present with refractory cases, and at this time surgical intervention can be used [3]. Unfortunately, refractory cases can occur quite often, and no treatment has been shown to work best. The purpose of this review is to outline both the conservative and surgical options for treatment of iliotibial band syndrome in athletes.

2. Methods

In order to find the most current treatment options for ITB syndrome in athletes, a literature search was conducted in the PubMed database. Criteria for inclusion in this review were papers that primarily (but not exclusively) focused on the athletic population, achieved a level III or greater level of evidence, addressed therapeutic options for ITB syndrome (conservative or surgical), and were written in English. An initial search of iliotibial band syndrome yielded 176 results. After limiting the results to those articles that discussed treatment options, and focused on the athletic population, 10 articles were reviewed. Figure 1 outlines the sequence of the literature search.

TABLE 1: Conservative treatment.

Study	Number of participants	Study type	Therapeutic regimen (all groups)	Group specific therapy	Comparison between groups	Outcomes, conclusions
Schwellnus et al. [10]	43 runners	RCT	Day 0–7: rest ice and medication, daily stretching Days 3, 5, and 7 DTFM	Group 1: placebo 2: anti-inflammatory (Voltaren) 3: anti-inflammatory/analgesic combo (Myprodol)	Group 3 had less pain and increased running time/distance from day 0 to 7	All treatments are effective; analgesic/anti-inflammatory is superior
Gunter and Schwellnus [11]	18 runners	RCT	No running for 14 days after injection and ice for 30 min every 12 hrs.	Group 1: corticosteroid injection (methylprednisolone acetate 40 mg) Group 2: placebo injection	Using a visual analogue scale for pain perception, significant ($P = 0.01$) decrease in pain during running in group 1	Local corticosteroid infiltration effectively decreases pain during running in the first 2 wks of treatment of ITBS Group 1 avg. of 53.6% decreases in pain from day 0 to 14
Pinshaw et al. [12]	24 runners	Case series	Softer running shoes, correct leg-length discrepancies, reduce training distance, ice 30 min. BID		Response to treatment was variable, even some who followed treatment judiciously did not benefit	After 8 weeks, 44% were 100% cured, 22% were 75% cured, and 34% were 50% or less cured
Fredericson et al. [2]	24 (10 M 14 F) injured runners, 30 (16 M 14 F) controls	Case series	Injured runners enrolled in a 6-week rehab to strengthen gluteus medius	Statistically significant ($P < 0.05$) higher hip abductor torque in control group compared to injured runners.	After rehab females increased hip abductor torque 34.9%, males 51.4%	22/24 athletes were pain-free and able to return to running, with recurrence at 6 months

3. Results

3.1. Conservative Treatment. There are many different conservative treatment modalities for IT band syndrome. Many of these treatment modalities have been geared toward the runner population, and certain guidelines to return to sport (running) have been suggested [3]. Table 1 illustrates four studies that outlined conservative treatment modalities.

In a randomized controlled trial (RCT), Schwellnus et al. investigated the effect of initial treatment (day 0–7: rest, ice application, and medication) in 43 patients with unilateral ITBS. All subjects received physical therapy consisting of ultrasound, deep transverse friction massages on days 3, 5, and 7 and daily stretching of the IT band. Medication was delivered over the 7 days in a double-blind, placebo-controlled fashion with group 1 taking a placebo anti-inflammatory, group 2 an anti-inflammatory (Voltaren), and group 3 an anti-inflammatory/analgesic (Myprodol). Compared with the other groups, group 3 had less pain during running from day 3 onward, and their running time/distance on the treadmill significantly increased from day 0 to 7 [10].

In another randomized controlled trial, 18 runners with acuteonset ITB syndrome (<14 days' duration) were randomly assigned into two groups: group 1 received a corticosteroid injection and group 2 received a placebo injection. Subjects were instructed not to run for 14 days following the injection and to apply ice to the area for 30 minutes every 12 hours. Running pain was significantly decreased in the group that received the corticosteroid injection [11].

In a case series of 196 running injuries, Pinshaw et al. found ITBS to the third most common injury (12%) behind peripatellar pain syndrome (22%) and posterior tibial stress syndrome (18%). In those with ITBS a four-step conservative approach was used for treatment. These steps included running shoes: change to softer shoes, use of in-shoe support and shoe alterations, and/or removal of the outside heel flare of the shoe for the injured side. Leg-length discrepancies: adapt shoe of the shorter leg by adding material to the mid-sole to ensure 100% correction at the heel, 50% correction in the mid-sole, and 25% correction at the ball of the foot. Training methods: if appropriate, reduce training distance and decrease running speed and amount of hill running. Also, incorporate a sufficient number of days for recovery. Ice application: apply ice to the injured area for 30 minutes twice a day [12].

Finally, in a case series done at the Stanford Sports Medicine Clinic, 24 runners (10 M, 14 W) with ITBS completed a 6-week rehabilitation program, which consisted of local application of ultrasound with corticosteroid gel for the first two sessions. All patients were instructed to stretch the IT band three times a day, and hip abduction exercises and pelvic drop sets to strengthen the gluteus were increased throughout the program with a goal of 3 sets of 30 repetitions. Nonsteroidal anti-inflammatory drugs were prescribed until the patients were free of pain during daily activities. The investigators found a mean increase of 34.9% and 51.4% in the injured leg of the hip abductor torque for females and males, respectively. Twenty-two of the 24 athletes (91.7%) of the athletes were able to return to running at the end of the 6-week program [2].

These four studies demonstrate how diverse conservative treatment for ITBS can be. From clinical experience, rest is the best treatment for the acute cases. This treatment becomes less useful as it becomes a more chronic condition when bursal and periosteal changes have set in. There is limited evidence to support one specific approach to the treatment of ITBS; however, when looking at the desired goal of return to sport, a combination of rest (2–6 weeks), stretching, pain management, and modification of running habits produces a high return to sport rate.

3.2. Surgical Treatment. Surgery is often reserved for refractory cases that have failed other avenues of conservative management. However, in the athletic population, return to sport is a common concern, and multiple, long absences from sport due to trials of various conservative treatment approaches are often not ideal.

There are differing viewpoints as to when surgical treatment should be implemented. Martens et al. suggests that conservative treatments should be maintained for an average of 9 months before consideration of surgical intervention [13]. Others have based their decision for surgical intervention on the observation that at 30 degrees flexion, the posterior fibers of the ITB are tighter against the lateral femoral epicondyle than are the more anterior fibers, in which case a surgical release in the posterior fibers is needed to correct the problem [14, 15].

In one study, 36 athletes with a resistant ITBS were treated with a standard arthroscopic technique, limited to the resection of lateral synovial recess. The patients had suffered from ITBS for an average of 18 months (1–7 years). Thirty-three patients (mean age 31.1 years) were available for followup at least 6 months postoperatively. Prior to surgery, all patients had been treated conservatively for at least 6 months with rest, correction of training error, shoe modification, physical therapy and local infiltration with steroids. Thirty-two patients had good or excellent results based on subjective functional results at followup. All patients went back to sports after 3 months. In 2 patients a meniscal lesion was found, which required treatment, and an associated cartilage lesion of the femoral condyle was found in the one patient that reported a fair outcome at followup. The author concluded that arthroscopic resection of the lateral synovial recess in resistant ITBS is a valid option with a consistently good outcome, which also allows excluding or treating other intra-articular pathology [16].

A retrospective study on athletes in Norway looked at 45 patients who failed conservative management of ITBS. The surgical procedure of choice for these resistant ITBS cases was transection of the posterior half of the iliotibial band where it passes over the lateral epicondyle of the femur. With a mean age of 27 (14–46) years, 38 (84.4%) had excellent or good results, 6 (13.3%) had fair results, and 1 (2.3%) had a poor result [17]. Return to sport was not documented in this study, but 75.6% of patients reported that they would have the operation again [17].

Bursectomy has also been explored as a surgical treatment option for ITBS. In a recent study a single surgeon performed 11 open iliotibial band bursectomies on 11 patients (7 M, 4 W). Each patient presented with persistent (>6 months) symptoms despite conservative treatment, with an average age at onset of 29 (24–41) years [18]. After a minimum of 20-month followup, all patients were able to return to their preinjury Tegner activity levels, and all reported less pain (11-point visual analogue scale score decreased by 6 points) [18]. Nine of the 11 patients said that knowing what they know now they would have the surgery performed again for the same problem. This population, however, was a mix of athletic and the general population, and the study did not separate out the results of each population.

4. Discussion

Iliotibial band syndrome (also called iliotibial band friction syndrome) is a common problem encountered in the knees' of athletes, especially endurance athletes whose sport requires repetitive knee flexion. ITBS can often recur in the athletic population, causing significant morbidity and delay in return to sport [19]. There is debate on whether iliotibial band syndrome is truly a friction syndrome where the ITB itself is pathologic or whether a pathologic bursa forms between the ITB and the lateral femoral condyle, causing the pain. This is an important concept because successful surgical treatment of the syndrome must address the underlying pathological causes [18].

Regardless of stance on the pathophysiology, conservative management is the first line of therapy for ITBS. However, both conservative and surgical therapies play a major role in recalcitrant cases. A combination of therapies (rest, pain relief, stretching, strength training, and running habit modification) works best for returning athletes to their preinjury level and reducing their symptoms. However, a systematic regimen involving all aspects of conservative therapy has not been established. A recent systematic review on iliotibial band syndrome in runners concluded that there is limited evidence to support one specific approach to the diagnosis and treatment of ITBS, suggesting that additional research is needed to elucidate an optimal treatment regimen [20]. In our review, conservative therapy alone was found to have a 44% complete cure rate with return to sport at 8 weeks and a 91.7% return to sport rate at 6 months [2, 12].

ITB syndrome pathophysiology plays a key role in guiding surgical treatments. Most surgeons who have published in the literature ascribe to the iliotibial friction band syndrome theory, and numerous procedures that excise or release this supposedly pathologic portion of the ITB have been described. Cortisone injections should still be used first in these scenarios, as ITBS is considered an inflammatory friction syndrome. However, as the duration of symptoms increases and conservative measures fail, surgical treatment may be needed for resolution of symptoms. Three of these procedures have been described above, all in athletes, with a return to sport rate of 100% at an average of 3 months [16] and 7 weeks [13]. One study did not report return to sport rate [17]. Furthermore, Fairclough et al. did not find a bursa in either the 6 cadaveric specimens they dissected or the 2 symptomatic patients on whom they performed an MRI [21]. In patients with iliotibial band syndrome MRI findings of the ITB can be normal. In a study of 16 patients with ITBS, 31% had a discrete fluid collection medial to the ITB, with a normal looking ITB. However, it was hypothesized that this collection likely arose from chronic inflammation beneath the ITB, resulting in the formation of a secondary or adventitious bursa rather than from the inflammation of an existing primary bursa [22].

There are also those that ascribe to the theory that the ITB itself is not pathological in patients with iliotibial band syndrome, but rather the pain and functional deficits are generated by a pathological bursa that forms beneath the ITB due to compression of that underlying tissue rather than a friction mechanism. In the study performed by Hariri et al. described above, they consistently found what appears to be an inflamed bursa underlying a benign-appearing ITB [18]. This study, however, was not done solely on the athletic population whereas the ones described which favor the friction theory of iliotibial band syndrome were. Surgical intervention is often only utilized after patients have failed conservative management for ITBS, making return to preinjury level a difficult task. Although there are two theories on the pathophysiology of ITBS, when looking at return to sport rate in the athletic population, resection of the lateral synovial recess, after failure of conservative therapy provides an excellent return to sport rate.

5. Conclusion

Iliotibial band syndrome is a common cause of lateral knee pain in the athlete, especially runners and other endurance athletes [23]. Both conservative and surgical approaches are viable treatment options, and both need to be considered during treatment planning. While the majority of cases resolve with conservative management, resistant cases are seen in many athletes, requiring surgical intervention. The cases that require surgical intervention are often chronic in nature, and it is important to recognize the duration of symptoms so that surgical treatment can be initiated early. Despite many options for both surgical and conservative treatment, there has yet to be consensus on one standard of care. Further research is needed to delineate the true pathology behind iliotibial band syndrome in athletes, as well as the optimal treatment regimen.

References

[1] S. P. Messier, D. G. Edwards, D. F. Martin et al., "Etiology of iliotibial band friction syndrome in distance runners," *Medicine and Science in Sports and Exercise*, vol. 27, no. 7, pp. 951–960, 1995.

[2] M. Fredericson, C. L. Cookingham, A. M. Chaudhari, B. C. Dowdell, N. Oestreicher, and S. A. Sahrmann, "Hip abductor weakness in distance runners with iliotibial band syndrome," *Clinical Journal of Sport Medicine*, vol. 10, no. 3, pp. 169–175, 2000.

[3] M. Fredericson and A. Weir, "Practical management of iliotibial band friction syndrome in runners," *Clinical Journal of Sport Medicine*, vol. 16, no. 3, pp. 261–268, 2006.

[4] S. P. Messier and K. A. Pittala, "Etiologic factors associated with selected running injuries," *Medicine and Science in Sports and Exercise*, vol. 20, no. 5, pp. 501–505, 1988.

[5] J. E. Taunton, M. B. Ryan, D. B. Clement, D. C. McKenzie, D. R. Lloyd-Smith, and B. D. Zumbo, "A retrospective case-control analysis of 2002 running injuries," *British Journal of Sports Medicine*, vol. 36, no. 2, pp. 95–101, 2002.

[6] J. W. Orchard, P. A. Fricker, A. T. Abud, and B. R. Mason, "Biomechanics of iliotibial band friction syndrome in runners," *American Journal of Sports Medicine*, vol. 24, no. 3, pp. 375–379, 1996.

[7] J. C. Gose and P. Schweizer, "Iliotibial band tightness," *Journal of Orthopaedic and Sports Physical Therapy*, vol. 10, no. 10, pp. 399–407, 1989.

[8] G. Nishimura, M. Yamato, K. Tamai, J. Takahashi, and M. Uetani, "MR findings in iliotibial band syndrome," *Skeletal Radiology*, vol. 26, no. 9, pp. 533–537, 1997.

[9] E. F. Ekman, T. Pope, D. F. Martin, and W. W. Curl, "Magnetic resonance imaging of iliotibial band syndrome," *American Journal of Sports Medicine*, vol. 22, no. 6, pp. 851–854, 1994.

[10] M. P. Schwellnus, L. Theunissen, T. D. Noakes, and S. G. Reinach, "Anti-inflammatory and combined anti-inflammatory/analgesic medication in the early management of iliotibial band friction syndrome: a clinical trial," *South African Medical Journal*, vol. 79, no. 10, pp. 602–606, 1991.

[11] P. Gunter and M. P. Schwellnus, "Local corticosteroid injection in iliotibial band friction syndrome in runners: a randomised controlled trial," *British Journal of Sports Medicine*, vol. 38, no. 3, pp. 269–272, 2004.

[12] R. Pinshaw, V. Atlas, and T. D. Noakes, "The nature and response to therapy of 196 consecutive injuries seen at a runners' clinic," *South African Medical Journal*, vol. 65, no. 8, pp. 291–298, 1984.

[13] M. Martens, P. Libbrecht, and A. Burssens, "Surgical treatment of the iliotibial band friction syndrome," *American Journal of Sports Medicine*, vol. 17, no. 5, pp. 651–654, 1989.

[14] C. A. Noble, "Iliotibial band friction syndrome in runners," *American Journal of Sports Medicine*, vol. 8, no. 4, pp. 232–234, 1980.

[15] C. A. Noble, "The treatment of iliotibial band friction syndrome," *British Journal of Sports Medicine*, vol. 13, no. 2, pp. 51–54, 1979.

[16] F. Michels, S. Jambou, M. Allard, V. Bousquet, P. Colombet, and C. De Lavigne, "An arthroscopic technique to treat the iliotibial band syndrome," *Knee Surgery, Sports Traumatology, Arthroscopy*, vol. 17, no. 3, pp. 233–236, 2009.

[17] J. O. Drogset, I. Rossvoll, and T. Grøntvedt, "Surgical treatment of iliotibial band friction syndrome: a retrospective study of 45 patients," *Scandinavian Journal of Medicine and Science in Sports*, vol. 9, no. 5, pp. 296–298, 1999.

[18] S. Hariri, E. T. Savidge, M. M. Reinold, J. Zachazewski, and T. J. Gill, "Treatment of recalcitrant iliotibial band friction syndrome with open iliotibial band bursectomy: indications, technique, and clinical outcomes," *American Journal of Sports Medicine*, vol. 37, no. 7, pp. 1417–1424, 2009.

[19] C. A. Lucas, "Iliotibial band friction syndrome as exhibited in athletes," *Journal of Athletic Training*, vol. 27, no. 3, pp. 250–252, 1992.

[20] M. P. van der Worp, N. van der Horst, A. de Wijer, F. J. Backx, and M. W. Nijhuis-van der Sanden, "Iliotibial band syndrome in runners: a systematic review," *Journal of Sports Medicine*, vol. 42, no. 11, pp. 969–992, 2012.

[21] J. Fairclough, K. Hayashi, H. Toumi et al., "Is iliotibial band syndrome really a friction syndrome?" *Journal of Science and Medicine in Sport*, vol. 10, no. 2, pp. 74–76, 2007.

[22] C. Muhle, J. M. Ahn, L. Yeh et al., "Iliotibial band friction syndrome: MR imaging findings in 16 patients and MR arthrographic study of six cadaveric knees," *Radiology*, vol. 212, no. 1, pp. 103–110, 1999.

[23] M. Fredericson and C. Wolf, "Iliotibial band syndrome in runners: innovations in treatment," *Sports Medicine*, vol. 35, no. 5, pp. 451–459, 2005.

4

Validation of the Continuum of Care Conceptual Model for Athletic Therapy

Mark R. Lafave,[1] **Dale Butterwick,**[2] **and Breda Eubank**[1]

[1]*Department of Health and Physical Education, Mount Royal University, 4825 Mount Royal Gate SW, Calgary, AB, Canada T3E 6K6*
[2]*Faculty of Kinesiology, University of Calgary, 2400 University Drive NW, Calgary, AB, Canada T2N 1N4*

Correspondence should be addressed to Mark R. Lafave; mlafave@mtroyal.ca

Academic Editor: S. John Sullivan

Utilization of conceptual models in field-based emergency care currently borrows from existing standards of medical and paramedical professions. The purpose of this study was to develop and validate a comprehensive conceptual model that could account for injuries ranging from nonurgent to catastrophic events including events that do not follow traditional medical or prehospital care protocols. The conceptual model should represent the continuum of care from the time of initial injury spanning to an athlete's return to participation in their sport. Finally, the conceptual model should accommodate both novices and experts in the AT profession. This paper chronicles the content validation steps of the Continuum of Care Conceptual Model for Athletic Therapy (CCCM-AT). The stages of model development were domain and item generation, content expert validation using a three-stage modified Ebel procedure, and pilot testing. Only the final stage of the modified Ebel procedure reached a priori 80% consensus on three domains of interest: (1) heading descriptors; (2) the order of the model; (3) the conceptual model as a whole. Future research is required to test the use of the CCCM-AT in order to understand its efficacy in teaching and practice within the AT discipline.

1. Introduction

Injury is common in sport. Specifically, sport-related injuries have been ranked as second only to home and leisure accidents for injury occurrence and third in terms of severity after traffic accidents and violence [1]. The spectrum of injuries that arise can range from catastrophic events to those that are less urgent. This spectrum of events results in the need for a structured injury care model that can be used to manage sport injuries regardless of severity.

Athletic therapists/trainers (i.e., ATs herein) are professional caregivers that are often hired to provide on-site care in the management of sport-related injuries, which is a key competency for working in a field environment [2]. ATs must fulfill a spectrum of competencies that begin when an injury is often witnessed and end when an athlete safely returns to participation.

ATs often adopt emergency care protocols and standards of care for injured athletes from existing standards of medical and paramedical professions [3–6].

The adoption of emergency care protocols for catastrophic and urgent conditions (such as managing an unconscious athlete) seems quite appropriate for the AT profession since there are no specialized standards or expectations for patient care with these conditions. However, anecdotal experiences suggest that the majority of injuries managed by ATs are nonurgent and non-life-threatening (e.g., sprains, strains, and contusions), thus requiring a different paradigm of assessment, management, and treatment [4]. The care provided to an athlete who suffered prolonged loss of consciousness as compared to one who has a first degree ankle sprain would require evaluation and management strategies that are quite different. The former would require the AT to call emergency medical services (EMS) and to evaluate, assess, immobilize, and stabilize the athlete until assistance arrives. The AT may also need to package the athlete in preparation for transportation to the hospital due to the urgent nature of an unconscious athlete. In the ankle sprain example, the evaluation and management are not as clearly defined using emergency care models found in the literature. If an AT were to follow the existing emergency care model to care for a sprained ankle, the AT would need to call emergency medical services, immobilize the athlete, and wait until EMS arrived. This is not likely the most practical nor ideal way to manage injuries of this calibre. ATs are trained to evaluate the type and severity of injuries and are competent to recognize and manage injuries on-field accordingly. Therefore, a model of care must be able to allow for flexibility across the spectrum of injuries; support decision making from the time the AT begins their evaluation to the point where they decide on the best management protocol; and make use of the skill-set of the caregiver. Currently, there are no such models that have strong levels of evidence that exist in the literature for relatively simple neuromusculoskeletal injuries.

ATs are often faced with a number of challenges and variables associated with managing injuries at both ends of this injury severity spectrum in a real-life environment. Expert ATs should be able to handle these challenges and variables proficiently. However, novice or student ATs learning this material for the first time may require a tool such as a conceptual model to facilitate the learning process. Conceptual models are often used for teaching novice learners complex concepts, which ensures that their interactions are accurate, consistent, and complete [7]. A Continuum of Care Conceptual Model for Athletic Therapy (CCCM-AT) may assist the complex relationship between knowledge and the ability to apply knowledge appropriately.

There are a number of definitions of conceptual models in the literature. Mayer defined a conceptual model as "words or diagrams that are intended to help learners build mental models of the system being studied: a conceptual model highlights the major objects and actions in a system as well as causal relations among them" [8, page 43]. Greca and Moreira defined a conceptual model as "an external representation created by researcher, teachers, engineers, and so forth, that facilitates the comprehension or the teaching of systems" [9, page 5]. Conceptual models have been employed successfully to facilitate learning across a variety of disciplines: (a) computer programming content [10]; (b) electricity principles [11]; (c) nursing critical thinking skills [12, 13]; (d) accounting principles [14]; (e) athletic training therapeutic modality decision making [15].

Although conceptual models are popular outside of the AT discipline, there does not appear to be a conceptual model in the literature that comprehensively represents the full spectrum of nonurgent to urgent conditions within the AT discipline. There were some linear models that outlined the primary and secondary survey comprehensively [4, 6, 16, 17] and one circular model that outlined an interdisciplinary and generic approach to care [18]. None of the models, in their entirety, were applicable to the full AT scope of practice.

The purpose of this study was to develop and validate a comprehensive conceptual model that could account for injuries ranging from nonurgent to catastrophic events including events that do not follow traditional medical or prehospital care protocols. The conceptual model should provide a framework for the management of injuries by an AT regardless of severity.

2. Methods

2.1. Content Validation of the Conceptual Model. Traditionally, content validation processes such as the modified Ebel procedure have been employed to establish content validity of a measurement tool or instrument [19–21]. In the current study, a modified Ebel procedure was employed to establish the heading descriptors in the Continuum of Care Conceptual Model for Athletic Therapy/Training (CCCM-AT). The modified Ebel procedure consists of three stages: (1) simple validation; (2) initial validation; (3) final consensus or removal of items for validation if necessary [22–24]. The first stage consisted of simple validation (or face validity). It was a process whereby a local/regional group reviewed the literature, interacted, and conceived the content of the model. Materials from all existing models were used to build an AT-specific model of health care delivery as part of the simple validation process [4, 6, 16–18].

The initial CCCM-AT was designed, created, and underwent simple validation with the authors of this paper and four other athletic therapists from the University of Calgary and Mount Royal University. This first version of the CCCM-AT was pilot tested for approximately six months with the ATs who participated in the simple validation process. Pilot testing consisted of ATs working in the field mentally envisioning the headings of the CCCM-AT in conditions across the urgent to nonurgent spectrum.

In the second stage of the modified Ebel procedure, the authors identified a group of experts ($n = 20$) external to the University of Calgary and Mount Royal University. These potential validators were educated in both Canada and the United States.

Potential validators were contacted to confirm interest and availability for the project. The final group of validators ($n = 11$) were self-selected and had expertise in caring for community, collegiate, elite, and professional athletes. Further, they were active educators and examiners in accredited Canadian Athletic Therapists' Association (CATA) programs. This group included 11 certified ATs and one AT/physiotherapist. The sample size of validators was consistent with content validation methodology [25].

The 11 validators were informed about the purpose of the project and sent a marking grid through electronic mail. Validators were asked to rate the importance of keeping each heading descriptor, the order of the model, and the conceptual model as a whole using a marking rubric or importance scale (very important, important, and not important) as part of the second stage. Eighty percent consensus was the target for one of the three categories: very important; important; and not important [22–25]. If that target was achieved, it meant the validators agreed with the content of the conceptual model for use by ATs. If 80% was not achieved, a third and final stage of face-to-face discussion would ensue on the importance of keeping the heading descriptors, the order of the model, and the conceptual model as a whole [22–25]. During the face-to-face discussion each item required 80% consensus for inclusion in the final model.

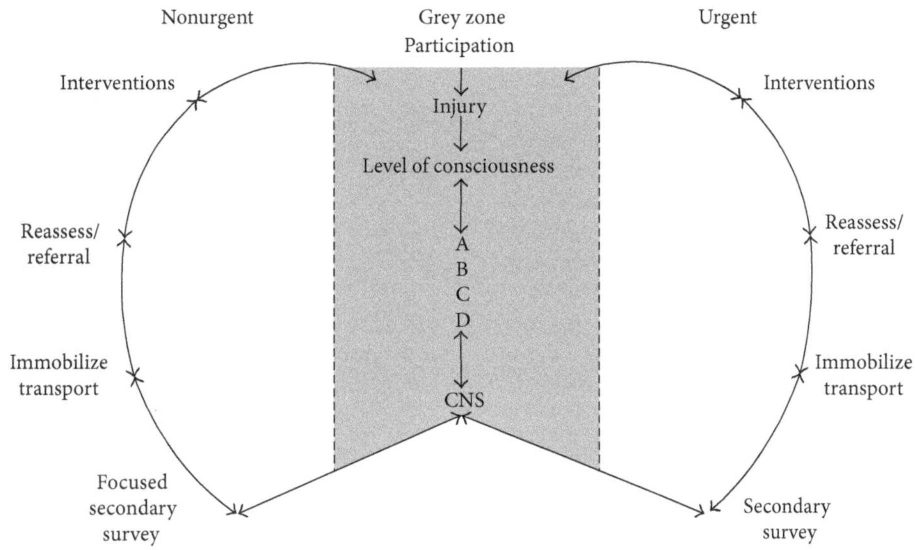

Figure 1: The Continuum of Care Conceptual Model for Athletic Therapy.

3. Results

The simple validation committee during stage one of the modified Ebel procedure produced a model that was presented to the validators in the second stage. The second stage did not achieve 80% consensus for the three major domains: (1) heading descriptors; (2) the order of the model; and (3) the conceptual model as a whole. However, the third stage's face-to-face discussion did achieve 80% consensus for all three major domains. The final result of the Continuum of Care Conceptual Model for Athletic Therapy/Training (CCCM-AT) is presented in Figure 1. The dramatic change in agreement from stage two to stage three was the result of concrete examples employed to illustrate how the model could be employed.

It was agreed that the CCCM-AT be divided into three major regions: grey, urgent, and nonurgent zones. The face-to-face discussion that ensued and ultimately resulted in agreement for all aspects of the model is central to the results of this paper. Some of the face-to-face discussion included differentiating between the three regions of the model and how they may be different or the same as a traditional emergency care protocol taught in prehospital care educational programs. Below is a synopsis of the discussion that transpired and that is central to the results of this paper.

All injury assessment begins at the top of the grey zone. The grey zone is the time to rapidly gather information about the nature of the injury and assess the patient's vital functions in order to establish which treatment pathway to enter.

Metaphorically, it is grey due to the initial uncertainty about the extent and/or severity of the injury, and the undefined interventions required. For example, if an athlete is unconscious and not breathing, the appropriate management protocol is to activate EMS (i.e., call 911). This is a simple, black and white case to manage, continuing with the color metaphor. However, the majority of other conditions are not as simple, thus requiring greater critical thought on the best management techniques. The traditional prehospital care model employs linear approach to management of conditions where the care provider should complete the ABC's of a primary survey. However, in the AT discipline, we would contend that the evaluation and management should not be simply to complete the linear evaluation outlined in the primary survey. Rather, there may be times for the AT discipline to appropriately and very rapidly (i.e., 5 seconds) evaluate the primary survey and move directly into a focused secondary survey. For example, if a running back in football made a cut and immediately dropped to the ground writhing in pain, grasping their knee *without* contacting an opposition player, an AT may quickly surmise the athlete's airway (A), breathing (B), and circulation (C) are functioning normally. Again, it may be obvious to the AT that the athlete's airway, breathing and circulation are clear because they are screaming in pain and the mechanism of injury did not support external or internal deadly bleeding (D). As a result of the ABC's being clear, the AT may skip to a focused secondary survey or football player's knee injury more quickly. This plan of action is supported with advanced level of emergency care through the International Trauma Life Support (ITLS) for Prehospital Care Providers [26], but not at lower levels of emergency care standards such as those in the Canadian Red Cross [27]. The lower levels of advanced first aid would expect a thorough and complete primary followed by a secondary survey (i.e., head to toe examination). The validator group was given this example and agreed that it accurately represented a common scenario they may be confronted with regularly in their practice. Perhaps more importantly, the validators told the research team that this is the way they currently manage these types of injuries, which further validated the functionality of the model.

In contrast, there may be an athlete who fell to the ground without another player touching them and was lying motionless: no distinct and clear mechanism of injury. An urgent life-threatening injury may be in the AT's mind and a traditional emergency care model should be implemented since there was little explicit information of why this player was lying motionless without obvious cause. In this case, an AT would more carefully and purposefully move through the grey region to ensure the ABC's are evaluated and treated prior to moving into the urgent side of the model (i.e., the right side). Again, the validator group was given this example and all agreed that it could be representative of similar situations where careful and purposeful primary and secondary survey (i.e., not focused) were more appropriate than the first example provided.

These contrasting injuries provide an example of how differently an AT may manage conditions based on seeing the mechanism of injury occur. The examples also illustrate how quickly or slowly one may go through the grey area and move into either the right side (urgent) or left side (nonurgent). To reiterate, if the injury is determined to be urgent, the right side of the conceptual model is the recommended method of management. It incorporates the use of traditional emergency care algorithms found in the literature [4, 6, 16–18]. It also incorporates the notion of a focused secondary survey accepted at the ITLS level of care [26]. The purpose of this model is not to propose any new standards of care if an athlete suffers from an urgent condition. Rather, the purpose of this model is to more accurately represent what transpires in actual practice for ATs.

The utility of the CCCM-AT is both the speed at which one can move from the grey region (centre) to either right or left sides and the speed at which one can focus on the specific injury at hand. The AT scope of practice manages many more non-life-threatening or nonurgent conditions than urgent conditions in everyday practice. This is one of the key differences in the scope of practice between the AT discipline and the prehospital care professional. Prehospital care professionals likely find a bigger balance between urgent and nonurgent conditions, while the AT profession primary deals with nonurgent conditions but has to be prepared to deal with either. When given the option to have a model that captured both urgent and nonurgent conditions so fluidly, the validation group agreed and validated the model provided the arrows were not one directional and linear.

The final but critical aspect of the model that was validated was the use of two-way arrows. It was important to recognize that, at any given stage, athletes (or patients) could suffer an injury that could be classified in the grey, urgent, or nonurgent zones and need to revert one or more steps backwards. The example one validator provided was with the same example of the football running back that was not contacted, thus making the assumption that the injury was nonurgent. However, if that same athlete had the comorbidity of asthma and the athlete went into shock due to pain, it is possible that this athlete's condition could worsen compromising their airway, breathing, and/or circulation. In this case, it would be important to revert back to the evaluation and management procedures outlined in previous, urgent condition steps in the grey zone and quickly move from the left side of the model to the grey zone (center) and then onto the right side of the model. It should be noted that the rest of the CCCM-AT on both the right side and left side after the secondary or focused secondary survey achieved consensus with very little discussion. These examples of the scenarios helped the validators agree and ultimately content validate the CCCM-AT as presented in Figure 1.

4. Discussion

In the AT profession, a thorough search of the literature revealed that no conceptual models existed that outlined a continuum of care from the point of initial injury to full return to sport or activity. Additionally, there were no conceptual models that allowed for flexibility in protocols for managing a full spectrum of injury severity. As a result, a new conceptual model was proposed and validated in the current study. The AT discipline is a unique profession whereby the scope of practice may include managing injuries immediately following an injury in a sport or recreational environment. In addition, another unique feature of the AT discipline is the careful guidance and supervision of the athlete after their injury, particularly when the athlete returns to participation in their sport or activity. A conceptual model to help capture this wide scope of practice is important from a teaching, learning, and practice perspective. It can be overwhelming for a novice or student AT to learn, organize and plan the full spectrum of steps from immediate onset of an injury straight through to the eventual return to play due to vast number of steps between those two end points. Placing the entire continuum of care from initial injury to the return to participation into context may be helpful in managing all the steps and variables necessary between each of the major categories outlined in the CCCM-AT, particularly for a novice AT.

Conceptual models have been employed in a number of other disciplines to successfully teach complex concepts and relationships between those concepts.

None of the conceptual models employed in teaching other disciplines reported a similar process of content validation as the process employed in the current study.

However, it seems to be logical to ensure that the conceptual model being proposed actually represents what it is intended to represent: content validity.

The use of conceptual models to teach is supported within a theoretical framework of human cognition. In essence, a novice builds meaning of ideas, concepts, or the steps in a conceptual model by organizing and making connections between those principles [28]. This theory is supported by Ausubel: "If existing cognitive structure is clear, stable and suitably organized, it facilitates the learning and retention of a new subject matter. If it is unstable, ambiguous, disorganized, or chaotically organized, it inhibits learning and retention" [29, page 217]. Theoretically, the conceptual model proposed in the current study is thought to create a "clear, stable, and suitably organized" structure to facilitate learning of the many steps under each major category in the CCCM-AT. It is clear that novices process information differently and move through varying levels of detail differently than experts [30]. A conceptual model, if taught to students early in their learning process, can act like a compass or a guide directing them and contextualizing their learning much like an Advance Organizer or Graphical Organizer [31]. Experts may move through an urgent or nonurgent situation quickly and make, what may appear to a novice, quantum leaps from one conceptual model descriptor to another (i.e., from primary survey to secondary survey) with ease and seemingly little thought [32]. However, an expert has likely lived through a number of experiences that have contributed to their current comfort level with a particular injury or scenario. An expert may be able to negotiate both large steps like those outlined in the CCCM-AT, while also managing the smaller steps that would naturally be embedded under each of those categories. The point of this conceptual model is not to replace those smaller steps under each category listed in the CCCM-AT, but rather to supplement or provide a larger map that helps chart the pathway from the time an athlete injures himself or herself until the point where they return to play. Part of the utility of the CCCM-AT is its simplicity when classifying the complex spectrum of injuries from nonurgent to urgent into one of the three regions.

Schmidt and Boshuizen hypothesized that experts begin to accumulate "illness scripts" over time, which are injuries or conditions that have a similar pattern and thus permit efficiency in an expert's decision making [33, 34]. Fadde suggested that breaking the entire performance down into its pieces and then practicing those pieces may help to hasten the transition from novice to expert [32]. Therefore, it is postulated that this conceptual model could act as a bridge between novices and experts. The model could guide and anchor learning based on a student's perception of the descriptors identified in the CCCM-AT.

One very unique aspect of the CCCM-AT that differentiates it from emergency care models is the concept of a focused secondary survey (FSS) [17, 35]. In the FSS, the urgent pathway of care has been ruled out and a complete secondary survey, including vitals assessment and monitoring, is rarely required. However, advanced first aid education teaches that a head-to-toe examination is necessary to eliminate other sources of injury or potentially life-threatening conditions [27]. This methodology of patient evaluation is one of the differential diagnoses whereby if you eliminate all other things, it must be the one injury or condition remaining that should be the focal point. However, in sport environments or where an AT typically works, it is rare that a condition is ever something more than what the athlete is overtly presenting. If we were to examine this closer using the same example provided in the results above (i.e., the football player who has a suspected noncontact knee injury), in a traditional medical model, the secondary survey would consist of the care provider going through a long, thorough primary survey followed by a head-to-toe examination. It may also require taking vital signs early in the process long before the caregiver ever addressed the athlete's main concern: their knee. To the ATs who were part of the validation group, they thought this type of care for an athlete would be incongruent with the way they practiced or what they wanted to see novices taught or practicing. It is possible for more serious conditions to be present in cases like the athlete's condition regressing due to breathing difficulty, for example. However, in circumstances when complications of a minor injury arise (e.g., shock), the circular nature of the CCCM-AT requires one to return to management strategies as dictated by the grey zone.

The conceptual model in this study has been content validated and needs to undergo future testing and research to determine its efficacy in learning the principles of field-based care in the AT discipline. Research on other conceptual models across other disciplines may provide a foundation for the thesis that this model will help to facilitate learning. Seel demonstrated that students learned economic concepts better when they were exposed to a conceptual model as compared to those students who were not exposed to the conceptual model [36]. Kern achieved more success with teaching an important accounting principle to students using a conceptual model when compared to students who did not use a conceptual model [14]. The question remains whether the results from other disciplines who have had success in teaching using conceptual models are generalizable to the AT discipline and this new model.

5. Summary

The athletic therapy discipline is unique with a combination of both clinical and field practice. The profession may be one of the few that is required to manage an athletic injury at both ends of an injury continuum: from the initial injury to return to participation. There were no current models of care in the literature that outlined this unique scope of practice across the full spectrum. The current study adopted the relevant prehospital care professionals' scope of practice and merged it with the AT discipline and scope of practice.

Generally, conceptual models have not been content validated prior to testing their efficacy in teaching and learning. Considering that no models in the AT discipline existed, it seemed appropriate to go through this process prior to testing the conceptual model in an educational environment. Employing conceptual models to teach in other disciplines such as basic science, computer information systems, nursing, accounting, and economics has been successfully implemented. Future research should employ the use of the CCCM-AT to understand its efficacy in teaching within the AT discipline.

Conflict of Interests

The authors declare that there is no conflict of interests regarding the publication of this paper.

References

[1] R. Dekker, J. Kingma, J. W. Groothoff, W. H. Eisma, and H. J. T. Duis, "Measurement of severity of sports injuries: an epidemiological study," *Clinical Rehabilitation*, vol. 14, no. 6, pp. 651–656, 2000.

[2] Canadian Athletic Therapists Association, *CATA Competencies*, 2005.

[3] B. D. Browner, A. N. Pollak, and C. L. Gupton, *Emergency Care and Transportation of the Sick and Injured*, Jones and Bartlett, Toronto, Canada, 8th edition, 2008.

[4] W. Prentice, "On the field acute care and emergency procedures," in *Arnheim's Principles of Athletic Training: A Competency-Based Approach*, p. 342, McGraw-Hill Higher Education, New York, NY, USA, 13th edition, 2009.

[5] R. Rehberg, *On Location*, Train Cond, 1998.

[6] C. Starkey, S. D. Brown, and J. Ryan, *Examination of Orthopedic and Athletic Injuries*, F.A. Davis, Philadelphia, Pa, USA, 3rd edition, 2010.

[7] C. Wu, N. B. Dale, and L. J. Bethel, "Conceptual models and cognitive learning styles in teaching recursion," *ACM SIGCSE Bulletin*, vol. 30, no. 1, pp. 292–296, 1998.

[8] R. Mayer, "Models for understanding," *Review of Educational Research*, vol. 59, no. 1, p. 43, 1989.

[9] I. M. Greca and M. A. Moreira, "Mental models, conceptual models, and modelling," *International Journal of Science Education*, vol. 22, no. 1, pp. 1–11, 2000.

[10] P. Bayman and R. E. Mayer, "Using conceptual models to teach BASIC computer programming," *Journal of Educational Psychology*, vol. 80, no. 3, pp. 291–298, 1988.

[11] J. M. Royer and G. W. Cable, "Illustrations, analogies, and facilitative transfer in prose learning," *Journal of Educational Psychology*, vol. 68, no. 2, pp. 205–209, 1976.

[12] S. Desanto-Madeya, "Using case studies based on a nursing conceptual model to teach medical-surgical nursing," *Nursing Science Quarterly*, vol. 20, no. 4, pp. 324–329, 2007.

[13] Y.-C. Huang, H.-H. Chen, M.-L. Yeh, and Y.-C. Chung, "Case studies combined with or without concept maps improve critical thinking in hospital-based nurses: a randomized-controlled trial," *International Journal of Nursing Studies*, vol. 49, no. 6, pp. 747–754, 2012.

[14] B. B. Kern, "Enhancing accounting students' problem-solving skills: the use of a hands-on conceptual model in an active learning environment," *Accounting Education*, vol. 11, no. 3, pp. 235–256, 2002.

[15] C. Starkey, *Therapeutic Modalities*, FA Davis, Philadelphia, Pa, USA, 4th edition, 2013.

[16] D. Magee, *Orthopedic Physical Assessment*, Saunders, Toronto, Canada, 5th edition, 2008.

[17] National Association of Emergency Medical Technicians, *PHTLS, Basic and Advanced Prehospital Trauma Life Support*, Mosby, St. Louis, Mo, USA, 7th edition, 2011.

[18] M. Miller and D. Berry, *Emergency Trauma Management for Athletic Trainers*, Lippincott Williams & Wilkins, Baltimore, Md, USA, 1st edition, 2011.

[19] J. A. Cantor, "A validation of Ebel's method for performance standard setting through its application with comparison approaches to a selected criterion-referenced test," *Educational and Psychological Measurement*, vol. 49, no. 3, pp. 709–721, 1989.

[20] R. Ebel and D. Frisbie, *Essentials of Educational Measurement*, vol. 4, Prentice Hall, Englewood Cliffs, NJ, USA, 1986.

[21] C. Violato, A. Marini, and D. McDougall, *Assessment of Classroom Learning*, Detselig Enterprises, Calgary, Canada, 1998.

[22] D. J. Butterwick, D. M. Paskevich, N. G. Lagumen, A. L. C. Vallevand, and M. R. Lafave, "The development of content-valid technical skill assessment instruments for athletic taping skills," *Journal of Allied Health*, vol. 35, no. 3, pp. 147–155, 2006.

[23] M. R. Lafave, D. J. Butterwick, B. Lau, R. Murray, and T. Freeman, "Content validation of the rodeo SCAT," *International Journal of Sports Medicine*, vol. 34, no. 2, pp. 170–175, 2013.

[24] M. Lafave, L. Katz, and D. Butterwick, "Development of a content-valid standardized orthopedic assessment tool (SOAT)," *Advances in Health Sciences Education*, vol. 13, no. 4, pp. 397–406, 2008.

[25] M. R. Lynn, "Determination and quantification of content validity," *Nursing Research*, vol. 35, no. 6, pp. 382–385, 1986.

[26] J. E. Campbell, *International Trauma Life Support for Prehospital Care Providers*, Pearson Education, Saddle River, NJ, USA, 7th edition, 2013.

[27] Canadian Red Cross Society, *Canadian Red Cross Emergency Care*, Canadian Red Cross Society, Ontario, Canada, 2012.

[28] D. Ifenthaler, I. Masduki, and N. M. Seel, "The mystery of cognitive structure and how we can detect it: tracking the development of cognitive structures over time," *Instructional Science*, vol. 39, no. 1, pp. 41–61, 2011.

[29] D. Ausubel, "Cognitive structure and the facilitation of meaningful verbal learning," *Journal of Teacher Education*, vol. 14, article 217, 1963.

[30] C. L. Carraccio, B. J. Benson, L. J. Nixon, and P. L. Derstine, "From the educational bench to the clinical bedside: translating the dreyfus developmental model to the learning of clinical skills," *Academic Medicine*, vol. 83, no. 8, pp. 761–767, 2008.

[31] J. W. Alba and L. Hasher, "Is memory schematic?" *Psychological Bulletin*, vol. 93, no. 2, pp. 203–231, 1983.

[32] P. Fadde, "Look 'ma, no hands: part-task training of perceptual-cognitive skills to accelerate psychomotor expertise," in *Proceedings of the Interservice/Industry Training, Simulation, and Education Conference*, Paper No 100065:1, Orlando Fla, USA, 2010.

[33] H. G. Schmidt, G. R. Norman, and H. P. A. Boshuizen, "A cognitive perspective on medical expertise: theory and implications," *Academic Medicine*, vol. 65, no. 10, pp. 611–621, 1990.

[34] H. G. Schmidt and H. P. A. Boshuizen, "On acquiring expertise in medicine," *Educational Psychology Review*, vol. 5, no. 3, pp. 205–221, 1993.

[35] S. M. Campbell, M. O. Roland, and S. A. Buetow, "Defining quality of care," *Social Science & Medicine*, vol. 51, no. 11, pp. 1611–1625, 2000.

[36] N. M. Seel, "Epistemology, situated cognition, and mental models: 'like a bridge over troubled water'," *Instructional Science*, vol. 29, no. 4-5, pp. 403–427, 2001.

5

Effects of Cooling on Ankle Muscle Strength, Electromyography, and Gait Ground Reaction Forces

Amitava Halder,[1] Chuansi Gao,[1] and Michael Miller[2]

[1] *Division of Ergonomics and Aerosol Technology, Department of Design Sciences, Faculty of Engineering, Lund University, P.O. Box 118, 221 00 Lund, Sweden*
[2] *Division of Physiotherapy, Department of Health Science, Faculty of Medicine, Lund University, P.O. Box 157, 221 00 Lund, Sweden*

Correspondence should be addressed to Amitava Halder; amitava.halder@design.lth.se

Academic Editor: Adrian W. Midgley

The effects of cooling on neuromuscular function and performance during gait are not fully examined. The purpose of this study was to investigate the effects of local cooling for 20 min in cold water at 10°C in a climate chamber also at 10°C on maximal isometric force and electromyographic (EMG) activity of the lower leg muscles. Gait ground reaction forces (GRFs) were also assessed. Sixteen healthy university students participated in the within subject design experimental study. Isometric forces of the tibialis anterior (TA) and the gastrocnemius medialis (GM) were measured using a handheld dynamometer and the EMG was recorded using surface electrodes. Ground reaction forces during gait and the required coefficient of friction (RCOF) were recorded using a force plate. There was a significantly reduced isometric maximum force in the TA muscle ($P < 0.001$) after cooling. The mean EMG amplitude of GM muscle was increased after cooling ($P < 0.003$), indicating that fatigue was induced. We found no significant changes in the gait GRFs and RCOF on dry and level surface. These findings may indicate that local moderate cooling 20 min of 10°C cold water, may influence maximal muscle performance without affecting activities at sub-maximal effort.

1. Introduction

Temperature is considered to be significant determinant of skeletal muscle function and performance [1, 2]. Muscle force generation and power output vary with changes in body temperature. An optimal temperature range at which the best performance of muscle isometric contraction occurs has been described [3, 4]. It has also been demonstrated that muscle contraction forces and rate of force development were impaired at low muscle temperatures [5, 6] and voluntary muscular force production capabilities were reported to be affected below 27°C without core temperature change [2]. In fact, Rutkove showed that even a low degree of cooling decreased the rate of muscular force production [7].

Various peripheral cooling protocols have been used to explore the effects on muscle performance. De Ruiter et al. [1] investigated the effect of temperature on the rate of isometric force development in the lower arm following 20 min immersion in water baths at 37°, 31°, 25°, and 22°C and found that isometric force was reduced below 25°C. Cold water immersion of a limb causes a higher rate of heat loss compared to other environmental cooling. There are various sports and recreational activities both in water and land, where exposure to cold environments may affect power generation [3]. A recent study by Cè et al. [8] showed that both fatigue and muscle cooling decreased nerve conduction velocity. Local vasoconstriction in tissues exposed to cold is likely to decrease oxygen extraction and impair the oxidative reactions [9]. It has also been reported that muscle fatigue due to high intensity dynamic work developed earlier when the muscle temperature was decreased [10].

Several experiments that have been performed in humans and in rats show that muscle shortening velocity and isometric muscle tension were altered by decreasing temperature [11]. Drinkwater and Behm found that the rate of isometric twitch and tension force development declined by 50% and 46%, respectively, when the plantar flexors were cooled to 22°C [12]. Davies et al. [13] reported that local cooling to 24°C of the triceps muscle reduced its maximal voluntary contraction (MVC). Oksa et al. [14] found reduced maximal muscle performance during dynamic exercise performed at a lowered room air temperature (10°–5°C) and Ranatunga et al. [15] summarized that maximum voluntary tension remained relatively stable on cooling to 25°C but varied by about 30% on cooling to 12°–15°C. However, Meigal et al. [16] reported that exposure to cold room air (10°C) for 30 min did not impair the MVC during isometric elbow flexion.

Studies have also shown that ankle dorsiflexion (DF) and plantar flexion (PF) strengths are strongly correlated to walking speed [17]. During gait the reciprocal activity of agonist and antagonist muscles is important for the production of optimal force and for coordination [18]. Oksa et al. [19] argued that muscle activation changes, due to cooling and rewarming, are centrally regulated due to muscle agonist/antagonist pattern changes followed by cooling. As muscle function is affected by cooling, one may assume that postural balance and gait performance may also be affected. Local leg cooling techniques using water immersion have been used to induce some degree of foot sole anesthesia and the effects on postural control have been examined. Eils et al. [20] and Stål et al. [21] used ice water as a cooling method to assess the effects on muscle function during gait by using data from force plates and electromyography. However, few studies have investigated electromyographic activity and ground reaction forces specifically during gait following local muscle cooling by water immersion. Petrofsky and Lind [22], Bigland-Ritchie et al. [23], and De Luca [24] investigated the effect of cooling on EMG frequency during isometric and submaximal exercise. The results showed increased amplitude of surface EMG but decreased center frequency power spectra with lower muscle temperature and also revealed evidence of muscle fatigue through cooling the muscles in water from 40° to 10°C [22].

Biomechanics of gait can be affected due to cooling of lower extremity muscles [20]. As a result, one may have poor coordination or may even slip and fall. The required coefficient of friction (RCOF) has been used in several studies to ascertain the minimum friction required at the foot or shoe and floor interface as an important biomechanical parameter for evaluating slips and falls [25]. To the best of our knowledge, the effects of lower leg muscle cooling on both EMG and RCOF have not been well documented. Neither has ankle muscle strength, ground reaction forces during gait, and EMG activity following lower leg muscle cooling been adequately investigated. Therefore, further exploration of muscle performance in cold environments is required [2].

The objectives of this study were to assess the effects of lower leg cooling on maximum ankle DF and PF muscle forces, EMG, GRF, and RCOF during gait in healthy young subjects. It was primarily hypothesized that, as a consequence of cooling the muscles of the lower leg, maximum isometric force would be reduced and changes may occur in the muscle EMG recordings. It was hypothesized primarily that consequences of cooling would reduce maximum isometric force and affect muscle electrical activities of the lower extremities. The secondary hypothesis was that local cooling would modify the gait strategies in anterior-posterior and vertical components of the ground reaction forces, the required coefficient of friction, and the electromyographic properties during walking.

2. Materials and Methods

2.1. Participants. Sixteen university students participated in the within subject design study, 8 males and 8 females. Physical and anthropometric characteristics of the participants were age, 27.0 ± 2.9 years; body mass, 66.3 ± 9.8 kg; height, 169.5 ± 7.8 cm, and body mass index (BMI) 23.0 ± 2.5. All volunteer participants signed an informed consent form. All participants were clinically healthy, no neurological or musculoskeletal abnormalities and no previous history of lower limb injuries which might influence normal walking and balance ability. Subjects were requested to abstain from alcoholic beverages and intensive physical exercise 24 hours prior testing. A complete explanation of the purpose of the study and experimental procedures was described and the participants were also informed of the risk of experiencing some discomfort. The study was approved by the regional ethical review board in Lund (EPN) and performed according to declaration of Helsinki for research involving human subjects.

2.2. Experimental Design. A repeated measure of the same subject design was used with two independent variables by using two experimental stations. One of them was in a "room temperature environment" (air temperature was about 21°C) where the walkway with force plate was installed. The other experimental station was the "cold climate chamber" at 9.5°C, which is 0.5°C lower than target water temperature 10°C with a chair and two 60 liter plastic water baths in front of the chair in order to immerse both lower legs while sitting. The purpose of the cold chamber was to maintain cold water temperature at 10°C during the 20 min immersion period [1, 20, 26]. A physical examination bench was also placed inside the climate chamber to accommodate lying position for the dynamometer measures. Skin temperatures were measured using an infrared thermometer (Agema Infrared Systems, model-TPT64P, Germany).

2.3. Experiment Protocol. See Figure 1.

2.4. Cooling and Temperature Measurements

2.4.1. Before Cooling. EMG electrodes were attached to the muscle belly of the GM muscle and the TA muscle. Afterwards, pre cooling (Tsk-pre) skin temperature was measured on GM and TA muscle bellies next to the EMG electrodes. Isometric ankle DF and PF dynamometer testing was performed on dominant leg in the supine position with the knee straight. Gait over the force plate and EMG measurements were performed immediately after the dynamometer testing.

2.4.2. Muscle Cooling. Water-resistant adhesive tape was applied over the EMG electrodes to prevent water influx into electrodes. In the cold chamber, the subjects were dressed in light winter jackets with the trousers folded up above both knees, and gloves and thin woolly caps were provided upon individual demands. The cold water volume

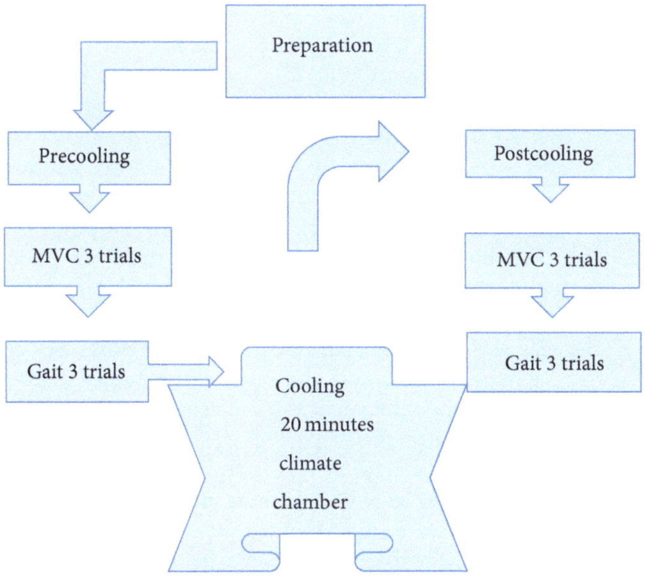

FIGURE 1: The procedure of experimental study: each subject performed 3 maximal voluntary contractions (MVCs) and 3 gait trails during the pre- and postcooling stages. The subjects performed precooling trials, followed by 20 min of cold water immersion at 10°C, followed by the trials immediately after cooling.

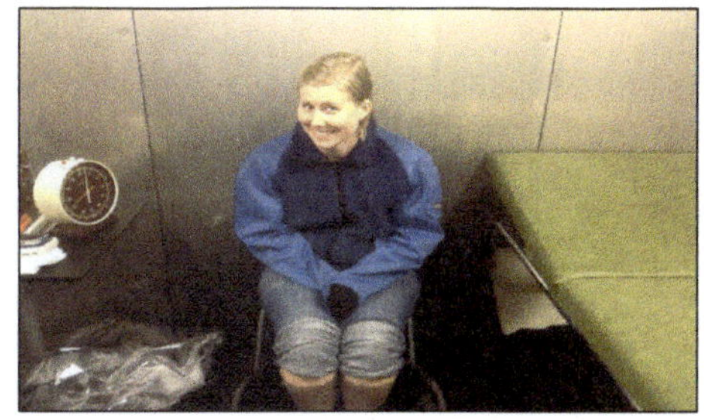

FIGURE 2: Subject's both legs were immersed in a cold water bath in the cold climate chamber.

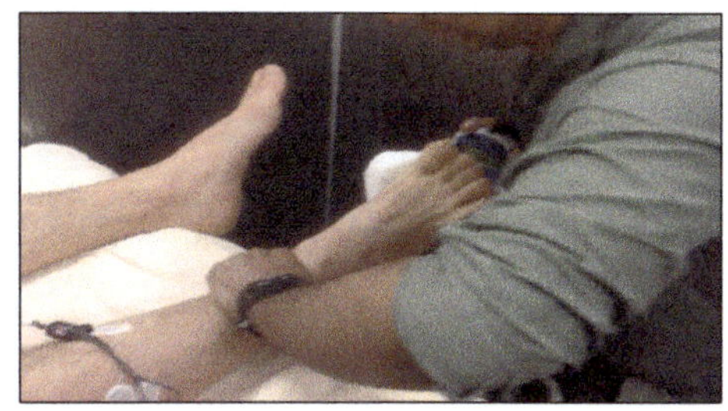

FIGURE 3: Measuring plantar flexion force using the hand held dynamometer.

was approximately four times more than leg volume to maintain a temperature of 9.5 to 10.5°C (Figure 2).

2.4.3. After Cooling. Again skin temperature (Tsk-post 1) was obtained from the same locations that were dried quickly with a towel; then the isometric DF and PF tests were performed. Immediately after the isometric tests, the Tsk-post 2 was recorded with the subjects still being in the 9.5°C cold chamber. The postcooling walking trials were then performed at ambient room temperature on the force plate walkway in the laboratory. Finally, the Tsk-post 3 was taken at room temperature after the gait trials.

2.5. Instrumentation

2.5.1. Dynamometer. Maximum isometric voluntary force measurements were performed using the Lafayette Handheld Dynamometer, model LA-01163, IN, US.

Dynamometer Procedure. All the dynamometer PF and DF, MVC tests were carried out by the same assessor. In the supine position, the subjects were instructed to fixate themselves by firmly gripping the sides of the bench and maintain the hips and knees extended. The assessor stabilized the lower leg by manual fixation proximal to the ankle joint to minimize substitution movements [17] (Figure 3). To measure DF force, the dynamometer was applied against the dorsal surface of the foot just proximal to the metatarsal heads. For PF measurement, the dynamometer was applied to the sole of the foot just proximal to the metatarsal heads. An extra soft towel was placed between the dynamometers contact plate and the subjects' feet for comfort. To standardize the positions for the isometric tests, PF testing was performed at maximal subtalar end range of DF and the DF tests were performed at comfortable subtalar end range of PF. The ankle joint (talocrural) was positioned at midrange of motion in each direction. Before the force measurements the subjects practiced the two movements in order to avoid confusion and minimize the training effect during the actual dynamometer tests. Three consecutive MVCs of the ankle DF and PF were registered using the "make" technique, where the examiner held the dynamometer stationary while the subject exerts a maximal force against it [17, 27]. Subjects were asked to build their force to maximum as hard as possible up to two-second period. By increasing force gradually in this manner it was easier for the tester to hold the dynamometer stationary against the subject's exertion. Subjects thereafter continue at a maximum effort for another 4-5 seconds until the "beep" sound from the dynamometer. A brief pause allowed for about 30 seconds of recovery between contractions to avoid fatigue. Strong verbal encouragement was given during each contraction. If the difference between scores was within 3 kilograms, the test was considered complete; otherwise, the test was repeated.

2.5.2. Walkway and Force Plate

Walkway. The laboratory wooden walkway with a vinyl surface was of the following dimensions, 0.6 m wide and 7.2 m long (Figure 4).

Force Plate. A force plate Kistler 9281B (Switzerland) (Figure 4) was incorporated into the walkway. The DAQ System 5695A1 and Amplifier type 9865A with BioWare Software

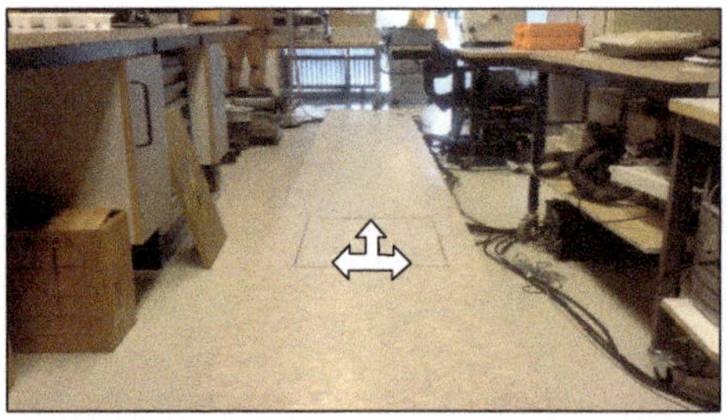

FIGURE 4: Force plate installed in laboratory walkway.

(version 4.1.0.2, type 2812A-04) were used for data collection. The force plate was placed in the walkway at 4.1 m and was also layered with vinyl sheet and lay flush with the walkway.

Gait Protocol. Each subject was instructed to walk barefooted at a comfortable habitual pace and not to focus on the force plate. Each subject was first given the opportunity to become familiar with the walkway by walking across the force plate so that the dominant foot struck the force plate area.

2.5.3. EMG. The Megawin (ME6000-T16 Mega Electronics, Kuopio, Finland) System Biomonitor and Software "Megawin" version 3.1-b10 were used to record and analyze surface EMG data. The sampling rate was set at 1024 Hz. The skin was prepared by shaving if necessary then lightly abraded with fine sand paper and cleaned with isopropyl alcohol to minimize impedance. The pregelled bipolar surface electrodes (Ambu Neuroline 720) were placed adjoining in the fiber direction at the upper third portion of the GM and TA muscles. The ground electrodes were fixed over noncontractile tissue. Water-proof adhesive tape was also applied. The same investigator attached all electrodes using the SENIAM recommendations.

2.6. Data Processing and Analysis

2.6.1. Strength Measurements. The means of the three maximum voluntary of contractions (MVCs) for each muscle pre- and postcooling were calculated and used in the statistical analysis.

2.6.2. EMG. The raw EMG signal was processed in the following way: the DC offset using the inbuilt Megawin software was applied. The raw EMG signal was digitally band pass filtered (20–400 Hz); a notch filter 50 Hz was also applied to clean the signal from eventual artifacts from the surrounding electrical appliances: the signal was then full-wave rectified and root mean square (RMS) averaging was applied. From the processed signals the peak and median values in μV were obtained. The mean of the three highest EMG peaks for each MVC trial for each muscle pre-and postcooling was calculated. Markers on the EMG recording were used to identify the period of onset and end of each gait trial and the median EMG for each period was recorded. The mean values of the medians pre- and postcooling were used in the analysis. The peak EMG values for each muscle and subject were used to normalize the EMG values from the gait tests [28].

2.6.3. Ground Reaction Forces. Three forces from the force plate, namely, vertical force (F_z), lateral shear force (F_x), and anterior-posterior shear force (F_y), were obtained using 8 channels. The GRF data were processed using a zero lag low-pass Butterworth 4th order filter with a cut-off frequency of 100 Hz and then normalized to each subject's body weight. Time was normalized to 100% of the stance phase with 0% being heel strike (HS) and 100% representing toe-off (TO) [29, 30]. The body weight was weighed on the force plate in order to normalize the ground reaction forces (N) to the subjects' respective body weights (N).

The stance period was identified as follows: onset began when F_z exceeded 10 N and the end of the stance phase was determined when the vertical force dropped below 10 N. The force plate stance phase period was divided into two percentage subphases (HS and TO) from the midpoint of stance phase using the time slice options in the "Bioware". The HS and TO phases were associated with the actions of the DF and PF. The average of HS and TO peaks from the three trials was calculated for each subject and the mean values of all sixteen subjects were compared for the pre- and postcooling conditions.

2.6.4. Required Coefficient of Friction (RCOF). The ratio of shear to normal ground reaction force, termed the required coefficient of friction (RCOF) [29], was calculated for each trial by dividing longitudinal anterior-posterior force by vertical force (F_y/F_z). According to Chang et al. [25] RCOF was generally accepted to be the value of the third peak of the RCOF versus time curve, as shown in (Figure 5) below. The third peak was scrutinized from GRF curve by selecting the time period from 20 milliseconds to 200 milliseconds after heel contact (when F_z reached 10 N); however, on a few occasions the third peak was unclear so the second peak was used instead.

2.7. Statistical Analysis. Paired two-tailed t-tests were used to test for differences between pre- and postcooling for the maximal strength measurements, mean EMG from the maximal strength measurements, the median EMG during gait trials, and the mean of the peak GRFs and the RCOF. When the normality was challenged for the EMG data, Wilcoxon Signed-Rank Test was also performed. However, the statistical results were in essence similar to the t-test results (Table 1). Significance was set at $P \leq 0.05$ throughout and exact P values are given above 0.05. All data were processed and analyzed using SPSS v.20, IBM Corp., US.

3. Results

3.1. Cooling of Lower Legs. All sixteen subjects successfully completed 20 minutes of cooling on both legs in cold water at 10°C in the cold chamber. The average skin temperatures over the two muscles (TA and GM) decreased by about 15.7°C and 15.6°C, respectively, after 20 minutes of cooling. Most of the subjects reported reduced sensation after 20 minutes cooling at 10°C, which were gradually regained during walking trials. Skin temperatures gradually increased by about 2.9 and 2.2°C for TA and GM, respectively, after postcooling MVC tests,

TABLE 1: The means and standard deviations (mean ± SD) of the three MVC trials as well as the mean EMG amplitude during the three MVC trials and normalized mean of the three median EMG values from the three gait trials are given for the TA and GM muscles before and immediately after cooling ($n = 16$).

	Dorsiflexion (TA muscle)			Plantar flexion (GM muscle)		
	Precooling	Postcooling	t-test	Precooling	Postcooling	t-test
MVC (Kg)	23.8 ± 2.7	21.3 ± 2.7	<0.001	30.6 ± 4.5	29.7 ± 3.0	0.221
EMG during MVC (μV)	446.4 ± 218.2	443.4 ± 250.7	0.939	284.8 ± 128.3	705.5 ± 487.7	0.003
Normalized EMG in gait trials (%)	11.3 ± 5.3	13.1 ± 7.3	0.158	13.6 ± 10.3	19.8 ± 11.9	<0.001

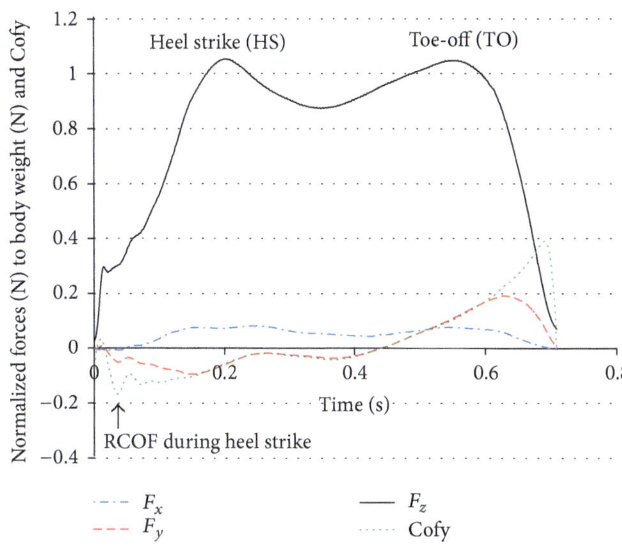

FIGURE 5: Example of GRFs and RCOF used for analysis, the vertical force (F_z), longitudinal shear force (F_y), and transverse force (F_x) during the HS and TO phases. The second peak of Cofy indicated by an arrow at the bottom represents the RCOF during heel strike.

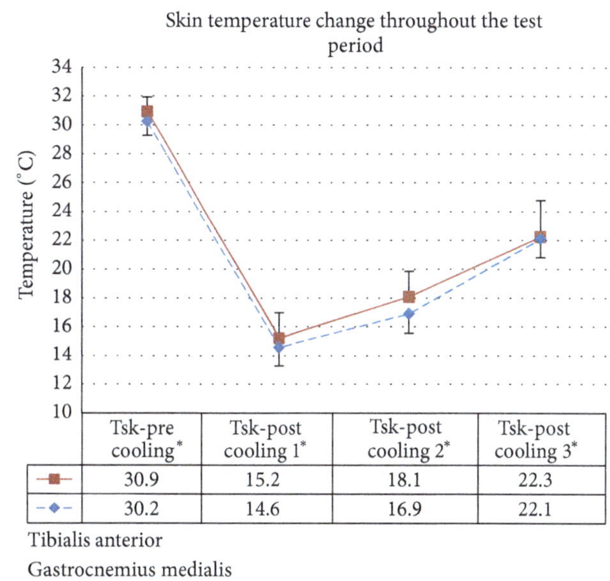

FIGURE 6: Mean skin temperature over the two muscles (TA and GM) for four measurement phases. Tsk-pre: before cooling, Tsk-post cooling 1: immediately after cooling, Tsk-post cooling 2: after the postcooling MVC test, and Tsk-post cooling 3:end of gait trials.

even though the tests were performed in the cold chamber. At the end of all gait trials, skin temperatures increased by about 4 to 5°C. The skin temperature changes over the two muscles throughout the test period are shown in Figure 6.

3.2. The Effects of Cooling on Strength MVC. There was a significantly reduced isometric maximum force in TA muscle ($P < 0.001$) after cooling, and the GM muscle force difference was not significant (Table 1).

3.3. The Effects of Cooling on EMG during MVC. The mean EMG amplitude of GM muscle was significantly increased by approximately 400 μV after cooling ($P < 0.003$). There was no difference for the TA muscles (Table 1).

3.4. The Effects of Cooling on the EMG of Gait Muscles. The average of the median for the three gait trials after cooling was significantly higher in the GM ($P < 0.001$) compared to the precooling value. There was no difference for the TA muscles (Table 1).

3.5. The Effects of Cooling on Gait Ground Reaction Forces. We found no differences in the GRFs between pre- and post-cooling. Neither did the third peak of coefficient of friction result in a significant difference ($P = 0.851$) (Table 2).

4. Discussion

The present study investigated the effects of cooling on ankle muscle maximum isometric force, ground reaction forces, and EMG activity of the TA and GM during MVC trials and gait trials. The main findings showed that cooling decreased maximum force of the TA but not the GM muscle. The study also showed that cooling increased the EMG amplitude significantly of the GM but not the TA muscle during the maximum voluntary contractions and gait trials.

4.1. The Cooling Effect on Ankle Muscle Strength. A significant decrease in MVC strength in the order of 10% was recorded in the TA after cooling; however, there was no change for the GM. Several studies have shown that cooling with water decreases isometric strength in superficial muscles [1, 13]. Holewijn and Heus [5] also monitored a drop in maximal handgrip force after 30 min local cooling at 15°C. Comeau et al. [31] evaluated the effects of environmental cooling on force production in the thigh muscles and registered a significant force drop in the quadriceps and hamstrings at temperatures 10°C or below. We have only found in the

TABLE 2: Vertical and longitudinal GRFs (normalized by body weight in Newton) (mean ± SD) during heel strike and toe-off in relation to DF and PF, respectively, and RCOF before and after cooling ($n = 16$).

	Heel strike (HS) phase			Toe-off (TO) phase		
	Precooling	Postcooling	t-test	Precooling	Postcooling	t-test
Peak vertical (F_z)	1.14 ± 0.11	1.17 ± 0.10	0.140	1.15 ± 0.08	1.14 ± 0.06	0.186
Peak longitudinal (F_y)	0.21 ± 0.05	0.21 ± 0.06	0.903	0.24 ± 0.03	0.23 ± 0.03	0.129
Required coefficient of friction (RCOF)*	0.26 ± 0.04	0.26 ± 0.05	0.851			

*RCOF during heel strike phase was included in the analysis.

present study that the TA significantly decreased in MVC performance. One possible explanation for this discrepancy may be the morphological differences of the muscles. The TA muscle has a much lesser volume than the GM muscle; however, the muscle fiber length is almost the double. The internal cooling of the muscles could not be measured in this study and cooling may have been greater in the TA and thus nerve conduction and the contraction process at sarcomere level may be more affected [2, 6, 7, 23]. Furthermore, the common peroneal nerve that innervates the TA is very superficial and therefore quite exposed to the cold water which may result in lower conductibility [8, 32] and thereby possible lesser force production in accordance with findings by Hsu and Stevenson [33]. Moreover, the TA has a muscle fiber length twice the length of GM, which allows for a more favorable force generation compared with the plantar flexors [34]. One other factor is that the deep soleus muscle also contributes to plantar flexor strength and it is quite possible that the soleus was less affected by the cooling resulting in a less affected force production. Despite the fact that surface skin temperature did decrease significantly, more invasive techniques are required to register the core muscle temperature. Another possible criticism may be the limitations of using a handheld dynamometer; however, the hand held dynamometer has been demonstrated reasonably reliable and valid to measure the foot and ankle strength of young and old adults [17, 35, 36].

4.2. The Cooling Effect on EMG Values. We found a significant and large increase in the mean EMG amplitude for the GM muscle during the MVC trials after cooling and we also found similar results in the normalized median EMG during the gait trials (Table 1). It is known that EMG amplitude of the fatigued and cooled muscles increases on isometric and submaximal exercise due to altered motor unit recruitment and activation [22, 23, 37]. It is possible that the cooling effect in this experiment induced an EMG fatigue response of the GM. Previous studies have revealed that PF was more prone to fatigue after a prolonged level running; however DF is less subjected to fatigue during a prolonged five-hour hilly running than that of PF studied by Fourchet et al. [38]. Taken together, for the TA we found a lower maximal force production immediately after cooling but no difference in the mean EMG, and for the GM we found no difference in maximal force production after cooling but a very large and significant increase in the mean EMG amplitude.

4.3. Muscle Cooling and Ground Reaction Forces during Gait. The analysis of ground reaction forces showed no significant alterations on peak vertical and longitudinal ground reaction forces. Other studies have shown that cooling of the feet to numbness with ice water close to 0°C did produce force changes such as, a delay in the force distributions during heel strike [20, 21]. In our study the cooling temperature was 10°C; thus cutaneous sensation on the soles of the feet may not have been functionally impaired. Hreljac reported that the DF muscles perform at or near maximum capacity when a transition of speed is required and this may make the muscle susceptible to overexertion [39]. Neptune et al. [40] argued that the muscle TA is primarily responsible for helping to toe-off in early swing, while the plantar flexors support the body during propulsion and at swing initiation in late stance.

RCOF is the ratio of F_y over F_z and is used to assess slip risk. If available coefficient of friction in GRF is smaller than that of RCOF, a slip will occur. Reductions in the relative magnitude of the shear forces were more than the vertical forces resulting in the overall effect of a decrease in the peak RCOF [29]. Again, we found no difference in RCOF values between pre- and postcooling which may also be explained by the low gait speed in a secure environment. Since the average peak vertical ground reaction force was not significantly changed, the time component was primarily responsible for the nonsignificant decrease in vertical impulse. In other words, either the extra time necessary to produce force following cooling or the muscle contraction time is slower [6, 41]. One probable explanation to the nonsignificant results for the force plate values is that the gait task used in this study was not demanding enough. Gait speed, although not measured, was relatively slow in the confines of the laboratory with a short 3.5 m approach to the force plate and moreover, the slip risk on dry vinyl floor surface was relatively small.

Cold water exposure has been demonstrated to increase joint stiffness due to increased viscosity of the joints' synovial fluid [42–44]. Increased joint stiffness may also alter postural control and muscle force production. However, some researchers have found that the muscle cooling itself has no effect on force production and that a decrease in nerve conduction velocity is a primary contributor to the decrease in isometric maximal performances [45–47].

To increase our knowledge of EMG, muscle force, and ground reaction force changes, further studies need to be performed with more extreme cooling and at more vigorous and prolonged duration of muscle intensity and repetitive activities. Mean power frequency and the ratio between MVC and EMG (MVC/EMG) of the TA and GM could be further analyzed. In application to injury management, the results from this study imply that the treatment of injuries by cooling may affect muscular performance immediately after treatment. The results also indicate that neuromuscular control and/or muscular homeostasis regulation may be negatively affected by the degree of cooling described in this laboratory study and may have implications for motor performance during cold exposure in recreational, sports, and occupational activities. The findings may assist researchers in evaluating physical performance after cold exposure. The cooling procedure described may be applied in studies of sportsmen and workers who need to perform in wet and cold conditions.

5. Conclusion

Cooling of both lower legs in cold water at 10°C and in a climate chamber with an air temperature of 10°C for 20 minutes resulted in a decrease of the maximal isometric voluntary force in the TA muscles but not in the GM muscles in young healthy individuals. The mean EMG amplitude during the maximal force tests was unchanged in the TA muscle but significantly increased in the GM perhaps indicating an induced fatigue response. Force plate reaction forces and RCOF during gait were not affected on a dry and level walkway. In conclusion, 20 min cooling in cold water at 10°C can influence our maximum muscle performance, but the cooling may not be severe enough to have some impact on daily submaximal activities.

Conflict of Interests

The authors declare that there is no conflict of interests regarding the publication of this paper.

Acknowledgments

The authors wish to acknowledge the financial assistance of AFA Insurance, Sweden, for the Project "Slip and fall accidents, friction requirement and balance ability" ID no. 100026 and all participants for their contribution.

References

[1] C. J. De Ruiter, D. A. Jones, A. J. Sargeant, and A. De Haan, "Temperature effect on the rates of isometric force development and relaxation in the fresh and fatigued human adductor pollicis muscle," *Experimental Physiology*, vol. 84, no. 6, pp. 1137–1150, 1999.

[2] E. Drinkwater, "Effects of peripheral cooling on characteristics of local muscle," *Medicine and Sport Science*, vol. 53, pp. 74–88, 2008.

[3] G. C. Crowley, A. Garg, M. S. Lohn, N. Van Someren, and A. J. Wade, "Effects of cooling the legs on performance in a standard Wingate anaerobic power test," *British Journal of Sports Medicine*, vol. 25, no. 4, pp. 200–203, 1991.

[4] J. S. Petrofsky, R. L. Burse, and A. R. Lind, "The effect of deep muscle temperature on the cardiovascular responses of man to static effort," *European Journal of Applied Physiology and Occupational Physiology*, vol. 47, no. 1, pp. 7–16, 1981.

[5] M. Holewijn and R. Heus, "Effects of temperature on electromyogram and muscle function," *European Journal of Applied Physiology and Occupational Physiology*, vol. 65, no. 6, pp. 541–545, 1992.

[6] S. Zhou, M. F. Carey, R. J. Snow, D. L. Lawson, and W. E. Morrison, "Effects of muscle fatigue and temperature on electromechanical delay," *Electromyography and Clinical Neurophysiology*, vol. 38, no. 2, pp. 67–73, 1998.

[7] S. B. Rutkove, "Effects of temperature on neuromuscular electrophysiology," *Muscle and Nerve*, vol. 24, no. 7, pp. 867–882, 2001.

[8] E. Cè, S. Rampichini, L. Agnello, E. Limonta, A. Veicsteinas, and F. Esposito, "Combined effects of fatigue and temperature manipulation on skeletal muscle electrical and mechanical characteristics during isometric contraction," *Journal of Electromyography and Kinesiology*, vol. 22, no. 3, pp. 348–355, 2012.

[9] T. Shiojiri, M. Shibasaki, K. Aoki, N. Kondo, and S. Koga, "Effects of reduced muscle temperature on the oxygen uptake kinetics at the start of exercise," *Acta Physiologica Scandinavica*, vol. 159, no. 4, pp. 327–333, 1997.

[10] U. Bergh, "Human power at subnormal body temperatures," *Acta Physiologica Scandinavica, Supplement*, vol. 478, pp. 1–39, 1980.

[11] K. W. Ranatunga, "Temperature-dependence of shortening velocity and rate of isometric tension development in rat skeletal muscle," *Journal of Physiology*, vol. 329, pp. 465–483, 1982.

[12] E. J. Drinkwater and D. G. Behm, "Effects of 22°C muscle temperature on voluntary and evoked muscle properties during and after high-intensity exercise," *Applied Physiology, Nutrition and Metabolism*, vol. 32, no. 6, pp. 1043–1051, 2007.

[13] C. T. M. Davies, I. K. Mecrow, and M. J. White, "Contractile properties of the human triceps surae with some observations on the effects of temperature and exercise," *European Journal of Applied Physiology and Occupational Physiology*, vol. 49, no. 2, pp. 255–269, 1982.

[14] J. Oksa, H. Rintamäki, and S. Rissanen, "Muscle performance and electromyogram activity of the lower leg muscles with different levels of cold exposure," *European Journal of Applied Physiology and Occupational Physiology*, vol. 75, no. 6, pp. 484–490, 1997.

[15] K. W. Ranatunga, B. Sharpe, and B. Turnbull, "Contractions of a human skeletal muscle at different temperatures," *Journal of Physiology*, vol. 390, pp. 383–395, 1987.

[16] A. Y. Meigal, J. Oksa, L. I. Gerasimova, E. Hohtola, Y. V. Lupandin, and H. Rintamäki, "Force control of isometric elbow flexion with visual feedback in cold with and without shivering," *Aviation Space and Environmental Medicine*, vol. 74, no. 8, pp. 816–821, 2003.

[17] M. J. Spink, M. R. Fotoohabadi, and H. B. Menz, "Foot and ankle strength assessment using hand-held dynamometry: reliability and age-related differences," *Gerontology*, vol. 56, no. 6, pp. 525–532, 2010.

[18] J. Oksa, H. Rintamäki, T. Mäkinen, V. Martikkala, and H. Rusko, "EMG-activity and muscular performance of lower leg during stretch-shortening cycle after cooling," *Acta Physiologica Scandinavica*, vol. 157, no. 1, pp. 71–78, 1996.

[19] J. Oksa, H. Rintamäki, S. Rissanen, S. Rytky, U. Tolonen, and P. V. Komi, "Stretch- and H-reflexes of the lower leg during whole body cooling and local warming," *Aviation Space and Environmental Medicine*, vol. 71, no. 2, pp. 156–161, 2000.

[20] E. Eils, S. Behrens, O. Mers, L. Thorwesten, K. Völker, and D. Rosenbaum, "Reduced plantar sensation causes a cautious

walking pattern," *Gait and Posture*, vol. 20, no. 1, pp. 54–60, 2004.

[21] F. Stål, P. A. Fransson, M. Magnusson, and M. Karlberg, "Effects of hypothermic anesthesia of the feet on vibration-induced body sway and adaptation," *Journal of Vestibular Research: Equilibrium and Orientation*, vol. 13, no. 1, pp. 39–52, 2003.

[22] J. S. Petrofsky and A. R. Lind, "The influence of temperature on the amplitude and frequency components of the EMG during brief and sustained isometric contractions," *European Journal of Applied Physiology and Occupational Physiology*, vol. 44, no. 2, pp. 189–200, 1980.

[23] B. Bigland-Ritchie, E. F. Donovan, and C. S. Roussos, "Conduction velocity and EMG power spectrum changes in fatigue of sustained maximal efforts," *Journal of Applied Physiology Respiratory Environmental and Exercise Physiology*, vol. 51, no. 5, pp. 1300–1305, 1981.

[24] C. J. De Luca, "Myoelectrical manifestations of localized muscular fatigue in humans," *Critical Reviews in Biomedical Engineering*, vol. 11, no. 4, pp. 251–279, 1984.

[25] W.-R. Chang, S. Matz, and C.-C. Chang, "A comparison of required coefficient of friction for both feet in level walking," *Safety Science*, vol. 50, no. 2, pp. 240–243, 2012.

[26] C. J. De Ruiter and A. De Haan, "Similar effects of cooling and fatigue on eccentric and concentric force-velocity relationships in human muscle," *Journal of Applied Physiology*, vol. 90, no. 6, pp. 2109–2116, 2001.

[27] P. W. Stratford and B. E. Balsor, "A comparison of make and break tests using a hand-held dynamometer and the Kin-Com," *Journal of Orthopaedic and Sports Physical Therapy*, vol. 19, no. 1, pp. 28–32, 1994.

[28] C. Gao, J. Oksa, H. Rintamäki, and I. Holmér, "Gait muscle activity during walking on an inclined icy surface," *Industrial Health*, vol. 46, no. 1, pp. 15–22, 2008.

[29] R. Cham and M. S. Redfern, "Changes in gait when anticipating slippery floors," *Gait and Posture*, vol. 15, no. 2, pp. 159–171, 2002.

[30] I. C. Sacco, P. M. Akashi, and E. M. Hennig, "A comparison of lower limb EMG and ground reaction forces between barefoot and shod gait in participants with diabetic neuropathic and healthy controls," *BMC Musculoskeletal Disorders*, vol. 11, article 24, 2010.

[31] M. Comeau, J. Potteiger, and L. Brown, "Effects of environmental cooling on force production in the quadriceps and hamstrings," *The Journal of Strength & Conditioning Research*, vol. 17, no. 2, pp. 279–284, 2003.

[32] E. Herrera, M. C. Sandoval, D. M. Camargo, and T. F. Salvini, "Effect of walking and resting after three cryotherapy modalities on the recovery of sensory and motor nerve conduction velocity in healthy subjects," *Revista Brasileira de Fisioterapia*, vol. 15, no. 3, pp. 233–240, 2011.

[33] M. Hsu and F. Stevenson, "Reduction in muscular motility by selective focused cold therapy: a preclinical study," *Journal of Neural Transmission*, vol. 121, no. 1, pp. 15–20, 2014.

[34] R. R. Neptune and K. Sasaki, "Ankle plantar flexor force production is an important determinant of the preferred walk-to-run transition speed," *Journal of Experimental Biology*, vol. 208, no. 5, pp. 799–808, 2005.

[35] K. J. Rose, J. Burns, M. M. Ryan, R. A. Ouvrier, and K. N. North, "Reliability of quantifying foot and ankle muscle strength in very young children," *Muscle and Nerve*, vol. 37, no. 5, pp. 626–631, 2008.

[36] C.-Y. Wang, S. L. Olson, and E. J. Protas, "Test-retest strength reliability: hand-held dynamometry in community-dwelling elderly fallers," *Archives of Physical Medicine and Rehabilitation*, vol. 83, no. 6, pp. 811–815, 2002.

[37] J. Oksa, M. B. Ducharmeand, and H. Rintamäki, "Combined effect of repetitive work and cold on muscle function and fatigue," *Journal of Applied Physiology*, vol. 92, no. 1, pp. 354–361, 2002.

[38] F. Fourchet, G. P. Millet, K. Tomazin et al., "Effects of a 5-h hilly running on ankle plantar and dorsal flexor force and fatigability," *European Journal of Applied Physiology*, vol. 112, no. 7, pp. 2645–2652, 2012.

[39] A. Hreljac, "Determinants of the gait transition speed during human locomotion: kinematic factors," *Journal of Biomechanics*, vol. 28, no. 6, pp. 669–677, 1995.

[40] R. R. Neptune, S. A. Kautz, and F. E. Zajac, "Contributions of the individual ankle plantar flexors to support, forward progression and swing initiation during walking," *Journal of Biomechanics*, vol. 34, no. 11, pp. 1387–1398, 2001.

[41] S. J. Kinzey, M. L. Cordova, K. J. Gallen, J. C. Smith, and J. B. Moore, "The effects of cryotherapy on ground-reaction forces produced during a functional task," *Journal of Sport Rehabilitation*, vol. 9, no. 1, pp. 3–14, 2000.

[42] A. J. Sargeant, "Effect of muscle temperature on leg extension force and short-term power output in humans," *European Journal of Applied Physiology and Occupational Physiology*, vol. 56, no. 6, pp. 693–698, 1987.

[43] J. S. LeBlanc, "Impaired of manual dexterity in the cold," *Journal of Applied Physiology*, vol. 9, no. 1, pp. 62–64, 1956.

[44] C. Sekihara, M. Izumizaki, T. Yasuda, T. Nakajima, T. Atsumi, and I. Homma, "Effect of cooling on thixotropic position-sense error in human biceps muscle," *Muscle and Nerve*, vol. 35, no. 6, pp. 781–787, 2007.

[45] D. G. Burke, S. A. MacNeil, L. E. Holt, N. C. MacKinnon, and R. L. Rasmussen, "The effect of hot or cold water immersion on isometric strength training," *Journal of Strength and Conditioning Research*, vol. 14, no. 1, pp. 21–25, 2000.

[46] B. M. Hatzel and T. W. Kaminski, "The effects of ice immersion on concentric and eccentric isokinetic muscle performance in the ankle," *Isokinetics and Exercise Science*, vol. 8, no. 2, pp. 103–107, 2000.

[47] K. M. Cross, R. W. Wilson, and D. H. Perrin, "Functional performance following an ice immersion to the lower extremity," *Journal of Athletic Training*, vol. 31, pp. 113–116, 1996.

6

Immediate Effects of Neurodynamic Sliding versus Muscle Stretching on Hamstring Flexibility in Subjects with Short Hamstring Syndrome

Yolanda Castellote-Caballero,[1] Maríe C. Valenza,[2] Emilio J. Puentedura,[3] César Fernández-de-las-Peñas,[4] and Francisco Alburquerque-Sendín[5]

[1] *Hospital Virgen de las Nieves, Servicio Andaluz de Salud, Avenida de las Fuerzas Armadas 2, 18014 Granada, Spain*
[2] *Department of Physical Therapy, Universidad de Granada, Avenida del Hospicio s/n, 18071 Granada, Spain*
[3] *Department of Physical Therapy, School of Allied Health Sciences, University of Nevada Las Vegas, 4505 Maryland Parkway, P.O. Box 453029, Las Vegas, NV 89154-3029, USA*
[4] *Department of Physical Therapy, Occupational Therapy, Rehabilitation and Physical Medicine, Universidad Rey Juan Carlos, Avenida de Atenas s/n, Alcorcon, 28922 Madrid, Spain*
[5] *Department of Physical Therapy, Universidad de Salamanca, Patio de Escuelas, 137008 Salamanca, Spain*

Correspondence should be addressed to Emilio J. Puentedura; louie.puentedura@unlv.edu

Academic Editor: Gabriel Ng

Background. Hamstring injuries continue to affect active individuals and although inadequate muscle extensibility remains a commonly accepted factor, little is known about the most effective method to improve flexibility. *Purpose*. To determine if an isolated neurodynamic sciatic sliding technique would improve hamstring flexibility to a greater degree than stretching or a placebo intervention in asymptomatic subjects with short hamstring syndrome (SHS). *Study Design*. Randomized double-blinded controlled trial. *Methods*. One hundred and twenty subjects with SHS were randomized to 1 of 3 groups: neurodynamic sliding, hamstring stretching, and placebo control. Each subject's dominant leg was measured for straight leg raise (SLR) range of motion (ROM) before and after interventions. Data were analyzed with a 3 × 2 mixed model ANOVA followed by simple main effects analyses. *Results*. At the end of the study, more ROM was observed in the Neurodynamic and Stretching groups compared to the Control group and more ROM in the Neurodynamic group compared to Stretching group. *Conclusion*. Findings suggest that a neurodynamic sliding technique will increase hamstring flexibility to a greater degree than static hamstring stretching in healthy subjects with SHS. *Clinical Relevance*. The use of neurodynamic sliding techniques to improve hamstring flexibility in sports may lead to a decreased incidence in injuries; however, this needs to be formally tested.

1. Introduction

Injuries to the hamstring musculature are commonplace in many mainstream sports and occupations involving physical activity [1, 2]. They have not declined in recent times and the high rate of recurrence suggests that the current understanding of such injuries remains incomplete [3]. Hamstring muscle strains/tears account for 13–15% of injuries in Australian football [4, 5], 11% of injuries in elite New Zealand cricketers [6], 12–14% of injuries in professional soccer [7, 8], and up to 24% of injuries in Gaelic football [9]. Many predisposing factors for hamstring injury have been suggested within the literature, including insufficient warm-up [10], poor flexibility [11], muscle imbalances [12], neural tension [13], fatigue [14], and previous injuries [15].

Inadequate flexibility within the posterior thigh compartment appears to be one of the more commonly accepted causes of hamstring injuries [2, 16]; however, the evidence for decreased hamstring flexibility as a risk factor remains equivocal [11, 17]. A recent Cochrane review found no evidence for stretching as a sole intervention for prevention of hamstring injury [18], and this has led to the suggestion that decreased flexibility is but one factor in the multifactorial etiology of hamstring strain injury [19].

Despite varying theories for the observed increases in muscle flexibility after the application of stretching, we are lacking in evidence for any credible explanation. In a recent review article, Weppler and Magnusson [20] suggested that such increases in tissue flexibility may result, not from affecting the mechanical properties of the muscle being stretched, but from changes in the individual's perception of stretch or pain. They suggested that the point of limitation in hamstring range may increase, not because of changes within the muscle structure itself but rather because the individual experiencing the stretching may adopt a "new stop point" for limitation in hamstring range based on altered perceptions of stretch and pain. They referred to this as the "sensory theory" and proposed that increases in muscle flexibility after stretching were likely due to the modified sensation [20]. Changes in the mobility of the nervous system (neurodynamics) achieved through movement and stretching could modify such sensations [21–23].

Decreased hamstring flexibility as evidenced by limited range in the passive straight leg raise test (SLR) could be due to altered neurodynamics affecting the sciatic, tibial, and common fibular nerves [24]. Altered posterior lower extremity neurodynamics could arguably influence resting muscle length and lead to changes in the perception of stretch or pain [25]. Providing movement or stretching could lead to changes in the neurodynamics and modification of sensation and could help to explain the observed increase in flexibility.

The mechanosensitivity of the neural structures in the posterior leg, thigh, buttock, and vertebral canal may play a part in determining the flexibility of the hamstring muscles. Protective muscle contraction of the hamstring muscles found in the presence of neural mechanosensitivity [26, 27] may account for hamstring tightness and thereby predispose the muscle to subsequent strain injury. Neurodynamic sliding interventions are thought to decrease neural mechanosensitivity [26, 28, 29] and it is possible that the inclusion of these interventions in the management of hamstring flexibility could be beneficial.

In a recent pilot study involving 28 male soccer players, our research team was able to demonstrate that a neurodynamic sliding intervention led to a short-term increase in hamstring flexibility [30]. Findings from that study were limited by a small sample size, inclusion of young males only, and also because the experimental group was compared to a control group that received no intervention. Despite these shortcomings, the study did suggest that neurodynamic treatment can significantly increase hamstring flexibility in a young male athletic population and proposed that future research compares neurodynamic techniques with other interventions in a broader population of subjects.

Therefore, the aim of this study was to examine the immediate effects of a neurodynamic sciatic sliding technique, hamstring stretching, and placebo control intervention in asymptomatic subjects with decreased hamstring flexibility or short hamstring syndrome. We hypothesized that an isolated neurodynamic sciatic sliding technique would improve range of motion, assessed by passive straight leg raise test (SLR), greater than hamstring stretching or placebo in the short term. Findings from this study may provide further the evidence for the relevance of neural tissues in determining range of motion and may indicate benefits for adding neural mobilization techniques to the rehabilitation and/or prevention of hamstring injuries.

2. Methods

2.1. Subjects. We recruited a sample of 120 subjects (60 female; mean age 33.4 ± 7.4, range 20–45) who exhibited bilateral short hamstring syndrome (SLR test = 80° or less) [31–33]. Sample size was calculated using Ene 3.0 software (Autonomic University of Barcelona, Spain) and calculations were based on detecting between-group mean differences of 7° at postdata [30]. Assuming a standard deviation of 8° when comparing 2 means, an alpha level of 0.05, and desired power of 90%, a sample size of 29 subjects per group was generated. We increased the sample size by 25% (40 per group) to increase statistical power. Exclusion criteria were hamstring injury within the past year, exceeding 80° in the initial SLR test, verbal report of performing regular lower extremity muscle stretching exercises, history of neck trauma (whiplash), neck symptoms, history of fracture in any part of the body, history of growth disorders, history of neurological or orthopedic disorders, diagnosis of herniated disk, low back pain in the last 6 months, and body mass index (BMI) lower than 20 Kg/cm^2 or higher than 30 Kg/cm^2. We chose the BMI range as an exclusion criterion to allow for better identification of body landmarks and introduce some degree of homogeneity for subject body type. Subjects were recruited from the general population via advertisements in local newspapers. All subjects signed an informed consent before they were included in the study, and all procedures were conducted according to the Declaration of Helsinki. The period of recruitment was from January 2009 to June 2011. Figure 1 provides a flowchart of subject recruitment during the study.

2.2. Measurement of Hamstring Flexibility. All physical measurements were obtained by a pair of trained examiners who were blinded to each subject's group allocation. The passive SLR test was used to determine changes in hamstring muscle flexibility and has demonstrated high interobserver reliability (0.94–0.96) [34, 35]. Each test was performed with the subject supine wearing shorts or underwear, and the following bony landmarks were identified and labeled with a marker: the anterior superior iliac spine (ASIS), greater trochanter and lateral epicondyle of the femur, and the head of the fibula and the fibular malleolus. The passive SLR test was recorded 3 times for each subject using a universal goniometer. One examiner performed the passive SLR by keeping the knee in full extension and the ankle in neutral plantarflexion-dorsiflexion. Full ankle dorsiflexion was avoided to prevent calf muscle stiffness or pain (gastrocnemius and soleus) from confounding the sensation of hamstring stiffness and pain

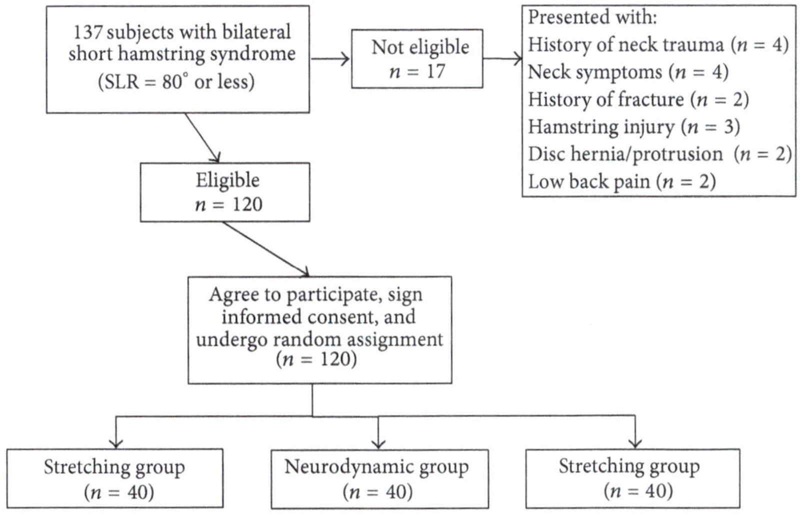

FIGURE 1: CONSORT flow diagram of patient recruitment and retention.

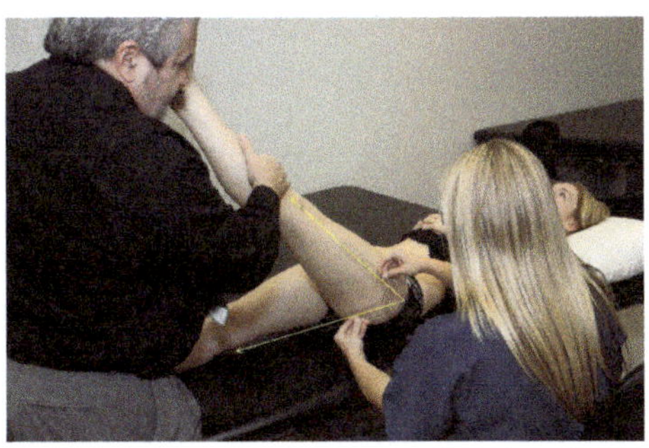

FIGURE 2: Measurement of range during passive straight leg raise test was performed by trained examiners who were blinded to subject group assignment.

which would signal the limit of the SLR test. The examiner would hold the talus and avoid any hip rotation during flexion of the hip as they lifted the subject's lower limb until he or she first complained of stiffness or pain in the region of the thigh, bent his/her knee, or began to swing into a posterior pelvic tilt (noted as movement of the ASIS). The second examiner placed the axis of the goniometer over the mark on the greater trochanter of the femur. The stationary arm of the goniometer was placed parallel to the table and checked with a level, and the moving arm was placed in the line between the head of the fibula and the fibular malleolus, and the degree of elevation of the straight leg was then noted (Figure 2). Within-session intra-rater reliability was established on the first 10 subjects as sufficient for clinical measurement (ICC = 0.96); and although less relevant to calculation of responsiveness data and subsequent interpretation of the study findings, between-session intra-rater reliability was similarly established as sufficient (ICC = 0.94). The average of 3 measurements was obtained for each subject and used to determine changes in hamstring muscle flexibility.

2.3. Randomization. Subjects were randomly divided into 3 blocks of 40, using a simple random distribution (http://www.randomization.com/) into the 3 intervention groups: Stretching, Neurodynamic, and Control. The Stretching group would receive static passive stretches to their hamstring muscles; the Neurodynamic group would receive neurodynamic sliders; and the Control group would receive passive mobilization of their intrinsic foot joints as placebo. These interventions were performed on each subject's dominant leg; the duration of each intervention was standardized, and all interventions were provided by a therapist who remained blinded to the SLR measurements. Subjects were informed that the intervention being provided to them was a relaxation technique that was thought to improve SLR comfort and range.

2.4. Interventions

2.4.1. Passive Stretching Technique. Subjects in the Stretching group received passive stretching of the hamstring muscles in their dominant leg. While lying supine, a researcher who was blinded to SLR test measures would passively position the subject into the SLR position (hip in flexion, knee in extension, and ankle in neutral) without pain/discomfort to the point where resistance to movement was first noted (Figure 3). This position was then maintained for 30 seconds [36, 37] and repeated further 5 times. During the 30 second stretches, the therapist monitored the subjects to ensure they did not make any compensation that could modify the stretching position. Each subject had a total of 180 seconds of stretching on their lower extremity.

2.4.2. Neurodynamic Sliding Technique. Subjects in the Neurodynamic group received sciatic neurodynamic sliders, performed in supine. The objective of the technique is to produce a sliding movement of neural (sciatic) structures relative to their adjacent tissues [21, 38]. Sliders involve the application of movement/stress to the nervous system proximally while

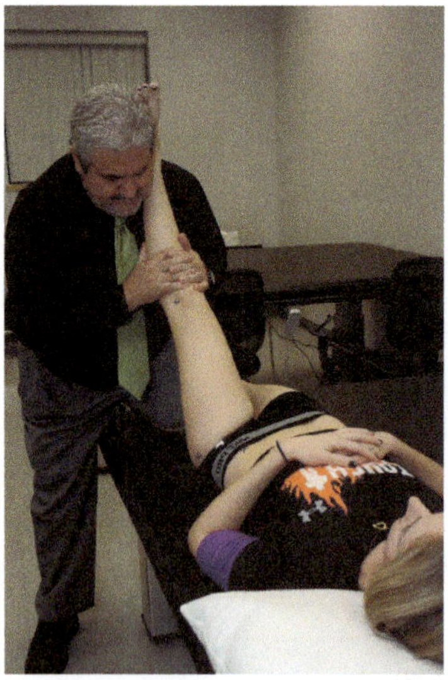

Figure 3: Static stretching of the hamstring muscles was performed for 30 seconds, 6 times on their dominant leg for a total stretching time of 180 seconds.

releasing movement/stress distally and then reversing the sequence. Recent research has shown that sliders actually result in greater excursion than simply stretching the nerve [39]. Subjects were supine with their neck and thoracic spine supported in a forward flexed position. Concurrent hip and knee flexion were alternated dynamically with concurrent hip and knee extension (Figure 4). The therapist alternated the combination of movement depending on the tissue resistance level. This combination of movements was performed for 180 seconds on their dominant lower extremity [40].

2.4.3. Placebo Technique. Subjects in the Control group received passive mobilization of the intrinsic foot joints while being in the supine position. This was chosen as placebo intervention due to the absence of anatomic and/or physiological relations between this region and technique and the hamstring muscles and their stretching positions. Passive movements applied in a randomized order were supination, pronation, abduction, adduction, flexion, and extension (Figure 5). Subjects were given 180 seconds of mobilization to their dominant foot.

As well as standardizing the total treatment times for subjects in each group, preservation of blinding for the study was maintained by standardizing the interval between the SLR assessments for all subjects. No subject reported any persistent discomfort or pain associated with their participation in the study.

2.5. Statistical Analysis. Descriptive statistics (mean, standard deviation, 95% CI) were calculated for pretest and posttest SLR averaged values for the 3 groups. SLR responsiveness data were calculated using the between-session ICC established in this study (ICC = 0.96) and the formulae $\text{SEM} = \text{SD} \times \sqrt{(1 - \text{ICC})}$ [41] and $\text{MDC}_{95} = 1.96 \times \sqrt{2} \times \text{SEM}$ [42]. To analyze the difference in pre-/postintervention between groups on hamstring extensibility (SLR), a 3×2 mixed model ANOVA was performed, with groups (Stretching, Neurodynamic and Control) as the between-subjects variable, and time (time: pre and post) as the within-subjects variable. The hypothesis of interest was the group × time interaction. Simple main effects analyses with a Bonferroni corrected alpha would be utilized if an interaction was observed. Within-group effect size was calculated using Cohen d coefficient (d) [43]. An effect size greater than 0.8 was considered large, around 0.5 was moderate, and less than 0.2 was small. All statistical analyses were performed using SPSS version 21.

3. Results

There were no significant differences in baseline characteristics between groups at the beginning of the study (Table 1). Descriptive statistics are provided in Table 2. Standard deviations for SLR measurements ranged from 3.7 to 8.0°. This allowed us to calculate a range of SEM from 1.1 to 2.4° and subsequently a range for the MDC_{95} of 3.1–6.6°. The Neurodynamic group had a pretest mean range of 59.8° (95% CI: 58.1–61.3°) and posttest mean range of 69.7° (95% CI: 68.5–70.9°). The Stretching group had a pretest mean range of 59.9° (95% CI: 57.7–62.2°) and posttest mean range of 65.5° (95% CI: 62.9–68.0°). Finally, the Control group had a pretest mean range of 59.4° (95% CI: 57.5–61.2°) and posttest mean range of 59.4° (95% CI: 57.6–61.1°). The before and after differences in mean SLR values exceeded the upper limit of this MDC_{95} range for the Neurodynamic group (9.9°) but not for the Stretching group (5.5°) or the Control group (0.03°) (Table 2).

A statistically significant interaction was observed, $F(2, 117) = 313.715$, $P < 0.001$ ($\eta_p^2 = 0.843$) (Figure 6). There was no difference between the 3 groups at the start, $P = 0.893$; however, at the end of the study, the groups were significantly different. Mean SLR values were significantly higher for both the Neurodynamic and Stretching groups compared to the Control group ($P < 0.001$) and for the Neurodynamic group compared to the Stretching group ($P = 0.006$). Both the Neurodynamic and Stretching groups significantly improved ROM compared to their baseline values ($P < 0.001$), whereas there was no significant improvement noted for the Control group ($P = 0.800$). The effect sizes were large for Neurodynamic group ($d = 2.36$), moderate for Stretching group ($d = 0.73$), and very small for Control group ($d < 0.01$).

4. Discussion

Results from this study show that an isolated neurodynamic intervention provides a greater immediate increase in passive SLR range of motion than static hamstring stretching in subjects with short hamstring syndrome. Although both interventions were more effective in increasing SLR range than the placebo control, only the neurodynamic intervention group demonstrated before and after differences in mean SLR which exceeded the MDC_{95} upper limit of 6.6°.

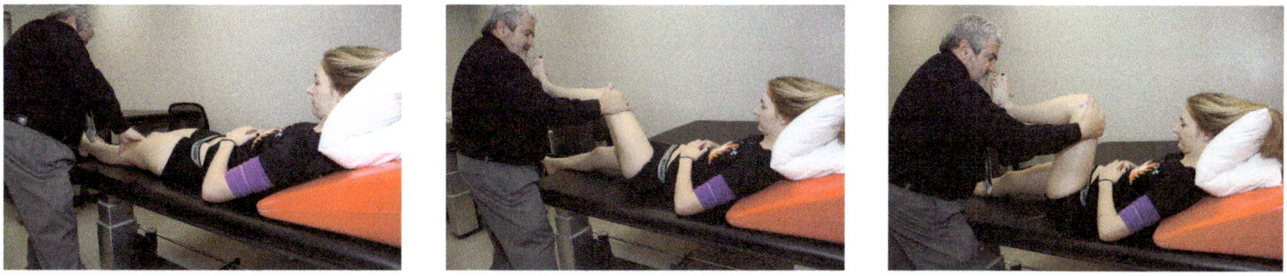

FIGURE 4: Neurodynamic sciatic slider technique was performed by alternating hip flexion, knee flexion, and ankle dorsiflexion with hip extension, knee extension, and ankle plantarflexion while the subject's cervical and thoracic spine were maintained in flexion. Movements were performed for 180 seconds on their dominant leg.

TABLE 1: Baseline sample characteristics.

	Stretching group $n = 40$	Neurodynamic group $n = 40$	Control group $n = 40$	P values
Gender (female)	20 (50%)	20 (50%)	20 (50%)	1.00[a]
Age (years)	33.9 ± 7.44	33.7 ± 7.68	32.7 ± 7.08	0.75[b]
Weight (kg)	69.8 ± 12.93	68.9 ± 11.09	68.4 ± 10.98	0.87[b]
Height (cm)	170.9 ± 7.75	171.4 ± 7.17	170.7 ± 6.46	0.88[b]
BMI (kg/cm^2)	23.7 ± 2.63	23.3 ± 2.10	23.3 ± 2.28	0.72[b]

Values are expressed as mean ± standard deviation.
[a]Chi-square.
[b]ANOVA.
BMI: Body mass index.

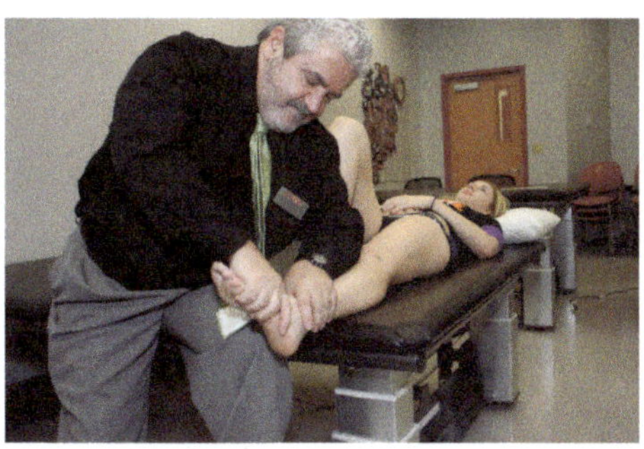

FIGURE 5: Passive mobilization of the intrinsic foot joints with the subject in supine lying. Passive movements were applied for 180 seconds to the dominant foot.

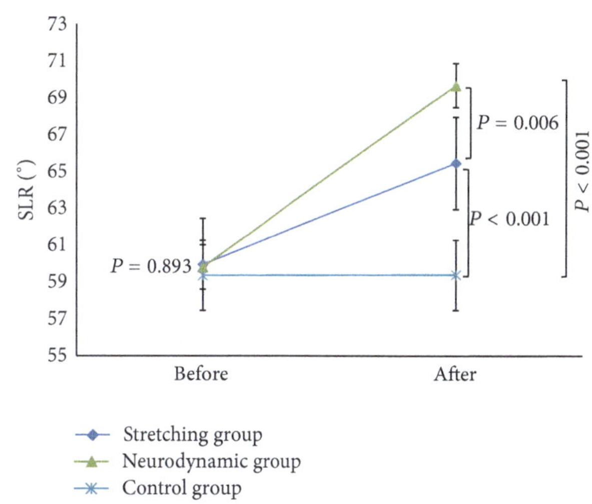

FIGURE 6: Before and after mean straight leg raise (SLR) values (°) with 95% confidence intervals of hamstring extensibility among the three groups.

The results confirmed our initial hypothesis that an isolated neurodynamic sciatic sliding technique would provide a greater immediate improvement in hip flexion, assessed by passive SLR, than hamstring stretching or placebo.

Increasing hamstring flexibility has been suggested as an important factor in the treatment and prevention of lower extremity overuse injuries [44, 45]. Much of the research on increasing hamstring flexibility has focused on the varying modes of stretching, such as proprioceptive neuromuscular facilitation (PNF) [46, 47], static stretching [46–48], plyometric stretching, and ballistic stretching [49]. They have also compared differing stretch intensities [25] and frequencies [50]. Very few studies have examined the effect of neurodynamic interventions on hamstring flexibility [24, 30, 40] and the results of this study can be seen as adding further evidence for the potential role of neural tissue mechanosensitivity in limiting the SLR.

A new conceptual model showing an interrelationship between the different factors involved in hamstring strains may provide a better understanding of this multifactorial

TABLE 2: Mean passive straight leg raise test (SLR) values pre- and postintervention for each of the 3 groups with associated standard deviations, mean differences over time, and associated 95% confidence intervals (CI).

Intervention	Time	Mean ± SD	Difference between before and after ± SD	95 % CI of the difference	
				Lower bound	Upper bound
Neurodynamic group	Pre	59.8 ± 4.70	9.86 ± 2.51*	9.07	10.68
	Post	69.7 ± 3.69			
Stretching group	Pre	59.9 ± 6.99	5.50 ± 1.62*	4.98	6.02
	Post	65.5 ± 7.97			
Control group	Pre	59.4 ± 5.68	0.03 ± 0.62	−0.17	0.22
	Post	59.4 ± 5.45			

All measurements are in degrees.
*$P < 0.001$.

injury and therefore improve its prevention and prediction methods [51]. Neural tissue mechanosensitivity presenting clinically as tightness in the hamstrings is a plausible yet only retrospectively studied potential risk factor for and/or potential differential diagnosis to be considered in, hamstring strain injury [52]. The "sensory theory" proposed by Weppler and Magnusson suggests that muscle flexibility and its response to sudden stretch have more to do with perceptions of stretch and pain (sensation) than the biomechanical effects on muscle tissue itself [20].

This proposal was supported in a study by Aparicio and others which demonstrated that a suboccipital muscle inhibition technique altered hamstring muscle flexibility when compared to a placebo intervention [53]. The authors measured hamstring flexibility in 3 ways (forward flexion distance test, straight leg raise test, and popliteal angle test) and found significant before and after differences on all 3 measures for the suboccipital muscle inhibition technique but not for the placebo intervention. The fact that such a distant technique (suboccipital region) could have an immediate effect on the flexibility in the hamstrings may lend support to the "sensory theory" limiting flexibility of the posterior thigh structures. It seems reasonable to attribute the observed increase in hamstring tissue flexibility following the suboccipital muscle inhibition technique to changes in the subjects' perceptions of stretch or pain associated with the 3 flexibility measures.

The results of this study demonstrate a mean increase in the hip flexion range of the SLR for the neurodynamic group of 9.86° which compares favorably with other studies. Castellote-Caballero and others reported mean increases in SLR of 9.4° following a similar neurodynamic slider technique [30], and Aparicio et al. reported mean increases of 5.9° for the right SLR and 5.5° for the left SLR following application of the suboccipital muscle inhibition technique [53]. Mendez-Sanchez and others completed a pilot study on young healthy male soccer players and found mean increases of only 3.7° in the right SLR and 2.2° in the left SLR after sustained hamstring stretching intervention [40]. When they added a neurodynamic slider technique to the sustained hamstring stretching intervention, they found greater mean increases of 6.2° in the right SLR and 6.3° in the left SLR [40]. Finally, Hopper et al. reported mean increases of only 4.7° in SLR after the application of massage techniques to the hamstring musculature [54].

It has been suggested that stretching of the hamstring musculature to improve tissue flexibility may reduce the number of leg overuse injuries after exercise [44], although further high quality studies are needed [55]. While some theories explaining the therapeutic effects of muscle stretching suggest there is alteration of the viscoelastic properties of muscles, studies have shown the importance of distinguishing between real and apparent increases in muscle flexibility [37, 56]. Observed changes in SLR following interventions may be more associated with increased tolerance to the uncomfortable stretch sensation rather than true changes to muscle elasticity [56]. Although the results from this study do not provide information on the mechanisms for the observed changes, they do suggest that neurodynamic interventions can significantly increase SLR more than static stretching in the short term in healthy subjects with short hamstring syndrome.

4.1. Limitations. This study only examined immediate effects of a single episode and the lack of longer term follow-up should be considered. It is not known how long the observed increase in hamstring flexibility might have lasted. Furthermore, it is not known if repetition and an appropriate dosage of the neurodynamic interventions over time might lead to longer lasting effects. Finally, we did not conduct any long-term follow-up to determine if the observed changes in flexibility might have resulted in any change in incidence of hamstring injuries in these subjects with short hamstring syndrome.

5. Conclusion

Findings from this study indicate that a neurodynamic sliding intervention will increase short-term hamstring flexibility as measured by the passive SLR to a greater degree than static hamstring stretching in healthy subjects with short hamstring syndrome. Future research should look at longer term results and assess the effect of combining neurodynamic techniques with other interventions.

Ethical Approval

The study was approved by the Office for the Protection of Research Subjects at the University of Granada, Granada, Spain.

Conflict of Interests

The authors declare that there is no conflict of interests regarding the publication of this paper.

References

[1] R. Bahr and I. Holme, "Risk factors for sports injuries—a methodological approach," *British Journal of Sports Medicine*, vol. 37, no. 5, pp. 384–392, 2003.

[2] D. S. Davis, P. E. Ashby, K. L. McCale, J. A. McQuain, and J. M. Wine, "The effectiveness of 3 stretching techniques on hamstring flexibility using consistent stretching parameters," *Journal of Strength and Conditioning Research*, vol. 19, no. 1, pp. 27–32, 2005.

[3] D. A. Opar, M. D. Williams, and A. J. Shield, "Hamstring strain injuries: factors that lead to injury and re-injury," *Sports Medicine*, vol. 42, no. 3, pp. 209–226, 2012.

[4] J. Orchard and H. Seward, "Epidemiology of injuries in the Australian Football League, seasons 1997–2000," *British Journal of Sports Medicine*, vol. 36, no. 1, pp. 39–44, 2002.

[5] B. Gabbe, C. Finch, H. Wajswelner, and K. Bennell, "Australian football: injury profile at the community level," *Journal of Science and Medicine in Sport*, vol. 5, no. 2, pp. 149–160, 2002.

[6] W. L. Frost and D. J. Chalmers, "Injury in elite New Zealand cricketers 2002–2008: descriptive epidemiology," *British Journal of Sports Medicine*, 2012.

[7] J. Ekstrand, M. Hägglund, and M. Waldén, "Injury incidence and injury patterns in professional football: the UEFA injury study," *British Journal of Sports Medicine*, vol. 45, no. 7, pp. 553–558, 2011.

[8] G. Henderson, C. A. Barnes, and M. D. Portas, "Factors associated with increased propensity for hamstring injury in English Premier League soccer players," *Journal of Science and Medicine in Sport*, vol. 13, no. 4, pp. 397–402, 2010.

[9] J. C. Murphy, E. O'Malley, C. Gissane, and C. Blake, "Incidence of injury in Gaelic football: a 4-year prospective study," *The American Journal of Sports Medicine*, vol. 40, no. 9, pp. 2113–2120, 2012.

[10] M. R. Safran, W. E. Garrett Jr., A. V. Seaber, R. R. Glisson, and B. M. Ribbeck, "The role of warmup in muscular injury prevention," *The American Journal of Sports Medicine*, vol. 16, no. 2, pp. 123–129, 1988.

[11] E. Witvrouw, L. Danneels, P. Asselman, T. D'Have, and D. Cambier, "Muscle flexibility as a risk factor for developing muscle injuries in male professional soccer players: a prospective study," *The American Journal of Sports Medicine*, vol. 31, no. 1, pp. 41–46, 2003.

[12] J.-L. Croisier, "Factors associated with recurrent hamstring injuries," *Sports Medicine*, vol. 34, no. 10, pp. 681–695, 2004.

[13] S. E. Turl and K. P. George, "Adverse neural tension: a factor in repetitive hamstring strain?" *Journal of Orthopaedic and Sports Physical Therapy*, vol. 27, no. 1, pp. 16–21, 1998.

[14] U. M. Kujala, S. Orava, and M. Järvinen, "Hamstring injuries. Current trends in treatment and prevention," *Sports Medicine*, vol. 23, no. 6, pp. 397–404, 1997.

[15] G. M. Verrall, J. P. Slavotinek, P. G. Barnes, G. T. Fon, and A. J. Spriggins, "Clinical risk factors for hamstring muscle strain injury: a prospective study with correlation of injury by magnetic resonance imaging," *British Journal of Sports Medicine*, vol. 35, no. 6, pp. 435–439, 2001.

[16] L. C. Decoster, R. L. Scanlon, K. D. Horn, and J. Cleland, "Standing and supine hamstring stretching are equally effective," *Journal of Athletic Training*, vol. 39, no. 4, pp. 330–334, 2004.

[17] L. Hennessy and A. W. S. Watson, "Flexibility and posture assessment in relation to hamstring injury," *British Journal of Sports Medicine*, vol. 27, no. 4, pp. 243–246, 1993.

[18] E. F. Goldman and D. E. Jones, "Interventions for preventing hamstring injuries," *Cochrane Database of Systematic Reviews*, no. 1, Article ID CD006782, 2010.

[19] T. W. Worrell and D. H. Perrin, "Hamstring muscle injury: the influence of strength, flexibility, warm-up, and fatigue," *Journal of Orthopaedic and Sports Physical Therapy*, vol. 16, no. 1, pp. 12–18, 1992.

[20] C. H. Weppler and S. P. Magnusson, "Increasing muscle extensibility: a matter of increasing length or modifying sensation?" *Physical Therapy*, vol. 90, no. 3, pp. 438–449, 2010.

[21] D. S. Butler, *The Sensitive Nervous System*, Noigroup Publications, Adelaide, Australia, 2000.

[22] M. Shacklock, "Improving application of neurodynamic (neural tension) testing and treatments: a message to researchers and clinicians," *Manual Therapy*, vol. 10, no. 3, pp. 175–179, 2005.

[23] M. Shacklock, "Neurodynamics," *Physiotherapy*, vol. 81, no. 1, pp. 9–16, 1995.

[24] C. Kornberg and P. Lew, "The effect of stretching neural structures on grade one hamstring injuries," *Journal of Orthopaedic and Sports Physical Therapy*, vol. 10, no. 12, pp. 481–487, 1989.

[25] P. W. M. Marshall, A. Cashman, and B. S. Cheema, "A randomized controlled trial for the effect of passive stretching on measures of hamstring extensibility, passive stiffness, strength, and stretch tolerance," *Journal of Science and Medicine in Sport*, vol. 14, no. 6, pp. 535–540, 2011.

[26] T. Hall, M. Zusman, and R. Elvey, "Adverse mechanical tension in the nervous system? Analysis of straight leg raise," *Manual Therapy*, vol. 3, no. 3, pp. 140–146, 1998.

[27] B. S. Boyd, L. Wanek, A. T. Gray, and K. S. Topp, "Mechanosensitivity of the lower extremity nervous system during straight-leg raise neurodynamic testing in healthy individuals," *Journal of Orthopaedic and Sports Physical Therapy*, vol. 39, no. 11, pp. 780–790, 2009.

[28] A. I. De-la-Llave-Rincon, R. Ortega-Santiago, S. Ambite-Quesada et al., "Response of pain intensity to soft tissue mobilization and neurodynamic technique: a series of 18 patients with chronic carpal tunnel syndrome," *Journal of Manipulative and Physiological Therapeutics*, vol. 35, no. 6, pp. 420–427, 2012.

[29] C. L. Brown, K. K. Gilbert, J.-M. Brismee, P. S. Sizer, C. R. James, and M. P. Smith, "The effects of neurodynamic mobilization on fluid dispersion within the tibial nerve at the ankle: an unembalmed cadaveric study," *Journal of Manual and Manipulative Therapy*, vol. 19, no. 1, pp. 26–34, 2011.

[30] Y. Castellote-Caballero, M. C. Valenza, L. Martin-Martin, I. Cabrera-Martos, E. J. Puentedura, and C. Fernández-de-las-Peñas, "Effects of a neurodynamic sliding technique on hamstring flexibility in healthy male soccer players. A pilot study," *Physical Therapy in Sport*, vol. 14, no. 3, pp. 156–162, 2013.

[31] V. Ferrer, *Repercusiones de la Cortedad Isquiosural Sobre la Pelvis y el Raquis Lumbar*, Universidad de Murcia, Murcia, Spain, 1998.

[32] V. Ferrer, F. Santonja, M. Carrion, and L. Martinez, "Comparacion de dos tests (E.P.R. y Popliteo) para el diagnostico del sindrome de isquiosurales cortos," *Archivos de Medicina del Deporte*, vol. 11, no. 43, pp. 247–254, 1994.

[33] R. L. Gajdosik, C. K. Hatcher, and S. Whitsell, "Influence of short hamstring muscles on the pelvis and lumbar spine in standing and during the toe-touch test," *Clinical Biomechanics*, vol. 7, no. 1, pp. 38–42, 1992.

[34] S. S.-C. Hui and P. Y. Yuen, "Validity of the modified back-saver sit-and-reach test: a comparison with other protocols," *Medicine and Science in Sports and Exercise*, vol. 32, no. 9, pp. 1655–1659, 2000.

[35] F. Santonja and I. Martínez, *Valoración Médico-Deportiva del Escolar*, Secretariado de Publicaciones, Universidad de Murcia, Murcia, Spain, 1992.

[36] W. D. Bandy, J. M. Irion, and M. Briggler, "The effect of time and frequency of static stretching on flexibility of the hamstring muscles," *Physical Therapy*, vol. 77, no. 10, pp. 1090–1096, 1997.

[37] J. P. K. Halbertsma, I. Mulder, L. N. H. Göeken, and W. H. Eisma, "Repeated passive stretching: acute effect on the passive muscle moment and extensibility of short hamstrings," *Archives of Physical Medicine and Rehabilitation*, vol. 80, no. 4, pp. 407–414, 1999.

[38] P. Mintken, E. Puentedura, and A. Louw, "Neurodynamic interventions and physiological effects: clinical neurodynamics in neck and upper extremity pain," in *Neck and Arm Pain Syndromes*, C. Fernández-de-las-Peñas, J. Cleland, and P. Huijbregts, Eds., pp. 496–515, 2011.

[39] M. W. Coppieters and D. S. Butler, "Do "sliders" slide and "tensioners" tension? An analysis of neurodynamic techniques and considerations regarding their application," *Manual Therapy*, vol. 13, no. 3, pp. 213–221, 2008.

[40] R. Méndez-Sánchez, F. Alburquerque-Sendín, C. Fernández-de-las-Peñas et al., "Immediate effects of adding a sciatic nerve slider technique on lumbar and lower quadrant mobility in soccer players: a pilot study," *Journal of Alternative and Complementary Medicine*, vol. 16, no. 6, pp. 669–675, 2010.

[41] J. P. Weir, "Quantifying test-retest reliability using the intraclass correlation coefficient and the SEM," *Journal of Strength and Conditioning Research*, vol. 19, no. 1, pp. 231–240, 2005.

[42] P. W. Stratford, "Getting more from the literature: estimating the standard error of measurement from reliability studies," *Physiotherapy Canada*, vol. 56, no. 1, pp. 27–30, 2004.

[43] J. Cohen, *Statistical Power Analysis for the Behavioural Sciences*, Lawrence Erlbaum Associates, Hillsdale, NJ, USA, 1988.

[44] D. E. Hartig and J. M. Henderson, "Increasing hamstring flexibility decreases lower extremity overuse injuries in military basic trainees," *The American Journal of Sports Medicine*, vol. 27, no. 2, pp. 173–176, 1999.

[45] N. Malliaropoulos, S. Papalexandris, A. Papalada, and E. Papacostas, "The role of stretching in rehabilitation of hamstring injuries: 80 athletes follow-up," *Medicine and Science in Sports and Exercise*, vol. 36, no. 5, pp. 756–759, 2004.

[46] E. J. Puentedura, P. A. Huijbregts, S. Celeste et al., "Immediate effects of quantified hamstring stretching: hold-relax proprioceptive neuromuscular facilitation versus static stretching," *Physical Therapy in Sport*, vol. 12, no. 3, pp. 122–126, 2011.

[47] H. W. Wallmann, C. B. Gillis, and N. J. Martinez, "The effects of different stretching techniques of the quadriceps muscles on agility performance in female collegiate soccer athletes: a pilot study," *North American Journal of Sports Physical Therapy*, vol. 3, no. 1, pp. 41–47, 2008.

[48] H. W. Wallmann, J. A. Mercer, and J. W. McWhorter, "Surface electromyographic assessment of the effect of static stretching of the gastrocnemius on vertical jump performance," *Journal of Strength and Conditioning Research*, vol. 19, no. 3, pp. 684–688, 2005.

[49] M. N. Samuel, W. R. Holcomb, M. A. Guadagnoli, M. D. Rubley, and H. Wallmann, "Acute effects of static and ballistic stretching on measures of strength and power," *Journal of Strength and Conditioning Research*, vol. 22, no. 5, pp. 1422–1428, 2008.

[50] J. B. Feland and H. N. Marin, "Effect of submaximal contraction intensity in contract-relax proprioceptive neuromuscular facilitation stretching," *British Journal of Sports Medicine*, vol. 38, no. 4, article E18, 2004.

[51] J. Mendiguchia, E. Alentorn-Geli, and M. Brughelli, "Hamstring strain injuries: are we heading in the right direction?" *British Journal of Sports Medicine*, vol. 46, no. 2, pp. 81–85, 2012.

[52] B. J. Gabbe, C. F. Finch, K. L. Bennell, and H. Wajswelner, "Risk factors for hamstring injuries in community level Australian football," *British Journal of Sports Medicine*, vol. 39, no. 2, pp. 106–110, 2005.

[53] É. Q. Aparicio, L. B. Quirante, C. R. Blanco, and F. A. Sendín, "Immediate effects of the suboccipital muscle inhibition technique in subjects with short hamstring syndrome," *Journal of Manipulative and Physiological Therapeutics*, vol. 32, no. 4, pp. 262–269, 2009.

[54] D. Hopper, S. Deacon, S. Das et al., "Dynamic soft tissue mobilisation increases hamstring flexibility in healthy male subjects," *British Journal of Sports Medicine*, vol. 39, no. 9, pp. 594–598, 2005.

[55] S. M. Weldon and R. H. Hill, "The efficacy of stretching for prevention of exercise-related injury: a systematic review of the literature," *Manual Therapy*, vol. 8, no. 3, pp. 141–150, 2003.

[56] H. Folpp, S. Deall, L. A. Harvey, and T. Gwinn, "Can apparent increases in muscle extensibility with regular stretch be explained by changes in tolerance to stretch?" *Australian Journal of Physiotherapy*, vol. 52, no. 1, pp. 45–50, 2006.

7

Strength Gains as a Result of Brief, Infrequent Resistance Exercise in Older Adults

James Fisher,[1] James Steele,[1] Pat McKinnon,[2] and Stephen McKinnon[2]

[1] *Southampton Solent University, East Park Terrace, Southampton SO14 0YN, UK*
[2] *Abstract Bodyworks, Precision Exercise, Newbury RG14 5BY, UK*

Correspondence should be addressed to James Fisher; james.fisher@solent.ac.uk

Academic Editor: Karim Chamari

Chronological aging is associated with a decrease in skeletal muscle mass and bone mineral density, an increase in fat mass, frequency of falls and fractures, and the likelihood of obesity, diabetes, and coronary heart disease. Resistance exercise has been shown to counter all of these effects of aging and, in turn, reduce the risk of all-cause mortality. However, variables such as volume and frequency have become contentious issues, with recent publications suggesting that similar physiological adaptations are possible with both high- and low-volume approaches. The aim of this research was to consider strength increases as a result of brief, infrequent resistance exercise. The present study offers data from 33 (14 male and 19 female) older adults ($M = 55$ years) who underwent brief (<15 minutes per exercise session), infrequent (2×/week), resistance exercise to a high intensity of effort (6-repetition maximum) at a controlled repetition duration (10 seconds concentric : 10 seconds eccentric) on 5 resistance machines (chest press, leg press, pull-down, seated row, and overhead press). Data is presented for training interventions of 12 weeks (male) and 19 weeks (female). Significant strength increases were identified for all exercises. With the detailed health benefits obtainable, the present study suggests that resistance exercise can be efficacious in much smaller volumes than previously considered.

1. Introduction

The natural homeostatic processes in the human body often result in a physical decline with age. We lose bone mineral density (BMD), muscle mass, and strength and we have an increase in fat mass, ultimately resulting in reduced physical performance [1–4]. As such, with aging there is generally an increased risk of acute and chronic conditions including greater frequency of bone fractures, obesity, diabetes, coronary heart disease, and cancers [5]. However, by performing resistance training (RT) a person can improve their strength [6], muscle size [7], cardiovascular fitness [8], metabolic health [9], and BMD [10]. As a result, people can decrease the potential for injuries through strengthening their joints, tendons, and ligaments [11, 12]. Hurley and Roth [13] comment that the data suggests that "*~2 decades of age-associated strength loss can be regained in ~2 months of resistance exercise.*" Indeed, reduced strength has been shown to be a strong risk factor for all-cause mortality independently of muscle mass [14]. Melov et al. [15] reported reversal in mitochondrial deterioration to the extent that participants with an average age of 68 years showed mitochondrial characteristics similar to those of persons with a mean age of 24 years following 6 months of resistance exercise. Succinctly, resistance exercise appears to reverse aging in skeletal muscle. Indeed, the evidence supports that resistance exercise reduces the risk of all-cause mortality [14–17].

Previous publications have suggested that greater loads result in greater increases in strength for older adults [18–21]. However, these studies failed to accurately control intensity of effort. Previous reviews in asymptomatic individuals of younger and middle age people have suggested that when intensity of effort is controlled, research does not support the superiority of a particular load and/or repetition range for increasing muscular strength [6] and size [7]. Other publications have discussed that differences in low and high loads can be equated in intensity of effort and thus negated by increasing repetition duration of low load training groups [22].

Research in young adults has supported this proposition showing similar strength and hypertrophic increases when using low loads (50–60% 1-repetition maximum (1 RM)) for longer repetition duration (3 seconds concentric : 1 second isometric : 3 seconds eccentric (3 : 1 : 3)) compared to higher loads (80–90% 1 RM) at shorter repetition durations (1 second concentric : 1 second eccentric (1 : 1)) [23, 24]. More recently van Roie et al. [25] have also reported nonsignificant differences in strength increases between low (20–40% 1 RM) and high (80% 1 RM) training loads in older adults when exercise is taken to a point of muscular failure. Certainly this is of important consideration since exercise ~1 RM produced an orthopaedic injury prevalence of ~20% in older adults [26]. In addition heavy loads/shorter repetition duration appear more likely to cause muscle soreness [27] which appears counterintuitive to persons wishing to improve their quality of life. We should also consider that near maximal loads are simply not representative of normal daily function.

Previous research has concluded that single sets of an exercise, performed to momentary muscular failure, produce similar strength gains to multiple sets [6, 28, 29]. This remains a contentious issue in the field [30]; however, there is limited research which has implemented and evaluated a single set approach with older adults. Indeed, a recent meta-analysis of resistance exercise in older adults [31] reported that all included studies used a multiple-set method. In fact, Westcott et al. [32] assessed a single set approach using 13 resistance exercises, 2-3×/week with older adults and reported significant strength increases favouring a group training at long repetition duration (10 seconds concentric : 4 seconds eccentric) compared to a group training at a more moderate repetition duration (2 seconds concentric : 1 second isometric : 4 seconds eccentric). Theoretically, moving a load more slowly (for a longer repetition duration) decreases the potential for external forces such as momentum to interact, thus maintaining muscular tension and likely increasing intensity of effort. Evidence supports that fewer repetitions are possible when moving a load at a longer-compared to shorter-repetition duration [33–35].

van Roie et al. [25] also considered the use of a single set protocol with older adults but limited training and testing to lower body exercises only. In an aging population with only 10–15% of persons over 55 years of age performing any strengthening activities [36] it is important to consider time-efficient methods which might encourage exercise adherence. The present authors have previously recommended single sets of an exercise, performed infrequently (1-2×/week), to a high intensity of effort, using resistance machines through a full range of motion, at a repetition duration that maintains muscular tension as being optimal for increasing strength whilst efficiently using time and minimising risk of injury [6, 37].

Whilst data from Westcott et al. [32] supports this approach, the present study represents a further decreased volume of training. The authors have worked closely with a UK exercise facility which uses these recommendations, categorically clarifying that all exercise sessions will be completed in <15 minutes, whilst stringently recording all workout data. As such, the present study aims to retrospectively present the data from the members of that facility emphasizing the ecological validity of *real people in a real gym*, rather than a "*laboratory gym*" in which most research is undertaken and restricted by specific protocols and research questions.

Table 1: Participant demographic characteristics (Mean ± SD).

	Males	Females
Age (years)	55 ± 10	55 ± 11
Stature (cm)	177.6 ± 5.5	167.4 ± 5.8
Body mass (kg)	85.92 ± 12.50	71.43 ± 13.56
BMI	27.54 ± 4.11	25.63 ± 5.50

2. Methods

2.1. Study Design. This study was a retrospective analysis of strength outcomes of a cohort of members from a private UK based exercise facility. The facility uses standardised training protocols with members with all sessions being supervised by the same trainers who make meticulous records of every session allowing for analysis of load progression as a measurement of strength gains as a result of the training protocol administered. Participants training records were examined from the period beginning from January 2013 through to April 2014. The study design was approved by the relevant ethics committee at the author's institution.

2.2. Participants. Participants were required to have no medical condition for which RT is contraindicated to participate. Participant demographics are given in Table 1. Participants were existing members at the facility who provided written informed consent for their training data from their first session until their most recent to be released for analysis in this study. Power analysis of research using low volume RT in untrained participants was conducted to determine participant numbers (n) using an effect size (ES), calculated using Cohen's d [38] of ~1.0 [39] for the improvements in strength. Participant numbers were calculated using equations from Whitley and Ball [40] revealing a required 16 participants to meet required power of 0.8 at an alpha value of $P \leq 0.05$ for detecting changes.

2.3. Equipment. Strength was measured using MedX (USA) torso arm (pull down), chest press, seated row, overhead press, and leg press resistance machines. These were also used for the RT intervention in addition to MedX (USA) leg extension, leg curl, bicep curl, torso flexion, hip extension, chest fly, seated dip, abdominal isolator, and lumbar extension resistance machines, as well as a pull-over (Nautilus, USA).

2.4. Participant Training. Throughout the time period analysed participants attended the facility to participate in supervised RT sessions ~2×/week. All participants performed a single set of torso arm (pull down), chest press, seated row, overhead press, and leg press exercises in this order throughout their training period and some occasionally performed 1-2 additional exercises using the other resistance machines noted. Each exercise was completed using a load that allowed the participants to perform a self-determined 6 RM (meaning that they determined inability to complete further repetitions if attempted, i.e., predicted momentary muscular failure on the next repetition) through a full range of motion using repetition duration of 10 seconds concentric and 10 seconds eccentric. This equated to total repetition duration of 20 seconds and a total time under load of ~120 seconds. The trainer monitored participants repetition duration throughout each exercise using a stopwatch and advised participants to either speed up or slow down as appropriate to maintain this repetition duration. Load progression was provided based on the following characteristics as assessed by the trainer; (1) the ability to maintain the prescribed repetition duration of 10 : 10 within a margin of 2 seconds error (i.e., 8–12 : 8–12), (2) the ability to maintain interrepetition consistency to this repetition duration within the set, (3) and the quality of the participants form for the exercise. Once the trainer was confident the participant could exceed a 6 RM whilst meeting these criteria with their current load, a further 2–5 lbs was added in their next training session. This method of progression is consistent with previous research [32]. The trainers throughout this intervention encouraged very strict form during exercise; for example, controlled and continuous breathing frequency (without a valsalva manoeuvre) and attempting to keep muscles which are not the target of the exercise as relaxed as possible.

As a time efficient training approach participants were also encouraged to move from one exercise to the next without significant rest, generally <30 seconds. All machines were prepared for the clients prior to beginning each exercise session to make this possible. With an average of 5 exercises per session, at ~120 seconds per exercise, total workout time is approximately 12 minutes. Indeed the trainers and the exercise facility specifically advertise that sessions will not exceed 15 minutes in total time commitment per training session. This represents an ecologically valid approach to applying the aforementioned recommendations with stringent, yet practical methods of increasing load.

Mean (± SD) numbers of training sessions are presented in Table 2 which equate to study duration of $M = 12 \pm 6.7$ weeks for males and $M = 19 \pm 10.9$ weeks for females. The SDs suggest large differences in actual duration between participants. However, this is likely representative of *real people*, where some people train for extended periods whilst others cease exercise intermittently as a result of other commitments.

TABLE 2: Participant training session data.

Exercise	Number of training sessions (M ± SD)	
	Males	Females
Torso arm (pull down)	23 ± 12	37 ± 21*
Chest press	25 ± 16	40 ± 24
Seated row	24 ± 12	39 ± 23*
Overhead press	24 ± 12	34 ± 16
Leg press	24 ± 15	41 ± 25*
Exercises per session (number)	5 ± 1	5 ± 1

*Significant compared to males ($P < 0.05$).

2.5. Outcomes. Strength gains as progression in load used during exercise was the primary outcome for this study. As all participants had completed torso arm (pull down), chest press, seated row, overhead press, and leg press, load progression was examined for these exercises only. As participants continuously performed a standardised intervention, whereby the exercises were performed in the same order and used a self-determined 6 RM load (meaning that they determined inability to complete further repetitions if attempted that is, predicted momentary muscular failure on the next repetition) through a full range of motion using a repetition duration of 10 seconds concentric and 10 seconds eccentric throughout the training period, the increase in training load was considered to be adequate to determine strength gains as a result of the training completed. This was calculated as the training load in the most recent exercise session available for analysis minus the training load for the participants first training session.

2.6. Data Analysis. Training record data was available from 33 participants (male, $n = 14$; female, $n = 19$). Descriptive statistics including means and standard deviations were calculated for number of exercises performed each session, number of sessions completed for chest press, leg press, torso arm (pull down), seated row, and overhead press exercises, and load progression for these exercises. Data met assumptions of normality when examined using a Kolmogorov-Smirnov test. Gender comparisons were performed for demographic characteristics, number of exercises performed each session, number of sessions completed per exercise, and strength outcomes, including both absolute and relative change in training load and strength change relative to body mass, using an independent samples t-test. 95% confidence intervals (CI) were calculated in addition to ES using Cohen's d [38] for each absolute strength outcome to examine the significance and magnitude of effects where an outcome was considered to be significantly improved if the CI did not cross zero. Effect sizes (ESs) of 0.20–0.49 were considered as small, 0.50–0.79 as moderate and ≥0.80 as large.

3. Results

3.1. Participants. Participant baseline demographics are shown in Table 1. Age and BMI did not significantly differ between groups. Males had a significantly higher stature ($t_{(31)} = 5.106$, $P < 0.001$) and body mass ($t_{(29)} = 2.983$, $P = 0.005$) than females.

Table 3: Beginning training loads.

	Males	Females
Mean (±SD) training load (Kgs)		
Torso arm	61.23 ± 14.54	45.36 ± 10.34*
Chest press	43.16 ± 10.80	29.98 ± 7.17*
Seated row	47.66 ± 14.87	36.48 ± 9.48*
Overhead press	33.29 ± 8.02	22.92 ± 6.31*
Leg press	63.50 ± 13.35	47.56 ± 7.58*

*Significant compared to males ($P < 0.05$).

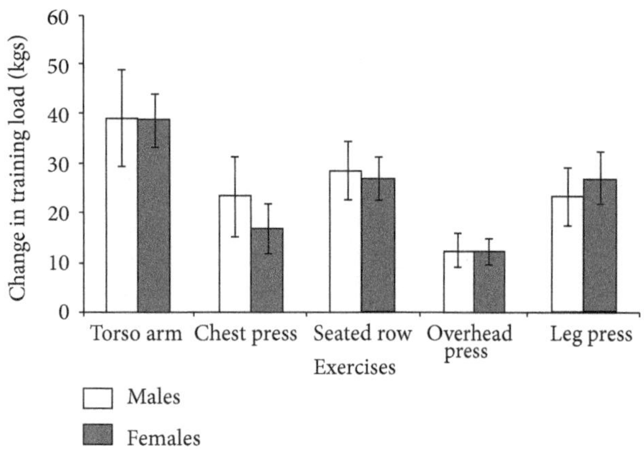

Figure 1: Mean change in absolute training load with 95% CIs for males and females.

3.2. Training Sessions. Training session data including number of training sessions per exercise and exercises per sessions are presented in Table 2. Females had performed significantly more sessions than males for torso arm ($t_{(31)} = -2.301$, $P = 0.028$), seated row ($t_{(31)} = -2.238$, $P = 0.033$), and leg press ($t_{(30)} = -2.126$, $P = 0.026$) exercises. There was no difference in number of exercises performed per session between males and females.

3.3. Strength Outcomes. Beginning training loads are presented in Table 3. Males had a significantly higher absolute training load at baseline than females for torso arm ($t_{(31)} = 3.488$, $P = 0.002$), chest press ($t_{(31)} = 4.215$, $P < 0.001$), seated row ($t_{(30)} = 2.603$, $P = 0.014$), overhead press ($t_{(30)} = 4.087$, $P < 0.001$), and leg press ($t_{(30)} = 3.898$, $P = 0.001$) exercises. Strength relative to body mass did not differ at baseline between males and females for any exercise. Figure 1 presents changes in absolute training load from first to last training sessions for each exercise for males and females. Change in absolute training load did not significantly differ between males and females for any exercise. 95% CIs suggest significant improvements in absolute strength for every exercise with large ESs for both males and females, respectively, of 2.14 and 3.31 for torso arm, 1.59 and 1.59 for chest press, 2.67 and 2.84 for seated row, 2.01 and 2.20 for overhead press, and 2.19 and 2.36 for leg press exercises. Relative increases in training load did not differ between males and females, respectively, for torso arm (68.7 ± 40.1% versus 90.8 ± 38.1%), chest press (55.8 ± 39.4% versus 59.0 ± 39.9%), seated row (65.0 ± 29.3 versus 81.2 ± 40.3%), and overhead press (39.0 ± 20.4% versus 58.0 ± 30.0%) exercises but was significantly greater for females for the leg press exercise (38.4 ± 18.2% versus 59.0 ± 28.6%; $t_{(30)} = -2.297$, $P = 0.018$). Figure 2 presents changes in training load relative to body mass from first to last training sessions for each exercise for males and females. Changes in training load relative to body mass did not differ between genders for torso arm, chest press, seated row, or overhead press; however, they were significantly greater for females for the leg press exercise ($t_{(30)} = -2.091$, $P = 0.045$).

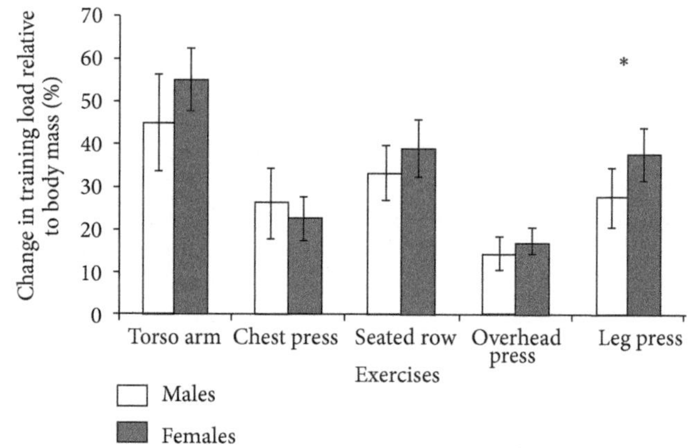

Figure 2: Mean change in training load relative to body mass with 95% CIs for males and females; *significant compared to males ($P < 0.05$).

4. Discussion

This study presents data from a retrospective single arm trial of resistance training in older adults. Previous recommendations (e.g. [6]) have suggested single sets of an exercise to a high intensity of effort performed 1-2×/week as producing the same strength adaptations as larger training volumes/frequencies and yet presenting far greater time efficiency. Training interventions of similar methodology in a similar population sample have reported significant strength gains [32]. However, the present study examined an approach which used an average of two training sessions per week consisting of ~5 exercises to activate most muscle groups, equating to a total time commitment of approximately 30 minutes per week, a significantly lower volume of exercise than Westcott et al. [32]. Previous research has suggested that the addition of single-joint (SJ) to multijoint (MJ) exercises does not increase muscle hypertrophy beyond that of MJ exercises alone [41]. Further research has reported similar strength and hypertrophy increases when comparing SJ and MJ exercises independently [42]. The efficiency of performing only 5 exercises compared to larger volumes suggests practical benefits if the same adaptations are obtainable.

Participants within the present study showed significant meaningful increases in both absolute and relative to body mass strength (6 RM) as evidenced by 95% CIs (Figures

1 and 2) and large ESs for all exercises tested. Female participants reported similar increases in absolute load to male participants albeit with a greater number of training sessions, for example, a longer training duration. However, female participants also showed a significantly greater relative increase in strength, and increase relative to body mass, for the leg press exercise than males and qualitatively greater relative increases for all other exercises. Evidence has supported a greater magnitude of improvement in upper body compared to lower body strength between males and females [43] and also a potentially smaller age related decline in lower body strength and muscle quality in females compared to males [44]. However, there appears no prior evidence supporting the present data that females show greater relative increases in lower-body strength than males. We suggest these differences in relative strength increase may be a result of the significant strength differences at baseline between males and females and also that females engaged in a longer duration of training than males in the present study.

We have previously discussed that intensity of effort, and intent to maximally recruit muscle fibres appears to be the most significant variable affecting strength and hypertrophic increases (e.g., training to momentary muscular failure (MMF)) [6, 7]. However, the present data suggests that untrained older adults can make significant increases in strength by training to RM, which might best be thought of as volitional fatigue. Self-determined RM does not represent a quantifiable measure of intensity of effort as is evidenced by trained participants providing poor estimates at the number of repetitions possible before MMF [45]. As such, RM might not be scientifically meaningful regarding intensity of effort compared to MMF. However, training to volitional fatigue represents a very pragmatic approach, especially in the present population group. The data herein represents "*real people, doing real resistance exercise*" from which they are intending to acquire the aforementioned health and fitness benefits. We might surmise that their aims are to function more efficiently and for greater longevity in their day-to-day life. As the discomfort and debilitation associated with delayed onset muscle soreness (DOMS) which might arise as a result of high volume and/or very high intensity of effort (e.g., MMF) resistance exercise seems counterintuitive to a person wishing to have a more functional life.

Previous research suggests that perceived difficulty and misinformation about expected outcomes are barriers to older persons performing resistance exercise [36]. This study presents data from a UK based exercise facility where sessions are performed on a 1 : 1 basis (client : trainer). The study shows that resistance training need not be time consuming, dauntingly complex, or overly difficult, and that considerable increases in strength can be achieved. A potential limitation to this approach might be the financial expense and practicality of a 1 : 1 (trainer to client) session. Certainly the significant improvements seen within this intervention and other resistance training research might be a result of the individual coaching and motivation received by each participant. In considering transference from research to practical application, improvements to the same degree might not be possible in most health clubs/gyms and so forth, where this ratio is expensive/inappropriate. However, future research might consider the efficacy of small group resistance exercise sessions (e.g., 2–5 participants : 1 trainer). Previous research has shown significant improvements in function as a result of group exercise ($n = \sim 23$ and $n = 16$–20 persons) in studies where mean age = 65 years [46] and 74 years [47]. However, Gentil and Bottaro [48] reported greater increases in upper and lower body strength in high supervision (1 : 5; trainer to athlete ratio) compared to a low supervision (1 : 25) group. Certainly improvements to the magnitude shown within the present study are possible from such a low frequency and volume of training suggests that there is scope to further evaluate this approach.

In the interests of transparency we have previously discussed that publishing data which does not identify control/clarity of variables potentially offers little to trainers or trainees with regard to how they might optimise training adaptations [49]. However, the protocol reported herein is highly standardised between participants and we offer the present findings to highlight the concept of undertaking this protocol and similar ones given the ecological validity of the study.

In summary our data suggests that when training to RM significant strength increases are possible from brief (<15 minutes/~5 exercises per workout), infrequent 1-2×/week, resistance exercise sessions. As previous research has indicated that strength is an independent risk factor for all-cause mortality [14], these results are meaningful for reducing this risk in the population examined. Previous research has shown that resistance exercise in older adults can significantly increase strength, muscle mass, and bone mineral density, improve gene expression and mitochondrial characteristics, and reduce the risk of falls, obesity, and type 2 diabetes and, as noted, reduce the risk of all-cause mortality. Since the present data suggest that strength can be significantly increased by following the aforementioned protocol, future research should consider whether other health markers such as blood pressure and glycemic control respond to the same low volume stimulus.

Conflict of Interests

The authors have no conflict of interests to declare.

References

[1] L. Warming, C. Hassager, and C. Christiansen, "Changes in bone mineral density with age in men and women: a longitudinal study," *Osteoporosis International*, vol. 13, no. 2, pp. 105–112, 2002.

[2] D. B. Burr, "Muscle strength, bone mass, and age-related bone loss," *Journal of Bone and Mineral Research*, vol. 12, no. 10, pp. 1547–1551, 1997.

[3] I. Janssen, S. B. Heymsfield, Z. Wang, and R. Ross, "Skeletal muscle mass and distribution in 468 men and women aged 18-88yr," *Journal of Applied Physiology*, vol. 89, no. 1, pp. 81–88, 2000.

[4] I. Janssen, S. B. Heymsfield, and R. Ross, "Low relative skeletal muscle mass (sarcopenia) in older persons is associated with

functional impairment and physical disability," *Journal of the American Geriatrics Society*, vol. 50, no. 5, pp. 889–896, 2002.

[5] K. Strong, C. Mathers, S. Leeder, and R. Beaglehole, "Preventing chronic diseases: how many lives can we save?" *Lancet*, vol. 366, no. 9496, pp. 1578–1582, 2005.

[6] J. Fisher, J. Steele, S. Bruce-Low, and D. Smith, "Evidence-based resistance training recommendations," *Medicina Sportiva*, vol. 15, no. 3, pp. 147–162, 2011.

[7] J. Fisher, J. Steele, and D. Smith, "Evidence-based resistance training recommendations for muscular hypertrophy," *Medicina Sportiva*, vol. 17, no. 4, pp. 217–235, 2013.

[8] J. Steele, J. Fisher, D. McGuff, S. Bruce-Low, and D. Smith, "Resistance training to momentary muscular failure improves cardiovascular fitness in humans: a review of acute physiological responses and chronic physiological Adaptations," *Journal of Exercise Physiology Online*, vol. 15, no. 3, pp. 53–80, 2012.

[9] J. O. Holloszy, "Invited review: exercise-induced increase in muscle insulin sensitivity," *Journal of Applied Physiology*, vol. 99, no. 1, pp. 338–343, 2005.

[10] G. A. Kelley, K. S. Kelley, and Z. V. Tran, "Resistance training and bone mineral density in women: a meta-analysis of controlled trials," *The American Journal of Physical Medicine and Rehabilitation*, vol. 80, no. 1, pp. 65–77, 2001.

[11] M. H. Stone, "Muscle conditioning and muscle injuries," *Medicine and Science in Sports and Exercise*, vol. 22, no. 4, pp. 457–462, 1990.

[12] J. B. Lauersen, D. M. Bertelsen, and L. B. Andersen, "The effectiveness of exercise interventions to prevent sports injuries: a systematic review and meta-analysis of randomised controlled trials," *British Journal of Sports Medicine*, vol. 48, no. 11, pp. 871–877, 2014.

[13] B. F. Hurley and S. M. Roth, "Strength training in the elderly: effects on risk factors for age-related diseases," *Sports Medicine*, vol. 30, no. 4, pp. 249–268, 2000.

[14] A. B. Newman, V. Kupelian, M. Visser et al., "Strength, but not muscle mass, is associated with mortality in the health, aging and body composition study cohort," *Journals of Gerontology—Series A Biological Sciences and Medical Sciences*, vol. 61, no. 1, pp. 72–77, 2006.

[15] S. Melov, M. A. Tamopolsky, K. Bechman, K. Felkey, and A. Hubbard, "Resistance exercise reverses aging in human skeletal muscle," *PLoS ONE*, vol. 2, no. 5, article e465, 2007.

[16] J. R. Ruiz, X. Sui, F. Lobelo et al., "Association between muscular strength and mortality in men: prospective cohort study," *British Medical Journal*, vol. 337, p. a439, 2008.

[17] E. G. Artero, D.-C. Lee, J. R. Ruiz et al., "A prospective study of muscular strength and all-cause mortality in men with hypertension," *Journal of the American College of Cardiology*, vol. 57, no. 18, pp. 1831–1837, 2011.

[18] O. Seynnes, M. A. F. Singh, O. Hue, P. Pras, P. Legros, and P. L. Bernard, "Physiological and functional responses to low-moderate versus high-intensity progressive resistance training in frail elders," *Journals of Gerontology Series A: Biological Sciences and Medical Sciences*, vol. 59, no. 5, pp. 503–509, 2004.

[19] H. T. Rabelo, R. J. Oliveira, and M. Bottaro, "Effects of resistance training on activities of daily living in older women," *Biology of Sport*, vol. 21, no. 4, pp. 325–336, 2004.

[20] I. G. Fatouros, A. Kambas, I. Katrabasas et al., "Strength training and detraining effects on muscular strength, anaerobic power, and mobility of inactive older men are intensity dependent," *The British Journal of Sports Medicine*, vol. 39, no. 10, pp. 776–780, 2005.

[21] S. Steib, D. Schoene, and K. Pfeifer, "Dose-response relationship of resistance training in older adults: a meta-analysis," *Medicine and Science in Sports and Exercise*, vol. 42, no. 5, pp. 902–914, 2010.

[22] J. Fisher and D. Smith, "Attempting to better define "intensity" for muscular performance: is it all wasted effort," *European Journal of Applied Physiology*, vol. 112, no. 12, pp. 4183–4185, 2012.

[23] M. Tanimoto and N. Ishii, "Effects of low-intensity resistance exercise with slow movement and tonic force generation on muscular function in young men," *Journal of Applied Physiology*, vol. 100, no. 4, pp. 1150–1157, 2006.

[24] M. Tanimoto, K. Sanada, K. Yamamoto et al., "Effects of whole-body low-intensity resistance training with slow movement and tonic force generation on muscular size and strength in young men," *Journal of Strength and Conditioning Research*, vol. 22, no. 6, pp. 1926–1938, 2008.

[25] E. van Roie, C. Delecluse, W. Coudyzer, S. Boonen, and I. Bautmans, "Strength training at high versus low external resistance in older adults: effects on muscle volume, muscle strength, and force-velocity characteristics," *Experimental Gerontology*, vol. 48, no. 11, pp. 1351–1361, 2013.

[26] M. L. Pollock, J. F. Carroll, J. E. Graves et al., "Injuries and adherence to walk/jog and resistance training programs in the elderly," *Medicine and Science in Sports and Exercise*, vol. 23, no. 10, pp. 1194–1200, 1991.

[27] P. M. Tiidus and C. D. Ianuzzo, "Effects of intensity and duration of muscular exercise on delayed soreness and serum enzyme activities," *Medicine and Science in Sports and Exercise*, vol. 15, no. 6, pp. 461–465, 1983.

[28] R. N. Carpinelli and R. M. Otto, "Strength training: single versus multiple sets," *Sports Medicine*, vol. 26, no. 2, pp. 73–84, 1998.

[29] R. A. Winett, "Meta-analyses do not support performance of multiple sets or high volume resistance training," *Journal of Exercise Physiology Online*, vol. 7, no. 5, pp. 10–20, 2004.

[30] R. M. Otto and R. N. Carpinelli, "A critical analysis of the single versus multiple set debate," *Journal of Exercise Physiology*, vol. 9, no. 1, pp. 32–57, 2006.

[31] N. L. Silva, R. B. Oliveira, S. J. Fleck, A. C. Leon, and P. Farinatti, "Influence of strength training variables on strength gains in adults over 55 years-old: a meta-analysis of dose-response relationships," *Journal of Science and Medicine in Sport*, vol. 17, no. 3, pp. 337–344, 2014.

[32] W. L. Westcott, R. A. Winett, E. S. Anderson et al., "Effects of regular and slow speed resistance training on muscle strength," *Journal of Sports Medicine and Physical Fitness*, vol. 41, no. 2, pp. 154–158, 2001.

[33] P. F. Lachance and T. Hortobagyi, "Influence of cadence on muscular performance during push-up and pull-up exercises," *Journal of Strength and Conditioning Research*, vol. 8, pp. 76–79, 1994.

[34] M. C. Morrissey, E. A. Harman, P. N. Frykman, and K. H. Han, "Early phase differential effects of slow and fast barbell squat training," *The American Journal of Sports Medicine*, vol. 26, no. 2, pp. 221–230, 1998.

[35] A. Sakamoto and P. J. Sinclair, "Effect of movement velocity on the relationship between training load and the number of repetitions of bench press," *Journal of Strength and Conditioning Research*, vol. 20, no. 3, pp. 523–527, 2006.

[36] R. A. Winett, D. M. Williams, and B. M. Davy, "Initiating and maintaining resistance training in older adults: a social

cognitive theory-based approach," *The British Journal of Sports Medicine*, vol. 43, no. 2, pp. 114–119, 2009.

[37] J. Fisher, J. Steele, M. Brzycki, and B. DeSimone, "Primum non nocere: a commentary on avoidable injuries and safe resistance training techniques," *Journal of Trainology*, vol. 3, pp. 31–34, 2014.

[38] J. Cohen, "A power primer," *Psychological Bulletin*, vol. 112, no. 1, pp. 155–159, 1992.

[39] M. Fröhlich, E. Emrich, and D. Schmidtbleicher, "Outcome effects of single-set versus multiple-set training—an advanced replication study," *Research in Sports Medicine*, vol. 18, no. 3, pp. 157–175, 2010.

[40] E. Whitley and J. Ball, "Statistics review 4: sample size calculations," *Critical Care*, vol. 6, no. 4, pp. 335–341, 2002.

[41] P. Gentil, S. R. S. Soares, M. C. Pereira et al., "Effect of adding single-joint exercises to a multi-joint exercise resistance-training program on strength and hypertrophy in untrained subjects," *Applied Physiology, Nutrition and Metabolism*, vol. 38, no. 3, pp. 341–344, 2013.

[42] P. Gentil, S. Soares, and M. Bottaro, "Single vs. Multi-joint resistance exercise: effects on muscle strength and hypertrophy," *Asian Journal of Sports Medicine*. In press.

[43] A. E. J. Miller, J. D. MacDougall, M. A. Tarnopolsky, and D. G. Sale, "Gender differences in strength and muscle fiber characteristics," *European Journal of Applied Physiology and Occupational Physiology*, vol. 66, no. 3, pp. 254–262, 1993.

[44] R. S. Lindle, E. J. Metter, N. A. Lynch et al., "Age and gender comparisons of muscle strength in 654 women and men aged 20–93 yr," *Journal of Applied Physiology*, vol. 83, no. 5, pp. 1581–1587, 1997.

[45] D. A. Hackett, N. A. Johnson, M. Halaki, and C.-M. Chow, "A novel scale to assess resistance-exercise effort," *Journal of Sports Sciences*, vol. 30, no. 13, pp. 1405–1413, 2012.

[46] A. Barnett, B. Smith, S. R. Lord, M. Williams, and A. Baumand, "Community-based group exercise improves balance and reduces falls in at-risk older people: a randomised controlled trial," *Age and Ageing*, vol. 32, no. 4, pp. 407–414, 2003.

[47] L. Z. Rubenstein, K. R. Josephson, P. R. Trueblood et al., "Effects of a group exercise program on strength, mobility, and falls among fall-prone elderly men," *Journals of Gerontology Series A Biological Sciences and Medical Sciences*, vol. 55, no. 6, pp. M317–M321, 2000.

[48] P. Gentil and M. Bottaro, "Influence of supervision ratio on muscle adaptations to resistance training in nontrained subjects," *Journal of Strength and Conditioning Research*, vol. 24, no. 3, pp. 639–643, 2010.

[49] J. Fisher, "A critical commentary on the practical application of resistance training studies," *Journal of Trainology*, vol. 2, pp. 10–12, 2013.

8

A Structured and Flexible Language for Physical Activity Assessment and Characterization

Pedro Silva,[1] Maria Teresa Andrade,[2] Pedro Carvalho,[2] and Jorge Mota[1]

[1] *CIAFEL, Faculty of Sports, University of Porto, 4200-450 Porto, Portugal*
[2] *INESC Porto, University of Porto, 4200-450 Porto, Portugal*

Correspondence should be addressed to Pedro Silva; perrinha@gmail.com

Academic Editor: Adrian W. Midgley

Developing more accurate assessments of physical activity (PA) and sedentary behavior (SB) is an important public health research priority. Assessing PA and SB is challenging in all segments of the population, but it is especially difficult in children due to cognitive limitations and more sporadic and intermittent activity patterns. Moreover, they are influenced by several factors including temporal-spatial constraints and social conditions. To accurately assess PA and SB, it is essential to clearly define methods for describing all these factors. The goal of this paper is to potentiate advances in the field by proposing a base ontology for characterizing physical activity, sedentary behavior, and the context in which it occurs. The ontology would establish a flexible base language to facilitate standardized descriptions of these behaviors for researchers and public health professionals.

1. Introduction

Epidemiological studies have demonstrated that regular physical activity (PA) is truly a "medicine" with proven efficacy to reduce morbidity and mortality associated with chronic disease [1]. Being physically active is a major contributor to one's overall physical and mental well-being [2]. The literature indicates that PA is influenced by a large group of factors, including, environmental, social, psychological, and cultural ones [3–6]. However, methods are not available to systematically study the complex interactions that influence PA and sedentary behavior (SB). To advance public health research, it is important to develop more robust methodologies.

Measuring PA and characterizing the context under which the PA occurs are a challenging task. A number of studies have evaluated PA patterns with objective activity monitors, but few studies have examined contextual variation in PA and sedentary activity [7–9]. Recent research efforts have sought to overcome these limitations, and a number of different instruments have been used: daily logs; diaries; questionnaires; direct observation.

Different areas are needed to tackle the global pandemic of physical inactivity because multidisciplinary work are essential [10]. Moreover, as Hallal et al. [11] stated, "technological advancements that nudge us towards physical inactivity make it urgently necessary to take actions. More of the same (in terms of research and practice) will not be enough." The challenge is to turn these technological advancements from only user friendly to "health friendly." More recently, solutions based on global positioning system, (GPS) geographical information system, (GIS) smartphones, and electronic ecological momentary assessment (EMA) have been introduced as these approaches offer considerable advantages in terms of data processing and communication technologies. PA is one of many health behaviors that have the potential to change substantially as a result of increasing availability of information and communication technologies and of technology-based interventions [12].

While many methods have been tested, direct observation (DO) remains as a criterion (gold standard) measure for evaluating the context of PA and SB. Because behaviors are analyzed at the location by a trained observer, DO avoids some limitations of subjective methods (such as the recall of information) and objective methods (such as the reactivity to the devices) [13]. At this time, DO techniques provide the only approach that can objectively code both the behavior and the context in which it occurred. Despite the advantages, systematic observation methods are underused by researchers [14]. The main reason for this is the shortcomings associated with DO methods. The most significant limitation is the cost and burden associated with collecting and processing the data. This barrier typically leads to a limited scope or amount of observation data, bringing into question whether data from those samples are adequate for that setting or whether they can be generalizable. Another major limitation is that observers must be properly trained to be objective and nonjudgmental. Steps must be taken to ensure that they maintain their skills over time, and there is the possibility of observed people behaving differently when an observer is present (i.e., reactivity).

These limitations have proven difficult to overcome, but new advances in automated video-based processing techniques offer considerable promise in this area. Advances in sensor, communications, and computer technologies favor their introduction in the PA assessment problem. Comprehensive surveillance systems are crucial to advance public health. The development and introduction of such a comprehensive system pose challenges and are dependent on the capacities and resources available. Yet having such PA information will serve to improve investment of scarce resources, increase accountability, and help to make efficient and effective investments [10]. While the use of devices such as GPS or accelerometers has provided interesting results, their usage presents a burden to participants and has a number of significant limitations for field-based research. The most significant limitation is the inability to extract meaningful contextual information. Advanced video-based tracking systems have been shown to have considerable promise in surveillance and security applications, and these same techniques can be applied to enhance the monitoring of PA and SB. The video has the advantage of being nonintrusive and enabling more complete contextual characterizations. The introduction of new technologies has contributed to a finer temporal resolution of the observations while decreasing the burden in the human observer. Moreover, an increase in automation has improved the objectivity of the process and extended the type/diversity of gathered data. These attributes directly overcome some of the stated limitations of current DO tools. If similar technology is applied to PA and SB assessment, it would be possible to directly (and automatically) code these behaviors.

Before this can be done, it is necessary to first develop a systematic way to code the various classes and types of behavior. This is essential since the volume and diversity of collected data can only be adequately managed if the data can be properly represented, using well-established rules and formats. The absence of a common language to represent this information and interpret the individual behavior is presently an obstacle in this research field. Reinforced by the absence of standardized instruments suitable for international use by the researchers [15]. Its existence would foster the exchange of information between researchers and facilitate its reuse and analysis. This is particularly significant with the increased granularity of the supported classes.

Ontologies can be a solution to create a standard and interoperable language for specific application domains. According to Grüninger and Lee [16], the use of ontologies can serve three purposes: (1) to support communication, between machines, between humans, and between humans and machines; (2) for knowledge reuse as, for example, shared repositories of technical documentation; (3) for computational deduction, enabling the extraction of new knowledge from existing data as, for example, in internal structure analysis. The development of a clear ontology for capturing the context and diverse aspects of PA and SB is a priority for advancing the development of more automated DO tools. Continued improvement in monitoring behavior would help to guide development of policies and programs to increase activity levels and to reduce the burden of noncommunicable diseases [15]. To the author's knowledge, there is currently no ontology available to facilitate the systematic study of PA and SB. Therefore, the present paper will propose an ontology for assessing PA and SB (OPA ontology), containing concepts that can capture knowledge about the context in which the behavior is being performed. The goal is to establish a common ground for researchers assessing behavior and its context using different instruments.

2. Methods

2.1. PA and SB Categorization. An individual activity profile is characterized by a complex matrix of behaviors that take place in a range of social contexts, each with its own set of physiological, psychological, and sociological determinants and outcomes. Sallis et al. [17] stated that the wide range of correlates supports the application of ecological models of behavior to improve understanding of the influences on PA. Moreover, variables within individuals, such as psychological and biological factors, are widely studied, as are interpersonal variables. Environmental, policy, and global variables are less studied but are thought to have widespread effects. The combination and interaction of factors and at these levels are expected to influence PA [6]. Hence, PA behavior is best described as a profile rather than a single entity or indicator.

Figure 1 presents a profile that does not pretend to be a socioecological model, but rather a conceptual diagram to simplify the characterization of physical activity and sedentary behavior and its context. In the center, there are individual characteristics that shape self-behavior. The interception of the other domains provides the context where the behavior occurs and how the activity can be characterized or classified.

Another aim of the model (Figure 1) is to facilitate the assessment of PA and SB since it focuses on fundamental domains of these behaviors; that is, they are influenced by space, time, and social factors. It supports examination of problems similar to the way they occur in a natural setting, with simultaneous influences of multiple factors. Since physical activity is multifaceted, it makes good theoretical sense to evaluate those facets using these factors. DO methods are considered to be a gold standard for capturing PA and SB classification, but, as previously stated, they have important shortcomings. The need to observe the activity *in situ* requires a small number of classes of classification to enable the process. As a result, state-of-the-art methods cannot capture

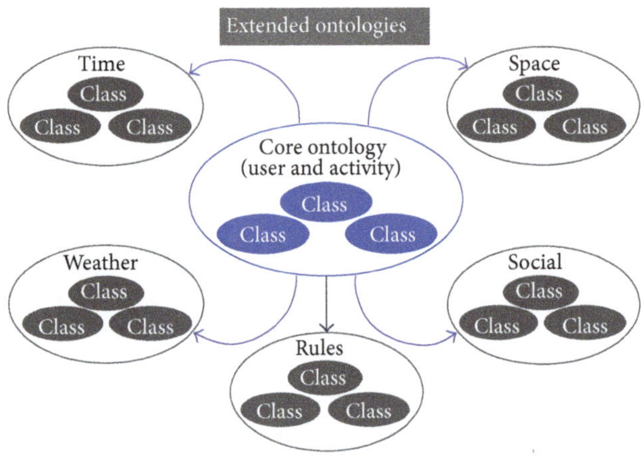

FIGURE 1: Conceptual profile of the factors influencing physical activity assessment and characterization.

all the factors involved. Therefore, monitoring individual level and microenvironment social inequalities is crucial for evaluating the effects of programs and policies and providing an insight into whether current efforts should be continued or modified [18]. The dilemma in examining PA in a theoretical framework is balancing parsimony with comprehensiveness [19]. Research needs improved measures of exposure (correlates), objective PA measures, prospective designs, and advanced data modelling to assess causal determinants rather than just associations between variables [6].

2.2. OPA: A Common Language for PA and SB Classification. To integrate all the previous concepts, we propose the OPA ontology. A useful conceptual definition of ontology can be consulted here [20]. The aim of an ontology is to capture and to create knowledge models that can be reused and shared between applications or groups of people [21]. The availability of a PA and SB ontology, defining a common vocabulary for researchers in this area, would provide an important tool for information sharing and reuse, thus increasing the opportunity for advances in the domain.

An ontology can be seen as collection of terms from a vocabulary, capturing into a formal model and enabling automated processing of that model, common understanding and knowledge about a given domain knowledge or real-world situation populated by resources. The fundamental blocks of an ontology are classes, individuals, and properties. A class represents a category or a group of resources sharing common characteristics. Individuals are specific resources that belong to a given category or class; that is, they are instances of classes. Finally, properties enable describing the resources. They can be used to establish relations between classes and individuals or between individuals and literal values associated with them [20]. In the present domain of knowledge—assessment of PA and SB—the resources in the ontology would be persons and groups or categories of persons and activities and categories of activities. Additionally, given the intention of characterizing the activity not only through its type (e.g., sitting, running, jumping, etc.) but also with the information about the context under which that type of activity is taking place, resources would also be concepts, and their instances are associated with the time, space, and social dimensions.

To develop an ontology, it is necessary to choose a language to represent it. One of the most commonly used languages is Web ontology language (OWL) [22, 23]. OWL is a standard specified by the World Wide Web Consortium (W3C) [24] adding new capabilities to the standards previously released by the W3C in pursuit of the Semantic Web paradigm, notably, Extensible Markup Language (XML), Resource Description Framework (RDF), and RDF Schema (RDFS). RDF is an XML-based language used to represent information on the Web. RDFS extends the scope of application of RDF, by enabling the development of specific metadata vocabularies and describing relationships among resources in terms of named properties and values. Comparing with RDFS, OWL extends the use of properties by enabling the use of statements regarding properties and by imposing restrictions on how properties behave. OWL was designed to allow any software or hardware system (or any human) to be able to process the information contained in the ontology, reason about it and unambiguously interpret it, and infer the original high-level concepts.

Based on these classes and on the model proposed in Figure 1, we define an ontology hierarchy to be used as a common language for researchers involved in PA and SB analysis and classification. Figure 2 presents the proposed OPA ontological model. The core ontology is composed of the defined generic classes for activity classification and for the individual conducting the activity. Those classes follow very closely the widely accepted compendium for PA by Ainsworth et al. [25]; the compendium is used globally in a variety of situations, for example, to quantify the energy cost of PA and SB in adults for surveillance activities [26]; in research studies and in clinical settings; to write PA recommendations; to assess energy expenditure in individuals. Connected to this base ontology, extended ontologies are used to allow capturing knowledge external to the activity but very likely to have a decisive impact on the way activity is conducted. These extended ontologies incorporate concepts that represent factors related to the dimensions "Time," "Space," and "Social." They can be seen as the representation of the context under which the activity is being performed and will permit standardized comparisons of correlates, with similar measures in high-income and low-income countries, that take into account strengths of different correlates and an investigation of cultural and country-level factors [6].

Each of the ontologies present in the OPA ontological model is further detailed in Figures 3–7. Figure 3 represents the attributes of the individual performing the activity (the complete profile). Figures 4–7 provide illustrations of the classes in the extended ontologies that represent the time, space, social, and weather dimensions, respectively.

We propose five main classes to characterize PA and SB because PA behaviors are affected by factors operating at several levels, which are broadly perceived as personal (such as biological and psychological attributes), social (family, affiliation group, and work factors, Figure 6), and environmental (contexts for different forms of activity and factors

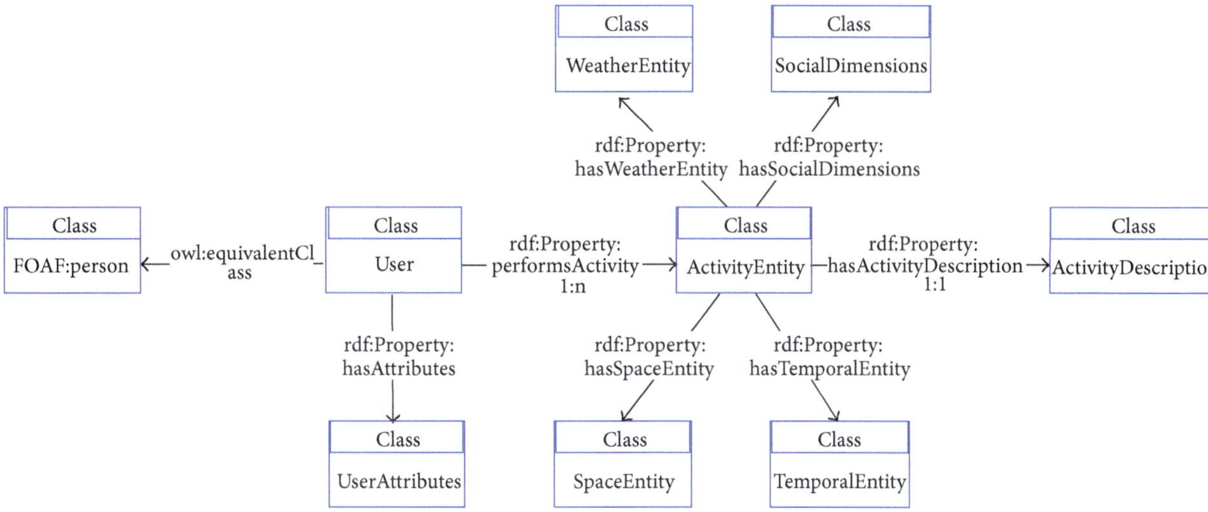

FIGURE 2: Conceptual diagram of the base classes intended for physical activity and inactivity classification.

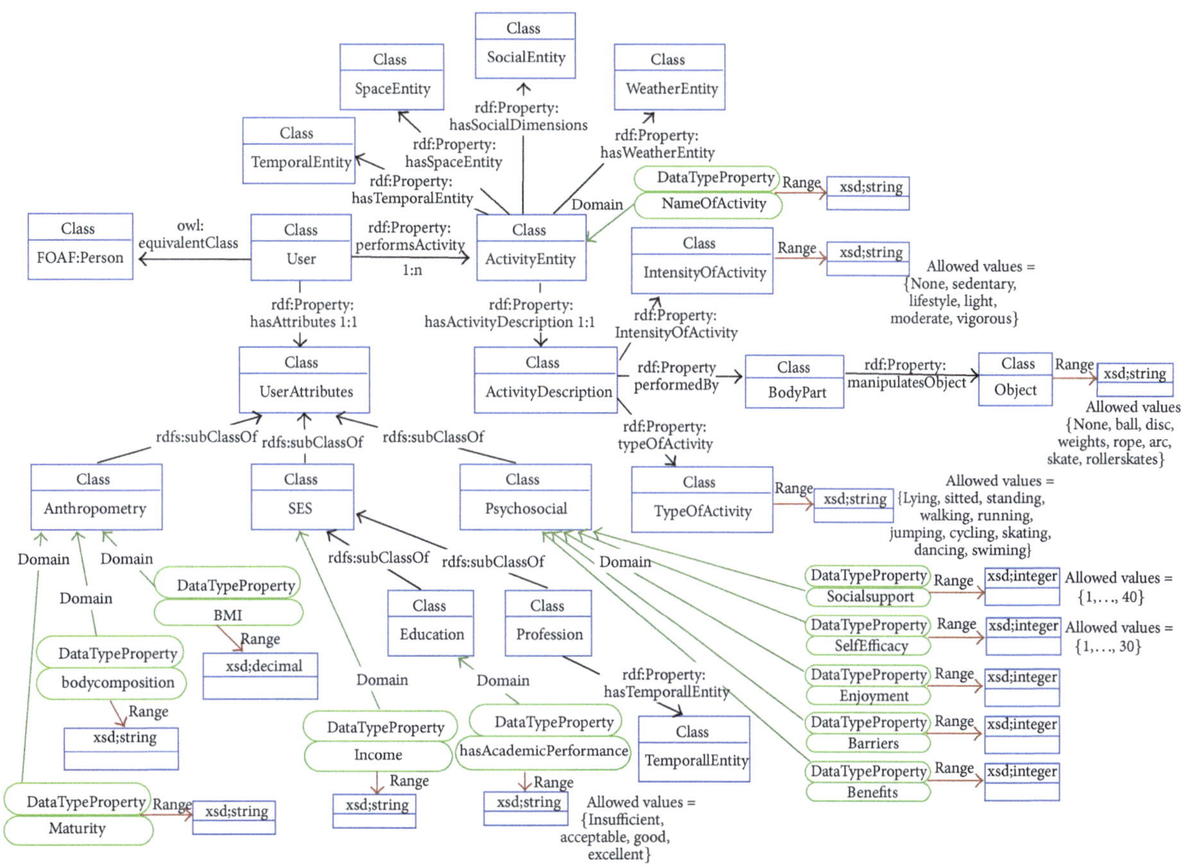

FIGURE 3: Conceptual diagram to characterize an individual performing physical activity.

that could determine availability of relevant settings and opportunities, Figures 4, 5, and 7) ones [27]. Hence, these five classes provide a good compromise between simplicity and complexity (i.e., sufficient ability to make distinctions). While more complex models are possible, they would have little value if they could not be easily applied. The five main classes represent distinct contexts, and each has a clear utility for describing PA and SB.

The models and concepts presented are in no way restrictive. Rather, we chose to define a set of base concepts and classes that can be flexibly and transparently extended, favored by the use of the proposed OPA ontology.

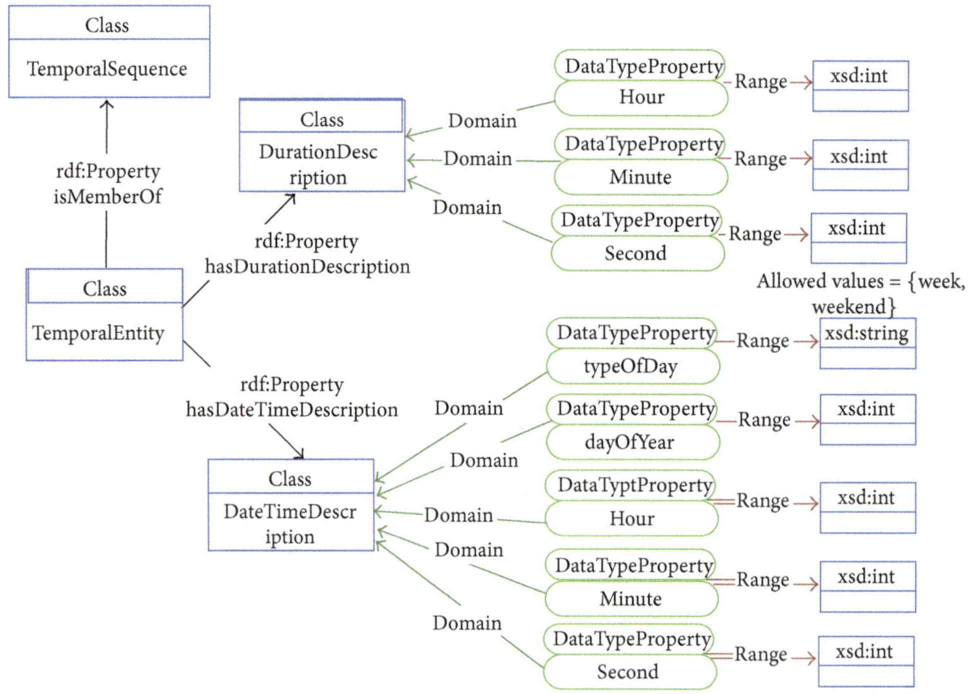

FIGURE 4: Conceptual diagram of the temporal information associated with the physical activity.

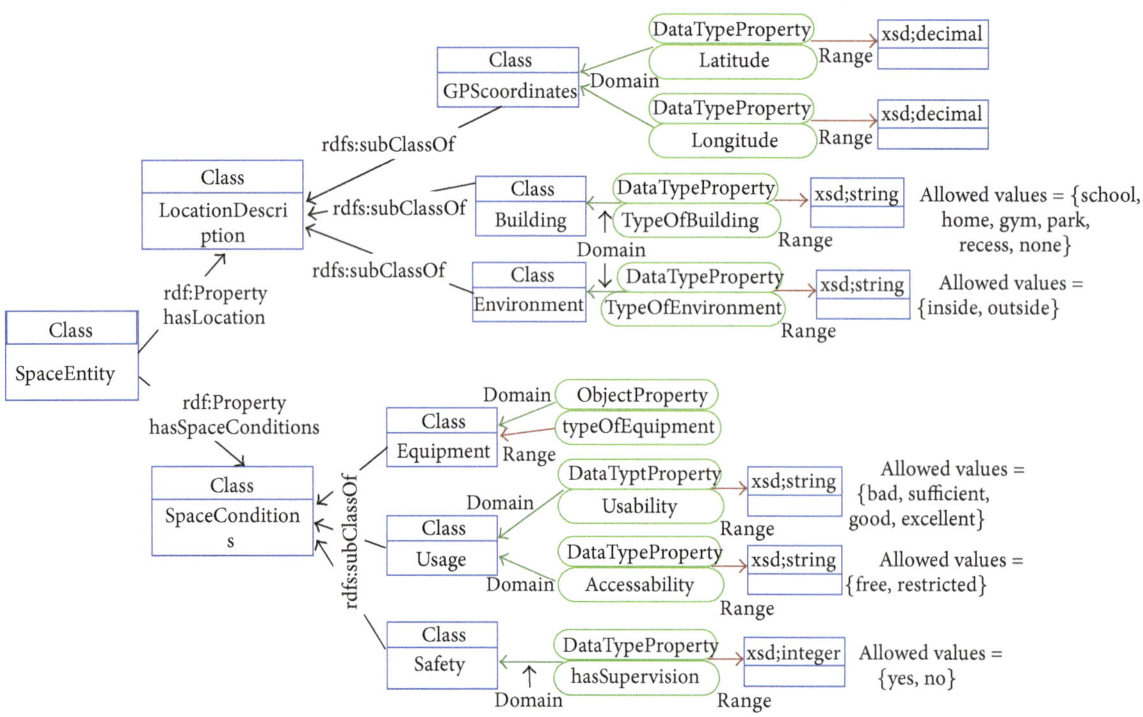

FIGURE 5: Conceptual diagram of information to characterize the space where the physical activity takes place.

2.3. Applying the OPA Ontology. A principle adopted in the design of the OPA ontology is to reuse existing ontologies, whenever required; concepts already exist in other well-established ontologies. Instead of reinventing the wheel, this procedure has the additional benefit of facilitating the exchange of data between the knowledge base of the OPA system and other knowledge bases. The external ontologies that are integrated into the OPA ontology are well-known ontologies, referred to by the W3C. Together with the concepts specifically introduced by the OPA ontology, they

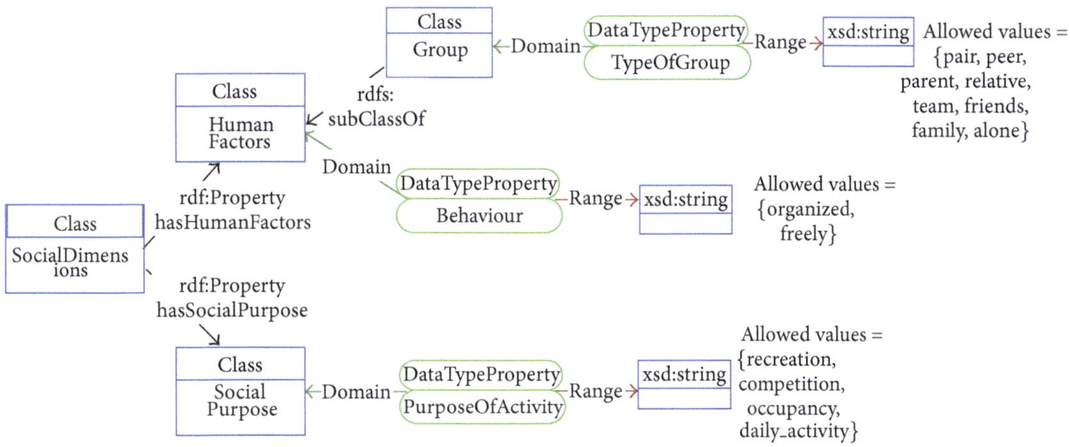

FIGURE 6: Conceptual diagram of information to characterize the social context associated with the physical activity.

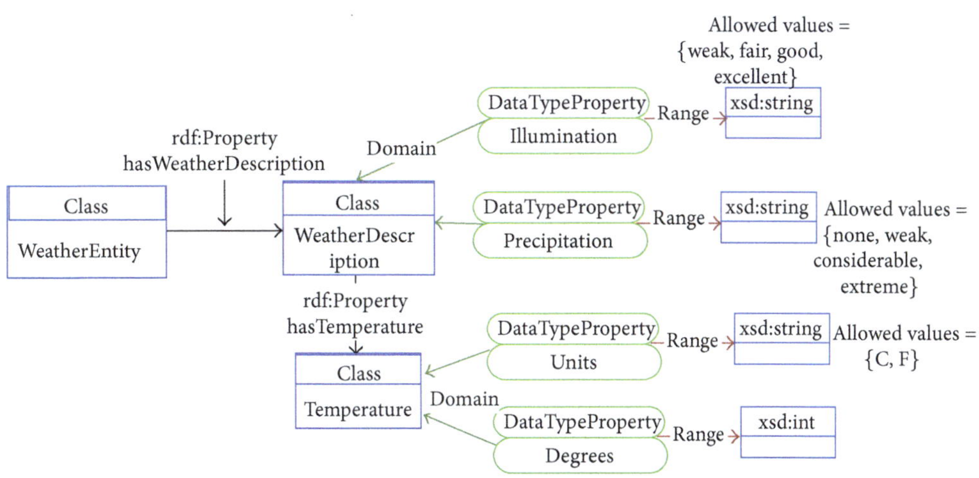

FIGURE 7: Conceptual diagram of information to characterize the weather context associated with the physical activity.

provide all the concepts required to obtain a detailed characterization of people, their physical activity, and associated context.

(i) FOAF (Friend of a Friend) (http://xmlns.com/foaf/spec/): the FOAF ontology is used to express metadata about persons: their names, addresses, their interests, pictures of them, and so forth. FOAF is formally specified in RDFS/OWL and was developed within the context of the social Web, to enable establishing links between people on the Web. In our work, we use specifically the class "Person" and some of its properties and relationships with other (sub) classes. Including the FOAF ontology within the OPA framework allows us to describe the performers of (in)activity through a well-established specification. Nonetheless, given that FOAF was developed with the purpose of establishing social relationships among people on the Web, it does not provide all the properties needed to qualify the performer of an activity. As such, we have defined additional properties, which we use together with original FOAF slots to describe the instances of the class FOAF: Person.

(ii) REL (RELATIONSHIP: vocabulary for describing relationships between people) (http://vocab.org/relationship/.html, http://www.xml.com/pub/a/2004/02/04/foaf.html): the REL ontology provides a way to formally express relationships between persons. It is currently used in diverse applications in conjunction with the FOAF ontology. In our work we use it to express the relationships between participants in the physical activity.

(iii) OWL-Time (http://www.w3.org/TR/owl-time/) is the successor of DAML-Time ontology. It was developed by the W3C to formally express and relate temporal concepts, aiming at describing temporal aspects and properties of Webpages and Web services.

To simulate the use of the OPA ontology, we will use the following example: "Catarina lives in Porto, Portugal, with her parents. Catarina's email address is catarina.costa@gmail.com. Catarina studies at the secondary school Garcia de Orta. She is on the 8th grade. She practices dance with some friends in a gym three times a week. Normally she walks everyday about 15 minutes in the morning to get to the school.

In the afternoons when she has dance she also walks to the gym, which is pretty close to her home (5 minutes away). During the days when she does not have dance, Catarina enjoys walking for about 30 minutes with her mother, Maria Costa, in the evening, along the park near their home, whenever the weather is good."

The OPA ontology can be used to describe this individual case and to enable systematic characterizations of the behavior. This requires creating instances of classes and providing values to the properties associated with the selected classes. Accordingly, the first step to formally describe the above case is to identify the required classes and the properties (or slots) associated with those classes that will be needed.

(1) Class FOAF: Person

(a) an instance will be created to represent "Catarina Costa;"

(b) the slots "name", "age," and "race" will be filled in with appropriate values;

(c) the class.

(2) Class OPA: UserAttributes

(a) given that the properties that exist in the ontology FOAF associated with the class Person are not sufficient for our purpose, an instance of the class UserAttributes, associated with the instance "Catarina Costa" through the relationship "has Attributes will be created;"

(b) one instance of each subclass of the UserAttributes class will be created (classes Anthropometry, Socio Economic Status (SES), and Psychosocial); corresponding slots will be filled in with appropriate values; it is assumed that these values are manually inserted or, otherwise, obtained automatically from a user profile database.

(3) Class OPA: Activity

(a) given that four different activities are mentioned in the text, four instances of the class Activity will be created ("walkToSchool," "Dance," "walkToGym," and "walkInPark"), related to the previous instance of Person, through the property "performsActivity". Each instance of the class Activity will be further characterized by the 5 specific dimensions:

(3.1) an instance of the class ActivityDescription to which it is connected through the property "hasActivityDescription"; each ActivityDescription instance has the subclasses "IntensityOfActivity", "TypeOfActivity" and "BodyPart"; the latter is further characterized by the type of equipment manipulated during the activity;

(3.2) an instance of the class TemporalEntity to which is connected through the property "hasTemporalEntity", with associated subclasses instantiated and corresponding slots appropriately filled in. These sub-classes and slots will capture the temporal information present in the text, associated to each different activity performed by Catarina in two dimensions: the actual date when the activity is performed and the duration of the activity;

(3.3) an instance of the class SpaceEntity to which is connected through the property "hasSpaceEntity", with associated subclasses instantiated and corresponding slots appropriately filled in. These slots will capture the spatial information that is provided in the text, associated to each different activity performed by Catarina;

(3.4) an instance of the class SocialEntity to which is connected through the property "hasSocialEntity", with associated subclasses instantiated and corresponding slots appropriately filled in. These slots will capture the social aspects associated to each different activity performed by Catarina, which information is included in the text;

(3.5) an instance of the class WeatherEntity to which is connected through the property "hasWeatherEntity", with associated subclasses instantiated and corresponding slots appropriately filled in. These slots will capture the weather aspects associated to each different activity performed by Catarina, which information is included in the text.

(4) Class FOAF: Person

(a) a second instance of this class will be created to represent Catarina's mother;

(b) the property "parentOf" borrowed from the REL ontology will be associated to this class.

(5) Class FOAF: Group

(a) an instance of this class will be created to represent the dance group in which Catarina participates.

3. Conclusion

Future research directions in the PA and SB fields should lead to gain further insights into the levels and the contexts, under which they occur, that have stronger impact on those behaviors. The use of current and emerging technologies such as GPS and intelligent video processing is expected to be an integral part of this research field and provide richer information. The increased quantity and granularity that these new technologies can provide require additional tools to support its processing, management, and exchange.

The availability of the OPA ontology defining a common vocabulary for researchers in this area would provide an important tool for information sharing and reuse, thus increasing the opportunity for advances in the domain. The OPA ontology can enable automatically capturing the semantics of relationships that may exist between the different concepts and resources involved in PA and SB and their context in various dimensions (space, time, social, etc.). Accordingly they can greatly assist the researcher to infer new knowledge and conclusions derived from the captured knowledge and established relationships. Ontologies are being seen as the next level towards the fulfillment of the Semantic Web paradigm, to achieve interoperability and automated use of any resource available on the Web. Many disciplines now develop standardized ontologies that domain experts can use to share and annotate information in their fields [20].

The strength of this proposal is the support of the Compendium of Physical Activities [25]. The current paper presents a language and ontology consisting of a set of base classes but can be easily extended to accommodate additional information. By using the compendium, the OPA ontology can aggregate the qualitative information with the quantitative one allowing a better discrimination and characterization of the behavior observed, resulting in a more complete individual activity profile (iAP).

It is our goal that this proposal will be well accepted by the researchers on this field and foster discussions and international development through the assistance of new technological tools. In view of the diversity between countries and populations in published work, results should be applicable to various settings and communities [27] since the ontology can incrementally become more flexible accommodating new information gathered from new scenarios. A systems' approach that focuses on populations and the complex interactions among the correlates of physical inactivity, rather than solely a behavioral science approach focusing on individuals, is the way forward to increase physical activity worldwide [10].

Acknowledgment

Pedro Silva is currently receiving a Grant (SFRH/BPD/71332/2010) from FCT and works at CIAFEL (PEst-OE/SAU/UI0617/2011).

References

[1] J. E. Fulton, M. T. McGuire, C. J. Caspersen, and W. H. Dietz, "Interventions for weight loss and weight gain prevention among youth: current issues," *Sports Medicine*, vol. 31, no. 3, pp. 153–165, 2001.

[2] P. Das and R. Horton, "Rethinking our approach to physical activity," *The Lancet*, vol. 380, no. 9838, pp. 189–190, 2012.

[3] J. Sallis and N. Owen, *Physical Activity & Behavioral Medicine*, vol. 3, Sage, Thousand Oaks, Calif, USA, 1999.

[4] J. F. Sallis, K. Kraft, and L. S. Linton, "How the environment shapes physical activity. A transdisciplinary research agenda," *American Journal of Preventive Medicine*, vol. 22, no. 3, p. 208, 2002.

[5] R. K. Dishman, R. W. Motl, R. Saunders et al., "Self-efficacy partially mediates the effect of a school-based physical-activity intervention among adolescent girls," *Preventive Medicine*, vol. 38, no. 5, pp. 628–636, 2004.

[6] A. E. Bauman, R. S. Reis, J. F. Sallis, J. C. Wells, R. J. Loos, and B. W. Martin, "Correlates of physical activity: why are some people physically active and others not?" *The Lancet*, vol. 380, no. 9838, pp. 258–271, 2012.

[7] P. Blatchford, P. Bassett, and P. Brown, "Teachers' and pupils' behavior in large and small classes: a systematic observation study of pupils aged 10 and 11 years," *Journal of Educational Psychology*, vol. 97, no. 3, pp. 454–467, 2005.

[8] S. J. Verstraete, G. M. Cardon, D. L. De Clercq, and I. M. De Bourdeaudhuij, "Increasing children's physical activity levels during recess periods in elementary schools: the effects of providing game equipment," *European Journal of Public Health*, vol. 16, no. 4, pp. 415–419, 2006.

[9] T. L. McKenzie, N. C. Crespo, B. Baquero, and J. P. Elder, "Leisure-time physical activity in elementary schools: analysis of contextual conditions," *Journal of School Health*, vol. 80, no. 10, pp. 470–477, 2010.

[10] H. W. Kohl III, C. L. Craig, E. V. Lambert et al., "The pandemic of physical inactivity: global action for public health," *The Lancet*, vol. 380, no. 9838, pp. 294–305, 2012.

[11] P. C. Hallal, A. E. Bauman, G. W. Heath, H. W. Kohl III, I. M. Lee, and M. Pratt, "Physical activity: more of the same is not enough," *The Lancet*, vol. 380, no. 9838, pp. 190–191, 2012.

[12] M. Pratt, O. L. Sarmiento, F. Montes et al., "The implications of megatrends in information and communication technology and transportation for changes in global physical activity," *The Lancet*, vol. 380, no. 9838, pp. 282–293, 2012.

[13] T. L. McKenzie, "The use of direct observation to assess physical activity," in *Physical Activity Assessments for Health-Related Research*, G. Welk, Ed., pp. 179–195, Human Kinetics, Champaign, Ill, USA, 2002.

[14] T. L. McKenzie, "2009 C. H. McCloy lecture seeing is believing: observing physical activity and its contexts," *Research Quarterly for Exercise and Sport*, vol. 81, no. 2, pp. 113–122, 2010.

[15] P. C. Hallal, L. B. Andersen, F. C. Bull, R. Guthold, W. Haskell, and U. Ekelund, "Global physical activity levels: surveillance progress, pitfalls, and prospects," *The Lancet*, vol. 380, no. 9838, pp. 247–257, 2012.

[16] M. Grüninger and J. Lee, "Ontology applications and design," *Communications of ACM*, vol. 45, no. 2, pp. 39–41, 2002.

[17] J. F. Sallis, W. C. Taylor, M. Dowda, P. S. Freedson, and R. R. Pate, "Correlates of vigorous physical activity for children in grades 1 through 12: comparing parent-reported and objectively measured physical activity," *Pediatric Exercise Science*, vol. 14, no. 1, pp. 30–44, 2002.

[18] R. E. Lee and C. Cubbin, "Striding toward social justice: the ecologic milieuof physical activity," *Exercise and Sport Sciences Reviews*, vol. 37, no. 1, pp. 10–17, 2009.

[19] P. Silva, R. Lott, K. A. Wickrama, J. Mota, and G. Welk, "Psychosocial correlates of physical activity in two cultural contexts: different pathways?" *Journal of Physical Activity & Health*, vol. 9, no. 4, pp. 581–593, 2012.

[20] N. Noy and D. Mcguinness, "Ontology development 101: a guide to creating your first ontology," Stanford Knowledge Systems Laboratory Technical Report KSL-01-05 and Stanford Medical Informatics Technical Report SMI-2001-0880, 2001.

[21] P. Abreu, M. Faria, L. P. Reis, and J. Gargarnta, "Knowledge representation in soccer domain: an ontology development," in *Proceedings of the 5th Iberian Conference on Information Systems and Technologies (CISTI '10)*, pp. 1–6, June 2010.

[22] D. McGuinness and F. van Harmelen, "Owl web ontology language review," W3C Recommendation, 2004.

[23] B. Motik, B. Grau, I. Horrocks, Z. Wu, A. Fokoue, and C. Lutz, "Owl 2 web ontology language profiles," W3C Recommendation, 2009.

[24] "(W3C) WWWC," http://www.w3.org/.

[25] B. E. Ainsworth, W. L. Haskell, S. D. Herrmann et al., "2011 compendium of physical activities: a second update of codes and MET values," *Medicine and Science in Sports and Exercise*, vol. 43, no. 8, pp. 1575–1581, 2011.

[26] C. Tudor-Locke, T. L. Washington, B. E. Ainsworth, and R. P. Troiano, "Linking the American Time Use Survey (ATUS) and the compendium of physical activities: methods and rationale," *Journal of Physical Activity and Health*, vol. 6, no. 3, pp. 347–353, 2009.

[27] G. W. Heath, D. C. Parra, O. L. Sarmiento et al., "Evidence-based intervention in physical activity: lessons from around the world," *The Lancet*, vol. 380, no. 9838, pp. 272–281, 2012.

9

Nutritional Considerations for Performance in Young Athletes

JohnEric W. Smith, Megan E. Holmes, and Matthew J. McAllister

Department of Kinesiology, Mississippi State University, P.O. Box 6186, Mississippi State, MS 39762, USA

Correspondence should be addressed to JohnEric W. Smith; johneric.smith@msstate.edu

Academic Editor: Adrian W. Midgley

Nutrition is an integral component to any athletes training and performance program. In adults the balance between energy intake and energy demands is crucial in training, recovery, and performance. In young athletes the demands for training and performance remain but should be a secondary focus behind the demands associated with maintaining the proper growth and maturation. Research interventions imposing significant physiological loads and diet manipulation are limited in youth due to the ethical considerations related to potential negative impacts on the growth and maturation processes associated with younger individuals. This necessary limitation results in practitioners providing nutritional guidance to young athletes to rely on exercise nutrition recommendations intended for adults. While many of the recommendations can appropriately be repurposed for the younger athlete attention needs to be taken towards the differences in metabolic needs and physiological differences.

1. Introduction

Current estimates suggest approximately 35 million youth between the ages of 5–18 years participate in organized sports each year [1]. While a majority of these young athletes are playing sports for the aspects of comradery and fun, a growing segment of young athletes train to enhance their opportunity to make a career of sport. While elite sport has long seen the presence of young athletes (Nadia Comaneci, 14 years of age (1976 Olympic Gold Medalist), Marjorie Gestring, 13 years of age (1936 Olympic Gold Medalist), and Dimitrios Loundras, 10 years of age (1896 Olympic Bronze Medalist)), the past few decades have experienced an expansion in the numbers of young athletes working to perform at higher levels as younger athletes. This expansion can be seen in the establishment of the many facilities open focusing specialized training for sports performance on not only elite athletes but also largely youth athletes.

While the increase in physical activity of youth is important we currently do not fully understand the effects such training has on the growth and development of youth. The American Academy of Pediatrics outlined potential risks associated with sports specialization in young athletes in a publication in 2000 [2]. Noted orthopedic surgeon, Dr. James Andrews, recently discussed the potential for negative effects of specialized training on developing bodies and the rise in youth sport injuries he experienced since around the same 2000 timeframe [3]. It is not within the scope of this review to discuss the ethical considerations of having youth focus their training on a singular sport, nor to discuss the potential for injury as related to overuse injuries. However, with the continual trend in younger athletes training for high level performance it appears that our current options are to continue to underscore the potential risks while at the same time work with the participants providing as much assistance as possible to enhance safety.

Proper nutrition is a fundamental component of athletes' training and performance plan. Proper nutrition ensures that an individual is amassing the fuels necessary for the energy production needs related to activity and recovery. One of the areas needing to be addressed is the unique nutritional needs associated with intense exercise stress. However, our understanding of the effects of strenuous physiological training and nutritional variations in combination with exercise stress in youth athletes is greatly limited. This limited knowledge is most likely due to the ethical considerations of withholding nutrients and physiologically overstressing a vulnerable population such as children and adolescents still in the process of growth and development.

Our knowledge regarding the nutritional needs of youth is based on the needs related to proper growth and development in healthy children or those suffering from illness. Most of the knowledge we possess related to the physiological adaptations to training, exercise performance, and sports nutrition is based on research conducted in college aged, middle aged, and older adult populations. Therefore, most sports nutrition recommendations promoted in youth sport are actually based on findings in adult populations. While this is a starting point, research has shown that adolescent energy expenditure and metabolism can differ from those of their adult counterparts so many of these recommendations may not provide ideal insight into the nutritional needs of the youth athlete [4–6].

The goal of this review is to compile an overview of our understanding of the nutritional needs of the young athlete during training and competition. We will also identify the knowledge gaps that currently exist in our understanding of this vulnerable population's needs around physiologically stressing occasions. Due to the limited research on the young athlete population, in many instances the knowledge gained through research on adult populations is the only means to provide recommendations for the young athlete.

Nutrition for healthy growth and maturation is governed by a variety of parameters, each essential in the development from child to adult. This paper emphasizes the importance of adolescent nutrition by first examining gross total caloric intake to better understand the energy requirements of adolescents. Total caloric intake must be sufficient to meet the additional demands of growth, which vary at different stages of growth and maturation and between individual children. Likewise, the proportion of calories allocated to each macronutrient is heavily dependent on the situational constraints of the individual child, which is further complicated by the physiological constraints of a given level of development. This paper emphasizes the importance of each macronutrient with specific focus on the physiological nuances of adolescent metabolism specifically focused around the young athlete. Similarly, micronutrient needs are driven by demands of growth and maturation as well as activity levels. Unique demands of the growing adolescent have highlighted a few select micronutrients in the literature which will be reviewed here following a general overview of micronutrient needs.

2. Growth and Development

Growth, maturation, and development are three constructs paramount in any discussion regarding youth. While these terms often manifest concurrently in youth, they refer to three different parameters. Growth simply refers to the quantifiable increase in size, whereas maturation refers to timing and tempo of progress toward the mature state. Timing and tempo refer to the age at which specific maturational events occur and rate at which an individual progresses through these events. Both timing and tempo vary considerably between children [8]. Development is considered a social construct that typically focuses on behaviors and attitudes. Behaviors and attitudes developed during childhood and adolescence provide the basis for adult behaviors and attitudes. Refinement of accepted behaviors in a society requires the development of competencies in an array of interrelated domains that ultimately shape a given behavior and attitude toward that behavior. Taken together, growth, maturation, and development synergistically influence an individual's general self-concept and self-esteem [8]. This holistic perspective is often overlooked when focused on specific pediatric topics, such as nutrition.

Much like business, calorie supply (i.e., energy intake) is dictated by demand (i.e., energy expenditure). Energy expenditure is represented by four major components in children and adolescents: basal/resting metabolic rate, thermic effect of food, thermic effect of activity, and the energy requirements of growth [8]. Basal and resting metabolic rates (BMR and RMR, resp.) vary chiefly on assessment methodology, but only marginally in amount of calories. For the purposes of this discussion, the term RMR will be used to represent both. In adults RMR increases proportionally with body mass, particularly lean body mass [9]. Similarly, RMR increases as children gain body mass. However, when RMR is examined per unit of body mass, RMR decreases as children progress to their adult size [10], which demonstrates the contribution of growth to RMR in children and adolescents. The thermic effect of food varies significantly by the proportion of macronutrients comprising the food consumed. On average, 6–8% of ingested calories are used in the digestive, absorptive, and storage processes of food. Thermic effect of activity is the most variable component of energy expenditure and refers to the calorie cost of movement. When estimating caloric requirements, activity levels are examined at three levels: light, moderate, and vigorous lifestyle physical activity. Given the significant participation in high energy demanding activities, vigorous lifestyle physical activity is exemplified in the youth athlete population. The energy cost of growth is examined in two parameters, the energy to synthesize tissue and the energy deposited in those tissues [7]. Growth varies according to the tempo of maturational development and is very rapid during infancy and early childhood and, thus, accounts for a greater proportion of caloric expenditure. Conversely, during late childhood and adolescence, growth accounts for 1-2%, which reflects a slower rate of growth [8]. With consideration to each of these four components, the FAO/WHO/UNU expert panel used typical weight gains per year to develop age specific and gender specific caloric recommendations [7]. Table 1 shows the caloric recommendations for boys and girls participating in vigorous lifestyles physical activity. Daily energy requirements increase with age and are similar between boys and girls until pubertal ages.

3. Protein

Protein is needed for normal cellular functioning as well as synthesis of various bodily tissues [11]. Athletes tend to have elevated demands for dietary protein intake compared to sedentary individuals [12]. As a general recommendation for maintaining health, current recommendations are between

TABLE 1: Age-specific energy requirements for boys and girls who participate in heavy physical activity levels.

Age (years)	Boys (kcals/day)	Girls (kcals/day)
6-7	1,800	1,650
7-8	1,950	1,775
8-9	2,100	1,950
9-10	2,275	2,125
10-11	2,475	2,300
11-12	2,700	2,475
12-13	2,925	2,625
13-14	3,175	2,725
14-15	3,450	2,855
15-16	3,650	2,875
16-17	3,825	2,875
17-18	3,925	2,875

Adapted from FAO/WHO/UNU, 2004 [7].

0.8 and 1.2 grams of protein per kg of body mass daily [13]. This recommendation is sufficient to meet the bodily demands of 97.5% of the population, which also accounts for variations in demographic BMI as well as gender [11]. A review by Nemet and Eliakim speculates these requirements are likely sufficient for children and youth athletes. The American College of Sports Medicine and American Dietetic Association recommend intakes between 1.2 and 1.8 g/kg of body mass for active adults [14, 15], which appears to be an adequate requirement for youth athletes [16, 17]. Protein synthesis is highest during infancy and, as such, during this time relative dietary protein intake is at an elevated demand [11]. The question of how much dietary protein is needed to maximize performance among athletes is a question that has been debated for more than 150 years [11, 18] and still remains a debate. Recent evidence suggests two to three times the RDA for protein intake may be optimal to enhance fat-free mass during periods of caloric restriction [19] which may be commonly practiced among athletic populations to achieve a body composition more favorable for performance. Investigation of dietary intakes for various youth age groups suggests that intakes this high are often achieved in normal dietary patterns [20], which indicates intake is sufficient to meet the elevated demands.

Many athletes make dietary modifications in attempt to maximize performance and meet body weight requirements for competitive classes [21]. Several studies have shown increased dietary protein intake accompanied by exercise intervention may aid in weight loss as well as preservation of lean body mass typically associated with reduced body weight [22–25]. Some suggest the mechanism may be partially attributed to increased thermogenesis and satiety associated with elevated protein intake. When compared to fat and carbohydrate, protein has a greater thermic effect that is likely only significant enough to result in weight loss when the high protein diet is maintained over the course of several months [26]. Additional research is needed to fully investigate this hypothesis. Several studies have demonstrated satiating effects of high protein diets [27–29], which may better elucidate a mechanism of weight loss with this dietary intervention. Branched chain amino acids found in protein-rich foods are known to assist in preservation of lean body mass [30], which has significant implications for athletes particularly during periods of weight loss. Leucine specifically is one branched chain amino acid that is strongly associated with protein synthesis [31]. This amino acid can be ingested in supplement form; however, when determining the safe tolerable upper intake level for leucine intake, trials in youth are limited. One study suggests the upper level for young males aged 20–35 years is 500 mg/kg/day or 35 g/day based on plasma and urinary ammonia and leucine concentrations [32]. This recommendation has not been examined in youth and caution of leucine at these high levels is warranted. However, food sources such as egg whites and dairy sources contain multiple amino acids and, as such, protein-rich foods should be emphasized to a greater extent than single amino acids alone.

The most significant question is whether or not youth athletes are obtaining the amount of protein needed for their elevated demands. It has been documented that youth athletes in general are achieving protein intakes much greater than the RDA [20]. Given this evidence, it is unlikely beneficial to promote increased protein intake in youth. A thorough dietary evaluation is suggested before promoting increased protein intake in youth athletes. However, as a general recommendation, athletes should ingest balanced protein feedings throughout the day [19] and emphasize whole foods as opposed to protein based supplements due to the lack of scientific support for protein based supplements in comparison to protein-rich whole foods [33].

As previously mentioned, athletes require higher protein intake to maintain protein synthesis [33]. Additionally, research has shown the ingestion of 20 g of protein following exercise helps maintain positive protein balance following exercise [34]. Evidence suggests that protein based supplements are not required to meet this increased demand [2]. Nonetheless, protein supplements remain one of the most common dietary supplements [35] purchased by athletes who seek to increase markers of performance such as speed, strength, power, and hypertrophy [36]. Several reports have documented athletes' perception that protein supplements are necessary to build muscle [37, 38] and achieve peak performance [39]. This notion has been well investigated in adults but also appears true in the limited research regarding youth athletes, specifically high school football players [33]. This misconception among youth is partially driven by the lack of formal knowledge in nutrition [40]. Youth athletes gain a significant amount of nutrition information from magazines, family members, and coaches [41] and, thus, may not be able to make appropriate, evidence based decisions regarding the use of protein supplements [33]. Considering the lack of scientific support for protein based supplements being superior to natural protein containing foods, youth athletes should be advised to consume their protein from whole foods as opposed to supplements.

4. Fat

Dietary lipids are essential for the absorption of vitamins A, D, E, and K, as well as synthesis of cholesterol and other sex hormones [42]. In terms of caloric requirements, most sources recommend lipid intake should be limited to 25–30% of total caloric intake [43], which is relatively the same for both sedentary and active individuals. It is important to consider caloric demands are increased in athletic populations; therefore, *absolute* lipid intakes are likely to be higher. The average adolescent consumes roughly one-third of their dietary intake as lipids [44]. It is important to restrict lipid intake to avoid excessive caloric intake; however, there is no health benefit in diets with less than 15% of calories from lipids [2]. In terms of athletic requirements, an increase of dietary carbohydrate should account for a majority of the increased caloric demands, rather than an increase of dietary lipid. Adequate calorie consumption to support periods of rapid growth is of greatest concern when considering nutrition to maximize performance of adolescent athletes [45]. Roughly fifty percent of adult body mass as well as skeletal mass is achieved during puberty. Large increases in lean and adipose tissue are also seen in males and females during the transition from child to adult as well [44]. During this time, dietary fat is especially important to aid in the synthesis of hormones and assist in normal bodily functioning as well as healthy growth and maturation [46]. Dietary lipid intakes beyond 30% are not advised since this could contribute to excessive weight gain [47]. However, acutely, excessive lipid intake can also result in postprandial oxidative stress, which is associated with impaired vascular and metabolic functioning [48, 49]. Elevated lipid intake is also potentially associated with the pathogenesis of cardiovascular disease [42] which is particularly relevant for youth athletes, given that the origins of CVD begin at an early age and progress into adulthood [48, 50, 51]. The organized group setting provides an ideal platform for discussion of nutrition and physical activity habits among individuals who already acknowledge their value.

Adolescents are more efficient in terms of substrate utilization, which has been shown both at rest and during graded exercise tests since younger children derive a higher percentage of energy from lipids as indicated by lower RER values at submaximal intensities [52]. Improved aerobic efficiency is related to increased dependency on lipids for ATP production commonly noted in youth [5]. This could potentially be the result of an adaptive response since infants and toddlers (under the age of 2) require a higher percentage of energy from lipids to support their increased caloric and growth demands [53]. Alterations in dietary lipid intake could contribute to changes of enzymatic activity as well as elevated lipid metabolism [54]. A lack of glycolytic enzyme activity could be another reason for the aforementioned increased dependency on lipid metabolism [4]. During exercise, carbohydrates and lipids are the main sources of skeletal muscle ATP production, with lipids serving as an important source of energy during low and moderate intensity [45]. Chronic exercise training results in favorable mitochondrial adaptations in adults, which favor enhanced lipid metabolism as well [55].

Upon investigation of differences in lipid oxidation among different age and gender groups in children, a review by Aucouturier et al. [4] reported only miniscule differences between age groups among male and female adolescents. These miniscule differences are likely associated with a change in body size (e.g., acquisition of skeletal and muscle mass) during periods of growth and maturation among different age groups and are more significant in males compared to females. However, Aucouturier et al. reported all children (in general) depend more readily on lipids in comparison to adults. This metabolic characteristic could depend on pubertal status, since it has been shown that 12-year-old females demonstrate elevated lipid metabolism during exercise performed at 70% $\dot{V}O_{2\ max}$ compared to 14-year-old females [56]. Similar findings have also been reported in boys aged 12 and 14 [57]. However, to our knowledge there is little to no evidence showing prepubescent males and females differ *significantly* in terms of relative fat and carbohydrate oxidation during submaximal exercise [4]. In comparison to adults, however, children lack the ability to sustain longer duration exercise, which may be related to a lack of the ability to store glycogen in children [58]. Generalizing substrate utilization during *prolonged* exercise is difficult given the paucity of experimental or quasi-experimental evidence which examines exercise testing in children for greater than one hour in duration [58], which is likely reflective of the general short and intermittent physical activity patterns and behaviors of that age group [59].

The composition of dietary fatty acids (e.g., chain length) can affect fat oxidation during submaximal exercise [54]. However, this response may vary among maturational levels of the young athlete since prepubescent males tend to have a higher percentage of fatty acid oxidation [60]. It is also important to consider the potential adaptations resulting from modifications of lipid intake. Short term elevations in lipid intake are likely to result in positive energy balance which may not be immediately matched with an increase in beta-oxidation [54]. However, trials in adult populations show that exercise can enhance lipid metabolism by stimulating mitochondrial biogenesis [61] as well as increasing activity of lipoprotein lipase [62] and carnitine palmitoyltransferase 1 [63]. The aforementioned adaptations can enhance lipid metabolism and contribute to an accommodated energy balance due to changes in fat metabolism [54]. This evidence is especially applicable to athletes since exercise training has been shown to accommodate the metabolic effects of short term high fat diets [64]. These adaptations, however, still do not constitute promotion of lipid intakes greater than 30% in youth athletes.

As mentioned earlier, factors such as the type of lipid ingested (i.e., composition of the hydrocarbon chain) can affect the subsequent metabolism [54] and potential storage [65, 66]. Piers et al. [67] demonstrated the substitution of saturated fat with monounsaturated fatty acids can potentially have a favorable effect on body composition. The contribution of saturated fatty acid intake to the development of CVD is important [42]; however, a meta-analysis by Siri-Tarino et al. [68] included twenty-one studies and reported no significant risk of coronary heart disease with elevated saturated fatty acid intake. It is important to note coronary heart disease is a *chronic, progressive* disease, the origins of which begin early in life. Thus, youth require appropriate dietary advice that may potentially become healthy behaviors in adulthood as a means of preventing or reducing disease risk. Further, these findings [68] may not be applicable to all individuals since intensity of activity and lipid composition both affect lipid metabolism [54]. Considering the evidence to date, dietary unsaturated fatty acids should not serve as exclusively the sole source of lipids. However, as a general recommendation, and in the interest of promoting long-term healthy behaviors, unsaturated fatty acids should be emphasized to a greater extent.

Some athletes may believe certain lipid based supplements may allow for an ergogenic effect given the limited findings suggesting supplementation may enhance lipid metabolism by decreasing dependency on glycogen/glucose for energy metabolism [69]. Commercial marketing is based on the premise some lipid based dietary supplements can thereby increase aerobic capacity and performance, improve lipid metabolism, and reduce inflammatory damage [70]. Fish oil and conjugated linoleic acid (CLA) are two lipid based supplements that have been investigated in relation to potential ergogenic effects.

Fish oil contains two essential fatty acids (eicosapentaenoic acid [EPA] and docosahexaenoic acid [DHA]). Increased dietary intake of these essential fatty acids has been associated with decreased prevalence of cardiovascular diseases [71, 72], as well as reduced markers of inflammation [73, 74]. In regard to physical performance, a variety of trials failed to demonstrate an ergogenic effect of EPA and DHA [75–77]; Tartibian et al. [78] reported improved pulmonary functioning in young wrestlers [78]. In terms of the ability to improve athletic performance, the majority of data demonstrate a lack in ergogenic effect of fish oil ingestion on athletic performance in well trained athletes [76, 79, 80]. The overwhelming scientific support for fish oil supplementation highlights improvements in cardiovascular health and decreases markers of inflammation which *could* contribute to decreased recovery time between exercises as speculated by Macaluso et al. [69]. However, this has not yet been supported in literature. Furthermore, the majority of clinical trials utilize extremely high doses (>3 g/day) [69, 77, 81], which is difficult to achieve without dietary supplementation of fish oil.

Other benefits of fish oil consumption have been noted including improved cognitive function and reduced ADHD symptoms in children [82]. A meta-analysis by Yang et al. [83] indicated dietary fish and/or fish oil supplementation is also associated with a reduced prevalence of asthma in children [83]. However, additional trials in youth (specifically with athletic samples) are warranted as this population has not been investigated to our knowledge. Given the gap in the literature examining youth athletes, clear recommendations for fish oil consumption cannot be made and warrant further investigation.

CLA is another lipid based dietary supplement that has been proposed to improve athletic performance [69]. CLA is found naturally occurring in beef, lamb, and dairy products such as milk and cheese [84] but is also available in supplement form. Animal studies utilizing CLA administration have demonstrated potentially favorable effects on body composition [85]. However, this may not be applicable to humans since Zambell et al. [86] failed to show a change in energy expenditure and lipid metabolism. A recent review by Macaluso et al. [69] reported fish oil and CLA supplementation can *potentially* have a favorable effect on anabolic effects of exercise which could be related to increased testosterone synthesis. However, given the strong relationship between growth, maturation, and anabolic hormone levels in youth, the demands for youth athletes to intentionally manipulate hormone levels are not advised.

5. Carbohydrate

Human metabolism relies primarily on the oxidation of fats and carbohydrates as its fuel sources. As physiological intensity increases from rest to vigorous there is a transition from fat functioning as the primary fuel source to carbohydrate supplying a majority of the body's fuel for energy. The sources of carbohydrate for metabolism are glycogen stores in the muscle, glycogen stores in the liver, and exogenous carbohydrate entering the blood stream through the ingestion of carbohydrate. Some confusion exists in athletes understanding of the specific carbohydrate needs and it has been suggested by Burke et al. to stem from the fact that many recommendations are based on percentage of total caloric intake which adds to the difficulty in understanding the dietary needs of carbohydrate in athletes that have caloric intakes which often exceed general recommendations [87].

General carbohydrate intake recommendations suggest adult athletes consume 5–12 grams of carbohydrate per kilogram per day dependent on their primary form of exercise/activity, activity intensity, sex, and environmental conditions [88]. The great variance that exists in the demands of sports, training, and level of play make it difficult to provide a single concise recommendation. As training duration and intensities increase carbohydrate requirements rise. Young athletes lack even the large range recommendations that are provided for adult athletes. The recommendations for young athletes suggest at least 50% of young athletes diet should be in the form of carbohydrate [89] or between 3 and 8 grams [90] of carbohydrate per kilogram of body mass dependent primarily on exercise intensity.

The role of carbohydrate ingestion around active occasions is an area of intense study. Early research into carbohydrate's role in exercise performance examined the effect of blood glucose levels and physiological state following prolonged exercise [91, 92]. Additional research investigated muscle glycogen's role in muscle fatigue [93, 94]. Subsequent research investigated the role of carbohydrate ingestion following exercise to restore muscle glycogen stores following the depletion related to exercise stress [95]. More recently the research focus has shifted to explore the role of carbohydrate ingestion during exercise stress in sustaining exercise intensity and improve performance [96–98].

It is commonly suggested that normal body stores of carbohydrate can be a significant fuel source for approximately 90–120 minutes of moderate to vigorous exercise. While this statement is accurate in many exercise settings where individuals are exercising at moderate-vigorous intensities typically associated with endurance exercise, more detailed investigation would demonstrate exercise intensity is a vital component in understanding glycogen depletion rates. Significant glycogen depletion can occur anywhere from ~10 minutes with supramaximal intensities to greater than 3 hours at low exercise intensities [99]. This oversimplification needs to be considered as we look at the findings from carbohydrate research. Many of the research investigations providing our understanding of carbohydrate needs around exercise are based on endurance type exercise. As we consider the sports typically involving young athletes some of our understanding may not fully translate.

As stated previously part of our limited understanding in the nutritional needs of young athletes is the result of proper research ethics. The research described above with adults involved muscle biopsies, exercise to failure, and exercise resulting in "poor" physiological states. This type of request would be inappropriate to make to children. Therefore most of our understanding of youth athletes comes from the utilization of less invasive techniques. Young athletes have been shown to have a lower respiratory exchange ratio (RER) during exercise at similar relative submaximal intensities ($\%\dot{V}O_{2\ max}$) as their adult counterparts [4]. Based on the RER changes resulting from the shift from fat as a primary fuel source to increasing carbohydrate utilization, this would suggest young athletes are better able to utilize fat as a fuel or are potentially limited in their maximal performance as a result of not being able to utilize carbohydrate readily enough at higher intensities.

Research has shown that increasing glycogen stores will enhance exercise performance [100] and reductions in muscle glycogen content correspond with increasing levels of fatigue. Unfortunately, young athletes have been shown to store less glycogen than adults [4]. During prolonged exercise and exercise at elevated intensities reduced glycogen levels will lead to early onsets of fatigue. Due to their lower glycogen stores, young athletes will likely experience accelerated rates of fatigue. This accelerated fatigue is a result of the inability of the body to maintain sufficient blood glucose levels to meet the young athletes elevated glucose needs of the brain as compared to adults [4].

With reduced muscle glycogen stores the need for exogenous sources of carbohydrate becomes increasingly more important in the maintenance of exercise intensity. Much of our understanding regarding the role of carbohydrate ingestion in exercising youth is the result of the work of the researchers in the Children's Exercise and Nutrition Centre at McMaster University. Riddell demonstrated adolescent athletes utilized lower absolute amounts of exogenous glucose as compared to values reported in adults [101]. However, exogenous carbohydrate utilization has been demonstrated as a greater relative contributor to total energy utilization in the young athlete even with lower absolute utilization rates [58, 101].

Current research foci have shifted more towards the improvement of health and wellness as opposed to performance. However recent research continues to demonstrate the ergogenic effects of carbohydrate ingestion on youth sport. Dougherty et al. demonstrated performance improvements with basketball skills test with carbohydrate compared to water ingestion [102]. Batatinha et al. demonstrated gymnasts experienced a reduction in the number of falls from a balance beam with carbohydrate ingestion during a session [103]. Smith et al. demonstrated performance was improved with carbohydrate ingestion during football skill performance [104].

While the need for carbohydrate is recognized as important, the differences between youth and adult are still not fully understood. Research has shown carbohydrate ingestion spares endogenous carbohydrate stores in exercising youth while at the same time youth seem to be unable to utilize carbohydrate at rates similar to those seen in adults [101]. Research in adults has led to the establishment of guidelines suggesting carbohydrate ingestion during activities lasting 45 minutes or longer provides an ergogenic effect with doses varying from "small amounts including mouth rinse" up to 90 g/h [88]. Currently, specific recommendations similar to what exists for adults are not available for the youth athlete.

For performance enhancement young athletes will benefit from the ingestion of carbohydrate during exercise. Without specific rates recommended for the young athletes, we must rely on the recommendations of adults and refine carbohydrate intakes during exercise based on trial and error methods. These recommendations suggest athletes should ingest simple sugars at a rate of 30–60 g/h for exercise lasting longer than 60 minutes. Additionally, athletes should ingest 1–1.5 g/kg of body mass in the 30 minutes following cessation of prolonged exercise [15]. The ingestion of carbohydrate during exercise should be considered an equally significant component of the training plan as the skill aspects of sport.

6. Water

As with their adult counterparts hydration status during sport is important to performance in young athletes. It could be argued that, due to their increased susceptibility to succumb to heat stressors, due to their greater body surface areas to body mass ratio, hydration is a more important consideration in young athletes [105]. In addition to an increased body surface area to body mass ratio, adolescents have been shown to have diminished sweat rates as compared to their adult counterparts [106]. Diminished sweat rates are advantageous as a result of their protection of body water status but are disadvantageous due to the reduced ability to dissipate heat. Added importance of hydration is due to the fact that, in addition to performance decrements, hypohydration has been shown to lead to increased physiological strain, increased risk of heat injury/illness, and increased perceived exertion at similar workloads [15, 107].

As a result of hypohydration, the body experience fluid shifts resulting in increased cardiovascular strain as plasma volume declines [108, 109]. Additionally, the impaired cardiovascular function also leads to diminished skin blood flow resulting in a decline in the ability to dissipate heat to the environment [110]. Hypohydration also leads to an increase in the perception of exertion required to maintain a steady work rate. Research investigating the role of hydration on exercise performance has shown fluid ingestion and the maintenance of proper hydration status improve performance [102, 111].

To add to the physiological strain associated with dehydration inherent with physical activity, most athletes have been found to arrive to practice in a hypohydrated state [106, 112]. Even with education emphasizing the need for proper hydration, preactivity hydration assessments of athletes involved in sport have demonstrated significant percentages of the population to be hypohydrated [113]. Kavouras et al. reported that educational interventions significantly improved preexercise hydration status, however following education regarding hydration 66% of the youth athletes reported to practice in a hypohydrated state [114].

While unlikely to be a broad risk in youth sport, attention must also be drawn to the potential to ingest fluids at excessive levels resulting in the risk of hypernatremia and potentially death. Since the first reports in the literature of hyponatremia in endurance events greater focus has continued to grow regarding the risks associated with over drinking [115]. Hyponatremia has been reported to be as high as 51% in ultramarathons performed under hotter ambient temperatures [115]. The incidence of hyponatremia increases as duration of activity increases along with fluid ingestion. A potential means to reduce the rate of plasma sodium concentration decline is through the ingestion of sodium containing beverages [116]. It should be noted that very few beverages actually contain sodium levels sufficient to maintain plasma sodium levels; however the ingestion of sodium containing beverages will reduce the rate of decline.

The American College of Sports Medicine's Position Stand on Nutrition and Athletic Performance recommends athletes to consume 5–7 mL/kg of body mass 4 hours prior to exercise, enough fluid to reduce body mass changes to less than 2% during activity, and 450–675 mL for every 0.5 kg of body mass lost during exercise [15]. These recommendations do not account for age but are likely a good place to begin for youth athletes since they are based on body mass rather than absolute volumes. Hydration goals should be to minimize body mass losses associated with dehydration while ensuring fluid ingestion does not exceed sweat losses. This is easily assessed through body weight measures immediately prior to and immediately following activity. Increases in body mass would inform the athlete fluid ingestion was too high and significant decreases in body mass would inform the athlete fluid ingestion was insufficient. Additionally, in situations where repeated days of exercise are performed in the heat sodium ingestion rates should be increased to maintain plasma sodium levels. Flavored fluids have been repeatedly shown to aid in the maintenance of fluid intake reducing voluntary dehydration.

Equation for determining sweat rate is as follows:

$$\frac{\mathrm{BW}_0 + \mathrm{DF}_0 - \mathrm{BW}_E - \mathrm{DF}_E}{\text{Time (hrs)}}, \tag{1}$$

where BW_0 is body mass before exercise, DF_0 is mass of exercise food and drink before exercise, DF_E is body mass after exercise, and DF_E is mass of exercise food and drink after exercise.

7. Micronutrients

Micronutrients categorically refer to vitamins and minerals used by the body during normal physiological functions. Generally, it is accepted that a well-balanced diet of sufficient caloric intake will provide the adequate micronutrients to support normal growth and maturation. The American Medical Association (AMA) and the American Dietetic Association (ADA) recommend nutrients be obtained from food sources rather than supplements in healthy children [117]. Likewise, the American Academy of Pediatrics (AAP) does not endorse regular supplementation of vitamins and minerals in healthy children (with the exception of fluoride in unfluoridated areas). However, AAP has noted that some children are at increased risk of nutrient deficiencies. Specifically, AAP suggests that children and adolescents with anorexia or poor appetites, chronic diseases, and food insecurity are at greater risk for nutrient deficiencies. Youth who do not consume adequate amounts of dairy or have sufficient sun exposure may also be at risk for deficiencies [118].

The daily time constraints of an elite young athlete can make achieving a balanced diet difficult, thus putting these individuals at a potential increased risk for micronutrient deficiencies as well. These deficiencies are most commonly observed in girls rather than boys and in mineral intake rather than vitamin intake. Athletic youth may actually be more likely to achieve the recommended intake of vitamins than nonathletic youth due to their increased total caloric intake. Adequate intake of minerals appears to be a bigger challenge for youth, particularly girls [119]. Specifically, iron and calcium are frequently noted as common nutritional concerns among children and adolescents.

Iron deficiency and subsequent anemia are common in adolescents [120]. Increases in hemoglobin production, blood volume, and muscle mass are normal characteristics of growth and maturation and account for the majority of increased iron needs in developing adolescents. However, iron requirements become even greater for girls at the onset of menses. Iron-deficient anemia has significant, negative implications on performance in adults [121, 122] and youth [123–125]. Diminished performance is most apparent in iron-deficient anemic athletes participating in activities with higher aerobic demands (i.e., endurance event athletes) [124]. The recommended intake of iron for boys and girls aged 9–13 years is 18 mg per day. Boys and girls aged 14–18 years should consume 11 mg and 15 mg per day, respectively [126]. In accordance with AMA, ADA, and AAP guidelines, youth should improve their iron status through consumption of iron-rich foods at meals such as red meat, beans, and green vegetables. Athletes will likely find additional benefit by including other iron-rich foods such as peanuts and dried fruits and iron-fortified cereals as regular snacks. Furthermore, the inclusion of foods higher in ascorbic acid with these nonheme iron sources will improve iron absorption from these snacks [127].

Calcium requirements are greatest during adolescence, 1,300 mg per day for both boys and girls [128]. This higher requirement accommodates the prime opportunity for acquisition of bone mass that spans the pubertal ages. Availability of nutrients critical for bone development (e.g., calcium) and opportunity for increased bone loading (e.g., physical activity) prior to achieving skeletal maturation is critical in preventing osteoporosis later in life [129]. Despite the greater requirements and the clear benefits of consuming adequate amounts, United States children and adolescents' average intake falls below the minimum recommendations [130]. In the American diet, the majority of dietary calcium is obtained from milk and other dairy sources [131]. However, milk consumption has shown a general decline in this age group [132]. Given the perishability of most dairy products, young athletes face practicality issues scheduling regular consumption throughout the day. Breakfast consumption is associated with greater calcium intake among this age group [133] and should be strongly encouraged. Likewise, athletes should consume regular snacks that include rich sources of calcium (e.g., fortified orange juice, almonds, and broccoli), throughout the day. Furthermore, calcium absorption is dependent on adequate levels of vitamin D [128]. Thus, attention to sources of calcium fortified with vitamin D is warranted, particularly among individuals who are not likely to be exposed to sufficient sunlight to endogenously produce adequate vitamin D. While whole food sources are always preferred, the convenience of calcium supplements (often fortified with vitamin D) may make adequate intake a more viable possibility.

An additional consideration warranting attention in young athletes participating in large amounts of training and competition is the potential need to replenish sodium and potassium lost in sweat. The summation of the electrolyte loss resulting from sweat loss has been shown to be equivalent to daily intakes, even in young athletes [105]. Much of this additional loss in salt can be offset through the ingestion of sport drinks during practice and competition, which also partially addresses hydration concerns in the group.

8. Summary

Research regarding the nutritional needs of young competitive athletes is sparse and is primarily composed of investigations of youth-adult differences. In addition to the limited research, the majority of our current knowledge in the adult population is based on differences between typical adults compared to their more active counterparts. Research to date suggests similarities in the caloric and macronutrient needs of active adults and their younger counterparts; however, youth-adult differences in fuel utilization have also been clearly demonstrated. In addition to the energy needs of highly active youth, nutritional intake plays a critical role in the growth and development of young athletes and should be a principal emphasis at this stage in their lives. General guidelines for nutrition for active youth are summarized in Table 2. These guidelines serve as recommendations that support healthy growth and development and also account for the additional caloric needs of active youth. As emphasis on performance outcome goals continues to increase in youth athletics, active youth quickly become young athletes. Likewise, nutritional considerations move beyond increased caloric needs and promotion of healthy growth and development to nutritional strategies that can optimize performance. A summary of available performance-based nutritional strategies can be found in Table 3. The paucity of data examining the unique needs of young athletes draws attention to increased need for further investigations on this subject which consider the distinct nutritional requirements of growth and maturation at all age and skill levels. Given the popularity of youth sports and the increasing demand for performance outcomes, increased attention on this topic is warranted by the scientific community.

Table 2: General nutrition recommendations for maintaining health.

Protein	15–20% of total calories should come from protein; 0.8–1.2 g/kg/day derived from whole food sources
Fat	>15% and <30% of total calories should come from fat
Carbohydrate	>50% of total calories should come from carbohydrates, or 3–8 g/kg/day
Micronutrients	Regular supplementation is not recommended in healthy children and adolescents consuming a balanced diet

Table 3: Supplemental nutrition recommendations for athletes.

Protein	1.2–1.8 g/kg/day derived from whole food sources *After exercise*: 20 g of high quality protein shortly after exercise
Carbohydrate	*During exercise*: 30–60 g/hr for exercise lasting more than 1 hour *After exercise*: 1.0–1.5 g/kg of body mass within 30 minutes of exercise cessation
Fluid	*Before exercise*: 5–7 mL/kg 4 hrs prior to exercise *During exercise*: assess sweat rate and develop hydration plan to maintain body mass during exercise *After exercise*: 450–675 mL/0.5 kg and additional sodium consideration to account for loss through sweat
Micronutrients	*During exercise*: sodium to offset losses associated with sweat being lost in sweat

Conflict of Interests

The authors declare that there is no conflict of interests regarding the publication of this paper.

Authors' Contribution

Megan E. Holmes and Matthew J. McAllister are coauthors.

References

[1] V. Seefeldt and M. Ewing, "Youth sports in America, an overview," *President's Council on Physical Fitness and Sports Research Digest*, vol. 2, no. 11, pp. 1–10, 1997.

[2] American College of Sports Medicine and American Dietetic Association & Dietitians of Canada, "Joint Position Statement: nutrition and athletic performance," *Medicine & Science in Sports & Exercise*, vol. 32, no. 12, pp. 2130–2145, 2000.

[3] D. Manoloff, "Noted surgeon Dr. James Andrew wants your young athlete to stay healthy by playing less," 2013, http://www.cleveland.com/dman/index.ssf/2013/02/noted_surgeon_dr_james_andrews.html.

[4] J. Aucouturier, J. S. Baker, and P. Duché, "Fat and carbohydrate metabolism during submaximal exercise in children," *Sports Medicine*, vol. 38, no. 3, pp. 213–238, 2008.

[5] G. E. Duncan and E. T. Howley, "Substrate metabolism during exercise in children and the crossover concept," *Pediatric Exercise Science*, vol. 11, no. 1, pp. 12–21, 1999.

[6] J. S. Harrell, R. G. Mcmurray, C. D. Baggett, M. L. Pennell, P. F. Pearce, and S. I. Bangdiwala, "Energy costs of physical activities in children and adolescents," *Medicine and Science in Sports and Exercise*, vol. 37, no. 2, pp. 329–336, 2005.

[7] Food and Agriculture Organization of the United Nations, United Nations University, and World Health Organization, *Human Energy Requirements: Report of a Joint FAO/WHO/UNU Expert Consultation: Rome, 17–24 October 2001*, Food and Agricultural Organization of the United Nations, Rome, Italy, 2004.

[8] R. M. Malina, C. Bouchard, and O. Bar-Or, *Growth, Maturation, and Physical Activity*, Human Kinetics, Champaign, Ill, USA, 2nd edition, 2004.

[9] E. Ravussin and C. Bogardus, "Relationship of genetics, age, and physical fitness to daily energy expenditure and fuel utilization," *The American Journal of Clinical Nutrition*, vol. 49, supplement 5, pp. 968–975, 1989.

[10] S. M. Garn and L. C. Clark Jr., "The sex difference in the basal metabolic rate," *Child Development*, vol. 24, no. 3-4, pp. 215–224, 1953.

[11] D. Nemet and A. Eliakim, "Pediatric sports nutrition: an update," *Current Opinion in Clinical Nutrition and Metabolic Care*, vol. 12, no. 3, pp. 304–309, 2009.

[12] K. D. Tipton, A. E. Jeukendrup, and P. Hespel, "Nutrition for the sprinter," *Journal of Sports Sciences*, vol. 25, supplement 1, pp. S5–S15, 2007.

[13] E. Smit, J. Nieto, C. J. Crespo, and P. Mitchell, "Estimates of animal and plant protein intake in US adults: results from the Third National Health and Nutrition Examination Survey, 1988–1991," *Journal of the American Dietetic Association*, vol. 99, no. 7, pp. 813–820, 1999.

[14] S. M. Phillips and L. J. C. Van Loon, "Dietary protein for athletes: from requirements to optimum adaptation," *Journal of Sports Sciences*, vol. 29, supplement 1, pp. S29–S38, 2011.

[15] N. R. Rodriguez, N. M. Di Marco, and S. Langley, "American College of Sports Medicine position stand. Nutrition and athletic performance," *Medicine & Science in Sports & Exercise*, vol. 41, no. 3, pp. 709–731, 2009.

[16] N. Boisseau, M. Vermorel, M. Rance, P. Duché, and P. Patureau-Mirand, "Protein requirements in male adolescent soccer players," *European Journal of Applied Physiology*, vol. 100, no. 1, pp. 27–33, 2007.

[17] F. Meyer, H. O'Connor, and S. M. Shirreffs, "Nutrition for the young athlete," *Journal of Sports Sciences*, vol. 25, supplement 1, pp. S73–S82, 2007.

[18] P. W. Lemon, "Beyond the zone: protein needs of active individuals," *Journal of the American College of Nutrition*, vol. 19, supplement 5, pp. 513S–521S, 2000.

[19] C. H. Murphy, A. J. Hector, and S. M. Phillips, "Considerations for protein intake in managing weight loss in athletes," *European Journal of Sport Science*, vol. 15, no. 1, pp. 21–28, 2015.

[20] A. Jeukendrup and L. Cronin, "Nutrition and elite young athletes," *Medicine and Sport Science*, vol. 56, pp. 47–58, 2011.

[21] S. Mettler, N. Mitchell, and K. D. Tipton, "Increased protein intake reduces lean body mass loss during weight loss in athletes," *Medicine and Science in Sports and Exercise*, vol. 42, no. 2, pp. 326–337, 2010.

[22] D. K. Layman, R. A. Boileau, D. J. Erickson et al., "A reduced ratio of dietary carbohydrate to protein improves body composition and blood lipid profiles during weight loss in adult women," *Journal of Nutrition*, vol. 133, no. 2, pp. 411–417, 2003.

[23] D. K. Layman, E. Evans, J. I. Baum, J. Seyler, D. J. Erickson, and R. A. Boileau, "Dietary protein and exercise have additive effects on body composition during weight loss in adult women," *Journal of Nutrition*, vol. 135, no. 8, pp. 1903–1910, 2005.

[24] H. J. Leidy, N. S. Carnell, R. D. Mattes, and W. W. Campbell, "Higher protein intake preserves lean mass and satiety with weight loss in pre-obese and obese women," *Obesity*, vol. 15, no. 2, pp. 421–429, 2007.

[25] K. A. Meckling and R. Sherfey, "A randomized trial of a hypocaloric high-protein diet, with and without exercise, on weight loss, fitness, and markers of the metabolic syndrome in overweight and obese women," *Applied Physiology, Nutrition, and Metabolism*, vol. 32, no. 4, pp. 743–752, 2007.

[26] T. L. Halton and F. B. Hu, "The effects of high protein diets on thermogenesis, satiety and weight loss: a critical review," *The Journal of the American College of Nutrition*, vol. 23, no. 5, pp. 373–385, 2004.

[27] J. D. Latner and M. Schwartz, "The effects of a high-carbohydrate, high-protein or balanced lunch upon later food intake and hunger ratings," *Appetite*, vol. 33, no. 1, pp. 119–128, 1999.

[28] S. D. Poppitt, D. McCorMacK, and R. Buffenstein, "Short-term effects of macronutrient preloads on appetite and energy intake in lean women," *Physiology and Behavior*, vol. 64, no. 3, pp. 279–285, 1998.

[29] A. R. Skov, S. Toubro, B. Rønn, L. Holm, and A. Astrup, "Randomized trial on protein vs carbohydrate in *ad libitum* fat reduced diet for the treatment of obesity," *International Journal of Obesity*, vol. 23, no. 5, pp. 528–536, 1999.

[30] D. K. Layman, "Protein quantity and quality at levels above the RDA improves adult weight loss," *Journal of the American College of Nutrition*, vol. 23, no. 6, supplement, pp. 631s–636s, 2004.

[31] J. C. Anthony, T. G. Anthony, S. R. Kimball, and L. S. Jefferson, "Signaling pathways involved in translational control of protein synthesis in skeletal muscle by leucine," *Journal of Nutrition*, vol. 131, no. 3, pp. 856s–860s, 2001.

[32] R. Elango, K. Chapman, M. Rafii, R. O. Ball, and P. B. Pencharz, "Determination of the tolerable upper intake level of leucine in acute dietary studies in young men," *The American Journal of Clinical Nutrition*, vol. 96, no. 4, pp. 759–767, 2012.

[33] M. C. Duellman, J. M. Lukaszuk, A. D. Prawitz, and J. P. Brandenburg, "Protein supplement users among high school athletes have misconceptions about effectiveness," *Journal of Strength and Conditioning Research*, vol. 22, no. 4, pp. 1124–1129, 2008.

[34] M. Beelen, L. M. Burke, M. J. Gibala, and L. J. C. van Loon, "Nutritional strategies to promote postexercise recovery," *International Journal of Sport Nutrition and Exercise Metabolism*, vol. 20, no. 6, pp. 515–532, 2010.

[35] D. Nemet, B. Wolach, and A. Eliakim, "Proteins and amino acid supplementation in sports: are they truly necessary?" *Israel Medical Association Journal*, vol. 7, no. 5, pp. 328–332, 2005.

[36] K. Froiland, W. Koszewski, J. Hingst, and L. Kopecky, "Nutritional supplement use among college athletes and their sources of information," *International Journal of Sport Nutrition and Exercise Metabolism*, vol. 14, no. 1, pp. 104–120, 2004.

[37] B. H. Jacobson and S. G. Aldana, "Current nutrition practice and knowledge of varsity athletes," *The Journal of Strength & Conditioning Research*, vol. 6, no. 4, pp. 232–238, 1992.

[38] B. G. Wiita and I. A. Stombaugh, "Nutrition knowledge, eating practices, and health of adolescent female runners: a 3-year longitudinal study," *International Journal of Sport Nutrition and Exercise Metabolism*, vol. 6, no. 4, pp. 414–425, 1996.

[39] S. S. Jonnalagadda, C. A. Rosenbloom, and R. Skinner, "Dietary practices, attitudes, and physiological status of collegiate freshman football players," *Journal of Strength and Conditioning Research*, vol. 15, no. 4, pp. 507–513, 2001.

[40] C. A. Rosenbloom, S. S. Jonnalagadda, and R. Skinner, "Nutrition knowledge of collegiate athletes in a Division I National Collegiate Athletic Association institution," *Journal of the American Dietetic Association*, vol. 102, no. 3, pp. 418–420, 2002.

[41] B. H. Jacobson, C. Sobonya, and J. Ransone, "Nutrition practices and knowledge of college varsity athletes: a follow-up," *Journal of Strength and Conditioning Research*, vol. 15, no. 1, pp. 63–68, 2001.

[42] A. H. Lichtenstein, E. Kennedy, P. Barrier et al., "Dietary fat consumption and health," *Nutrition Reviews*, vol. 56, no. 5, part 2, pp. S3–S28, 1998.

[43] J. W. Smith and A. Jeukendrup, "Performance nutrition for young athletes," in *Nutrition and Enhanced Sports Performance: Muscle Building, Endurance, and Strength*, S. D. N. Bagchi and C. K. Sen, Eds., pp. 523–529, Elsevier, 2013.

[44] R. Wahl, "Nutrition in the adolescent," *Pediatric Annals*, vol. 28, no. 2, pp. 107–111, 1999.

[45] P. Bjorntorp, "Importance of fat as a support nutrient for energy: metabolism of athletes," *Journal of Sports Sciences*, vol. 9, pp. 71–76, 1991.

[46] B. A. Bushman, "Calorie requirements for young competitive female athletes," *ACSM's Health & Fitness Journal*, vol. 16, no. 5, pp. 4–8, 2012.

[47] E. Jequier, "Is fat intake a risk factor for fat gain in children?" *The Journal of Clinical Endocrinology & Metabolism*, vol. 86, no. 3, pp. 980–983, 2001.

[48] R. J. Bloomer, M. M. Kabir, K. E. Marshall, R. E. Canale, and T. M. Farney, "Postprandial oxidative stress in response to dextrose and lipid meals of differing size," *Lipids in Health and Disease*, vol. 9, article 79, 2010.

[49] K. H. Fisher-Wellman and R. J. Bloomer, "Exacerbated postprandial oxidative stress induced by the acute intake of a lipid meal compared to isoenergetically administered carbohydrate, protein, and mixed meals in young, healthy men," *Journal of the American College of Nutrition*, vol. 29, no. 4, pp. 373–381, 2010.

[50] C. Bouziotas, Y. Koutedakis, A. Nevill et al., "Greek adolescents, fitness, fatness, fat intake, activity, and coronary heart disease risk," *Archives of Disease in Childhood*, vol. 89, no. 1, pp. 41–44, 2004.

[51] L. T. Mahoney, T. L. Burns, W. Stanford et al., "Coronary risk factors measured in childhood and young adult life are associated with coronary artery calcification in young adults: the Muscatine study," *Journal of the American College of Cardiology*, vol. 27, no. 2, pp. 277–284, 1996.

[52] M. Máček and J. Vávra, "Prolonged exercise in 14-year-old girls," *International Journal of Sports Medicine*, vol. 2, no. 4, pp. 228–230, 1981.

[53] American Academy of Pediatrics and National Cholesterol Education Program, "Report of the expert panel on blood cholesterol levels in children and adolescents," *Pediatrics*, vol. 89, no. 3, part 2, pp. 525–584, 1992.

[54] J. A. Cooper, A. C. Watras, T. Shriver, A. K. Adams, and D. A. Schoeller, "Influence of dietary fatty acid composition and exercise on changes in fat oxidation from a high-fat diet," *Journal of Applied Physiology*, vol. 109, no. 4, pp. 1011–1018, 2010.

[55] R. J. Tunstall, K. A. Mehan, G. D. Wadley et al., "Exercise training increases lipid metabolism gene expression in human skeletal muscle," *The American Journal of Physiology—Endocrinology and Metabolism*, vol. 283, no. 1, pp. E66–E72, 2002.

[56] B. W. Timmons, O. Bar-Or, and M. C. Riddell, "Energy substrate utilization during prolonged exercise with and without carbohydrate intake in preadolescent and adolescent girls," *Journal of Applied Physiology*, vol. 103, no. 3, pp. 995–1000, 2007.

[57] B. W. Timmons, O. Bar-Or, and M. C. Riddell, "Influence of age and pubertal status on substrate utilization during exercise with and without carbohydrate intake in healthy boys," *Applied Physiology, Nutrition and Metabolism*, vol. 32, no. 3, pp. 416–425, 2007.

[58] B. W. Timmons, O. Bar-Or, and M. C. Riddell, "Oxidation rate of exogenous carbohydrate during exercise is higher in boys than in men," *Journal of Applied Physiology*, vol. 94, no. 1, pp. 278–284, 2003.

[59] G. J. Welk, C. B. Corbin, and D. Dale, "Measurement issues in the assessment of physical activity in children," *Research Quarterly for Exercise and Sport*, vol. 71, no. 2, pp. S59–S73, 2000.

[60] M. C. Riddell, V. K. Jamnik, K. E. Iscoe, B. W. Timmons, and N. Gledhill, "Fat oxidation rate and the exercise intensity that elicits maximal fat oxidation decreases with pubertal status in young male subjects," *Journal of Applied Physiology*, vol. 105, no. 2, pp. 742–748, 2008.

[61] J. O. Holloszy and E. F. Coyle, "Adaptations of skeletal muscle to endurance exercise and their metabolic consequences," *Journal of Applied Physiology Respiratory Environmental and Exercise Physiology*, vol. 56, no. 4, pp. 831–838, 1984.

[62] A. Raben, E. Mygind, and A. Astrup, "Lower activity of oxidative key enzymes and smaller fiber areas in skeletal muscle

of postobese women," *The American Journal of Physiology—Endocrinology and Metabolism*, vol. 275, no. 3, part 1, pp. E487–E494, 1998.

[63] P. M. Berthon, R. A. Howlett, G. J. F. Heigenhauser, and L. L. Spriet, "Human skeletal muscle carnitine palmitoyltransferase I activity determined in isolated intact mitochondria," *Journal of Applied Physiology*, vol. 85, no. 1, pp. 148–153, 1998.

[64] K. C. Hansen, Z. Zhang, T. Gomez, A. K. Adams, and D. A. Schoeller, "Exercise increases the proportion of fat utilization during short-term consumption of a high-fat diet," *The American Journal of Clinical Nutrition*, vol. 85, no. 1, pp. 109–116, 2007.

[65] P. J. H. Jones, J. E. Ridgen, P. T. Phang, and C. L. Birmingham, "Influence of dietary fat polyunsaturated to saturated ratio on energy substrate utilization in obesity," *Metabolism*, vol. 41, no. 4, pp. 396–401, 1992.

[66] J. C. Lovejoy, S. R. Smith, C. M. Champagne et al., "Effects of diets enriched in saturated (palmitic), monounsaturated (oleic), or trans (elaidic) fatty acids on insulin sensitivity and substrate oxidation in healthy adults," *Diabetes Care*, vol. 25, no. 8, pp. 1283–1288, 2002.

[67] L. S. Piers, K. Z. Walker, R. M. Stoney, M. J. Soares, and K. O'Dea, "Substitution of saturated with monounsaturated fat in a 4-week diet affects body weight and composition of overweight and obese men," *British Journal of Nutrition*, vol. 90, no. 3, pp. 717–727, 2003.

[68] P. W. Siri-Tarino, Q. Sun, F. B. Hu, and R. M. Krauss, "Meta-analysis of prospective cohort studies evaluating the association of saturated fat with cardiovascular disease," *The American Journal of Clinical Nutrition*, vol. 91, no. 3, pp. 535–546, 2010.

[69] F. Macaluso, R. Barone, P. Catanese et al., "Do fat supplements increase physical performance?" *Nutrients*, vol. 5, no. 2, pp. 509–524, 2013.

[70] A. E. Jeukendrup and S. Aldred, "Fat supplementation, health, and endurance performance," *Nutrition*, vol. 20, no. 7-8, pp. 678–688, 2004.

[71] É. E. Dewailly, C. Blanchet, S. Gingras et al., "Relations between n-3 fatty acid status and cardiovascular disease risk factors among Quebecers," *The American Journal of Clinical Nutrition*, vol. 74, no. 5, pp. 603–611, 2001.

[72] A. M. Hill, J. D. Buckley, K. J. Murphy, and P. R. C. Howe, "Combining fish-oil supplements with regular aerobic exercise improves body composition and cardiovascular disease risk factors," *The American Journal of Clinical Nutrition*, vol. 85, no. 5, pp. 1267–1274, 2007.

[73] P. M. M. Andrade, B. G. Ribeiro, M. T. Bozza, L. F. B. C. Rosa, and M. G. T. do Carmo, "Effects of the fish-oil supplementation on the immune and inflammatory responses in elite swimmers," *Prostaglandins, Leukotrienes & Essential Fatty Acids*, vol. 77, no. 3-4, pp. 139–145, 2007.

[74] T. H. Lee, R. L. Hoover, J. D. Williams et al., "Effect of dietary enrichment with eicosapentaenoic and docosahexaenoic acids on in vitro neutrophil and monocyte leukotriene generation and neutrophil function," *The New England Journal of Medicine*, vol. 312, no. 19, pp. 1217–1224, 1985.

[75] M. Bortolotti, L. Tappy, and P. Schneiter, "Fish oil supplementation does not alter energy efficiency in healthy males," *Clinical Nutrition*, vol. 26, no. 2, pp. 225–230, 2007.

[76] J. D. Buckley, S. Burgess, K. J. Murphy, and P. R. C. Howe, "DHA-rich fish oil lowers heart rate during submaximal exercise in elite Australian Rules footballers," *Journal of Science and Medicine in Sport*, vol. 12, no. 4, pp. 503–507, 2009.

[77] G. E. Peoples, P. L. McLennan, P. R. C. Howe, and H. Groeller, "Fish oil reduces heart rate and oxygen consumption during exercise," *Journal of Cardiovascular Pharmacology*, vol. 52, no. 6, pp. 540–547, 2008.

[78] B. Tartibian, B. H. Maleki, and A. Abbasi, "The effects of omega-3 supplementation on pulmonary function of young wrestlers during intensive training," *Journal of Science and Medicine in Sport*, vol. 13, no. 2, pp. 281–286, 2010.

[79] G. S. Oostenbrug, R. P. Mensink, M. R. Hardeman, T. De Vries, F. Brouns, and G. Hornstra, "Exercise performance, red blood cell deformability, and lipid peroxidation: effects of fish oil and vitamin E," *Journal of Applied Physiology*, vol. 83, no. 3, pp. 746–752, 1997.

[80] T. Raastad, A. T. Hostmark, and S. B. Stramme, "Omega-3 fatty acid supplementation does not improve maximal aerobic power, anaerobic threshold and running performance in well-trained soccer players," *Scandinavian Journal of Medicine and Science in Sports*, vol. 7, no. 1, pp. 25–31, 1997.

[81] C. Y. Guezennec, J. F. Nadaud, P. Satabin, F. Leger, and P. Lafargue, "Influence of polyunsaturated fatty acid diet on the hemorrheological response to physical exercise in hypoxia," *International Journal of Sports Medicine*, vol. 10, no. 4, pp. 286–291, 1989.

[82] M. J. Heilskov Rytter, L. B. B. Andersen, T. Houmann et al., "Diet in the treatment of ADHD in children-a systematic review of the literature," *Nordic Journal of Psychiatry*, vol. 69, no. 1, pp. 1–18, 2014.

[83] H. Yang, P. Xun, and K. He, "Fish and fish oil intake in relation to risk of asthma: a systematic review and meta-analysis," *PLoS ONE*, vol. 8, no. 11, Article ID e80048, 2013.

[84] H. B. MacDonald, "Conjugated linoleic acid and disease prevention: a review of current knowledge," *Journal of the American College of Nutrition*, vol. 19, no. 2, supplement, pp. 111s–118s, 2000.

[85] Y. W. Wang and P. J. Jones, "Conjugated linoleic acid and obesity control: efficacy and mechanisms," *International Journal of Obesity and Related Metabolic Disorders*, vol. 28, no. 8, pp. 941–955, 2004.

[86] K. L. Zambell, N. L. Keim, M. D. Van Loan et al., "Conjugated linoleic acid supplementation in humans: effects on body composition and energy expenditure," *Lipids*, vol. 35, no. 7, pp. 777–782, 2000.

[87] L. M. Burke, B. Kiens, and J. L. Ivy, "Carbohydrates and fat for training and recovery," *Journal of Sports Sciences*, vol. 22, no. 1, pp. 15–30, 2004.

[88] L. M. Burke, J. A. Hawley, S. H. S. Wong, and A. E. Jeukendrup, "Carbohydrates for training and competition," *Journal of Sports Sciences*, vol. 29, no. 1, pp. S17–S27, 2011.

[89] L. Bonci, "Sports nutrition for young athletes," *Pediatric Annals*, vol. 39, no. 5, pp. 300–306, 2010.

[90] P. M. Nisevich, "Sports nutrition for young athletes," *IDEA Fitness Journal*, pp. 65–67, 2008.

[91] B. Gordon, L. A. Kohn, S. A. Levine, M. Matton, W. M. Scriver, and W. B. Whiting, "Sugar content of the blood following a marathon race with especial reference to the prevention of hypoglycemia: further observations," *The Journal of the American Medical Association*, vol. 85, no. 7, pp. 508–509, 1925.

[92] S. A. Levine, B. Gordon, and C. L. Derick, "Some changes in the chemical constituents of the blood following a marathon race with special reference to the development of hypoglycemia," *The Journal of the American Medical Association*, vol. 82, no. 22, pp. 1778–1779, 1924.

[93] J. Bergstrom and E. Hultman, "A study of the glycogen metabolism during exercise in man," *Scandinavian Journal of Clinical & Laboratory Investigation*, vol. 19, no. 3, pp. 218–228, 1967.

[94] L. Hermansen, E. Hultman, and B. Saltin, "Muscle glycogen during prolonged severe exercise," *Acta Physiologica Scandinavica*, vol. 71, no. 2, pp. 129–139, 1967.

[95] D. L. Costill, W. M. Sherman, W. J. Fink, C. Maresh, M. Witten, and J. M. Miller, "The role of dietary carbohydrates in muscle glycogen resynthesis after strenuous running," *American Journal of Clinical Nutrition*, vol. 34, no. 9, pp. 1831–1836, 1981.

[96] E. F. Coyle and A. R. Coggan, "Effectiveness of carbohydrate feeding in delaying fatigue during prolonged exercise," *Sports Medicine*, vol. 1, no. 6, pp. 446–458, 1984.

[97] J. W. Smith, D. D. Pascoe, D. H. Passe et al., "Curvilinear dose-response relationship of carbohydrate (0–120 g.h(−1)) and performance," *Medicine & Science in Sports & Exercise*, vol. 45, no. 2, pp. 336–341, 2013.

[98] J. W. Smith, J. J. Zachwieja, F. Péronnet et al., "Fuel selection and cycling endurance performance with ingestion of [13C]glucose: evidence for a carbohydrate dose response," *Journal of Applied Physiology*, vol. 108, no. 6, pp. 1520–1529, 2010.

[99] P. D. Gollnick, K. Piehl, and B. Saltin, "Selective glycogen depletion pattern in human muscle fibres after exercise of varying intensity and at varying pedalling rates," *The Journal of Physiology*, vol. 241, no. 1, pp. 45–57, 1974.

[100] W. M. Sherman, D. L. Costill, W. J. Fink, and J. M. Miller, "Effect of exercise-diet manipulation on muscle glycogen and its subsequent utilization during performance," *International Journal of Sports Medicine*, vol. 2, no. 2, pp. 114–118, 1981.

[101] M. C. Riddell, O. Bar-Or, H. P. Schwarcz, and G. J. F. Heigenhauser, "Substrate utilization in boys during exercise with [^{13}C]-glucose ingestion," *European Journal of Applied Physiology*, vol. 83, no. 4-5, pp. 441–448, 2000.

[102] K. A. Dougherty, L. B. Baker, M. Chow, and W. L. Kenney, "Two percent dehydration impairs and six percent carbohydrate drink improves boys basketball skills," *Medicine & Science in Sports & Exercise*, vol. 38, no. 9, pp. 1650–1658, 2006.

[103] H. A. P. Batatinha, C. E. da Costa, E. de França et al., "Carbohydrate use and reduction in number of balance beam falls: implications for mental and physical fatigue," *Journal of the International Society of Sports Nutrition*, vol. 10, article 32, 2013.

[104] J. W. Smith, K. A. Lee, J. P. Dobson, T. J. Roberts, and A. E. Jeukendrup, "Fluid and carbohydrate ingestion improve performance in American football players," *Medicine & Science in Sports & Exercise*, vol. 45, no. 5, supplement, p. 549, 2013.

[105] H. J. Petrie, E. A. Stover, and C. A. Horswill, "Nutritional concerns for the child and adolescent competitor," *Nutrition*, vol. 20, no. 7-8, pp. 620–631, 2004.

[106] E. A. Stover, J. Zachwieja, J. Stofan, R. Murray, and C. A. Horswill, "Consistently high urine specific gravity in adolescent American football players and the impact of an acute drinking strategy," *International Journal of Sports Medicine*, vol. 27, no. 4, pp. 330–335, 2006.

[107] D. J. Casa, L. E. Armstrong, S. K. Hillman et al., "National athletic trainers' association position statement: fluid replacement for athletes," *Journal of Athletic Training*, vol. 35, no. 2, pp. 212–224, 2000.

[108] J. González-Alonso, R. Mora-Rodríguez, P. R. Below, and E. F. Coyle, "Dehydration markedly impairs cardiovascular function in hyperthermic endurance athletes during exercise," *Journal of Applied Physiology*, vol. 82, no. 4, pp. 1229–1236, 1997.

[109] S. J. Montain and E. F. Coyle, "Influence of graded dehydration on hyperthermia and cardiovascular drift during exercise," *Journal of Applied Physiology*, vol. 73, no. 4, pp. 1340–1350, 1992.

[110] R. Murray, "Dehydration, hyperthermia, and athletes: science and practice," *Journal of Athletic Training*, vol. 31, no. 3, pp. 248–252, 1996.

[111] L. B. Baker, D. E. Conroy, and W. L. Kenney, "Dehydration impairs vigilance-related attention in male basketball players," *Medicine and Science in Sports and Exercise*, vol. 39, no. 6, pp. 976–983, 2007.

[112] G. Arnaoutis, S. A. Kavouras, Y. P. Kotsis, Y. E. Tsekouras, M. Makrillos, and C. N. Bardis, "Ad libitum fluid intake does not prevent dehydration in suboptimally hydrated young soccer players during a training session of a summer camp," *International Journal of Sport Nutrition and Exercise Metabolism*, vol. 23, no. 3, pp. 245–251, 2013.

[113] N. R. Decher, D. J. Casa, S. W. Yeargin et al., "Hydration status, knowledge, and behavior in youths at summer sports camps," *International Journal of Sports Physiology and Performance*, vol. 3, no. 3, pp. 262–278, 2008.

[114] S. A. Kavouras, G. Arnaoutis, M. Makrillos et al., "Educational intervention on water intake improves hydration status and enhances exercise performance in athletic youth," *Scandinavian Journal of Medicine and Science in Sports*, vol. 22, no. 5, pp. 684–689, 2012.

[115] M. D. Hoffman, T. Hew-Butler, and K. J. Stuempfle, "Exercise-associated hyponatremia and hydration status in 161-km ultramarathoners," *Medicine and Science in Sports and Exercise*, vol. 45, no. 4, pp. 784–791, 2013.

[116] D. M. J. Vrijens and N. J. Rehrer, "Sodium-free fluid ingestion decreases plasma sodium during exercise in the heat," *Journal of Applied Physiology*, vol. 86, no. 6, pp. 1847–1851, 1999.

[117] American Dietetic Association, "Position of the American Dietetic Association: food fortification and dietary supplements," *Journal of the American Dietetic Association*, vol. 101, no. 1, pp. 115–125, 2001.

[118] American Academy of Pediatrics, Committee on Nutrition, and L. A. Barness, *Pediatric Nutrition Handbook*, American Academy of Pediatrics, Elk Grove Village, Ill, USA, 6th edition, 2009.

[119] T. Rankinen, M. Fogelholm, U. Kujala, R. Rauramaa, and M. Uusitupa, "Dietary intake and nutritional status of athletic and nonathletic children in early puberty," *International Journal of Sport Nutrition*, vol. 5, no. 2, pp. 136–150, 1995.

[120] World Health Organization, *Nutrition in Adolescence—Issues and Challenges for the Health Sector*, WHO, Geneva, Switzerland, 2005.

[121] B. Ekblom, A. N. Goldbarg, and B. Gullbring, "Response to exercise after blood loss and reinfusion," *Journal of Applied Physiology*, vol. 33, no. 2, pp. 175–180, 1972.

[122] P. S. Hinton, "Iron and the endurance athlete," *Applied Physiology, Nutrition, and Metabolism*, vol. 39, no. 9, pp. 1012–1018, 2014.

[123] J. Malczewska, G. Raczynski, and R. Stupnicki, "Iron status in female endurance athletes and in non-athletes," *International Journal of Sport Nutrition and Exercise Metabolism*, vol. 10, no. 3, pp. 260–276, 2000.

[124] R. A. Raunikar and H. Sabio, "Anemia in the adolescent athlete," *American Journal of Diseases of Children*, vol. 146, no. 10, pp. 1201–1205, 1992.

[125] T. W. Rowland, S. A. Black, and J. F. Kelleher, "Iron deficiency in adolescent endurance athletes," *Journal of Adolescent Health Care*, vol. 8, no. 4, pp. 322–326, 1987.

[126] Institute of Medicine (U.S.) Panel on Micronutrients, *Dietary Reference Intakes for Vitamin A, Vitamin K, Arsenic, Boron, Chromium, Copper, Iodine, Iron, Manganese, Molybdenum, Nickel, Silicon, Vanadium, and Zinc*, National Academy Press, Washington, DC, USA, 2001.

[127] J. D. Cook and M. B. Reddy, "Effect of ascorbic acid intake on nonheme-iron absorption from a complete diet," *The American Journal of Clinical Nutrition*, vol. 73, no. 1, pp. 93–98, 2001.

[128] A. C. Ross, J. E. Manson, S. A. Abrams et al., "The 2011 report on dietary reference intakes for calcium and vitamin D from the institute of medicine: what clinicians need to know," *Journal of Clinical Endocrinology and Metabolism*, vol. 96, no. 1, pp. 53–58, 2011.

[129] J.-P. Bonjour and T. Chevalley, "Pubertal timing, bone acquisition, and risk of fracture throughout life," *Endocrine Reviews*, vol. 35, no. 5, pp. 820–847, 2014.

[130] A. C. Looker, C. M. Loria, M. D. Carroll, M. A. McDowell, and C. L. Johnson, "Calcium intakes of Mexican Americans, Cubans, Puerto Ricans, non-Hispanic whites, and non-Hispanic blacks in the United States," *Journal of the American Dietetic Association*, vol. 93, no. 11, pp. 1274–1279, 1993.

[131] L. Gueguen and A. Pointillart, "The bioavailability of dietary calcium," *Journal of the American College of Nutrition*, vol. 19, no. 2, pp. 119S–136S, 2000.

[132] C. Cavadini, A. M. Siega-Riz, and B. M. Popkin, "U.S. adolescent food intake trends from 1965 to 1996," *Archives of Disease in Childhood*, vol. 83, no. 1, pp. 18–24, 2000.

[133] B. A. Barton, A. L. Eldridge, D. Thompson et al., "The relationship of breakfast and cereal consumption to nutrient intake and body mass index: the National Heart, Lung, and Blood Institute Growth and Health Study," *Journal of the American Dietetic Association*, vol. 105, no. 9, pp. 1383–1389, 2005.

10

A Meta-Analysis of Soccer Injuries on Artificial Turf and Natural Grass

Jay H. Williams, Emmanuel Akogyrem, and Jeremy R. Williams

Department of Human Nutrition, Foods and Exercise, Virginia Polytechnic Institute and State University, Blacksburg, VA 24060, USA

Correspondence should be addressed to Jay H. Williams; jhwms@vt.edu

Academic Editor: Adrian W. Midgley

The goal of this investigation was to determine if playing or training on third-generation artificial turf (AT) surfaces increases the incidence rate of injuries compared to natural grass (NG) surfaces. This was accomplished by a meta-analysis performed on previously published research. Eight studies met the criteria of competitive soccer players, participation on both surfaces, and presentation of both exposure time and injury occurrence. Exposure time and injury incidence values were used to generate injury rate ratios (IRRs, AT/NG) for all injuries as well as specific injuries. Subgroup analyses were also performed by condition (match or training), gender, and age (youth or adult). The overall IRR was 0.86 ($P < .05$) suggesting a lower injury risk on AT than NG. However, there was considerable heterogeneity between studies. Analyses of individual injuries and subgroups found that in many cases IRR values were significantly less than 1.0. In no case was the IRR significantly greater than 1.0. Based on this, it appears that the risk of sustaining an injury on AT under some conditions might be lowered compared to NG. However, until more is known about how issues such as altered playing styles affect injury incidence, it is difficult to make firm conclusions regarding the influence of AT on player safety.

1. Introduction

Unfortunately, acute injuries are far too common in the sport of soccer. Sprains and ruptures of the ligaments supporting the ankle and knee joints as well as muscle strains occur quite often. In some cases, joint injuries are sustained through contact with another player. A classic example occurs when one player collides with another, applying excessive force to the lateral side of the opponent's knee. This often results in damage to the medial collateral ligament, lateral meniscus, and the anterior cruciate ligament (ACL). However, a substantial number of soccer injuries occur through noncontact mechanisms. In these cases, an athlete may plant his or her foot then stop, cut, or turn. As the body changes direction while the foot is stationary, the knee and/or ankle experiences torque. As a result, ligament structures can be strained or ruptured.

Researchers have identified a number of risk factors for noncontact injuries. These include intrinsic factors such as proprioception, muscular strength, ligament properties, and biomechanics as well as extrinsic factors such as the playing surface and other environmental conditions. Several studies have focused on this latter factor as important, specifically the use of artificial turf playing surfaces. They suggest that the added friction between the shoe and the surface increases the torque experienced by the ankle and knee [1, 2]. This, in turn, raises the risk of a ligament injury. In fact, early studies on the first-generation artificial turf (AT) fields ("Astroturf-type" surfaces) did show an increased injury risk compared to natural grass (NG) [3, 4]. However, the nature of AT has changed over the past 10 years. The short-pile carpet laid over a thin pad has been replaced by a surface that contains long "grass-like" fibers that are embedded with granules of crushed rubber, sand, and/or silica and laid over a thick pad. This results in a more compliant surface and one that results in a considerably lower shoe-surface coefficient of friction [1]. Manufacturers of third-generation AT surfaces argue that such a design may lower the risk of noncontact joint injury. On the other hand, many coaches, trainers, and athletes remain concerned that playing on AT increases injury risk.

Whether or not third-generation AT alters the risk of noncontact injury remains unresolved. Several recent studies have focused on comparing injury incidence rates in soccer players who train and/or play matches on both AT and NG. Unfortunately, the results are somewhat variable, with some studies showing reduced risk of some injuries on AT and others showing no difference or slightly increased risk. Thus, the purpose of this investigation was to resolve this issue. To accomplish this, we used previous research and a meta-analytic approach to compare injury rates in soccer players performing on AT and NG.

2. Methods

PubMed and Google Scholar searches were used to identify individual studies. Key search terms were soccer, injury, grass, synthetic turf, and artificial turf. To be included in the meta-analysis, studies met several criteria: (1) focused on competitive soccer players, (2) compared acute injuries sustained during soccer matches and/or training on NG and on third-generation AT surfaces, (3) examined players who participated on both surfaces during the study period rather than teams that used one surface exclusively, (4) used the injury definition as described by Fuller et al. [5], (5) reported both exposure times and injury occurrences for play on AT and NG, and (6) written in English or an English translation.

The studies meeting our criteria were examined and exposure times, injury occurrences, and playing surface were recorded. In addition, the playing condition (match or training), gender, and age (youth or adult) were noted. Values for all acute injuries (regardless of type) were recorded. Chronic injuries were not considered as these could be attributed to both surfaces or to other causes. Acute knee injuries, ankle injuries, foot injuries, sprains, and muscle strains were recorded. These specific locations and types of injuries were selected because they were the most consistently defined across all of the included studies.

Crude injury rates were computed using the unweighted sum of total injuries and exposure times from all eight studies. Statistical analyses were performed on adjusted injury incidence rate ratios (IRRs, AT/NG) using the Mantel-Haenszel method for fixed effects. Upper and lower 95% confidence intervals were also computed. Significance was established at the 0.05 level. IRR values were first computed for entire data set. The data were then categorized based on condition (match or training), gender, and age (youth or adult).

3. Results

An initial literature search on PubMed returned more than 25 citations. Of those, eight studies met our criteria. These are shown in Table 1 along with key characteristics of each study. As can be seen, individual studies varied in terms of the number of players and teams examined. In addition, the period of investigation ranged from several months to several years resulting in varying exposure times. Three studies focused on either match or training injuries exclusively while five included both conditions. One study examined females exclusively and one did not categorize their data by gender. Five of the studies focused on adult players, generally college or professional players, whereas three studies focused on youth players that were 12 to 17 years of age.

The eight studies resulted in a total exposure time of 1,498,343 hours. Of that, 571,196 hours were played on AT (34.5%) and 981,147 on NG (65.5%). The amount of time spent in training and playing on AT and NG varied between studies. In the study by Soligard et al. [12], players competed on AT for less than 10% of the total time played. At the other end of the range, Ekstrand et al. [8] studied players who trained and competed on AT nearly three times as long as on NG. Matches accounted for 271,022 hours (18.1%) of total exposure time whereas training accounted for 1,227,321 hours (81.9%). Of the total exposure time, males accounted for 949,568 hours (66.1%) and females for 486,178 hours (33.9%). Soligard et al. [12] did not distinguish between male and female players and was not included in the analysis of gender.

A total of 9737 injuries were recorded with 2670 occurring on AT (27.4%) and 7067 on NG (75.6%). This resulted in crude injury incidence rates of 5.16 and 7.20 injuries per 1000 hours for AT and NG, respectively. Crude incidence rates for matches were 20.26 and 24.45 injuries per 1000 hours for AT and NG. For training injures on AT and NG, the incidence rates were 2.91 and 2.68 injuries per 1000 hours.

Figure 1 shows the injury IRRs for each of the studies examined along with the overall adjusted IRR of 0.86 (0.74–0.93, $P < 0.05$). This analysis included all reported injures and all categories examined. Five of the eight studies showed IRRs that were significantly lower than 1.0, indicating a lower incidence rate on AT [7–9, 12, 13], while the other three showed nonsignificant differences. The overall adjusted IRR was statistically significant with a lower incidence rate on AT.

Figure 2 shows the overall IRRs of specific injuries and locations. For knee, ankle, and foot injuries as well as sprains, incidence rates were significantly lower on AT compared to NG. The overall IRR for muscle strains was not significant.

The adjusted IRRs for the subcategory analyses are shown in Table 2. Analyses of male, female, youth, and adult subcategories for all injuries showed IRR values significantly lower than 1.0. For knee injuries, incidence rates on AT were lower for training injuries and adults. For sprains, incidence rates were lower on AT for females and adults. For muscle strains, incidence rates were lower on AT for match injuries, males, and both young and adult players. In no case was injury incidence increased on AT.

There was considerable heterogeneity across the studies examined. For the entire data set, including all injuries as well as both conditions, gender and age (Figure 1), the I^2 value was 80%. A portion of the heterogeneity was due to different injuries and locations. For specific injuries and sites (Figure 2), I^2 ranged between 43% and 74%. Condition, gender, and age also contributed as I^2 values for these categories ranged from 0 to 80%. We found that variations in exposure to AT accounted for some of the heterogeneity. Figure 3 shows a significant negative correlation between the relative amount of time spent on AT (AT exposure/NG exposure) and the IRR for each study. As can be seen, the two studies in which the greater exposure time on AT had the lowest IRR.

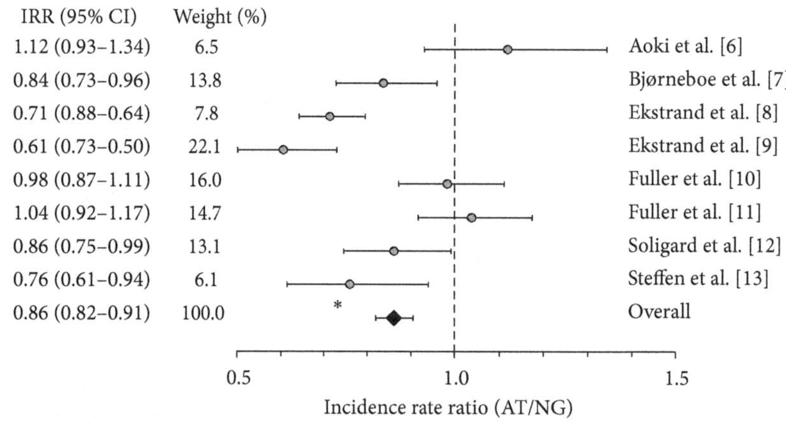

Figure 1: Injury incidence rate ratios for all injuries occurring on AT and NG (95% CI) $^{*}P < 0.05$.

Table 1: Descriptions of the studies used in the meta-analyses.

ID	Study	Condition	Gender	Age	Subjects	Study duration	Exposure (hr)	Injuries	Notes
1	Aoki et al. [6]	Both	Male	Youth	332 players	12 months	106,783	484	Ages 12–17 years. Injury location and type reported for training only.
2	Bjørneboe et al. [7]	Both	Male	Adult	14 clubs	4 seasons	261,541	1067	Professional teams in the Norwegian Tippeligaen.
3	Ekstrand et al. [8]	Both	Both	Adult	767 players	Followed teams for 4–38 months	246,475	1492	European elite players. Included “slight” injuries that required players to miss <1 day (~2% of total injuries). Since these could not be extracted, they were included in the present study.
4	Ekstrand et al. [9]	Both	Male	Adult	492 players	Followed teams for 4–32 months	82,874	449	European professional players. Compared two cohorts of players. The cohort of players that trained and played exclusively on grass were omitted from the current study.
5	Fuller et al. [10]	Match	Both	Adult	116 teams 126 teams	1st season 2nd season	79,253	1794	US College players. Utilized the NCAA Injury Surveillance System.
6	Fuller et al. [11]	Training	Both	Adult	116 teams 126 teams	1st season 2nd season	545,842	1592	US College players. Utilized the NCAA Injury Surveillance System.
7	Soligard et al. [12]	Match	Both	Youth	>68,000 players	4 occasions of a single tournament	62,597	2454	Norway Cup youth tournament. Matches played over six consecutive days. Ages 13–19 years. Data for male and female players were pooled.
8	Steffen et al. [13]	Both	Female	Youth	2020 players	8 months	113,023	405	Under-17 age group.

Table 2: Adjusted rate ratios for subcategory injuries (95% CI).

	ID	All injuries	Knee injuries	Ankle injuries	Foot injuries[1]	Sprains	Muscle strains
Match	1, 2, 3, 4, 5, 7, 8	0.97 (0.91–1.04)	1.04 (0.91–1.20)	0.98 (0.86–1.12)	0.82 (0.67–1.00)	0.97 (0.87–1.09)	0.85 (0.75–0.97)*
Training	1, 2, 3, 4, 6, 7, 8	1.04 (0.96–1.13)	0.77 (0.69–0.94)*	1.07 (0.92–1.24)	1.02 (0.75–1.38)	1.15 (0.99–1.30)	0.90 (0.78–1.03)
Male	1, 2, 3, 4, 5, 6, 7	0.87 (0.81–0.92)*	0.79 (0.69–1.03)	0.98 (0.87–1.11)	0.92 (0.74–1.15)	1.06 (0.96–1.17)	0.74 (0.66–0.83)
Female	3, 5, 6, 7, 8	0.85 (0.76–0.94)*	0.94 (0.77–1.16)	0.83 (0.67–1.02)	1.04 (0.73–1.49)	0.67 (0.56–0.79)*	0.84 (0.70–1.02)
Youth	1, 7, 8	0.90 (0.82–1.00)*	0.90 (0.66–1.23)	0.89 (0.74–1.08)	0.85 (0.57–1.28)	1.03 (0.84–1.26)	0.54 (0.36–0.81)*
Adult	2, 3, 4, 5, 6	0.85 (0.80–0.90)*	0.82 (0.72–0.92)*	0.89 (0.79–1.00)	0.96 (0.80–1.16)	0.89 (0.81–0.98)*	0.79 (0.72–0.87)*

$^{*}P < 0.05$. [1]Studies 1, 4, and 8 did not define foot injuries.

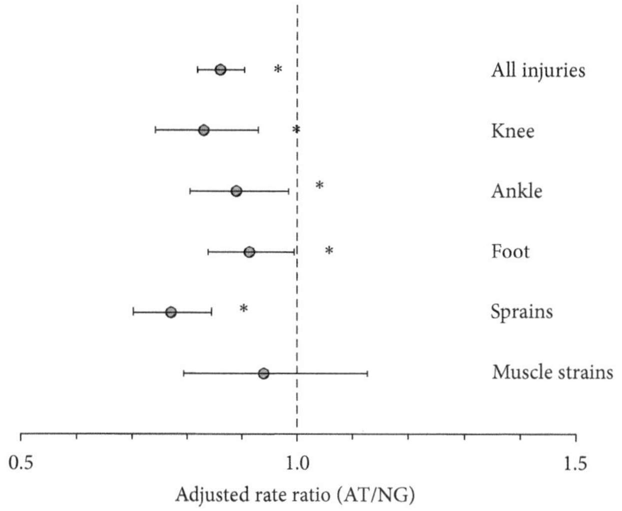

FIGURE 2: Incidence rate ratios for various injuries occurring on AT and NG (95% CI) $^*P < 0.05$.

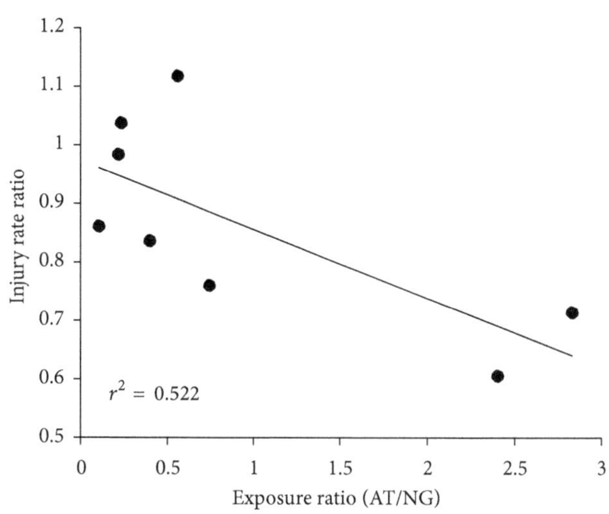

FIGURE 3: The correlation between the exposure ratio (exposure on AT/NG) and the injury incidence rate ratio. Each data point represents a single study.

4. Discussion

This meta-analysis examined eight studies that compared soccer injury rates occurring on AT and NG. In total, these studies report nearly 1.5 million hours of training and match play and almost 10,000 injuries. The adjusted IRR for all injures was significantly less than 1.0 indicating lower incidence rates for playing and training on AT. For specific categories and specific injuries, several IRR values were less than 1.0. In no case did we find an IRR value significantly greater than 1.0. Thus, the overall results of our analyses do not support the idea that playing or training on AT increases the risk of injury compared to NG. In fact, our analyses suggest that AT surfaces may reduce injury incidence for some types of injuries within specific categorizations.

There are several criticisms of our study that should be pointed out. First, despite the guidelines provided by Fuller et al. [5], the eight studies varied in terms of their injury descriptions. For example, Ekstrand et al. [8, 9] reported the incidence of injuries based on location and type (e.g., "knee sprains"), whereas Bjørneboe et al. [7], Fuller et al. [10, 11], Soligard et al. [12], and Steffen et al. [13] described injuries by location (e.g., "knee") or type (e.g., "sprain"). Only Ekstrand et al. [9] noted specific injuries such as "anterior cruciate ligament tears." Thus, our results are limited to the general classifications of location (knee, ankle, and foot) or type (sprains and muscle strains). Second, in one study [12], exposure and incidence values for males and females were pooled. This study was excluded from the subcategory analysis of gender. Third, the severity of injuries is categorized based on the number of training and match days missed. Unfortunately, there is inconsistency in this method between studies. For example, a "minor" or "mild" injury was defined as 1–7 days [7, 10, 11, 13], 4–7 days [8, 12], and 1–2 weeks [6] missed. Classification of severe injuries also varied from >21 to >28 days missed. Given these discrepancies, we were not confident using severity as a subcategory for analysis. Fourth, the studies failed to report environmental conditions such as temperature, wet/dry field conditions, or shoe type/cleat design. Finally, only three of the studies differentiated between contact and noncontact injuries [10, 11, 13]. This is an important limitation since contact injuries may or may not be directly attributable to playing surface.

Our results do not provide an explanation for possible reductions in injury risk on AT. Artificial turf surfaces provide a more consistent playing surface than NG, free of bare sports, ruts, and divots which could affect injury risk. However, the studies examined focused on teams competing at a high level, so it is likely that the NG surfaces were of high quality. Traditionally, physical characteristics of AT and frictional resistance at the shoe-surface interface have given rise to suggestions of greater injury risk on AT. However, laboratory experiments yield conflicting results regarding this idea. Several studies show greater rotational torque between the shoe and AT compared to NG [2, 14], whereas Cawley et al. [1] show higher values on NG. Livesay et al. [2] further argue that stiffness (the rate of change in torque) may play a role in injury risk. Yet, greater peak torque on AT does not result in increased stiffness. In human studies, Ford et al. [15] found different foot loading patterns during cutting maneuvers performed on AT and NG. On the other hand, Potthast [16] reported no differences in rear foot and ankle movements of the plant foot when goal kicking between NG and rubber-filled AT. McGhie and Ettema [17] found that impact forces experienced during cutting maneuvers on AT were not indicative of a hazardous condition. To further complicate this issue, torque and stiffness can be affected by the type of cleat worn on a particular surface as well as the temperature of the surface [2, 14]. Thus, it is difficult to conclude with confidence which of the physical characteristics of AT accounts for difference in injury incidence rates found in the present study.

It is possible that other factors may impact injury potential. For example, players seem to alter their style of play on AT. Match analyses show that the amount of time spent running at different intensities is similar between surfaces, but fewer slide tackles and shorter passes are executed on AT [18]. The reduction in slide tackles may stem from the fear of skin abrasions but may limit the number of "high risk" situations for injury, particularly contact injuries. Players also have more negative perceptions of playing on AT. They feel that heat as well as speed of play on AT requires greater physical effort compared to grass [18, 19]. However, these perceptions have been difficult to confirm as some controlled studies show increased energy expenditure while others show no differences in fatigue [20–23]. Ronkainen et al. [19] note that negative player perceptions of AT are stronger in those who have limited exposure to AT or are exposed to AT later in their careers. Figure 3 suggests that more time spent in training and competing on AT is associated with lower injury risk. Perhaps with increased exposure to AT, players develop a less aggressive play with fewer slide tackles that reduces injury risk. It should be pointed out, however, that this idea is speculative at this time. Clearly more research is needed regarding player movements, energy expenditure, and fatigue on AT and NG surfaces.

This study highlights several areas that need to be addressed before firm conclusions can be drawn. First, three of the eight studies focused only on male players [6, 7, 9]. Given the concern over the high incidence of ACL injuries in women, it seems reasonable to suggest that more information is needed regarding playing surface as a potential risk factor in females. Second, there is a need for uniformity in categorizing the severity of injury. Third, injury classification by location and type should be standardized and encouraged. More detailed classification would provide a better understanding of the risk of specific injuries. Fourth, more studies are needed on energy expenditure and fatigue on AT and NG, especially using activities that replicate match play. Given that fatigue can increase the risk of joint injury [24], it is important to understand if player perceptions of increased effort on AT have a physiological basis. Fifth, while preliminary studies suggest that players adjust their style of play on AT, it is not clear if this occurs across levels of play and across genders. Identifying specific movement patterns that either increase or decrease injury risk on AT could impact player training. Finally, more data are needed on young players. As the use of AT in club and school settings increases, a thorough understanding of safety and injury risks in youth and adolescent players is essential.

In this investigation, we found no evidence that playing matches or training on AT raises the risk of soccer players sustaining injury. In fact, the evidence suggests that the risk of some injuries and some subgroups might be lowered. However, until more is known about how issues such as altered playing styles affect injury incidence, it is difficult to make firm conclusions regarding the direct and indirect roles of AT in player safety.

References

[1] P. W. Cawley, R. S. Heidt Jr., P. E. Scranton Jr., G. M. Losse, and M. E. Howard, "Physiologic axial load, frictional resistance, and the football shoe-surface interface," *Foot and Ankle International*, vol. 24, no. 7, pp. 551–556, 2003.

[2] G. A. Livesay, D. R. Reda, and E. A. Nauman, "Peak torque and rotational stiffness developed at the shoe-surface interface: the effect of shoe type and playing surface," *The American Journal of Sports Medicine*, vol. 34, no. 3, pp. 415–422, 2006.

[3] K. D. Bowers Jr. and R. B. Martin, "Cleat surface friction on new and old astroturf," *Medicine and Science in Sports and Exercise*, vol. 7, no. 2, pp. 132–135, 1975.

[4] J. W. Powell and M. Schootman, "A multivariate risk analysis of selected playing surfaces in the National Football League: 1980 to 1989. An epidemiologic study of knee injuries," *The American Journal of Sports Medicine*, vol. 20, no. 6, pp. 686–694, 1992.

[5] C. W. Fuller, J. Ekstrand, A. Junge et al., "Consensus statement on injury definitions and data collection procedures in studies of football (soccer) injuries," *The British Journal of Sports Medicine*, vol. 40, no. 3, pp. 193–201, 2006.

[6] H. Aoki, T. Kohno, H. Fujiya et al., "Incidence of injury among adolescent soccer players: a comparative study of artificial and natural grass turfs," *Clinical Journal of Sport Medicine*, vol. 20, no. 1, pp. 1–7, 2010.

[7] J. Bjørneboe, R. Bahr, and T. E. Andersen, "Risk of injury on third-generation artifi cial turf in Norwegian professional football," *The British Journal of Sports Medicine*, vol. 44, no. 11, pp. 794–798, 2010.

[8] J. Ekstrand, M. Hägglund, and C. W. Fuller, "Comparison of injuries sustained on artificial turf and grass by male and female elite football players," *Scandinavian Journal of Medicine and Science in Sports*, vol. 21, no. 6, pp. 824–832, 2011.

[9] J. Ekstrand, T. Timpka, and M. Hägglund, "Risk of injury in elite football played on artificial turf versus natural grass: a prospective two-cohort study," *The British Journal of Sports Medicine*, vol. 40, no. 12, pp. 975–980, 2006.

[10] C. W. Fuller, R. W. Dick, J. Corlette, and R. Schmalz, "Comparison of the incidence, nature and cause of injuries sustained on grass and new generation artificial turf by male and female football players. Part 1: match injuries," *The British Journal of Sports Medicine*, vol. 41, supplement 1, pp. i20–i26, 2007.

[11] C. W. Fuller, R. W. Dick, J. Corlette, and R. Schmalz, "Comparison of the incidence, nature and cause of injuries sustained on grass and new generation artificial turf by male and female football players. Part 2: training injuries," *The British Journal of Sports Medicine*, vol. 41, supplement 1, pp. i27–i32, 2007.

[12] T. Soligard, R. Bahr, and T. E. Andersen, "Injury risk on artificial turf and grass in youth tournament football," *Scandinavian Journal of Medicine and Science in Sports*, vol. 22, no. 3, pp. 356–361, 2012.

[13] K. Steffen, T. E. Andersen, and R. Bahr, "Risk of injury on artificial turf and natural grass in young female football players," *The British Journal of Sports Medicine*, vol. 41, supplement 1, pp. i33–i37, 2007.

[14] M. R. Villwock, E. G. Meyer, J. W. Powell, A. J. Fouty, and R. C. Haut, "Football playing surface and shoe design affect rotational traction," *The American Journal of Sports Medicine*, vol. 37, no. 3, pp. 518–525, 2009.

[15] K. R. Ford, N. A. Manson, B. J. Evans et al., "Comparison of in-shoe foot loading patterns on natural grass and synthetic turf," *Journal of Science and Medicine in Sport*, vol. 9, no. 6, pp. 433–440, 2006.

[16] W. Potthast, "Motion differences in goal kicking on natural and artificial soccer turf systems," *Footwear Science*, vol. 2, no. 1, pp. 29–35, 2010.

[17] D. McGhie and G. Ettema, "Biomechanical analysis of surface-athlete impacts on third-generation artificial turf," *The American Journal of Sports Medicine*, vol. 41, no. 1, pp. 177–185, 2013.

[18] H. Andersson, B. Ekblom, and P. Krustrup, "Elite football on artificial turf versus natural grass: movement patterns, technical standards, and player impressions," *Journal of Sports Sciences*, vol. 26, no. 2, pp. 113–122, 2008.

[19] J. Ronkainen, P. Osei-Owusu, J. Webster, A. Harland, and J. Roberts, "Elite player assessment of playing surfaces for football," *Procedia Engineering*, vol. 34, pp. 837–842, 2012.

[20] R. di Michele, A. M. di Renzo, S. Ammazzalorso, and F. Merni, "Comparison of physiological responses to an incremental running test on treadmill, natural grass, and synthetic turf in young soccer players," *Journal of Strength and Conditioning Research*, vol. 23, no. 3, pp. 939–945, 2009.

[21] M. G. Hughes, L. Birdsey, R. Meyers et al., "Effects of playing surface on physiological responses and performance variables in a controlled football simulation," *Journal of Sport Science*, vol. 31, no. 8, pp. 878–886, 2013.

[22] M. Nédélec, A. McCall, C. Carling, F. le Gall, S. Berthoin, and G. Dupont, "Physical performance and subjective ratings after a soccer-specific exercise simulation: comparison of natural grass versus artificial turf," *Journal of Sport Science*, vol. 31, no. 5, pp. 529–536, 2013.

[23] A. Sassi, A. Stefanescu, P. Menaspa, A. Bosio, M. Riggio, and E. Rampinini, "The cost of running on natural grass and artificial turf surfaces," *Journal of Strength and Conditioning Research*, vol. 25, no. 3, pp. 606–611, 2011.

[24] S. G. McLean and J. E. Samorezov, "Fatigue-induced acl injury risk stems from a degradation in central control," *Medicine and Science in Sports and Exercise*, vol. 41, no. 8, pp. 1661–1672, 2009.

11

Functional Popliteal Artery Entrapment Syndrome: Poorly Understood and Frequently Missed? A Review of Clinical Features, Appropriate Investigations, and Treatment Options

Matthew Hislop,[1] Dominic Kennedy,[2] Brendan Cramp,[2] and Sanjay Dhupelia[2]

[1] *Brisbane Sports and Exercise Medicine Specialists Clinic, 87 Riding Road, Brisbane, QLD 4171, Australia*
[2] *Queensland X-Ray, Greenslopes Private Hospital, Brisbane, QLD 4120, Australia*

Correspondence should be addressed to Matthew Hislop; mhislop@bsems.com.au

Academic Editor: Adrian W. Midgley

Functional popliteal artery entrapment syndrome (PAES) is an important and possibly underrecognized cause of exertional leg pain (ELP). As it is poorly understood, it is at risk of misdiagnosis and mismanagement. The features indicative of PAES are outlined, as it can share features with other causes of ELP. Investigating functional PAES is also fraught with potential problems and if it is performed incorrectly, it can result in false negative and false positive findings. A review of the current vascular investigations is provided, highlighting some of the limitations standard tests have in determining functional PAES. Once a clinical suspicion for PAES is satisfied, it is necessary to further distinguish the subcategories of anatomical and functional entrapment and the group of asymptomatic occluders. When definitive entrapment is confirmed, it is important to identify the level of entrapment so that precise intervention can be performed. Treatment strategies for functional PAES are discussed, including the possibility of a new, less invasive intervention of guided Botulinum toxin injection at the level of entrapment as an alternative to vascular surgery.

1. Introduction

Functional popliteal artery entrapment syndrome (PAES) is an important and possibly underrecognized cause of exertional leg pain. It shares many features with other causes of exertional leg pain, and more than one condition can be present at once, confusing the clinical picture. An understanding of the typical presenting features of the common causes of exertional leg pain is essential, allowing the clinician to determine those suggestive of PAES and requiring further investigation.

Investigating functional PAES is fraught with potential problems and, if performed incorrectly, can result in false negative and false positive findings. The authors believe that currently accepted vascular investigations such as ankle-brachial indices and Doppler ultrasound performed at rest are not accurate in investigating functional PAES. Rather, a review of the literature would suggest that investigations such as provocative Doppler ultrasound and MRI angiography are performed as soon as possible after reproducing symptoms to "capture" the occlusion while it is occurring.

Once the diagnosis of functional PAES is confirmed, there are a number of treatment strategies available. Until recently, definitive intervention was only available in the form of vascular surgery with variable myotomies and releases. We provide information on a Pilot study suggesting a new less invasive intervention of guided botulinum toxin injection to the level of entrapment, as an alternative to surgical intervention.

2. Clinical Features and Differential Diagnosis of Exertional Leg Pain

PAES shares many clinical features with other causes of exertional leg pain, most of which are thought to be more

TABLE 1: Differential diagnosis and clinical features of exertional leg pain.

Condition	Incidence	Male/female preponderance	Unilateral/bilateral tendency	Site of pain	Pain present at rest	Pattern of pain
MTSS	13–42%	Possibly female	Bilateral	Posteromedial tibial border	Yes (on palpation)	Pain with activity can warm up and returns on cessation
Stress fracture	Unknown (0.7–20% exercising population)	Possibly female	Unilateral	Variable depending on site of stress fracture	Yes (on palpation)	Pain with impact activity
CECS	27–33%	Nil	Bilateral	Typically anterior and/or deep posterior compartments	No	Crescendo-decrescendo pattern: pain can last for minutes to hours on cessation
PAES (anatomical)	0.6–3.5% (rare)	Possibly male	Possibly unilateral	Typically superficial posterior compartment	Can be at rest (positional)	Crescendo-decrescendo pattern: pain can last for seconds to minutes on cessation
PAES (functional)	Unknown (possibly common and underrecognized)	Possibly female	Likely bilateral	Typically superficial posterior compartment	Can be at rest (positional)	Crescendo-decrescendo pattern: pain can last for seconds to minutes on cessation

common [1]. Adding to the complexity, more than one cause of exertional leg pain may be present in an individual patient at any one time. Chronic exertional compartment syndrome (CECS) in particular has many of the same features of PAES and the two conditions can be confused [2, 3]. Also, it is not possible to distinguish between anatomical and functional PAES on clinical symptoms alone. A detailed history and examination provide very useful information and help determine whether further investigation is warranted. An outline of the more common differential diagnoses of exertional leg pain and their features follows and a summary is provided in Table 1.

2.1. Medial Tibial Stress Syndrome (MTSS). This condition is thought to represent the most common cause of exertional leg pain [4] with an incidence between 13 and 42% [5]. Patients describe typically bilateral leg pain along a strip of the distal third of the posteromedial tibial border that comes on early with exercise and may warm up but usually will ache for some time after stopping [6]. The pain is also impact related [7]. Examination at rest will usually reveal palpable tenderness along the distal third of the posteromedial tibial border and pain with hopping [6]. Some studies suggest a possible predisposition of MTSS in females [8].

2.2. Stress Fractures. While stress fractures are not common in the nonexercising population, they are thought to represent 0.7–20% of sports medicine clinic presentations [6]. Patients typically complain of pain that is focal and palpable (unless the site is covered by a significant muscle layer where symptoms can be vague and nondescript). With lower limb stress fractures, pain often presents early with impact related exercise and is worse during the landing phase of running [7]. Stress fractures are typically unilateral and can affect any bone in the lower limbs, although the tibia is most common [1, 9]. Female athletes are thought to be at greater risk of developing stress fractures than males [8] and Bennell et al. suggest that menstrual disturbances, caloric restriction, lower bone density, muscle weakness, and leg length differences are important risk factors for stress fracture [10].

2.3. CECS. CECS is thought to have an incidence between 27 and 33% [5]. Patients by definition are pain-free at rest and develop a steadily worsening pain with exertion [11]. The pain will gradually build up over 10–20 minutes and is not rapid in onset (unlike some cases of PAES). The pain is typically isolated to one or more compartments, most commonly anterior and deep posterior, with the least most common being the superficial posterior compartment (where the majority of PAES pain is described) [5, 9]. Patients describe feelings of "hardness" in their affected compartment. The pain will typically dissipate slowly over minutes to hours but will return quickly if the patient attempts to return to exercise again. Fascial defects are more common but not diagnostic [1, 5]. The leg pain is overwhelmingly bilateral (although unilateral cases can present) and there is no difference in predisposition according to the sex of the individual [7, 11].

2.4. PAES. PAES can be further divided into two groups, anatomical and functional. In the case of anatomical PAES, there is a clearly defined anatomical lesion that directly leads to entrapment and subsequent occlusion of the popliteal artery. The second and larger subgroup of anatomically "normal" or functional PAES is particularly poorly understood [2]. In functional PAES, there is evidence of popliteal artery occlusion and subsequent claudicant symptoms, but no defined lesion can be found that directly causes the occlusion.

Anatomical and functional PAES most likely present in a similar fashion. Patients with anatomical PAES are thought to be older and more sedentary while functional PAES patients are thought to be younger, more commonly female, and more active [3]. Baltopoulos et al. suggest that functional PAES may be bilateral in 25–76% of cases [12]. The true incidence of functional PAES is unknown, and it is described as being rare [8, 13, 14]. However, it is possible that this condition is underreported [15] and the incidence may be greater than previously recognized. The pain is often vague and poorly localized. It occurs most commonly in the "back of the calf" but it can be anterior and lateral especially if the anterior tibial artery is involved [2, 16]. Patients can have pain with minimal exertion or provocative leg positioning and occasionally at rest. Symptoms such as coldness and paraesthesia have also been reported [17]. Running or walking on an incline can occasionally bring on symptoms [3]. The pain follows a claudicant pattern similar to CECS but unlike CECS will resolve more quickly on cessation of exercise [18]. However, an ache may persist for hours. Provocative manoeuvres may result in the development of a reduced peripheral pulses and/or a popliteal bruit on auscultation of the popliteal fossa [7] although this may also be possible in the "asymptomatic occluder" group as outlined later.

3. Examination Findings in Functional PAES

When examining patients with suspected functional PAES, it is important to diagnose and/or exclude other causes of exertional leg pain. Examination includes palpation and percussion over the lower limb to look for signs of bone stress, be it focal at the site of a stress fracture or along a strip of the distal posteromedial tibial border in the case of MTSS. Some authors suggest that PAES must have a combination of pain with hopping, in conjunction with the development of ischaemic signs like pallor, coldness, and reactive hyperaemia [18]. In our experience, pain with hopping more likely indicates some form of bone stress, and the development of physical signs of ischaemia in younger individuals with suspected functional PAES is extremely uncommon.

3.1. Clinical Vascular Provocation Test. A validated clinical provocation test for PAES has not been described in the literature. Some authors describe physical examination as unreliable [7] and rely on clinical suspicion as justification for progressing to vascular investigations. Some do not describe their clinical assessment [2], while others attempt to provoke symptoms by encouraging the patient to hop or climb stairs, followed by a cursory physical examination [18]. Most will assess resting peripheral pulses [12, 18] which should be examined at true rest. The popliteal fossa should be auscultated to determine the presence of a resting bruit. In general, bruits are not audible until an artery is approximately 50% occluded [19]. The sound increases in pitch as the lumen becomes more narrowed to a critical size. Thereafter, the sound may no longer be detectable as the volume of blood flow becomes greatly reduced [19]. If pulses are reduced or a bruit is present at rest, than this would indicate an underlying vascular malformation or significant luminal narrowing (such as in advanced atherosclerosis) and further radiological imaging is indicated.

We have developed a simple clinical test that can be performed in the consulting rooms. After assessing for a popliteal fossa bruit and examining peripheral pulses at rest, the patient is required to perform 15–20 single leg eccentric heel drops off the edge of a step, while asking about any developing or worsening leg pain. Immediately after the test is performed, the popliteal fossa is again auscultated for a bruit, and peripheral pulses are examined for any reduction. In our experience, it is worth auscultating for a number of minutes after exertion, as more significant cases (with complete occlusion) may initially have no bruit, or at least delayed onset of a bruit as flow reestablishes.

We believe that if patients do not develop pain or discomfort with this test, or if a bruit and/or pulse reduction is not evident, then it is unlikely that the patient is suffering from PAES. Unfortunately, the development of pain/bruit/pulse reduction does not mean the patient has PAES, as it is possible that they may fall into the asymptomatic occluder group. Provided that the patient has clinical features suggestive of PAES, a positive result warrants further vascular investigation.

4. Investigations in Functional PAES

Despite PAES being a well-defined condition, no clear-cut consensus regarding the diagnostic work-up of these patients exists [20]. The general population can be divided into four groups, including asymptomatic nonoccluders, who presumably will not present for assessment or investigation. Therefore, the three symptomatic groups that investigation must distinguish are

(1) anatomical PAES,

(2) asymptomatic occluder (i.e., exertional leg pain due to another cause, but in whom the artery can incidentally occlude),

(3) symptomatic occluder, that is, functional PAES.

4.1. Ankle Brachial Indices (ABIs). The ABI is calculated by dividing the systolic blood pressure at the ankle by that at the arm. Measures below 0.8 suggest at least moderate peripheral vascular disease. Some authors recommend the use of ankle brachial indices in standard work-up for functional PAES [3]. However, as occlusion in functional PAES occurs during exertion, testing after exercise is likely to result in a false negative result [20]. There are also difficulties in obtaining ABI measurements during exercise [18] and Pillai suggests that ABIs during forceful plantarflexion are difficult to interpret and not as helpful when assessing graded compression of a patent artery [17]. We agree that ABIs are unreliable for investigating functional PAES.

4.2. Compartment Pressure Testing. Some authors will routinely perform compartment pressure studies in addition to vascular studies in the work-up of suspected PAES [3]. This seems to be excessive and our review of the literature could find no compelling reason as to why this should be mandatory. For this reason we do not recommend routine compartment pressure studies, unless symptoms and history are strongly suggestive of possible concomitant CECS.

4.3. Doppler Ultrasound. Doppler ultrasound provides a relatively cheap, noninvasive, and accessible procedure to assess flow through the popliteal artery, and it is generally recommended that this be the first line investigation for PAES [20, 21]. Despite this, a review of the literature shows no definite consensus on how to perform Doppler ultrasound in investigating PAES [20]. Some authors suggest hand held Doppler units to complement clinical assessment in the rooms. This assesses loss of the posterior tibial artery distal pulse during sustained passive dorsiflexion and plantarflexion of the foot [12]. Doppler ultrasound is user dependent, which can affect reliability. Also, there is a risk of overcalling entrapment with movement of the artery, muscles, or probe during exercise giving the illusion of occlusion [21], but technique variations can usually overcome this.

4.3.1. Provocative Doppler Protocols. Many authors researching PAES suggest that the most important feature in its diagnosis is the reproduction of symptoms with the help of provocative manoeuvres and verification by duplex ultrasonography [17, 18, 21]. Typically, investigations at rest will show a patent popliteal artery with normal distal pulses. In functional PAES, occlusion will often only occur during exertion and can resolve almost immediately. This can give the false impression of no pathology if the assessment is delayed. Even the 30–60 seconds taken from getting off a treadmill to an examination bed and applying the ultrasound probe can be enough for arterial occlusion to cease. Because occlusion can resolve very quickly, immediate assessment after reproduction of symptoms is essential [18]. The position of most occlusions occurs when the patient has their knee extended, and they hold active plantarflexion. It is not possible to hold this position for sustained periods during a MRI due to discomfort and fatigue [21]. Ultrasound is a useful modality, as it allows real time assessment whilst some form of provocation to reproduce symptoms is performed. Despite the agreement that provocation is necessary, a clear and detailed description of the protocols to do this is generally not provided [20]. Our protocols are included below for completeness.

We perform a resting anatomical study first, with the patient in the supine position. We record waveforms and velocities of the peripheral arteries as well as assess for evidence of intimal thickening or fixed arterial disease. The anatomy of the popliteal fossa is assessed, looking particularly for any popliteal artery or soft tissue structure variations or whether the anterior tibial artery has a high bifurcation.

4.4. Provocation. Hoffman et al. [22] found that the force of plantarflexion required to occlude the popliteal artery during provocative positioning is important, with the majority of asymptomatic occluders occluding the popliteal artery with sustained holding of ≥70% of maximal plantarflexion force [22]. For this reason, we use a graded ultrasound protocol progressing through

(1) prone patient holding a position of provocation (knee extension and plantarflexion) against no load,

(2) patient is prone and pushing against approximately 25% of maximal plantarflexion force (Figure 1(a)),

(3) dynamic loading by pushing against 50–100% of maximal plantarflexion force (Figure 1(b)).

Symptomatic patients who occlude in the first 2 categories are presumed to represent more severe cases of functional PAES. If the initial 2 assessments are negative, the patient is assessed in an erect weight-bearing position while cycling through range of motion. This is thought to represent somewhere between 50 and 100% maximal plantarflexion force and may more reliably represent what is occurring functionally during activity. If the erect assessment is negative, the patient may attempt similar exertion that elucidates symptoms in a normal training experience, until they are symptomatic.

At this point, we again assess the patient in an erect position as previously described. We will use cine loops to demonstrate the popliteal artery from resting patency through compression to occlusion and mark the site of compression on skin for MRI correlation. We feel that Doppler ultrasound does not adequately demonstrate the anatomy to rule out anatomical PAES and confirmation of occlusion in a symptomatic patient means the patient may be in either the anatomical or functional PAES groups.

4.5. MRI and MRI Angiography. MRI is a valuable noninvasive modality that allows optimal visualization of the popliteal artery as well as the surrounding structures [23, 24]. MRI can also distinguish intrinsic vascular disease from extrinsic compression. MRI can demonstrate a variety of findings including abnormal lateralized insertion of the medial head of gastrocnemius, medial displacement, and occlusion of the popliteal artery in the popliteal fossa and fat tissue filling the normal location of the medial head of gastrocnemius [23, 25]. In this way, anatomical PAES can be distinguished from functional PAES and the muscles and anatomical boundaries contributing can be accurately delineated [3]. This in turn can direct injection therapy (as discussed in Section 5) or the site of surgical intervention.

MRI angiography can demonstrate the level of occlusion, but limitations include the development of movement artifact with forceful plantarflexion positions and inability to hold such a position for prolonged periods [17]. This is a significant limitation as for reasons outlined earlier; investigating for

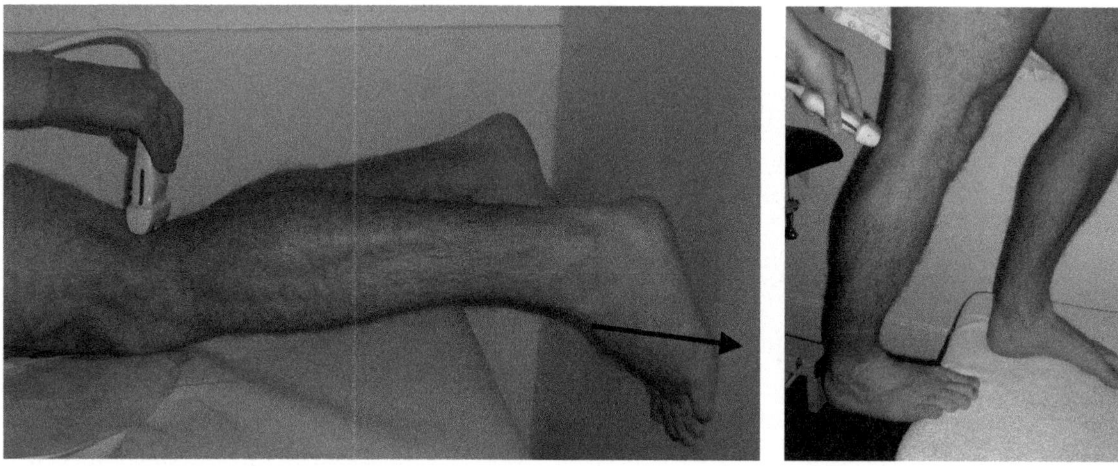

FIGURE 1: (a) Patient prone and pushing against a wall (in the direction of the arrow) at 25% maximum plantarflexion force. (b) Patient erect and plantarflexing against full body weight.

occlusion in functional PAES should occur during provocation. Most papers reviewed do not describe provocative manoeuvres with MRI angiography [23–25] while one suggests holding sustained forceful plantarflexion continuously for 20–29 seconds whilst the angiogram is performed [26]. Again for completeness we have provided our protocols below.

After positive ultrasound studies, a fiducial marker is placed on the patient's skin where the popliteal artery is being occluded to help correlate between the ultrasound and MRI site of occlusion. T1 weighted axial and coronal images are acquired to demonstrate the medial head and lateral heads of gastrocnemius, popliteus, and plantaris muscles and their alignment and associations with the femoral condyles and popliteal arteries and nerves. These images are acquired with the patient at rest.

Following these static images, the patient is instructed to dorsiflex and plantarflex their feet whilst acquiring T2 weighted 2D steady state images axially across the popliteal region. Before the final contrast MRI angiogram is performed, the patient is instructed to alternate a neutral ankle position with maximal plantarflexion force until they stimulate the pain that they usually experience (rather than a single sustained forceful contraction). Once they experience this pain, they keep their ankles in plantarflexion whilst we inject the contrast and perform the angiogram (Figure 2). One of the disadvantages of this technique is that there is an approximate 30-second delay before the contrast arrives at the popliteal artery and the angiogram can be performed and the artery may re-establish flow during this time. Patients quite often are in pain and or exhausted during this last series and may shake because of this.

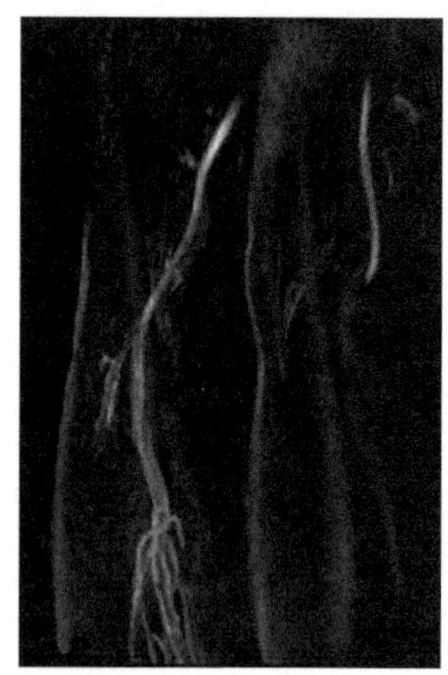

FIGURE 2: MRI angiogram of the popliteal fossa showing complete occlusion of the popliteal artery in the left leg.

5. Treatment

Based on our review of the literature, Figure 3 represents a decision-making flowchart in the assessment, work-up, and treatment of suspected PAES. Once confirmed, treatment depends on the type of PAES identified.

5.1. Anatomical PAES. Given the described rapid progression of arterial injury, it is recommended that anatomical PAES patients undergo surgery to remove the site of entrapment [17]. This typically involves exploration, limited fasciotomy, myotomy to varying degrees, and possible excision of occlusive fibrous bands [2, 17]. Results of popliteal fossa exploration, bypass, or muscle detachment, or a combination of these, and fossa decompression are generally good. Most series report a small number of patients, but >90% appear to return to activities in sports ≤ 3 months with resolution of all previous symptoms [17].

5.2. Functional PAES. The pathogenesis and progression of functionalPAES are uncertain, but it may be that these

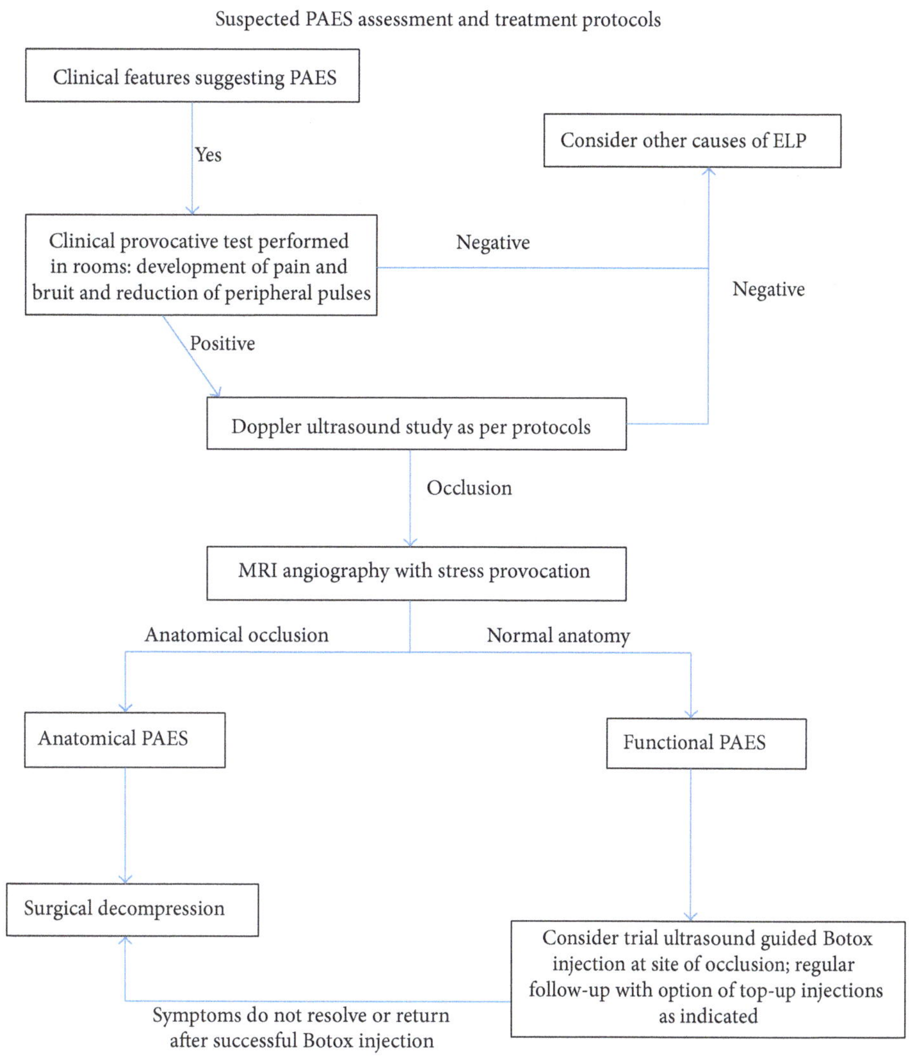

FIGURE 3: Assessment and treatment protocols for suspected PAES.

patients develop arterial injury more gradually with onset of more significant symptoms later in life [12]. Surgery has been recommended in functional occluders with significant repetitive and typical symptoms [17]. Turnipseed recommends resection of plantaris muscle and the crural band of soleus fascia that forms the outlet of the popliteal fossa as he feels that this fascial band is the fulcrum against which the neurovascular bundle is compressed in functional PAES [3].

However the site and amount of muscle necessary to be removed to prevent further occlusion is not always obvious. It is possible that a large segment of muscle will require excision. The popliteal artery will need exploration and there are increased risks of postoperative complications such as seroma (4.6%) and infection (2%) [2]. Also surgery for functional PAES does not seem to be as successful as that for anatomical PAES, with reports suggesting only 77% of patients after surgery reporting complete resolution of symptoms [14]. For this reason, a less invasive treatment option is desirable.

5.3. Guided Botulinum Toxin (Botox BTX-A) Injection Therapy. The use of botulinum injections for paralysis of muscles to manage medical conditions is well established. There are several descriptions of the use of botulinum in the treatment of muscle spasticity, particularly in cerebral palsy patients [27–29], and piriformis injection of BTX-A has been used successfully to treat sacral plexus and proximal sciatic nerve compression [30]. Bilici et al. described the use of BTX-A injection into a crus of the hemidiaphragm to treat renal artery stenosis [31].

The proposed mechanisms of action for intramuscular periarterial botulinum therapy for PAES are

(1) paralysis of the muscular slip of muscle responsible for the dynamic arterial occlusion,

(2) localised muscle atrophy caused by the botulinum which may increase space for the vessel and would explain the prolonged effect of botulinum on this

condition beyond the expected therapeutic effect of the medication,

(3) possible arterial smooth muscle relaxation of the popliteal artery resulting in vasodilatation.

Unfortunately, to date, there is no published data on the efficacy of botulinum injection in the management of functional PAES. We have commenced a pilot study using intramuscular periarterial injection of BTX-A to treat functional PAES with promising initial results. We hope to publish the outcomes as our cohort size increases, but at present this remains an unproven intervention.

6. Summary

Functional PAES is a condition that is possibly underrecognized and, if left untreated, can result in progressive arterial damage and the risk of developing lower limb ischaemia. It shares many features with other causes of exertional leg pain (especially chronic exertional compartment syndrome) and may coexist with one or more of these. A suggestive clinical history includes features of pain aggravated by exercise, but also possibly at rest with positions of knee extension and plantarflexion. The pain will typically resolve quickly once provocative manoeuvres are ceased, although an ache may persist for hours. Anatomical and functional PAES cannot be distinguished on clinical features alone, and possibly over half of the "normal" population can demonstrate some arterial occlusion with provocative manoeuvres. For this reason, specialized vascular investigations are indicated, particularly a Doppler ultrasound protocol performed at rest and during provocation and immediately after, which can demonstrate real time arterial occlusion and the level it is occurring at. Once occlusion is demonstrated, MRI can demonstrate the definitive anatomy of the popliteal fossa, whether anatomical PAES exists, and the site and extent of functional entrapment. From here, the best treatment can be provided, with consideration of guided Botox injection for functional PAES as a potential new intervention, or progression to surgical intervention.

Conflict of Interests

The authors declare that there is no conflict of interests regarding the publication of this paper.

Acknowledgments

The authors acknowledge Queensland X-ray for their assistance in providing high quality affordable investigations to their subjects.

References

[1] P. G. Blackman, "A review of chronic exertional compartment syndrome in the lower leg," *Medicine & Science in Sports & Exercise*, vol. 32, supplement, pp. S4–S10, 2000.

[2] W. D. Turnipseed, "Functional popliteal artery entrapment syndrome: a poorly understood and often missed diagnosis that is frequently mistreated," *Journal of Vascular Surgery*, vol. 49, no. 5, pp. 1189–1195, 2009.

[3] W. D. Turnipseed, "Popliteal entrapment in runners," *Clinics in Sports Medicine*, vol. 31, no. 2, pp. 321–328, 2012.

[4] S. B. Thacker, J. Gilchrist, D. F. Stroup, and C. D. Kimsey, "The prevention of shin splints in sports: a systematic review of literature," *Medicine and Science in Sports and Exercise*, vol. 34, no. 1, pp. 32–40, 2002.

[5] C. A. George and M. R. Hutchinson, "Chronic exertional compartment syndrome," *Clinics in Sports Medicine*, vol. 31, no. 2, pp. 307–319, 2012.

[6] N. Reshef and D. R. Guelich, "Medial tibial stress syndrome," *Clinics in Sports Medicine*, vol. 31, no. 2, pp. 273–290, 2012.

[7] T. T. Pham, R. Kapur, and M. I. Harwood, "Exertional leg pain: teasing out arterial entrapments," *Current Sports Medicine Reports*, vol. 6, no. 6, pp. 371–375, 2007.

[8] M. Reinking, "Exercise Related Leg Pain (ERLP): a review of the literature," *North American Journal of Sports Physical Therapy*, vol. 2, no. 3, pp. 170–180, 2007.

[9] M. Hislop, P. Tierney, P. Murray, M. O'Brien, and N. Mahony, "Chronic exertional compartment syndrome: the controversial "fifth" compartment of the leg," *The American Journal of Sports Medicine*, vol. 31, no. 5, pp. 770–776, 2003.

[10] K. Bennell, G. Matheson, W. Meeuwisse, and P. Brukner, "Risk factors for stress fractures," *Sports Medicine*, vol. 28, no. 2, pp. 91–122, 1999.

[11] M. Hislop and M. E. Batt, "Chronic exertional compartment syndrome testing: a minimalist approach," *British Journal of Sports Medicine*, vol. 45, no. 12, pp. 954–955, 2011.

[12] P. Baltopoulos, D. K. Filippou, and F. Sigala, "Popliteal artery entrapment syndrome: anatomic or functional syndrome?" *Clinical Journal of Sport Medicine*, vol. 14, no. 1, pp. 8–12, 2004.

[13] J. W. Love and T. J. Whelan, "Popliteal artery entrapment syndrome," *The American Journal of Surgery*, vol. 109, no. 5, pp. 620–624, 1965.

[14] S. Sinha, J. Houghton, P. J. Holt, M. M. Thompson, I. M. Loftus, and R. J. Hinchliffe, "Popliteal entrapment syndrome," *Journal of Vascular Surgery*, vol. 55, no. 1, pp. 252.e30–262.e30, 2012.

[15] L. J. Levien and M. G. Veller, "Popliteal artery entrapment syndrome: more common than previously recognized," *Journal of Vascular Surgery*, vol. 30, no. 4, pp. 587–598, 1999.

[16] E. Mavili, H. Dönmez, G. Kahriman, A. Özaşlamaci, N. Özcan, and K. Taşdemir, "Popliteal artery branching patterns detected by digital subtraction angiography," *Diagnostic and Interventional Radiology*, vol. 17, no. 1, pp. 80–83, 2011.

[17] J. Pillai, "A current interpretation of popliteal vascular entrapment," *Journal of Vascular Surgery*, vol. 48, pp. 61S–65S, 2008.

[18] R. Lane, T. Nguyen, M. Cuzzilla, D. Oomens, W. Mohabbat, and S. Hazelton, "Functional popliteal entrapment syndrome in the sportsperson," *European Journal of Vascular and Endovascular Surgery*, vol. 43, no. 1, pp. 81–87, 2012.

[19] R. D. Hill and R. Smith, "Examination of the extremities: pulses, bruits, and phlebitis," in *Clinical Methods: The History, Physical, and Laboratory Examinations*, H. K. Walker, W.D. Hall, and J. W. Hurst, Eds., pp. 148–152, Butterworths, Boston, Mass, USA, 1990.

[20] U. Altinatis, U. Helgstrand, and M. Hansen, "Popliteal artery entrapment syndrome: ultrasound imaging, intra-operative findings and clinical outcome," *Vascular and Endovascular Surgery*, vol. 47, no. 7, pp. 513–518, 2013.

[21] L. S. Erdoes, J. J. Devine, V. M. Bernhard, M. R. Baker, S. S. Berman, and G. C. Hunter, "Popliteal vascular compression in a normal population," *Journal of Vascular Surgery*, vol. 20, no. 6, pp. 978–986, 1994.

[22] U. Hoffmann, J. Vetter, L. Rainoni, A. J. Leu, and A. Bollinger, "Popliteal artery compression and force of active plantar flexion in young healthy volunteers," *Journal of Vascular Surgery*, vol. 26, no. 2, pp. 281–287, 1997.

[23] S. Atilla, E. T. Ilgit, S. Akpek, C. Yücel, E. Turgut Tali, and S. Iik, "MR imaging and MR angiography in popliteal artery entrapment syndrome," *European Radiology*, vol. 8, no. 6, pp. 1025–1029, 1998.

[24] A. W. Lambert and D. C. Wilkins, "Popliteal artery entrapment syndrome," *The British Journal of Surgery*, vol. 86, no. 11, pp. 1365–1370, 1999.

[25] U. Özkan, L. Oğuzkurt, F. Tercan et al., "MRI and DSA findings in popliteal artery entrapment syndrome," *Diagnostic and Interventional Radiology*, vol. 14, pp. 106–110, 2008.

[26] E. Di Cesare, L. Marsili, G. Marino et al., "Stress MR imaging for evaluation of popliteal artery entrapment," *Journal of Magnetic Resonance Imaging*, vol. 4, no. 4, pp. 617–622, 1994.

[27] I. S. Corry, A. P. Cosgrove, E. G. Walsh, D. McClean, and H. K. Graham, "Botulinum toxin A in the hemiplegic upper limb: a double blind trial," *Developmental Medicine and Child Neurology*, vol. 39, no. 3, pp. 185–193, 1997.

[28] D. Fehlings, "The use of botulinum toxin in paediatric hypertonia," *Paediatrics and Child Health*, vol. 10, no. 7, pp. 379–381, 2005.

[29] L. A. Koman, J. F. Mooney III, B. P. Smith, A. Goodman, and T. Mulvaney, "Management of spasticity cerebral palsy with botulinum—a toxin: report of a preliminary, randomized, double-blind trial," *Journal of Pediatric Orthopaedics*, vol. 14, no. 3, pp. 299–303, 1994.

[30] S. J. Yoon, J. Ho, H. Y. Kang et al., "Low-dose botulinum toxin type A for the treatment of refractory piriformis syndrome," *Pharmacotherapy*, vol. 27, no. 5, pp. 657–665, 2007.

[31] A. Bilici, M. Karcaaltincaba, A. T. Ilica, Y. Bukte, and A. Senol, "Treatment of hypertension from renal artery entrapment by percutaneous CT-guided botulinum toxin injection into diaphragmatic crus as alternative to surgery and stenting," *The American Journal of Roentgenology*, vol. 189, no. 3, pp. W143–W145, 2007.

12

Validity and Reliability of Farsi Version of Youth Sport Environment Questionnaire

Mohammad Ali Eshghi,[1] Ramin Kordi,[2] Amir Hossein Memari,[2] Ahmad Ghaziasgar,[2] Mohammad-Ali Mansournia,[3] and Seyed Hojjat Zamani Sani[4]

[1]*Exercise Physiology Research Center, Baqiyatallah University of Medical Sciences, Tehran, Iran*
[2]*Sports Medicine Research Center, Tehran University of Medical Sciences, P.O. Box 14395-578, Tehran, Iran*
[3]*Department of Epidemiology and Biostatistics, School of Public Health, Tehran University of Medical Sciences, Tehran, Iran*
[4]*Faculty of Physical Education and Sport Sciences, Shahid Beheshti University, Tehran, Iran*

Correspondence should be addressed to Amir Hossein Memari; amirmemari@farabi.tums.ac.ir

Academic Editor: Laura Guidetti

The Youth Sport Environment Questionnaire (YSEQ) had been developed from Group Environment Questionnaire, a well-known measure of team cohesion. The aim of this study was to adapt and examine the reliability and validity of the Farsi version of the YSEQ. This version was completed by 455 athletes aged 13–17 years. Results of confirmatory factor analysis indicated that two-factor solution showed a good fit to the data. The results also revealed that the Farsi YSEQ showed high internal consistency, test-retest reliability, and good concurrent validity. This study indicated that the Farsi version of the YSEQ is a valid and reliable measure to assess team cohesion in sport setting.

1. Introduction

Team cohesion is one of the key concepts within sport teams that has received substantial research attention over the last three decades [1, 2]. Team cohesion is defined as a dynamic process addressing the propensity for a team to bond together and remain integrated in chasing their purposes [3]. Team cohesion is directly associated with other main sport measures such as collective efficacy, performance, and achievement. Carron et al. [4] presented the first conceptual model of team cohesion in Group Environment Questionnaire (GEQ) including two categories: team integration and individual attraction to the team. Each category was divided into two subcategories known as social cohesion and task cohesion. Social cohesion was related to the extent team athletes adhere together to show appropriate social relationships, while task cohesion is indicative of joint effort among team members in order to reach specific team goals [5, 6].

The usefulness of the GEQ has been frequently examined. Researchers have assessed factor structure and construct validity of the GEQ across different cultures [7–9]. Results have questioned the validity of the GEQ for young individuals as whether the GEQ is generalizable to young athletes' population [10]. Seeking to answer the question, researchers examined the appropriateness of the GEQ items for youth athletes and revised questions to outfit if necessary. Accordingly, Eys et al. [11] developed a cohesion questionnaire for exclusively investigating young athletes (≤17) named the Youth Sport Environment Questionnaire (YESQ). Eys et al. [11] and other researchers believed that original conceptualization of GEQ might not be relevant to the young population [12, 13]. Since the developmental variables play a critical role in perceptions of youth about their peer interactions and relationships, team experiences in young athletes become increasingly diverse, complex, and integrated through developmental process [14]. Consequently and of relevance to the current study, Eys et al. [11] believed that young athletes may not perceive group unity from two aspects of team integration and individual attraction to the team but instead identify an unidimensional model of team cohesion. Furthermore, Eys et al. [11] emphasized item wording to increase readability and decrease response bias in younger individuals. Eys et al. [15]

also reported that certain individual characteristics (e.g., age) may influence both the participant's ability to interpret mixed or negatively worded questions and the internal consistency values of the GEQ subscales.

In sum, the literature reviewed above highlights the existing question of whether the YSEQ is effective as a measure of cohesion across age, culture, and youth sport teams [2]. However there is a lack of research on team cohesion in young athletes particularly outside of English-spoken countries [7]. This gap stems from lack of a valid, reliable, and relevant measure of the cohesion construct for youth sport groups. Therefore, the purpose of the current study was to continue the validation procedure of a sound measure of cohesion in order to assess the perception of cohesion in members of youth (13–17 years of age) sport groups using the Farsi version of the YSEQ. To meet this goal a sample of Iranian young athletes was recruited for the study.

2. Methods

2.1. Participants. The studied sample included 455 healthy youths (253 male) with an average age of 15.1 years (SD = 1.8). A convenience sample of athletes was recruited from local sports leagues. Coaches were initially contacted and upon their approval researchers explained the study for all athletes. Volunteered male or female athletes were assigned to the study if they were 13–17 years old and participated on competitive levels in karate, basketball, volleyball, and soccer.

2.2. Measures. In order to collect descriptive information, participants were asked to fill a questionnaire that consisted of demographic information such as gender, occupation, and age as well as exercise information including type of sport, number of participations per week, and duration of training sessions.

2.3. The Youth Sport Environment Questionnaire. The YSEQ is a modified form (18-item) of the validated version of the GEQ. The YSEQ also measures the team cohesion of the participants on a 9-point Likert scale ranging from 1 (*strongly disagree*) to 9 (*strongly agree*) (see Supplementary Material available online at http://dx.doi.org/10.1155/2015/985283). Scoring in the YSEQ is the same as the GEQ, but the items have just been categorized into two dimensions of *social cohesion* and *task cohesion*.

2.4. Sport Competition Anxiety Test. To test the concurrent validity, the Sport Competition Anxiety Test (SCAT) was used to measure competitive trait-anxiety through 15 questions [16]. The questions begin with "Before I compete I feel. . ." and athletes were asked to respond to each statement by checking a box corresponding to the frequency (hardly ever, sometimes, or often). The test score ranges from 10 (low competitive trait-anxiety) to 30 (high competitive trait-anxiety).

2.5. Shortened Marlowe-Crowne Social Desirability Scale (SMCSDS). For assessing social desirability bias in participants' responses, a 13-item short form of the SMCSDS was applied [17]. Social desirability bias suggests that respondents tend to show socially favorable and acceptable image of themselves to others when answering self-evaluative questions. The correlation between the SMCSDS and the YSEQ was obtained to reveal if answers were affected by social desirability bias.

2.6. Procedure. The Farsi version of the YSEQ was translated from the original language (English) to Farsi by two different independent bilingual translators whose first languages were Farsi [18]. One of the translators was a psychologist experienced in translating sport psychology questionnaires; she was aware of the purpose and the concepts applied in the questionnaire. The other translator had no psychological background and was uninformed about the purpose of study. Both translators discussed differences between translations and resolved inconsistencies. Ultimately they made a final version of translation upon which both agreed. The back translation of the Farsi version to English was made by one bilingual translator whose mother tongue was English and was experienced in the field of psychology. Afterward, a multidisciplinary expert committee evaluated and reviewed the final Farsi translation and the back translation. The committee consisted of the translators, a sport researcher, a psychologist, and a statistician. The expert committee reviewed and evaluated all the translations and compared them to the original English version and concluded that translations were idiomatically, semantically, and culturally equivalent. They resolved discrepancies and reached to a consensus to form the prefinal version of the Farsi version of the YSEQ. After finalizing the last draft, it was pretested in a sample of 25 young athletes in order to assess the clarity of the statements and the questionnaire. Based on the feedback we received, changes were made to the semantics of some statements in order to ensure understandability of the questionnaire for the Iranian population.

The Institutional Review Board of the Tehran University of Medical Sciences approved ethical aspect of this research. The participants after completing an informed consent received three questionnaires including YSEQ, SCAT, and SMCSDS and a demographic information form. Participants were briefed that there is no wrong or right answer and they should respond based on their experience.

2.7. Statistical Analysis. We conducted a confirmatory factor analysis (CFA) on the 18-item version of the questionnaire examining the final two-factor model parallel to one-factor model suggested by Eys et al. [11] study. A maximum likelihood method of estimation by AMOS 17.0 was used for confirmatory factor analysis. The concurrent validity was assessed to verify if the Farsi version of the YSEQ measures is in line with other psychological measures in the sport context. Thus we correlated each subscale of the YSEQ with the SCAT scores using Spearman's rank correlation coefficient. Furthermore, to assess the social desirability bias in participants we used Pearson's product-moment correlation between the YSEQ subscales and the SMCSDS. Internal consistency was assessed using Cronbach's coefficient alpha. Additionally "Cronbach's alpha if item deleted" was reported. In the "item

Table 1: Descriptive statistics and standardized factor loadings for confirmatory factor analysis ($N = 455$).

Factor	Item	Loading	Range	Mean	SD
Social cohesion	2	0.69	2–9	6.45	2.09
	4	0.68	1–9	6.21	2.13
	7	0.67	2–9	5.98	1.98
	9	0.73	1–9	6.87	2.35
	11	0.71	1–9	6.98	2.47
	13	0.84	1–9	5.57	1.99
	15	0.86	1–9	5.37	2.15
	17	0.81	1–9	6.61	2.24
Task cohesion	1	0.59	2–9	7.05	2.16
	3	0.67	1–9	6.55	2.24
	5	0.76	1–9	6.84	2.18
	8	0.63	1–9	5.98	1.95
	10	0.84	2–9	6.37	2.04
	14	0.77	2–9	7.09	2.07
	16	0.82	1–9	6.79	1.89
	18	0.74	1–9	6.13	1.97

total correlation," high correlation between item and total score for the subscale represents that the item is a powerful item. The YSEQ was readministered to 60 participants after an interval of four weeks. The test-retest reliability was then evaluated using intraclass correlation coefficient. IBM SPSS software version 17 was used for analysis and an alpha value of 0.05 was considered as the statistical significance level.

3. Results

3.1. Confirmatory Factor Analysis. Descriptive statistics and standardized factor loadings of all items are presented in Table 1. CFA was conducted to test goodness of fit for each one-factor and two-factor model of the Farsi YSEQ. Goodness of fit summary for one- and two-factor models is shown in Table 2 and the correlation matrix on which these CFAs were based is presented in Table 3. *The fit indices for* one-factor structure *showed a poor* fit of the model: $\chi^2 = 543.356$ ($p < 0.001$), DF = 170, $\chi^2/\text{df} = 3.102$, TLI = 0.68, NFI = 0.75, CFI = 0.81, IFI = 0.78, and RMSEA = 0.084 with 90% CI = 0.075–0.093. However the two-factor structure (social and task cohesion) indicated adequate fit of the model to the data, with $\chi^2 = 313.425$ ($p < 0.001$), DF = 169, $\chi^2/\text{df} = 1.854$, TLI = 0.93, NFI = 0.89, CFI = 0.92, IFI = 0.94, and RMSEA = 0.051 with 90% CI = 0.043–0.062. The significant chi-square test was highly likely with large sample sizes. Furthermore, examination of the standardized factor loadings suggested that two items had a low value (i.e., 6 and 12; spurious negative items). These items had been added to detect invalidating response sets. Therefore those items were not included in the final model.

3.2. Reliability. The results showed a high internal consistency ($\alpha = 0.93$) of the YSEQ for the total items. The item total correlation for social subscale ranged from 0.67 to 0.78 and item deleted alpha coefficients varied from 0.83 to 0.87 while overall coefficient alpha for this subscale was 0.87. The item total correlation for task subscale was between 0.61 and 0.73 and item deleted alpha coefficients were ranging from 0.83 to 0.85 with internal consistency coefficient of 0.89. All of the items had adequate correlation in relation to each subscale. Analysis also showed a high test-retest reliability of the Farsi version of the YSEQ after one month; intraclass correlation coefficient for the social and task scores was 0.89 and 0.92, $p < 0.001$.

3.3. Concurrent Validity. When examining concurrent validity, the Farsi version of the YSEQ was significantly correlated with the SCAT scores. High negative correlations were found between SCAT and the YSEQ subscales for task scores ($r = -0.59$, $p < 0.001$) and social scores ($r = -0.48$, $p < 0.001$). Furthermore, correlation between each YSEQ subscale and the SMCSDS was very low, ranging from 0.015 to 0.18 and these results confirmed the participants' answers were not influenced by social desirability.

4. Discussion

The YSEQ is a self-report instrument that has been recently used for measurement of team cohesion [11]. This study aimed to evaluate validity and reliability of the Farsi version of the YSEQ. From proposed models, two-factor structure (task and social cohesion) of the scale shows better fit indices compared with one-factor structure.

4.1. Validity. The current study findings on cohesion are comparable to those in previous reports indicating that younger athletes showed a specific perception on team cohesion [2]. The YSEQ was initially based on a strong theoretical foundation provided by Carron and colleagues [4] that is supported by over two decades of research; but in the initial version of the YSEQ the youth's perception on constructs of the group integration and attractions to the group were not separated. However, task and social differences were still clearly distinguished both conceptually and statistically. This can be due to the level of complexity in which youths athletes conduct their interactions and relationships with others in a sport team [19]. Furthermore there are questions about the overall utility of examining individual perceptions related to a group in the cohesion research. The distinction between task and social issues in the YSEQ is in line with a number of previous group dynamics studies that have indicated these issues as two primary orientations for most populations [20–22]. Examining cohesion in other disciplines (such as work groups) also supported the differences between task cohesion and social cohesion [23]. Similar to the original work, and in addition to the task and social items, two false negative questions have been added to address concerns about the response agreement and negative versus positive wording of items. Addressing the readability of statements, in line with the original study, current study provided further support for the appropriateness of the language for a youth sample with a different culture.

TABLE 2: Correlation matrix of the 16 items used in the confirmatory factor analyses.

Item	2	4	7	9	11	13	15	17	1	3	5	8	10	14	16	18
Social 2	—	0.56	0.48	0.51	0.44	0.57	0.44	0.47	0.18	0.32	0.31	0.28	0.24	0.30	0.27	0.23
Social 4		—	0.49	0.58	0.53	0.52	0.49	0.51	0.21	0.33	0.26	0.28	0.27	0.30	0.32	0.19
Social 7			—	0.54	0.48	0.51	0.43	0.47	0.22	0.23	0.27	0.26	0.24	0.33	0.31	0.22
Social 9				—	0.47	0.43	0.46	0.38	0.15	0.21	0.31	0.16	0.18	0.24	0.19	0.20
Social 11					—	0.38	0.41	0.43	0.16	0.23	0.24	0.19	0.24	0.27	0.26	0.17
Social 13						—	0.53	0.49	0.28	0.14	0.19	0.23	0.22	0.31	0.25	0.15
Social 15							—	0.55	0.17	0.21	0.23	0.30	0.19	0.18	0.22	0.20
Social 17								—	0.21	0.25	0.28	0.24	0.19	0.26	0.30	0.22
Task 1									—	0.52	0.56	0.48	0.41	0.50	0.39	0.51
Task 3										—	0.55	0.49	0.39	0.47	0.46	0.49
Task 5											—	0.43	0.51	0.56	0.47	0.55
Task 8												—	0.44	0.55	0.50	0.47
Task 10													—	0.49	0.47	0.52
Task 14														—	0.45	0.53
Task 16															—	0.50
Task 18																—

TABLE 3: Goodness of fit summary for one- and two-factor models.

Model	χ^2	df	χ^2/df	IFI	TLI	NFI	CFI	RMSEA		
								Value	90% CI	p value
One-factor	543.356*	170	3.102	0.78	0.68	0.75	0.81	0.084	0.075–0.093	<0.001
Two-factor	313.425*	169	1.855	0.94	0.93	0.89	0.92	0.051	0.043–0.062	<0.001

* p value < 0.001.

Examining the concurrent validity of the Farsi version of the YSEQ, current study indicated a strong negative correlation between subscales of the Farsi version of the YSEQ and the SCAT scores. This result is in line with other studies in which authors argued that cohesion is influenced negatively by the anxiety and distress of athletes related to their competitions [24]. Examining the scores of the MCSDS in relation to the subscales of the YSEQ indicated a very weak correlation. This indicates that the YSEQ questions did not affect athletes to answer questions with a social desirability tendency. Thus their responses could be assumed as indicators of their real intention. This suggests that the YSEQ might not bias participants to overestimate their team abilities [2].

4.2. Reliability. Current study results have also reported a high internal consistency for the total score and each factor of the YSEQ, confirming the stability of the scale. We also showed that total item correlations for subscales were satisfactory and each subscale was internally stable. Furthermore, test-retest reliability revealed a high stability for the Farsi version of the YSEQ after four weeks.

4.3. Strengths and Limitations. The strength of our study was to study athletes from a wide range of sports [25]. This has led to a high validity, robust factor structure, and internal reliability of both task and social cohesion subscales. However, the validation of YSEQ will be continuing and future research should investigate the predictive function of the YSEQ for theory-based concepts related to a sport team. A limitation of this study, which might be addressed by future research studies, is about the concurrent validity where we used only one scale instead of multiple designs. It would be more advantageous to correlate the YSEQ with other sport team measures scales in Farsi (e.g., role clarity, collective efficacy) for assessing concurrent and discriminant validity [26]. However there are several individual variables associated with cohesion particularly variables as competitive anxiety. Anxiety as an affective-cognitive variable is associated with task cohesion and athletes in cohesive teams will experience less anxiety. Based on previous data, it could be assumed that competitive anxiety is a fitting outcome variable for team cohesion. Thus our findings on association between cohesion and anxiety could improve the predictive value for the YSEQ.

5. Conclusion

In conclusion, findings of the current study indicated that the Farsi version of the YSEQ is a sound measure to assess perceptions of cohesion among youth athletes (13–17 years of age) from a range of sport groups. From a practical standpoint, current findings imply that psychologists can use the Farsi version of the YSEQ to assess overall task or social group cohesion in their young athletes.

Conflict of Interests

The authors declare that there is no conflict of interests regarding the publication of this paper.

Acknowledgments

The authors want to thank the young athletes and their coaches for their contribution and supports of this study.

References

[1] A. V. Carron, S. R. Bray, and M. A. Eys, "Team cohesion and team success in sport," *Journal of Sports Sciences*, vol. 20, no. 2, pp. 119–126, 2002.

[2] M. A. Eys, E. Jewitt, M. B. Evans, S. Wolf, M. W. Bruner, and T. M. Loughead, "Coach-initiated motivational climate and cohesion in youth sport," *Research Quarterly for Exercise and Sport*, vol. 84, no. 3, pp. 373–383, 2013.

[3] C. S. Jacob and A. V. Carron, "The association between status and cohesion in sport teams," *Journal of Sports Sciences*, vol. 16, no. 2, pp. 187–198, 1998.

[4] A. V. Carron, W. N. Widmeyer, and L. R. Brawley, "The development of an instrument to assess cohesion in sport teams: the group environment questionnaire," *Journal of Sport & Exercise Psychology*, vol. 7, no. 3, pp. 244–266, 1985.

[5] F. M. Leo, P. A. Sánchez-Miguel, D. Sánchez-Oliva, D. Amado, and T. García-Calvo, "Analysis of cohesion and collective efficacy profiles for the performance of soccer players," *Journal of Human Kinetics*, vol. 39, no. 1, pp. 221–229, 2013.

[6] J. Midtgaard, M. Rorth, R. Stelter, and L. Adamsen, "The group matters: an explorative study of group cohesion and quality of life in cancer patients participating in physical exercise intervention during treatment," *European Journal of Cancer Care*, vol. 15, no. 1, pp. 25–33, 2006.

[7] L. M. Iturbide, P. Elosua, and F. Yanes, "A measure of team cohesion in sport. Spanish adaptation of Group Environment Questionnaire (GEQ)," *Psicothema*, vol. 22, no. 3, pp. 482–488, 2010.

[8] J. Senécal, T. M. Loughead, and G. A. Bloom, "A season-long team-building intervention: examining the effect of team goal setting on cohesion," *Journal of Sport and Exercise Psychology*, vol. 30, no. 2, pp. 186–199, 2008.

[9] J. Sindik and S. Misoni, "A comparison of two conative characteristics of top basketball and recreational table tennis players," *Collegium Antropologicum*, vol. 37, supplement 2, pp. 187–196, 2013.

[10] M. J. Mason, C. Schmidt, A. Abraham, L. Walker, and K. Tercyak, "Adolescents' social environment and depression: social networks, extracurricular activity, and family relationship influences," *Journal of Clinical Psychology in Medical Settings*, vol. 16, no. 4, pp. 346–354, 2009.

[11] M. Eys, T. Loughead, S. R. Bray, and A. V. Carron, "Development of a cohesion questionnaire for youth: the Youth Sport Environment Questionnaire," *Journal of Sport & Exercise Psychology*, vol. 31, no. 3, pp. 390–408, 2009.

[12] M.-J. Aarts, J. J. P. Mathijssen, J. A. M. Van Oers, and A. J. Schuit, "Associations between environmental characteristics and active commuting to school among children: a cross-sectional study," *International Journal of Behavioral Medicine*, vol. 20, no. 4, pp. 538–555, 2013.

[13] C. C. Borrego, L. Cid, and C. Silva, "Relationship between group cohesion and anxiety in soccer," *Journal of Human Kinetics*, vol. 34, no. 1, pp. 119–127, 2012.

[14] O. Kjørmo and H. Halvari, "Two ways related to performance in elite sport: the path of self-confidence and competitive anxiety and the path of group cohesion and group goal-clarity," *Perceptual and Motor Skills*, vol. 94, no. 3, pp. 950–966, 2002.

[15] M. A. Eys, A. V. Carron, S. R. Bray, and L. R. Brawley, "Item wording and internal consistency of a measure of cohesion: the group environment questionnaire," *Journal of Sport and Exercise Psychology*, vol. 29, no. 3, pp. 395–402, 2007.

[16] R. Martens, *Sport Competition Anxiety Test*, Human Kinetics Publishers, Champaign, Ill, USA, 1977.

[17] W. M. Reynolds, "Development of reliable and valid short forms of the Marlowe-Crowne social desirability scale," *Journal of Clinical Psychology*, vol. 38, no. 1, pp. 119–125, 1982.

[18] A. H. Memari, M. Shayestehfar, F.-S. Mirfazeli, T. Rashidi, P. Ghanouni, and S. Hafizi, "Cross-cultural adaptation, reliability, and validity of the autism treatment evaluation checklist in Persian," *Iranian Journal of Pediatrics*, vol. 23, no. 3, pp. 269–275, 2013.

[19] T. M. Karr, D. Davidson, F. B. Bryant, G. Balague, and A. M. Bohnert, "Sport type and interpersonal and intrapersonal predictors of body dissatisfaction in high school female sport participants," *Body Image*, vol. 10, no. 2, pp. 210–219, 2013.

[20] R. Kordi, M. Abdollahi, A.-H. Memari, and M. G. Najafabadi, "Investigating two different training time frames during Ramadan fasting," *Asian Journal of Sports Medicine*, vol. 2, no. 3, pp. 205–210, 2011.

[21] K. De Cocker, I. De Bourdeaudhuij, M. Teychenne, S. McNaughton, and J. Salmon, "Educational inequalities in TV viewing among older adults: a mediation analysis of ecological factors," *International Journal of Behavioral Nutrition and Physical Activity*, vol. 10, article 138, 2013.

[22] A. V. Carron, W. N. Widmeyer, and L. R. Brawley, "The measurement of cohesion in sports teams: the Group Environment Questionnaire," *Canadian Journal of Sport Sciences*, vol. 14, no. 1, pp. 55–59, 1989.

[23] P. Steca, A. N. Pala, A. Greco, D. Monzani, and M. D'Addario, "A psychometric evaluation of the Group Environment Questionnaire in a sample of professional basketball and soccer players," *Perceptual and Motor Skills*, vol. 116, no. 1, pp. 262–271, 2013.

[24] M. A. Eys, J. Hardy, A. V. Carron, and M. R. Beauchamp, "The relationship between task cohesion and competitive state anxiety," *Journal of Sport and Exercise Psychology*, vol. 25, no. 1, pp. 66–76, 2003.

[25] A.-H. Memari, R. Kordi, N. Panahi, L. R. Nikookar, M. Abdollahi, and A. Akbarnejad, "Effect of Ramadan fasting on body composition and physical performance in female athletes," *Asian Journal of Sports Medicine*, vol. 2, no. 3, pp. 161–166, 2011.

[26] T. Seif-Barghi, R. Kordi, A.-H. Memari, M.-A. Mansournia, and M. Jalali-Ghomi, "The effect of an ecological imagery program on soccer performance of elite players," *Asian Journal of Sports Medicine*, vol. 3, no. 2, pp. 81–89, 2012.

13

Physiological and Psychophysical Responses to Listening to Music during Warm-Up and Circuit-Type Resistance Exercise in Strength Trained Men

Hamid Arazi,[1] Abbas Asadi,[1,2] and Morteza Purabed[1]

[1]*Department of Exercise Physiology, Faculty of Physical Education and Sport Sciences, University of Guilan, Rasht, Iran*
[2]*Department of Physical Education and Sport Sciences, Payame Noor University, P.O. Box 19395-3697, Tehran, Iran*

Correspondence should be addressed to Abbas Asadi; abbas_asadi1175@yahoo.com

Academic Editor: Koichi Nakazato

The purpose of this study was to assess the effects of listening to music during warm-up and resistance exercise on physiological (heart rate and blood pressure) and psychophysical (rating of perceived exertion) responses in trained athletes. Twelve strength trained male participants performed warm-up and resistance exercise without music (WU+RE without M), warm-up and resistance exercise with music (WU+RE with M), WU with M and RE without M, and WU without M and RE with M, with 48 hours space between sessions. After completing each session, the rating of perceived exertion (RPE) was measured. Also, heart rate (HR), systolic (SBP) and diastolic blood pressure (DBP), mean arterial pressure (MAP), and rate pressure product (RPP) were assessed before, after, and 15, 30, 45, and 60 min after exercise. Results indicated that RPE was higher for WU+RE without M condition in comparison with other conditions. All conditions showed increases in cardiovascular variables after exercise. The responses of HR, SBP, and RPP were higher for WU+RE without M condition. Thus, using music during warm-up and resistance exercise is a legal method for decreasing RPE and cardiovascular responses due to resistance exercise.

1. Introduction

Resistance training is important not only for athletes but also for members of the general population [1]. Many people use the weight training to improve their performance. Maximizing effort in the weight room can improve performance. Due to this, the use of ergogenic aids has become common place in exercise programs and resistance training. Some ergogenic aids can increase the capacity for bodily performance by inhibiting symptoms of fatigue such as imagery, caffeine, and steroids [2].

Several researchers have focused on the ergogenic aid of music during warm-up, exercise, and cool-down to enhance performance [3–6]. Music is considered to have a positive effect on exercise performance. Some have chosen to use music as an aid to physiological performance. Listening to music during resistance exercise is the good kind of distraction and can induce ups in the athletes effort, put the athletes in the peak effort, and elevate mood state resulting in greater work in resistance exercise movements. On the other hand, music has the capacity to capture attention, lift spirits, generate emotion, change or regulate mood, evoke memories, increase work output, reduce inhibitions, and encourage rhythmic movement all of which have potential applications in sport and exercise [2]. The most common positive outcomes when combining music and resistance exercise appear to be a decreased rating of perceived exertion, increased performance measures, improved mood, and increased arousal resulting in higher ability of weight lifts during resistance training and consequently better physiological and performance gains [4–8].

Another effect of listening to music is physiological (heart rate and systolic and diastolic blood pressure). Edworthy and Waring [9] found a significant increase in heart rate (HR) while listening to fast music during exercise. Conversely, Schwartz et al. [10] did not find any difference in exercise HR.

Birnbaum et al. [11] reported that listening to fast music decreased the subjects' HR and blood pressure during steady-state treadmill exercise. In contrast, Jarraya et al. [12] investigated the effect of listening to music during warm up on short term supramaximal performance during the 30 s Wingate tests in athletes and found no significant changes in HR. Recently, Atan [3] examined effects of fast music tempo on HR and found no significant changes. The contradictory findings may be due in part to variations in experimental design, such as differences in exercise mode, intensity, and duration. The type of music selected and the manner in which it was selected have also varied among the studies. Additionally, subjects differed in age, health, and physical conditioning.

It is widely known that the autonomic nervous system is involved in control of HR and cardiovascular responses. That is, increased sympathetic neural activity plays a role in controlling the rate and contractility of the heart and in the caliber of resistance and capacitance vessels in the systemic circulation [13]. Music also appears to affect the autonomic nervous system [14]. Therefore, physiological reactions should result from changes in the autonomic nervous system triggered by music.

Although previous studies supported the hypothesis of the ergogenic effects of music on cardiovascular performance, it is important to examine music's effect with trained athletes and using music during warm-up and circuit-type resistance exercise. The effects of music played during an exercise task on athletic performance have been previously studied. Yet, these results are not applicable for well-trained athletes and using music during warm-up and circuit-type resistance exercise with emphasis on physiological aspects. Therefore, the aim of this study was to compare four conditions of combining music and resistance exercise on physiological and psychophysical responses in trained athletes.

2. Material and Methods

2.1. Participants. Twelve healthy well-trained resistance exercise males (Table 1) volunteered to participate in this investigation. None of the athletes were on any medication. All participants were free from any lower and upper body injuries and cardiovascular diseases and did not use anabolic or other drugs that enhance the performance for at least 6 months prior to involvement in this study. Inclusion criteria included (a) at least 5 years of experience with resistance training, (b) no history of lower and upper body injuries, (c) no lower and upper extremity reconstructive surgery in the past two years or unresolved musculoskeletal disorders, and (d) not using any ergogenic aids throughout the study. Before any measurements and starting the study, each athlete gave written informed consent to participate. All participants understood that they could withdraw from the study at any time. This study was approved by the Local Ethics Committee and procedures were conducted in accordance with ethical standards in sport and exercise science research [15].

2.2. Experimental Design. At least one week prior to starting the treatments, all athletes reported to the laboratory, and during this session their body weight and height were determined in a standardized fashion. Height was measured in centimeters using a stadiometer (Seca 222, Terre Haute, IN) and body mass was measured in kilograms using a digital scale (Tanita, BC-418MA, Tokyo, Japan). At this session, the participants understood the procedures and experimental approach of this study and performed selected resistance exercises for familiarization, and then the one repetition maximum for each exercise was measured following NSCA guidelines [16]. After the first session, the athletes reported to laboratory four times and performed each condition (treatment). Each exercise session took place at approximately the same time of day for each athlete and sessions were separated by at least 48 hours.

Table 1: Participants characteristics and resting cardiovascular parameters (mean ± SD).

Number of athletes	12
Age (y)	24 ± 2
Height (cm)	175.1 ± 6.4
Weight (kg)	83.7 ± 11.2
Strength training experience (y)	5.2 ± 1.3
Heart rate (bpm)	70.6 ± 6.8
Systolic blood pressure (mmHg)	120.1 ± 7.3
Diastolic blood pressure (mmHg)	79.7 ± 3.1

2.3. Procedures. The research design consisted of four experimental conditions. Each athlete was tested four times under the same laboratory conditions in a randomized manner. Condition 1 (WU+RE without M) consisted of performing warm-up and resistance exercise without music. For condition 2 (WU+RE with M) the athletes listened to music during warm-up and while performing resistance exercise. Condition 3 (WU with M+RE without M) consisted of performing warm-up with M and performing resistance exercise without M, and for condition 4 (WU without M+RE with M), the athletes performed warm-up without listening to music and listened to music during resistance exercise.

Total time of warm-up was 10 minutes including five minutes of cycling on a cycle-ergometer (Sport Art Fitness, C52u, Taiwan) at a self-selected workload and cadence and five minutes of various stretching exercises with the aim of preparing the joints for resistance exercises. Resistance exercises included the squat, military press, leg press, lat pull dawn, knee flexion, bench press, knee extension, biceps extension, calf raise, and arm curl. The athletes performed a set of 10 repetitions with 60% of one repetition maximum, continually and without rest between stations. Only one circuit was performed by each participant.

Due to the exercise type of resistance exercise and the relationship between arousal and sympathetic nervous system with resistance exercise, fast (130 beats per minute [bpm]) tempo music was chosen for this study. The selection criteria were based on the five recommendations of

Karageorghis and Terry [17]. The motivational effects of asynchronous music and an associated measure of the motivational qualities of music known as the Brunel Music Rating Inventory (BMRI), with regard to the authors who indicated the main characteristics of motivational music are that it has a fast tempo (>120 bpm) and strong rhythm, which increase energy and induce bodily action (3, 18, 22). Music was played from five speakers connected to a computer. For conditions 2, 3, and 4, the music was played during the specified period. For example, in the WU without M+RE with M (condition 4) warm-up was performed without any music and when the athletes performed the resistance exercise, the music was played until the participants completed the circuit.

The RPE was assessed using CR-15 RPE scale. The RPE scale has been shown to be a valid instrument in which to evaluate perceived exertion and quantification of resistance exercise intensity in a variety of populations. Citation numbers from 6 to 20 on the scale were used to rate the intensity of the entire workout session. A rating of 6 was associated with rest, and the highest rating, 20, referred to maximal effort. After completing a circuit of resistance exercises, the athlete was asked "How would you rate your effort?" The participants would verbally indicate a number to rate their overall effort based on score of 6 to 20 [18].

Heart rate and blood pressure were measured before starting the conditions in a seated position in a quiet and comfortable place (prevalue). After performing each condition, the athletes' heart rate and blood pressure were measured every 15 minutes for 60 minutes. During postexercise assessment, the participants maintained seated positions in a quiet and comfortable place. Heart rate (HR) was measured using a Polar S610i HR monitor (FIN, 90440, Finland).

Blood pressure was measured by the same experienced observer using a standard mercury sphygmomanometer (Missouri) and stethoscope (Rappaport GF Health Products, Northeast Parkway Atlanta). Systolic blood pressure (SBP) was determined as the appearance of Korotkoff sounds, while the point of disappearance of these sounds was considered to be the diastolic blood pressure (DBP). Mean arterial pressure (MAP) was calculated as DBP + [0.333 (SBP − DBP)]. The rate pressure product (RPP) was calculated as SBP × heart rate. It is considered a reliable predictor of myocardial oxygen demand [19].

2.4. Statistical Analysis. Data are presented as means ± SD. Prior to analysis, data normality was checked with the Kalmogorov-Smirnoff test. Repeated measures analysis of variance (ANOVA) was used for determining differences. When a significant F value was achieved, the Bonferroni post hoc test was used to analyze the RPE, HR, SBP, DBP, MAP, and RPP responses after different conditions to determine where the difference occurred. The level of significance was set at $p < 0.05$ for all statistical procedures. All analyses were conducted using SPSS version 16.0 (SPSS Inc., Chicago, IL, USA).

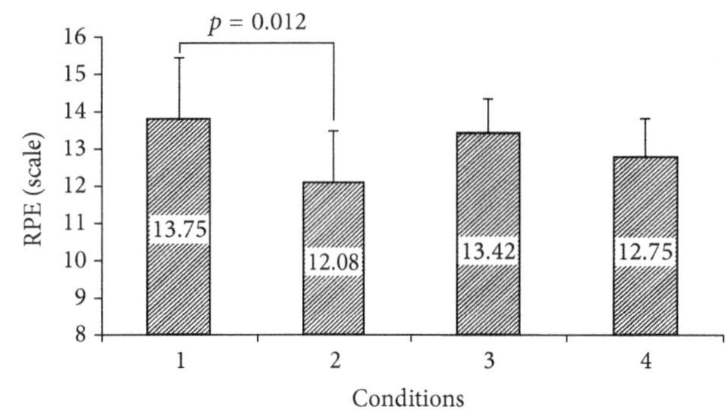

FIGURE 1: Rating of perceived exertion following 4 conditions; 1: WU+RE without M, 2: WU+RE with M, 3: WU with M+RE without M, and 4: WU without M+RE with M.

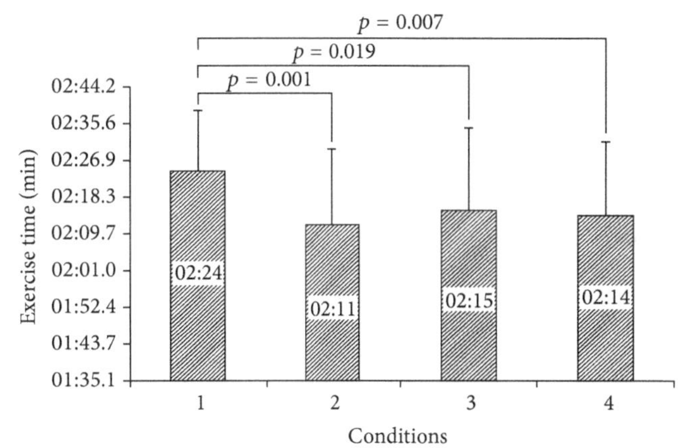

FIGURE 2: Completion time for a circuit resistance exercise (mean ± SD). 1: WU+RE without M, 2: WU+RE with M, 3: WU with M+RE without M, and 4: WU without M+RE with M.

3. Results

The repeated measures ANOVA showed a significant difference among the mean RPE values of the conditions ($F_{2.02,22.2} = 7.25$, $p = 0.004$) as condition 1 displayed an increase in perceived exertion greater than condition 2. RPE values are displayed in Figure 1.

Total time of completing a circuit of resistance exercise was higher for condition 1 compared to the other conditions ($F_{2.02,22.88} = 16.63$, $p = 0.001$) (Figure 2).

Heart rate, SBP, DBP, MAP, and RPP values for each condition are presented in Table 2. For HR, the main effect of resistance exercise was significant increases in HR postexercise and 15 minutes after exercise in all conditions. Likewise condition 1, condition 2, and condition 3 displayed these increases in HR until 30 minutes after circuit-type resistance exercise ($p = 0.001$). Only condition 1 showed incremental increases in HR until 45 minutes after exercise when compared to preexercise values ($p = 0.017$). There were no significant differences among conditions in HR at any time point after exercise ($F_{5.43,79.72} = 0.698$, $p = 0.639$).

No significant differences were observed at any time points of postexercise SBP ($F_{9.97,146.26} = 0.943$, $p = 0.496$),

TABLE 2: Heart rate (HR), systolic blood pressure (SBP), diastolic blood pressure (DBP), mean arterial pressure (MAP), and rate pressure product (RPE) responses to warm-up and resistance exercise with and without of music. Values are mean ± SD.

Conditions	Variable/time					
	HR (bpm)					
	Before	After*	15 min*	30 min†	45 min§	60 min
Condition 1	69.8 ± 7.7	133.9 ± 18.1	96.1 ± 9.8	80.5 ± 8.7	78.5 ± 9.3	75 ± 9.9
Condition 2	72.6 ± 10.5	138.8 ± 16.4	95.6 ± 9	78.5 ± 10.1	73.4 ± 8.6	69.5 ± 8.2
Condition 3	68 ± 8.4	131.5 ± 22.6	93.8 ± 14.6	79.3 ± 12	72.6 ± 10.6	69.5 ± 8.9
Condition 4	72 ± 7.1	134.3 ± 16.6	93.6 ± 11.8	77.8 ± 10.8	72.1 ± 8.4	70.6 ± 9.3
	SBP (mmHg)					
	Before	After*	15 min‡	30 min§	45 min	60 min
Condition 1	116.9 ± 6.7	142 ± 8.3	129.1 ± 10.1	124.4 ± 9.9	120.8 ± 7.3	115.9 ± 6.2
Condition 2	116.1 ± 6.7	141.9 ± 9.4	125.8 ± 9.9	120.1 ± 8	117.7 ± 6.8	115.8 ± 5.5
Condition 3	120.7 ± 8.1	146 ± 7.5	129.3 ± 7.7	126.4 ± 7.2	119.3 ± 6.3	119.2 ± 6.5
Condition 4	120.7 ± 8.1	149.5 ± 6.2	131.2 ± 9.5	122.9 ± 7.8	119.8 ± 6.8	119.5 ± 7.5
	DBP (mmHg)					
	Pre	Post	15-min	30-min	45-min	60-min
Condition 1	78.7 ± 3.1	84.7 ± 4.3	80.9 ± 2.1	81.2 ± 5.2	79.1 ± 3.2	79.5 ± 2.5
Condition 2	80 ± 2.1	85.4 ± 4.5	82.5 ± 3.9	80.2 ± 2.6	80 ± 2.1	79.5 ± 1.4
Condition 3	79.9 ± 1.7	85 ± 3.6	81.8 ± 3.2	81.6 ± 4.9	80 ± 2.1	79.7 ± 1.6
Condition 4	80.5 ± 3.9	84.8 ± 5.4	81.8 ± 3.2	82.2 ± 3.2	80.5 ± 1.5	80 ± 1
	MAP (mmHg)					
	Before	After*	15 min‡	30 min	45 min	60 min
Condition 1	97.8 ± 3.9	113.4 ± 5.6	104.8 ± 5.6	102.6 ± 6.2	92.4 ± 6.5	97.7 ± 3.5
Condition 2	98 ± 3.5	113.6 ± 5.9	104.1 ± 6.2	100.2 ± 4.4	99.9 ± 3.8	99.5 ± 3.8
Condition 3	100.3 ± 4.4	115.5 ± 4.4	105.5 ± 4.5	104.4 ± 5.2	99.6 ± 3.4	99.5 ± 3.3
Condition 4	100.6 ± 5.1	116.1 ± 3.6	106.5 ± 5.5	102.5 ± 4.4	100.2 ± 3.1	99.7 ± 3.7
	RPP (bpm × mmHg)					
	Before	After*	15 min*	30 min*	45 min‡	60 min
Condition 1	8190 ± 1224.4	19118 ± 3518.9	12434 ± 1784.4	10067 ± 1684.4	9512 ± 1422.7	8735 ± 1429
Condition 2	8449 ± 1348.6	19790 ± 3377.6	12077 ± 1854	9471 ± 1557	8665 ± 1286.9	8073 ± 1122
Condition 3	8245 ± 1319	19222 ± 3512.9	12567 ± 1741.2	10047 ± 1711.1	8698 ± 1523.4	8320 ± 1394.5
Condition 4	8707 ± 1175.5	19789 ± 2436.1	12305 ± 1878	9591 ± 1612.7	8674 ± 1313.5	8498 ± 1552.2

Condition 1: WU+RE without M, condition 2: WU+RE with M, condition 3: WU with M+RE without M, and condition 4: WU without M+RE with M. *Significant differences in comparison with prevalue for all conditions; †significant differences in comparison with prevalue for conditions 1, 2, and 3; ‡significant differences in comparison with prevalue for conditions 1 and 2; §significant differences in comparison with prevalue for condition 2.

DBP ($F_{9.70,142.4} = 0.366$, $p = 0.957$), MAP ($F_{5.02,73.76} = 0.741$, $p = 0.596$), and RPP ($F_{3.17,46.58} = 0.982$, $p = 0.413$) when the conditions were compared.

SBP and MAP increased significantly after exercise in comparison to before exercise ($p = 0.001$) for all conditions. Likewise, these increases for condition 1 ($p = 0.026$, $p = 0.023$) and condition 2 ($p = 0.018$, $p = 0.037$) continued until 15 minutes after exercise, respectively. Condition 1 showed incremental increases in SBP until 30 minutes after exercise when compared to preexercise values ($p = 0.015$).

The changes in DBP at all time points were not statistically significant for all conditions. For RPP, all conditions showed significant increases until 30 minutes after exercise when compared to preexercise values ($p = 0.001$), and only condition 1 maintained their increased RPP until 45 minutes after circuit-type resistance exercise ($p = 0.001$).

4. Discussion

The aim of this study was to examine the effects of listening to music on warm-up and circuit-type resistance exercise. The results showed that the rating of perceived exertion was higher for participants who performed both warm-up and resistance exercise without music in comparison with other conditions that played music for at least the warm-up or resistance exercise or both. There were significant differences between WU+RE without M and WU+RE with music in perceived exertion that support music as ergogenic aid. The results of the present study are consistent with those of previous studies that reported reduced RPE while listening to music. Nethery et al. [20], Potteiger et al. [7], Nethery [8], Yamashita et al. [4], and Dyer and McKune [5] reported a decrease in RPE when listening to music while exercising.

In contrast, Schwartz et al. [10], Caria et al. [21], Birnbaum et al. [11], and Chtourou et al. [22] did not find any significant differences in RPE when their subjects listened to music. These differences in findings could be at least partly attributed to differences in exercise intensity, duration, trained and untrained states of the participants, and the music selection process. Overall, with regard to the positive effects of listening to music in decreasing RPE in this study, enhancing arousal levels and facilitating motor coordination could be possible mechanisms for this effect. However, we did not measure these features specifically but previous studies reported this [4–8, 20]. With regard to significant differences between WU+RE without M and other conditions in completing a circuit resistance exercise time, it seems that increasing arousal during listening to music played a critical role in completing the resistance exercise session in minimal time. However, some authors reported no significant effects of music on completion time of exercise [5]. Consequently, further studies on the effect of music on exercise completion time are necessary.

To date, this study was the first investigation that examined the effects of music during warm-up or circuit-type resistance exercise on physiological or cardiovascular responses (HR, SBP, DBP, MAP, and RPP) in well-trained athletes. The results showed that postexercise HR, SBP, MAP, and RPP significantly increased in comparison with before exercise for all conditions. Likewise, RPP and HR were high until 15 minutes after exercise in all conditions. Moreover, HR, SBP, and RPP remained elevated until 30-to-45 min after exercise for the WU+RE without M condition. These findings revealed the ergogenic effect of music for decreasing cardiovascular responses to exercise. This is a surprising finding because of the common notion that music serves as a distraction from the exercise itself, and other investigators have reported an increase in HR and blood pressure due to stimulation of the sympathetic nervous system when listening to music while exercising [4, 11, 13, 14]. Edworthy and Waring [9] and Thornby et al. [23] observed a significant increase in HR when their subjects listened to fast music while exercising. Their studies used different exercise protocols and different music selection processes, which may account for the contradictory findings. The discrepancy between our findings and previous studies could be differences in exercise type (circuit-type resistance exercise versus treadmill or cycle), duration, training status of the subjects, and the music selection process (fast versus medium or low tempo).

The limitation of the study was the number of subjects. The limitations of this study include the low number of subjects which prevents generalization of the results. Additionally the results of the current investigation are based on nonsporting population, and further research is needed to determine if similar effects are obtained in the sporting population and during sport events. Moreover, there is no financial support for this project and we did not measure some of blood indicators, which can be a subject for further researches. In this study we used only one circuit and for further studies the researchers can increase number of circuits (i.e., 3 times).

5. Conclusions

In light of these study findings, fast tempo music (130 bpm) may decrease perceived exertion in well-trained individuals during a warm-up when completing circuit resistance exercise training. Likewise, music may be considered as a legal ergogenic aid for well-trained athletes during warm-up prior to resistance exercise and during resistance exercise for decreasing perceived exertion and minimizing training time. Thus, professional strength and conditioning coaches and practitioners interested in resistance exercise may be well advised to incorporate arousing music during warm-up and exercise sessions. Music may decrease physiological and/or cardiovascular responses in athletes while performing resistance exercise. Therefore, it can be recommend that coaches and strength and conditioning professionals use music during warm-up and resistance exercise for the decreases of RPE and cardiovascular responses.

Conflict of Interests

The authors declare that there is no conflict of interests regarding the publication of this paper.

References

[1] W. J. Kraemer and N. A. Ratamess, “Fundamentals of resistance training: progression and exercise prescription,” *Medicine and Science in Sports and Exercise*, vol. 36, no. 4, pp. 674–688, 2004.

[2] J. M. Davis, Z. Zhao, H. S. Stock, K. A. Mehl, J. Buggy, and G. A. Hand, “Central nervous system effects of caffeine and adenosine on fatigue,” *The American Journal of Physiology—Regulatory Integrative and Comparative Physiology*, vol. 284, no. 2, pp. R399–R404, 2003.

[3] T. Atan, “Effect of music on anaerobic exercise performance,” *Biology of Sport*, vol. 30, no. 1, pp. 35–39, 2013.

[4] S. Yamashita, K. Iwai, T. Akimoto, J. Sugawara, and I. Kono, “Effects of music during exercise on RPE, heart rate and the autonomic nervous system,” *Journal of Sports Medicine and Physical Fitness*, vol. 46, no. 3, pp. 425–430, 2006.

[5] B. J. Dyer and A. J. McKune, “Effects of music tempo on performance, psychological, and physiological variables during 20 km cycling in well-trained cyclists,” *Perceptual and Motor Skills*, vol. 117, no. 2, pp. 484–497, 2013.

[6] G. Atkinson, D. Wilson, and M. Eubank, “Effects of music on world-rate distribution during a cycling time trial,” *International Journal of Sports Medicine*, vol. 25, no. 8, pp. 611–615, 2004.

[7] J. A. Potteiger, J. M. Schroeder, and K. L. Goff, “Influence of music on ratings of perceived exertion during 20 minutes of moderate intensity exercise,” *Perceptual and Motor Skills*, vol. 91, no. 3, pp. 848–854, 2000.

[8] V. M. Nethery, “Competition between internal and external sources of information during exercise: influence on RPE and the impact of the exercise load,” *Journal of Sports Medicine and Physical Fitness*, vol. 42, no. 2, pp. 172–178, 2002.

[9] J. Edworthy and H. Waring, “The effects of music tempo and loudness level on treadmill exercise,” *Ergonomics*, vol. 49, no. 15, pp. 1597–1610, 2006.

[10] S. E. Schwartz, B. Fernhall, and S. A. Plowman, “Effects of music on exercise performance,” *Journal of Cardiopulmonary Rehabilitation*, vol. 10, no. 9, pp. 312–316, 1990.

[11] L. Birnbaum, T. Boone, and B. Huschle, "Cardiovascular responses to music tempo during steady-state exercise," *Journal of Exercise Physiology Online*, vol. 12, no. 1, pp. 50–57, 2009.

[12] M. Jarraya, H. Chtourou, A. Aloui et al., "The effects of music on high-intensity short-term exercise in well trained athletes," *Asian Journal of Sports Medicine*, vol. 3, no. 4, pp. 233–238, 2012.

[13] J. H. Mitchell and J. B. Wolffe, "Neural control of the circulation during exercise," *Medicine & Science in Sports & Exercise*, vol. 22, pp. 141–154, 1990.

[14] B. D. William and H. T. Michael, "The influence of preferred relaxing music on measures of state anxiety, relaxation and physiological responses," *Journal of Music Therapy*, vol. 26, pp. 168–187, 1989.

[15] D. J. Harriss and G. Atkinson, "Ethical standards in sport and exercise science research," *International Journal of Sports Medicine*, vol. 32, no. 11, pp. 819–821, 2011.

[16] D. E. Michel, *Music Therapy*, Charles C. Thomas Publisher, Springfield, Ill, USA, 1985.

[17] C. I. Karageorghis and P. C. Terry, "The psychophysical effect of music in sport and exercise: a review," *Journal of Sport Behavior*, vol. 20, pp. 54–68, 1997.

[18] H. Arazi, A. Asadi, M. Nasehi, and A. Delpasand, "Cardiovascular and blood lactate responses to acute plyometric exercise in female volleyball and handball players," *Sport Sciences for Health*, vol. 8, no. 1, pp. 23–29, 2012.

[19] H. Arazi, F. Rahmaninia, K. Hosseini, and A. Asadi, "Resting hormonal and cardiovascular responses to short term creatine supplementation and resistance exercises," *Science and Sport*, vol. 30, pp. 105–109, 2015.

[20] V. M. Nethery, P. A. Harmer, and D. R. Taaffe, "Sensory mediation of perveived exertion during submaximal exercise," *Journal of Human Movement Studies*, vol. 20, pp. 201–211, 1991.

[21] M. A. Caria, F. Tangianu, A. Concu, A. Crisafulli, and O. Mameli, "Quantification of Spinning bike performance during a standard 50-minute class," *Journal of Sports Sciences*, vol. 25, no. 4, pp. 421–429, 2007.

[22] H. Chtourou, A. Chaouachi, O. Hammouda, K. Chamari, and N. Souissi, "Listening to music affects diurnal variation in muscle power output," *International Journal of Sports Medicine*, vol. 33, no. 1, pp. 43–47, 2012.

[23] M. A. Thornby, F. Haas, and K. Axen, "Effect of distractive auditory stimuli on exercise tolerance in patients with COPD," *Chest*, vol. 107, no. 5, pp. 1213–1217, 1995.

14

Incidence and Time to Return to Training for Stress Fractures during Military Basic Training

Alexander M. Wood,[1] Richard Hales,[2] Andre Keenan,[3] Alexandra Moss,[3] Michael Chapman,[2] Trish Davey,[1] and Andrew Nelstrop[2]

[1] *Institute of Naval Medicine, Alverstoke, Hants PO12 2DL, UK*
[2] *Commando Training Centre Royal Marines, Lympstone, Devon EX8 5AR, UK*
[3] *Royal Army Medical Corps, Sandhurst GU15 4PQ, UK*

Correspondence should be addressed to Alexander M. Wood; drsandywood@googlemail.com

Academic Editor: Randy J. Schmitz

Currently, little is known about the length of time required to rehabilitate patients from stress fractures and their return to preinjury level of physical activity. Previous studies have looked at the return to sport in athletes, in a general population, where rehabilitation is not as controlled as within a captive military population. In this study, a longitudinal prospective epidemiological database was assessed to determine the incidence of stress fractures and the time taken to rehabilitate recruits to preinjury stage of training. Findings demonstrated a background prevalence of 5% stress fractures in Royal Marine training; femoral and tibial stress fractures take 21.1 weeks to return to training with metatarsal stress fractures being the most common injury taking 12.2 weeks. Rehabilitation from stress fractures accounts for 814 weeks of recruit rehabilitation time per annum. Stress fracture incidence is still common in military training; despite this stress fracture recovery times remain constant and represent a significant interruption in training. It takes on average 5 weeks after exercise specific training has restarted to reenter training at a preinjury level, regardless of which bone has a stress fracture. Further research into their prevention, treatment, and rehabilitation is required to help reduce these burdens.

1. Introduction

Stress fractures are well recognised in military training and athletes, with the first reported case being identified in 1855 by Breithaupt [1] and the first imaging of a stress fracture recorded by Stechow in 1897 [2].

The incidence of sustained stress fractures in military recruits can be as high as 12% [3], as compared with a rate of 21.1% of elite athletes [4] and 1% of the general population [5].

Trone et al. [6] suggest that recruits who sustain a stress fracture during basic training are over four times more likely to be discharged from training programmes, demonstrating that these injuries can be responsible for a significant portion of attrition in military training with consequent financial implication for military budgets.

Furthermore, after initial rehabilitation, recruits who suffered a stress fracture during basic training are at higher risk of sustaining stress fractures during subsequent training (10.6% incidence within one year of injury, versus 1.7% in injury-free recruits) [7], thereby increasing working days lost to injury and the accompanying financial burden.

Royal Marine training is conducted at the Commando Training Centre in Lympstone, Devon. Between 55 and 60 recruits join at fortnightly intervals throughout the year, excepting leave periods. Spanning 32 weeks, the basic training programme is the longest in the western world, with the average recruit taking a mean time of 37 weeks to complete the syllabus [8]. Training is progressively arduous over this period, culminating in the commando tests, comprising a 30-mile run cross-country, 9-mile run on roads, a 7-mile run cross-country (including through water and tunnels), an aerial assault course, and a week-long final exercise over difficult and varied terrain.

Any recruit who sustains an injury requiring longer than a week to rehabilitate is removed from training and placed in the rehabilitation company. This offers inpatient physiotherapy, remedial physical training, and ongoing military training until the recruit is deemed fit enough to return to mainstream training as a result of passing a predetermined set of "exit" criteria.

Currently, little is known about the length of time required to rehabilitate recruits from stress fractures and return them to their preinjury level of physical activity; previous studies have only looked at the return to sport in athletes, in a general population, where rehabilitation is not as controlled as within a captive military population [9].

We present the largest known study involving stress fractures and their controlled rehabilitation using a longitudinal prospective epidemiological database to determine the incidence of stress fractures and the time taken to rehabilitate patients to their preinjury stage of training.

2. Materials and Methods

All patients who were diagnosed with a stress fracture whilst undergoing commando training between April 2004 and April 2008 were treated in the rehabilitation unit with their diagnosis and rehabilitation time prospectively recorded. During this time 4200 Marines started commando training. Patients were diagnosed on plain radiograph taken at initial presentation, repeated at two weeks if symptomatic with an initial negative radiograph. Patients who had a second negative radiograph and were still symptomatic were referred for Magnetic Resonance Imaging to confirm the diagnosis.

Patients were removed from training upon initial presentation and placed into a rehabilitation company, where they initially underwent inpatient based physiotherapy and rehabilitation to recover from their injury and return to training.

The rehabilitation system was divided into two parts, with the first part focusing on the recovery from the initial injury (Group A). When patients were fully recovered from their condition they were moved to a second group (Group B) which focused on regaining fitness and military skills up to the required level for them to return back to training at their preinjury stage.

3. Results

During the study period there were 220 stress fractures sustained in 208 patients giving a background prevalence of 5%.

The most common stress fractures are as illustrated in Table 1.

The metatarsals were the most common bone type involved with the third metatarsal being the most likely bone to be fractured. The distribution of metatarsal fractures is as detailed in Table 2.

Table 1: Stress fracture type.

Fracture	Number
Metatarsals	143 (65%)
Tibia	52 (24%)
Femur	21 (10%)
Fibula	6 (3%)

Table 2: The distribution of metatarsal fractures.

Metatarsal	Number
1st	0
2nd	38
3rd	99
4th	5
5th	1

7.69% of patients with metatarsal stress fractures sustained multiple fractures in the same foot, with one patient having a concurrent stress fracture of his tibia.

81% (17 of 21) of the femoral stress fractures were located in the femoral neck, with the remaining 19% being located in the metaphysis of the femur.

Figure 1 demonstrates whether the fractures were sustained in the first part of second part of training, 53% (9/17) of the fractures found in the femoral neck occurred during the second half of the 32-week training program as compared to 78% (111/143) of metatarsal fractures ($P < 0.0001$). Only one metatarsal stress fracture occurred within the first 4 weeks of training.

Figure 2 demonstrates how long each fracture took to recover in the two stages of rehabilitation. The mean rehabilitation time was as follows: single metatarsal 12.2 (±1.3 95% CI) weeks (range 8–50 weeks); multiple metatarsal fractures 15.4 (±1.2 95% CI) weeks (range 12–18 weeks); tibia fractures 21.1 (±3.4 95% CI) weeks (range 10–47 weeks); fibula fractures 13.3 (±6.5 95% CI) (range 7–23 weeks); and femoral fractures 21.1 (±4.1 95% CI) weeks (range 11–43 weeks).

Stress fractures account for 814 weeks of recruit rehabilitation time per year.

20 (9.6%) of patients had other medical diagnosis at the same time as their stress fractures. The most common diagnosis (25%) was anterior knee pain, with 14/20 (70%) having another lower limb condition, 6/20 (30%) having an infection, 1/20 having a concurrent stress fracture, and 2/20 having an acute trauma fracture.

4. Discussion

During the 4-year study period there were 4200 recruits in Royal Marine training sustaining 220 stress fractures at a prevalence of 5%. Similar studies estimate the annual incidence of stress fractures among groups of athletes and military recruits to be between 5 and 30% [10]. Our rate of diagnosed stress fractures is at the lower end of previously reported incidences when compared with similar study groups. With the multifactorial etiology of stress fractures

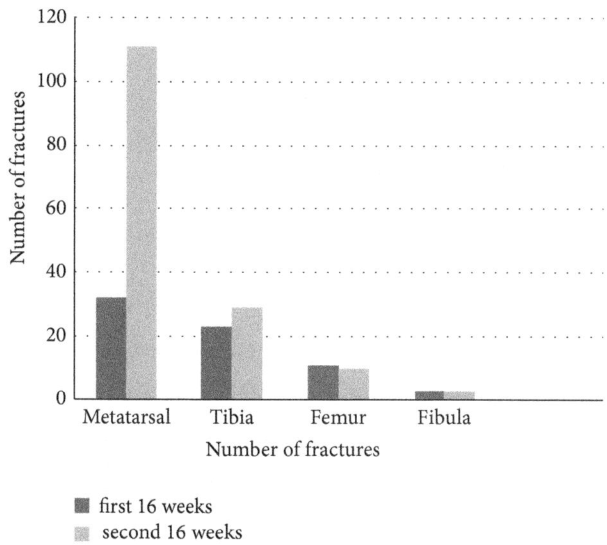

FIGURE 1: Time of occurrence of stress fracture and anatomical distribution.

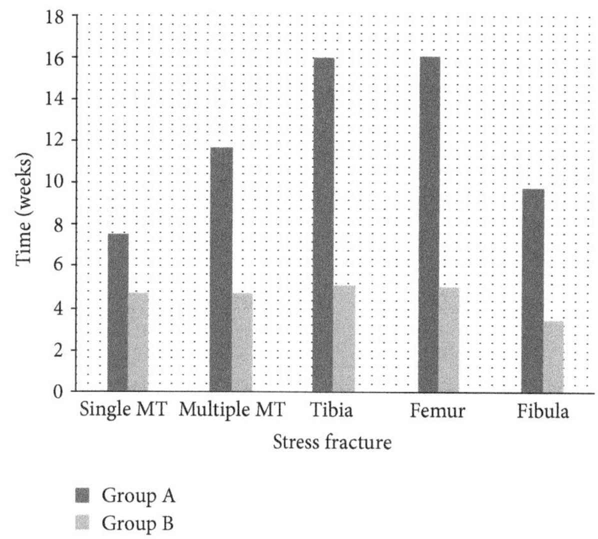

FIGURE 2: (Group A) Rehabilitation period from injury (Group B). Time in program for regaining fitness and military skills up to allow return to training at their preinjury stage.

[11] it is difficult to speculate on the precise reasons for the relatively low incidence within our group, although this may reflect a reluctance to present to the medical centre for fear of having to change their training group as a result of injury.

One possible explanation can be derived from a directly comparable study undertaken by Ross and Allsopp in 2002 [12]. This study looked at stress fracture rates in recruits undergoing basic training at the Commando Training Centre both before and after the installation of the Revised Common Recruit Syllabus (RCRS), commissioned to optimise the training programme with respect to reducing injury rates. Results demonstrated a statistically significant reduction in stress fracture rates with the more physiologically progressive RCRS syllabus (3.8%) versus the original training programme (7%), although in their study 30% of patients in the new syllabus were still in training when data collection was completed which may explain our slightly higher incidence of 5%.

Ross and Allsopp argued that RCRS has had a beneficial effect on the incidence of stress fractures; our results support a lower level of stress fractures than prior to the implementation of RCRS despite multiple changes to Royal Marine training since 2002.

Another possible reason for a low incidence of stress fractures is that most fractures were diagnosed by radiograph. It has been recognised that radiographs do not usually contain positive signs associated with stress fractures until two weeks after the onset of symptoms [13]. In this study recruits were diagnosed as having a stress fracture after symptomatic presentation with positive radiograph findings. If symptomatic with a negative initial radiograph, a further radiograph was taken at two weeks. Those who were symptomatic with two negative radiographs proceeded to Magnetic Resonance Imaging (MRI) to confirm the diagnosis. Whilst we have advocated the use of MRI as an initial investigative choice and this remains the UK military policy on suspected stress fractures [2] rapid access to MRI is not always possible, and as a result a pragmatic approach is applied. As a result of this approach, a significant period of time can elapse from presentation of symptoms until radiological diagnosis of stress fracture; however, as all recruits are treated symptomatically in Group A, regardless of diagnosis, a delay in obtaining a definite diagnosis does not cause delay in starting rehabilitation in our study, and we therefore believe that our results demonstrate accurate rehabilitation time for stress fractures.

Giladi et al. [13] advocate a high clinical index of suspicion and early referral for MRI to enable prompt diagnosis among at-risk populations, though definitive evidence is lacking as to whether early diagnostic MRI has significant effect on rehabilitation time from injury and further research into this is necessary.

The pattern of distribution of stress fractures in this study correlates well with previous studies; metatarsals sustain the greatest number of injuries in athletic and military populations [12, 14–17], with fractures of the third metatarsal being the most common although our results would suggest that a higher proportion of stress fractures are 3rd metatarsal (45%) than reported in other studies [12]. Previous research suggests that the third metatarsal is the most common site as a result of increased ligament support of the middle metatarsals resulting in relative resistance to movement, thereby increasing stress forces placed upon this bone [18, 19].

In 2006, Dixon et al. [20] undertook a study on Royal Marine recruits both with and without a history of third metatarsal stress fractures and discovered significant differences in dynamic biomechanical variables of the forefoot, concluding that future successful intervention to reduce the incidence of this injury will likely focus on this area; however, despite these findings, our results show that 3rd metatarsal stress fractures still represent a problem in military training.

Garcia et al. (1987) [21] demonstrated that a majority of metatarsal stress fractures occur in the first 3 weeks; the postulated reason for this is that during the early phase of bone remodeling excessive resorption temporarily decreases the ability for the bone to withstand force [21]. Our results demonstrate that metatarsal stress fractures occur later in training with less than 1% occurring in the first 4 weeks. This may be because Royal Marine training now has a gradual increase in intensity in the first few weeks, in order to allow more time for complete remodeling processes to occur, but in the second half of training there is a sudden increase in mileage as the recruits progress from basic infantry training to more arduous commando training.

Femoral stress fractures are uncommon [22, 23], representing only 10% of the fractures identified in this study. Of these 81% of them involved the neck of femur, with the remaining 19% being located in the metaphysis. A recent study undertaken on recruits based in Northallerton (2008) [22] documents a comparative femoral fracture rate of 8% of all diagnosed stress fractures, whilst Royal Marine training is longer; this does not appear to affect the proportion of femoral stress fractures when compared to other British military training.

Peak presentation time of femoral stress fractures has been debated, having been documented at weeks 13–16 of training [22] and weeks 4–7 of training [23]. Our study demonstrated that 53% of the diagnosed femoral stress fractures occurred during the second half of the training, indicating an equal spread of presentation throughout the 32-week course.

Femoral stress fractures, though less common than fractures at other lower limb locations, represent a more severe complication of training [2, 22, 24]. Unprotected, undisplaced fractures can lead to displaced femoral neck fractures, which carry a 63% complication rate even with optimum treatment [23]. Giladi et al. (1986) [13] showed that 10.6% of recruits who suffer a femoral stress fracture would sustain recurrent stress fractures within one year, demonstrating the gravity of the diagnosis.

The mean rehabilitation time in our study is similar to comparable studies [12]. A mean rehabilitation time for single metatarsal fractures was found to be 12.2 weeks, which increases to 15.4 for multiple stress fractures. There is a significant difference between rehabilitation time for metatarsals and stress fractures in the tibia and femur; however there was no significant difference between stress fractures in the tibia and femur both taking 21.1 weeks. Our results support previous findings with regard to total rehabilitation times [12].

Our results differ from previous studies [12] as we can identify when patients were able to return to activity specific training and also when they returned back to their previous training level. Recruits entered Group B when they were able to restart mainstream training activities and exited Group B back to recruit training after they had passed the appropriate fitness assessment for their level of preinjury training. Apart from fibula fractures where the numbers were quite small, the mean time in Group B ranged between 4.7 and 5.2 weeks, which probably represents the time required to regain cardiovascular and muscle strength fitness and is unrelated to type of stress fracture. Therefore, we believe that future research should be focused on trying to reduce the time required before activity specific training can be commenced.

Our results would suggest that the rehabilitation time required to recover from stress fractures has not decreased since the earlier studies [12] with the mainstay of treatment still being a period of rest from training sufficiently long enough so as to allow healing to occur. There is a requirement to investigate if patients can be physically loaded earlier in the recovery phase and if there are any pharmacological interventions, which can decrease rehabilitation time, in order to reduce the impact of stress fractures on patients sporting and military activities.

It is recognised that the prevention of stress fractures is difficult [13] due to the multifactorial nature of the injury. As such, the fundamental aspects of treatment remain early diagnosis, early identification of symptoms, and a sufficiently long pause in training so as to allow healing to occur [13, 22, 23, 25], Our results would suggest that stress fractures still remain relatively common in military training and that further studies into the prevention and causes of stress fractures are required.

5. Conclusion

Mean rehabilitation times vary with the location of the stress fracture. Effective treatment relies on a high index of clinical suspicion, early detection of symptoms, and early diagnosis to reduce rehabilitation time [26].

Despite awareness of the injury and relative lowincidence as compared to similar population groups', stress fractures represent a significant burden in RM training. Stress fractures account for approximately 814 weeks of recruit rehabilitation time per year at an estimated cost of £1500 per recruit per week, meaning that total costs exceed 1.2 million pounds [8] per annum warranting further research into their prevention, early detection, and improved recovery times.

Conflict of Interests

The authors declare that there is no conflict of interests regarding the publication of this paper.

References

[1] H. Lacroix and J. N. Keeman, "An unusual stress fracture of the fibula in a long distance runner," *Archives of Orthopaedic and Trauma*, vol. 111, no. 5, pp. 289–290, 2010.

[2] R. Thomas, A. M. Wood, J. Watson, C. H. Arthur, and A. M. Nicol, "Delay in diagnosis of neck of femur stress fracture in a female military recruit," *Journal of the Royal Naval Medical Service*, vol. 98, no. 2, pp. 3–5, 2012.

[3] R. R. Protzman and C. G. Griffis, "Stress fractures in men and women undergoing military training," *The Journal of Bone and Joint Surgery*, vol. 59, no. 6, p. 825, 1977.

[4] K. L. Bennell, S. A. Malcolm, S. A. Thomas et al., "Risk factors for stress fractures in track and field athletes: a twelve- month

prospective study," *The American Journal of Sports Medicine*, vol. 24, no. 6, pp. 810–818, 1996.

[5] I. I. I. Tornetta P, T. A. Einhorn, A. A. Schepsis, and B. D. Busconi, *Sports Medicine*, Orthopaedic Surgery Essentials, Lippincott Williams and Wilkins, Philadelphia, Pa, USA, 2006.

[6] D. W. Trone, J. P. Reis, C. A. Macera, and M. J. Rauh, "Factors associated with discharge during marine corps basic training," *Military Medicine*, vol. 172, no. 9, pp. 936–941.

[7] C. Milgrom, M. Giladi, R. Chisin, and R. Dizian, "The long-term followup of soldiers with stress fractures," *The American Journal of Sports Medicine*, vol. 13, no. 6, pp. 398–400, 1985.

[8] "Once A Marine, Always A Marine. What you could expect of Royal Marines Training from 1999," http://www.onceamarine-alwaysamarine.co.uk/trg99.htm.

[9] G. O. Matheson, D. B. Clement, and D. C. Mckenzie, "Stress fractures in athletes: a study of 320 cases," *The American Journal of Sports Medicine*, vol. 15, no. 1, pp. 46–58, 1987.

[10] J. D. Reeser, "Stress Fracture," eMedicine from WebMD, http://emedicine.medscape.com/article/309106-overview.

[11] C. N. Chatzipapas, G. I. Drosos, K. I. Kazakos, G. Tripslanis, C. Iatrou, and D.-A. J. Verettas, "Stress fractures in military men and bone quality related factors," *International Journal of Sports Medicine*, vol. 29, no. 11, pp. 922–926, 2008.

[12] R. A. Ross and A. Allsopp, "Stress fractures in Royal Marines recruits," *Military Medicine*, vol. 167, no. 7, pp. 560–565, 2002.

[13] M. Giladi, C. Milgrom, and H. Kashtan, "Recurrent stress fractures in military recruits: one-year follow-up of 66 recruits," *Journal of Bone and Joint Surgery B*, vol. 68, no. 3, pp. 439–441, 1986.

[14] M. Jansen, "March foot," *Journal of Bone and Joint Surgery*, vol. 8, no. 2, pp. 262–272, 1926.

[15] G. R. Krause and J. R. Thompson Jr., "March fracture, analysis of 200 cases," *The American Journal of Roentgenology*, vol. 52, pp. 281–290, 1944.

[16] D. G. Leavitt and H. W. Woodward, "March fracture: a statistical study of forty-seven patients," *Journal of Bone and Joint Surgery*, vol. 26, pp. 733–742, 1944.

[17] F. H. Tyner and W. T. Hileman, "March fracture: an analysis of 166 cases," *The American Journal of Roentgenology*, vol. 52, pp. 165–172, 1944.

[18] A. D. Perron, "Metatarsal Stress Fracture," eMedicine for WebMD, http://emedicine.medscape.com/article/85746-overview.

[19] R. Patel and F. Haddad, "Metatarsal Fractures," Sports Injury Bulletin, http://www.sportsinjurybulletin.com/archive/metatarsal-fractures.html.

[20] S. J. Dixon, M. W. Creaby, and A. J. Allsopp, "Comparison of static and dynamic biomechanical measures in military recruits with and without a history of third metatarsal stress fracture," *Clinical Biomechanics*, vol. 21, no. 4, pp. 412–419, 2006.

[21] J. E. Garcia, L. L. Grabhorn, and K. J. Franklin, "Factors associated with stress fractures in military recruits," *Military Medicine*, vol. 152, no. 1, pp. 45–48, 1987.

[22] J. C. Talbot, G. Cox, M. Townend, M. Langham, and P. J. Parker, "Femoral neck stress fractures in military personnel: a case series," *Journal of the Royal Army Medical Corps*, vol. 154, no. 1, pp. 47–50, 2008.

[23] A. Joshi, B. R. KC, B. C. Shah, P. Chand, B. B. Thapa, and N. Kayastha, "Femoral neck stress fractures in military personnel," *Journal of the Nepal Medical Association*, vol. 48, no. 174, pp. 99–102, 2009.

[24] J. T. Evans, P. M. Guyver, A. M. Kassam, and M. J. Hubble, "Displaced femoral neck stress fractures in royal marine recruits: management and results of operative treatment," *Journal of the Royal Naval Medical Service*, vol. 98, no. 2, pp. 3–5, 2012.

[25] J. Pegrum, T. Crisp, and N. Padhiar, "Diagnosis and management of bone stress injuries of the lower limb in athletes," *British Medical Journal*, vol. 344, no. 7854, Article ID e2511, 2012.

[26] S. Orava, A. Hulkko, S. Koskinen, and S. Taimela, "Stress fractures in athletes and military recruits: a review," *Orthopade*, vol. 24, no. 5, pp. 457–466, 1995.

15

The Injury/Illness Performance Project (IIPP): A Novel Epidemiological Approach for Recording the Consequences of Sports Injuries and Illnesses

Debbie Palmer-Green,[1] Colin Fuller,[2] Rod Jaques,[3] and Glenn Hunter[4]

[1] *University of Nottingham, Nottingham, UK*
[2] *F-MARC, Zurich, Switzerland*
[3] *English Institute of Sport, Bath, UK*
[4] *UK Sport, London, UK*

Correspondence should be addressed to Debbie Palmer-Green; debbie.palmer-green@nottingham.ac.uk

Academic Editor: S. John Sullivan

Background. Describing the frequency, severity, and causes of sports injuries and illnesses reliably is important for quantifying the risk to athletes and providing direction for prevention initiatives. *Methods.* Time-loss and/or medical-attention definitions have long been used in sports injury/illness epidemiology research, but the limitations to these definitions mean that some events are incorrectly classified or omitted completely, where athletes continue to train and compete at high levels but experience restrictions in their performance. Introducing a graded definition of performance-restriction may provide a solution to this issue. *Results.* Results from the Great Britain injury/illness performance project (IIPP) are presented using a performance-restriction adaptation of the accepted surveillance consensus methodologies. The IIPP involved 322 Olympic athletes (males: 172; female: 150) from 10 Great Britain Olympic sports between September 2009 and August 2012. Of all injuries (n = 565), 216 were classified as causing time-loss, 346 as causing performance-restriction, and 3 were unclassified. For athlete illnesses (n = 378), the majority ($P < 0.01$) resulted in time-loss (270) compared with performance-restriction (101) (7 unclassified). *Conclusions.* Successful implementation of prevention strategies relies on the correct characterisation of injury/illness risk factors. Including a performance-restriction classification could provide a deeper understanding of injuries/illnesses and better informed prevention initiatives.

1. Introduction

Recognition of the importance of injury and illness epidemiology research has grown in the last 10 years with international governing bodies of sport and the International Olympic Committee (IOC) regularly conducting surveillance studies at major sporting events [1–10]. The prevention of injuries and illnesses and the long-term protection of athletes' health are key factors influencing this growing interest [11]. In addition to the impact on an athlete's health, injuries and illnesses also impact on the athletes' ability to train and perform; these interruptions may affect their preparations for and availability to take part in competitions, which in turn impacts on their ability to achieve lifetime dreams and aspirations of sporting success. Information about the incidence, severity, and nature (location and type) of sports injuries and illnesses are all important, as together they quantify the overall risk of injury and illness to athletes and thus provide information that allows the prevention initiatives to be correctly prioritized [12].

The ability to describe the incidence, nature, and causes of injuries and illnesses reliably has been recognised through the development and publication of injury surveillance consensus statements [13–18]. The consensus statement for football defines an injury as "any physical complaint sustained by a player…irrespective of the need for medical-attention or time-loss from activities" [13], while for Olympic sports an injury/illness is defined as "any musculoskeletal complaint...that received medical attention regardless of the consequence with respect to absence from competition or training" [14]. Once the injury definition is set, subclassifications by consequence are used to determine what becomes a recordable event, such as (but not limited to) whether the injury/illness results in "tissue damage", "medical-attention" (without time-loss), "time-loss", and/or "missed match/competition".

Limitations with current consensus statements have been recognised for several years. For example, Fuller et al. [19] discussed how injury recurrences, reinjuries, and exacerbations could be recorded; Bahr [20] discussed how overuse injuries often limited athletic performance but were not recorded in injury surveillance systems if there was no time-loss; and Creighton et al. [21], discussed how injury severity was dependent on whether return-to-play decisions were based on an athlete's full return to sport without limitation or were based on limited return to training. Some injury surveillance studies have addressed the issue of continued participation or return-to-play under restricted performance conditions. Palmer-Green et al. [22] presented a methodology for recording impaired athlete availability and performance due to injury and illness in several sports during Great Britain Olympic team preparations for the Summer and Winter Olympics; Clarsen et al. [23] reported a methodology for recording over-use injuries of specific anatomical areas that resulted in restricted function of performance; and Jacobsson et al. presented a methodology for recording alterations in normal training due to the injury in athletics [24].

Most surveillance studies have focused on the etiology of "medical-attention" and/or "time-loss" definition of injury and illness incidents, but few epidemiological studies have related these events to an athlete's consequential training limitations. Regular training enables athletes to gain various sport-specific positive adaptations in skill development and physiological parameters designed to improve their performance [25]. Cessation or a marked reduction of the training stimulus can lead to a partial or complete reversal of a number of cardiovascular and musculoskeletal adaptations, [26, 27] and these reversals will ultimately compromise athletic performance. The magnitude of the detraining characteristics caused by injury/illness depends on the duration of training cessation (complete time-loss) and/or the duration of limited training (restriction) [28, 29]. The issue of impaired training and competitive performance, however, is not limited to overuse injuries, as limitations can also be associated with illness and acute, traumatic, gradual onset, and chronic injuries. The aim of this paper is to describe in detail (with illustrative data examples) an epidemiological recording system method based on the impact of injury/illness events on an athlete's capability to train/compete, previously reported briefly at the IOC World Conference of Prevention of Injury and Illness in Sport in Monaco in 2011 [22].

2. Methods

The following sections outline the background of the methodology developed and implemented in the summer of 2009 to monitor the injuries and illnesses sustained by Great Britain Olympic athletes in the period leading up to the 2010 Winter and 2012 Summer Olympics and which was used to quantify the impact of injury/illness on athletes' training and competition.

2.1. Injury/Illness Status (Time-Loss or Performance-Restriction?). While the majority of sports injury definitions encompass a time-loss classification the definitions are somewhat categorical in their use of the terms 'time-loss' or 'absence' from training or competition that is complete absence. Limitations attached to these definitions have been described by Bahr; [20] in particular, it was questioned as to how appropriate these definitions were when applied to sports such as swimming or athletics where there are few time-loss injuries but an abundance of overuse/chronic performance-limiting injuries [4, 5, 8]. Bahr [20] focussed his discussion on the causes of performance-limiting overuse injuries but, because many athletes continue to train (and even compete) at high levels when experiencing pain and loss of function through injury or illness [20, 23, 30], he also highlighted the need to develop scales for assessing function-limiting injuries. Subsequent papers began to propose alternate methods in injury recording around specific joints, overuse injury, and athletes' levels of impairment [23, 24]. The focus of the present study was to develop a methodology that provided a measure of the impact of both time-loss injuries/illnesses and injuries/illnesses that did not meet the definition of "time-loss" but resulted in a restriction or modification to an athlete's regular training (e.g., an upper respiratory tract illness lasting 20 days resulting in a 60% level of training capacity). If this latter type of illness was included as a recordable event according to most consensus methodologies, it would create an overestimation of the illness burden (because 20 full days of training were not lost). Conversely, if the strict "absence" criteria were applied, the event would not be recorded despite resulting in a significant impact on the athlete (i.e., 40% reduction in training capacity over a period of 20 days). The division between medical-attention (with no time-loss) and time-loss definitions is therefore blurred, with the potential for some injury/illness events to lie between the two extremes. Figures 1(a) and 1(b) provide a visual description of this situation with Figure 1(b) presenting a potential alternative hierarchy.

2.2. Time-Loss and Performance-Restriction Injuries/Illnesses and Restriction-Impact. Time-loss injuries/illnesses are regarded as those events resulting in 100% restriction (i.e., complete time-loss), with the severity of these injuries/illnesses measured from the date of onset of the injury/illness (DOI) to the date of return to "full fitness" (DOR). DOI was defined as the date of sudden onset, or, for gradual onset injuries/illnesses, the date the athlete was first unable to take a full part in training or competition; full fitness was defined as the athlete being able to complete his/her full and normal training/competition. Performance-restriction injuries/illnesses are those events that result in an athlete only being capable of a reduced level of performance (1 to 99% restriction). The severity of these injuries/illnesses is

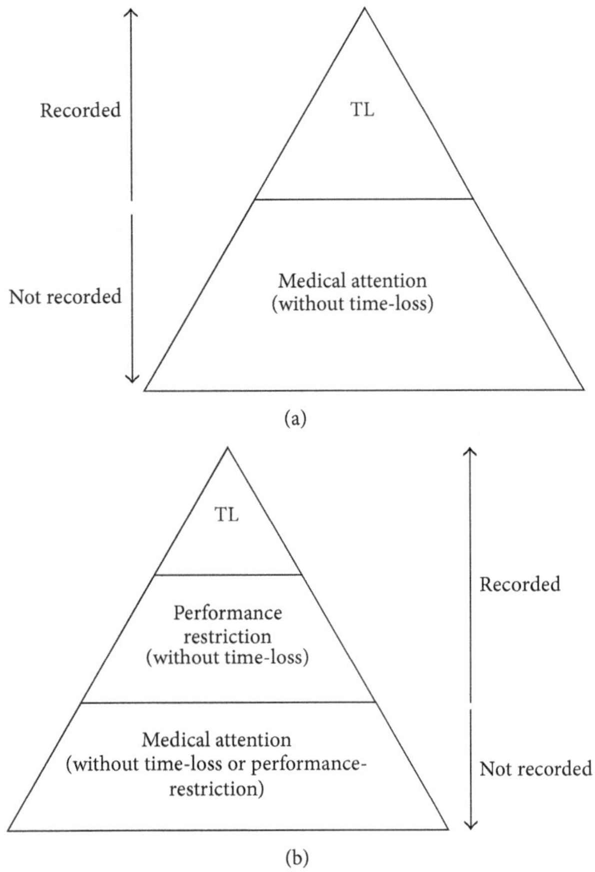

FIGURE 1: (a) Traditional hierarchy of injury/illness definition classification. (b) Alternative hierarchy of injury/illness definition classification. TL = time-loss; * classification of an injury or illness is based on the initial status of the injury and not on any subsequent change of status during the time course of its recovery and ** while injuries/illnesses are always required to be classified as either time-loss or medical-attention (or performance-restriction) is should be noted that there can and always will be overlap between categories.

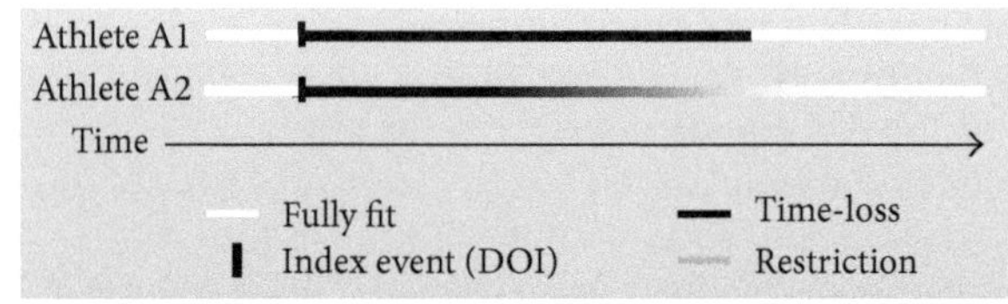

FIGURE 2: Traditional time-loss definition compared to the inclusion of a performance-restriction injury/illness classification and change of injury/illness status.

calculated using two parameters: (1) number of performance-restricted days of training/competition in the period between DOI and DOR and (2) percentage of performance-restriction in training/competition during the performance-restricted days. The percentage of performance-restriction (i.e., {100 – level of performance}) denotes the percentage of training/competition restriction compared to the athlete's normal training regimen each day/week. This parameter is meant to provide performance rather than clinical relevance and is a function of the restriction to both the athletes training volume and training intensity, with equal weighting given to decrements in each; for simplicity, percentage scores were denoted by 5% increments for medical staff to select on the report form (after discussion with the athlete/coach on the level). The percentage performance-restriction value multiplied by the duration of restricted performance provides a quantified measure of the impact of the injury/illness on the athletes performance, that is, the restriction-impact. As an example of the utility of this approach, two restriction injuries both lasting 10 days may appear to impact equally on an athlete; however, if the percentage of performance-restriction in the first case was mild (10%) and in the second case moderate (50%), the restriction-impacts of the two events would be full-time equivalent (FTE) severities of 1 day and 5 days, respectively, which reflects the greater impact of the latter injury on the athlete. All results for performance-restriction injury/illness severity are presented as restriction-impact full (FTE) days, in line with the traditional way of reporting time-loss days.

2.3. Changes in an Athlete's Injury/Illness Status. A 60-day time-loss injury implies that the athlete had 60 days absence from training/competition and returned to full training on day 61 (Figure 2, Athlete A1). In reality, there is more likely to be a graded return to normal full training comprised of increases in training intensity and volume (Athlete A2); in terms of athlete performance, the 60 days may therefore be an overestimation of the true impact of the injury/illness. Bahr [20] described the potential complexity of the time-line for an overuse injury and recommended that continuous or serial measurements should be made on an athlete's condition in order to monitor these changes; the situation is similar for all injuries and illnesses, including acute and chronic events. Hence, the proposal here is that any change of status (COS) in an athletes' ability to train/compete over time is recorded. This approach is particularly beneficial when tracking complex long-term injuries/illnesses, as it provides sensitive, real-time capture of information about the evolution of and recovery from an injury/illness. The date of change of status is simply taken when the athlete moves from complete time-loss to performance-restriction or vice versa. The total severity of an injury/illness is then calculated by summing the individual time-loss and restriction-impact (FTE) days.

The progression of an athlete's return to full fitness from a period of performance-restriction will depend on the level of performance-restriction at DOI and/or COS. Few injuries/illnesses display a truly linear return to fitness with time, and Figure 3 represents a conceptual schematic of this recovery relationship. The performance-restriction recovery envelope can be used to compare the recovery of an athlete experiencing (i) a rapid early progression followed by a final slower period of progression with an athlete experiencing (ii) a slow early progression followed by a rapid end-phase recovery to full fitness.

2.4. Athlete Pain Score. All athletes experience pain during their careers, whether through the normal rigors of training or as the result of injury [31]. Athletes often train and

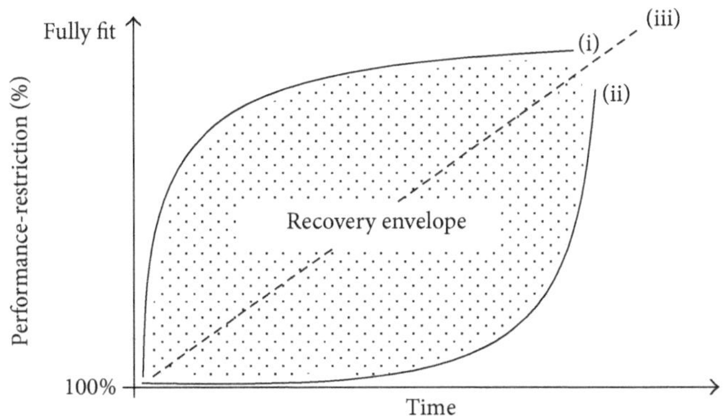

FIGURE 3: The performance-restriction injury/illness recovery envelope. (i) Fast/slow recovery; (ii) slow/fast recovery; and (iii) linear recovery.

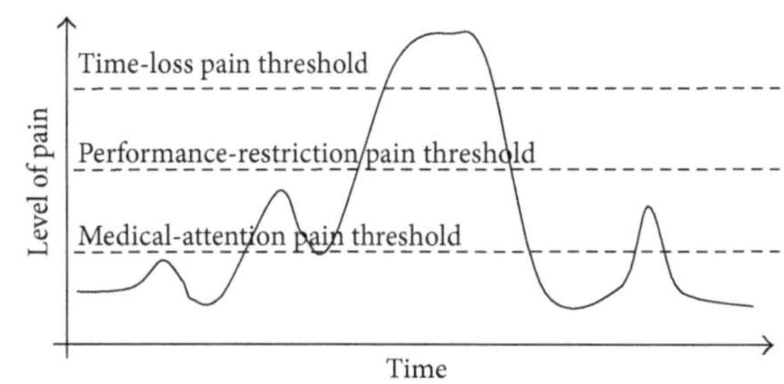

FIGURE 4: Theoretical model of pain and injury consequence (adapted from Bahr, [20]).

compete with injury/illness-related pain but how frequently this occurs and what the impact is on an athlete's ability to continue normal training are largely unknown. In two recent studies, it was reported that 52% of NFL players [32] and 60% of players at the 2010 FIFA football World Cup [33] used prescription pain killers during play. Although it has been recommended that surveillance methods should include the measurement of pain alongside days of absence [20], there is little other evidence on the need for recording pain [31] or that pain is being recorded within longitudinal surveillance studies. When athlete pain has been recorded alongside the incidence of injury, it has only been done retrospectively rather than prospectively at the time of injury [34]. It is proposed, as a component of injury surveillance, that pain could be used as an indicator of injury severity. Although there are no published data currently available, it is reasonable to assume that, at their onset, severe acute injuries such as fractures may elicit higher levels of pain for an athlete than chronic injuries such as a tendinopathy.

Multiple person-to-person physical and psychological factors and sport-to-sport sociological and environmental factors combine to determine an athlete's threshold and tolerance to pain, [31] and athletes may experience time-loss or restrictions to training/competition at different points along their own pain continuum. Figure 4 is an adaptation to the pain model presented by Bahr [20] that shows injury pain thresholds for an athlete moving from medical-attention through performance-restriction, complete time-loss, and recovery.

2.5. The Great Britain Injury/Illness Performance Project (IIPP). The current paper summarises the results recorded during the injury/illness surveillance study of Great Britain Olympic athletes conducted under the auspices of the UK Sport/English Institute of Sport Injury/Illness Performance Project (IIPP) and provides some illustrative example of the benefits of the proposed methodology. The IIPP methodology, which was based around the IOC, FIFA, and IRB injury/illness consensus statements, [13–15] included the methodological adaptations discussed above, and used the Sport Medicine Diagnostic Coding System [35]. The IIPP study involved 322 athletes (males: 172; female: 150) from 10 Great Britain Olympic sports (summer: 7; winter: 3), badminton (n = 21), canoe/kayak (n = 43), curling (n = 29), cycling (n = 61), football (women: n = 17), Judo (n = 35), modern pentathlon (n = 11), short track speed skating (n = 11), skeleton (n = 14), and swimming (n = 80). The study period covered September 2009 to August 2012, with data collected prospectively for each sport, each year, from the start of preseason training until the end of the competitive season (summer sports: September to August; winter sports: April to March). Medical staff working full time with centralised athletes recorded all the details of athlete injury/illness data, including full diagnosis, whenever a recordable event occurred. Standardised medical report forms were used with a questionnaire return compliance rate of 98%. Training and competition exposure data for all athletes were recorded on a weekly standardised report form by coaching and conditioning support staff but are not reported within the present paper.

The IIPP methodology defined any injury/illness that negatively impacted on an athlete's ability to undertake full and normal training as a recordable condition, irrespective of the athlete's ability to compete; "medical-attention" injuries/illnesses that did not impact on an athletes' ability to undertake full training/competition were not included. A recordable condition had two levels of subclassification: (i) time-loss, which was an injury/illness that caused an athlete's complete absence from all training/competition, and (ii) performance-restriction, which was an injury/illness where the athletes' training/competition continued but the volume and/or intensity were restricted or modified (e.g., a nonweight-bearing activity such as cycling replaced a weight-bearing activity such as running). The injury/illness initial status (i.e., time-loss or performance-restriction) was defined at the date of injury (DOI), irrespective of any subsequent change of status.

Severity data were reported in days for both time-loss and performance-restriction. Performance-restriction was reported as previously described as restriction-impact (FTE) days, with the number of performance-restricted days presented in superscript; for example, 18^{33} severity days means that the performance-restriction injury lasted for 33 days during which the level of restriction equated a restriction-impact of 18 full (FTE) days lost. Time-loss injuries that had a change of status to a period of performance-restriction also

TABLE 1: Injury and illness number (and severity mean days$^{\text{lasted-for}}$ in parenthesis), by status.

	Performance-restriction	Time-loss	Unclassified	Total
Competition	47 (18^{33})	50 (35^{54})	1 (11)	98 (26^{44})
Training	297** (9^{25})	163 (18^{30})	1 (14)	461 (12^{27})
Unclassified	2 (21^{62})	3 (55^{87})	1 (1)	6 (28^{66})
All injury	346 (10^{26})	216 (23^{36})	3 (9)	565 (15^{31})
All illness	101** (5^{11})	270 (7^{8})	7 (4^{9})	378 (6^{9})

** $P \leq 0.01$: significant difference between number of time-loss and performance-restriction injuries/illnesses.

display the number of days the injury lasted for (time-loss days added to performance-restricted days).

Significant differences were calculated using two-tailed Z tests [36]. Significance was accepted at $P \leq 0.05$ (equal variances assumed) and exact P values are reported throughout. Ethical approval for the study was obtained from the UK Sport (London) ethics advisory board.

3. Results

During the study, 565 injuries (competition: 98, training: 461, and unclassified: 6) and 378 illnesses were recorded. Of all injuries, 216 were classified as causing time-loss and 346 as causing performance-restriction (3 were not classified by medical staff at the time of recording) (Table 1). On average, each injury resulted in 15 days missed training (competition: 26 days; training: 12 days) and each illness 6 days, with time-loss injuries/illnesses more severe than performance-restriction injuries/illnesses. The numbers of time-loss (50) and performance-restriction (47) injuries occurring in competition were similar ($P = 0.57$); however, within training significantly more ($P < 0.01$) injuries resulted in performance-restriction (284) than time-loss (160). For athlete illnesses, the majority of events recorded ($P < 0.01$) resulted in complete time-loss (270) compared with performance-restriction (101) (7 unclassified).

By injury cause, 53% of all injuries were classified as overuse (gradual/sudden onset) and 47% as acute ($P = 0.19$). The majority of overuse injuries (72%) resulted in performance-restriction, while, conversely, 59% of acute traumatic injuries resulted in complete time-loss. Injuries to the knee, shoulder, and lumbar spine were most common, with more knee injuries resulting in time-loss but conversely more shoulder and lumbar spine injuries resulting in performance-restriction (Figure 5).

Figure 6 provides four examples of time lines of injuries/illnesses recorded within the IIPP study. Athlete A sustained a lower leg fracture initially causing complete time-loss from all competition and training, followed by a prolonged period of graduated training back to full fitness. Athlete B had a shoulder tendinopathy injury, which did not result in time-loss but impacted over an extended period of time on aspects of his training until his return to full fitness. Athlete C initially suffered a recurrence of a chronic lumbar spine disc injury causing the athlete to restrict her training; the athlete's condition began improving but there was a sudden exacerbation of the injury causing complete time-loss. As her condition improved once again, this athlete returned to restricted training where loads (intensity and volume) were progressively increased until she returned to full fitness. Athlete D presented a chronic fatigue illness with varying periods of complete time-loss and restricted training before returning to full fitness.

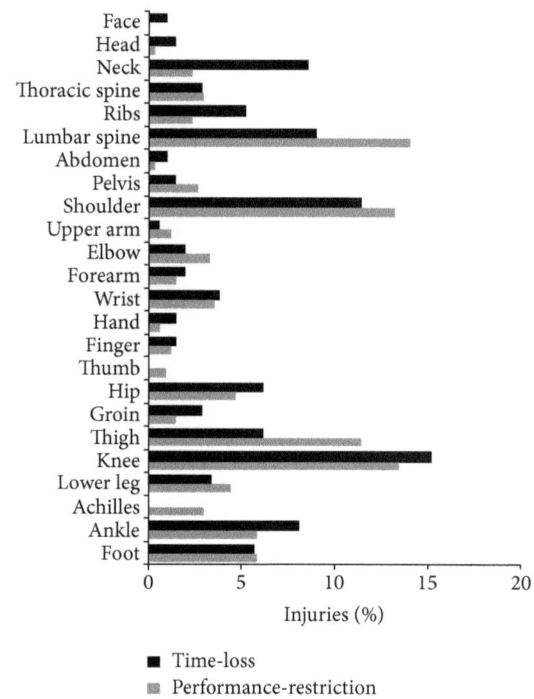

FIGURE 5: Percentage of injuries by location, as a function of injury status.

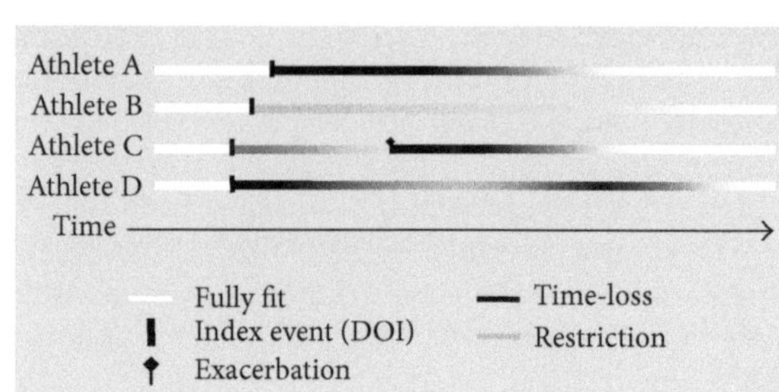

FIGURE 6: Examples of injury/illness occurrences collected during the IIPP based on time-loss and performance-restriction status.

The IIPP study methodology provided Great Britain sports with a summary of athletes' ongoing time-loss and

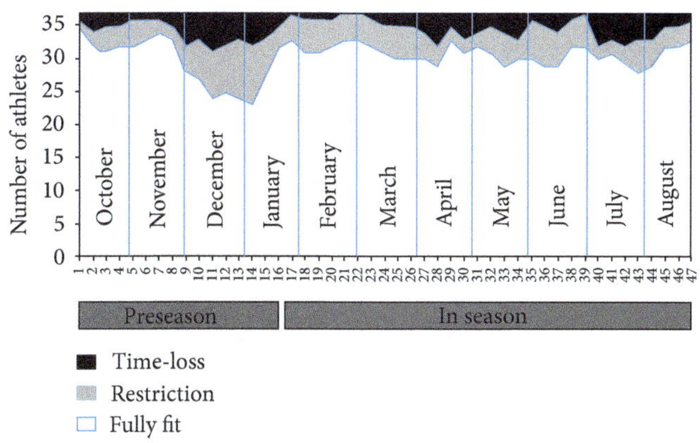

FIGURE 7: Great Britain sport (water-based) squad status 2010/11.

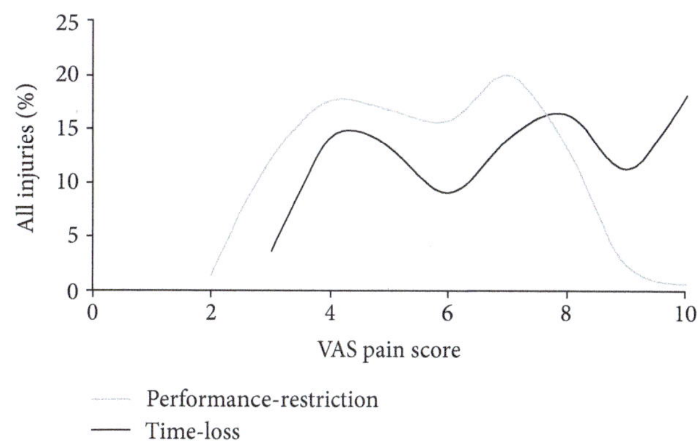

FIGURE 8: IIPP VAS pain score (at DOI) distribution for time-loss and performance-restriction injuries recorded between 2009 and 2012.

performance-restriction and the squad availability for training/competition. Figure 7 presents a sport's (water-based) squad data during the 2010/11 season; on average at any time during the season, 18% of the team were unavailable for full training/competition, with December and January posing the period of greatest impact on training as a consequence of injury or illness.

3.1. Pain. For all injuries reported in the IIPP study, athletes were asked to rate their pain at the initial date of injury (DOI) using a visual analogue scale (VAS) from 0 (no pain) to 10 (the worst pain). The athlete's pain scores were also recorded at each COS and DOR. All injured athletes reported having some level of pain at DOI (VAS: mean = 6.1; SD 2.1) and 39% some level of pain at DOR (VAS: mean = 1.8; SD 1.0). Figure 8 shows the distribution of pain levels at DOI for time-loss and performance-restriction injuries, with pain scores generally higher for time-loss compared with performance-restriction injuries. With the majority of time-loss injuries reported to be acute in nature and performance-restriction injuries to be overuse, this supports the theory proposed that acute injuries present more pain.

4. Discussion

When dealing with elite sport, the consequence of an athlete's injury/illness is often dependent on the sport involved. Injury and illness events may be of less consequence within team sports (because substitutes are normally used), some individual sports, where the format of competition is such that performance may be measured over an extended period of time (e.g., a season), and/or during particular times of the year that is preseason compared with in season. However, for athletes competing in many individual sports, the focus is on achieving peak performance at possibly one major event each year, for example, World Championship or Olympic Games. Injury/illness events are likely therefore to have a bigger influence on athletes competing in individual sports as these athletes must attain optimal conditioning and perform maximally at specific times, when winning margins are often measured in fractions of a second or millimeters.

Successful implementation of injury and illness prevention strategies relies on the correct characterisation of injury/illness risk factors, [37] and accurately assessing the consequences and severity of all sports injuries/illnesses is a crucial aspect in identifying the extent of the injury/illness problem. Hence, the addition of the proposed performance-restriction definition, alongside the traditional time-loss definition, provides an important additional layer of information that was previously unavailable. In the IIPP study, using the performance-restriction injury classification, an additional 346 injuries and 101 illnesses were recorded, equating to just over twice as many injuries and a quarter more illnesses reported compared to the traditional time-loss definition. This was similar to the findings by Clarsen et al. [23], who also reported that significantly more overuse injuries were recordable using a new overuse injury questionnaire compared with standard time-loss injury registration methods. In a subsequent paper, the same authors proposed adaptations to their overuse injury method to include the recording of all injuries and illnesses, again with similar more detailed results [38].

In addition to capturing more impactful injury/illness issues, the IIPP methodology allowed the use of standard days lost for reporting severity of performance-restriction so that data could be comparable with a time-loss definition. This provided more accurate information on the impact of injury and illness issues whereby potential overestimations were negated in terms of full-time equivalent days lost from training/competition compared with a pure time-loss definition. The use of full-time medical practitioners to record medical data including specific diagnoses also avoided reliability and validity issues related to athlete self-reporting.

For prevention initiatives to be effective, translation and implementation of research findings in a real-world setting are paramount [39]. Hence, full NGB/sporting body engagement is important not only for data returns compliance but also in provision and feedback of injury/illness data, so that information provided is acted upon and strategies adhered to. While not quantified in the present study currently, it is known that targeted prevention initiatives based on recommendations from biannual reports (and ad hoc NGB requested analyses) are being implemented by IIPP sports

NGB's with positive reductions in days lost to illness and injury. This was particularly evident in the run up to the London 2012 Olympic Games.

The inclusion of a performance-restriction classification also raises the possibility of examining the efficacy of current treatment and rehabilitation algorithms for injured/ill athletes from a different perspective. For example, is it better to allow an athlete to continue training at a restricted level, or should the athlete experience a complete break from training? It is reported that some of the negative effects of missed training can be avoided or limited by using reduced training strategies (e.g., reduced training volume), as long as the training intensity is maintained and the frequency of exposure is only reduced moderately [28]. Cross-training or a modified-training mode may also be beneficial in maintaining training-induced adaptations during periods of injury/illness [29].

Recording pain scores alongside performance-restriction injuries/illnesses will help provide a better description of those situations discussed by Bahr where athletes experience ongoing pain but do not sustain a time-loss injury [20]. The preliminary results presented here demonstrate the high proportion of athletes returning from injury to training/competition while still experiencing residual levels of pain; this supports the recent findings among NFL and football players where a large proportion of players were competing in pain [32, 33]. This type of information could be of great importance for studies of the consequences of long-term injuries experienced by many athletes (e.g., osteoarthritis). In addition, the distributions of pain scores for both time-loss and performance-restriction injuries in the current study show distinct bimodal responses. These distributions could arise for many reasons, the most common being that the distribution is made up of two unimodal distributions. If this was the case, it would suggest that there could be two different groups of athletes in terms of reporting or perceptions of pain, one with moderate (VAS: 3.0 to 5.0) and one with a higher (VAS: 6.5 to 8.5) level of pain. Conversely, this could represent the level of pain for two distinct groups of injuries, that is, the distribution of overuse injuries (the first peak) and acute injuries (the second peak). How the body reacts to pain is a complex process, [31] and the proposals for recording pain in epidemiological studies of sports injuries could provide opportunities to explore new perspectives in this area.

It is unlikely that a single universal system will be suitable for the needs of injury/illness studies in all populations and settings [40, 41], and one of the limitations of the proposed methodology is the additional time required of the medical staff to record the performance-restriction and pain score information. Therefore, the increased level of data collection proposed might not be appropriate for studies with large populations, for some contact sports where the incidences of injury are high and where full-time medical staff may not be available to collect the information. In addition, while clearly defined criteria are established for "medical-attention," "performance-restriction," and "time-loss" definition classifications, it is recognised that these thresholds may also still be blurred in real-world settings, for example, "medical-attention" classified injuries/illnesses may result in some restriction to training/competition but these restrictions may go unreported.

In the IIPP study, semiquantitative measures of training intensity and volume were used. Although research suggests that greater weight should be attached to a reduction in intensity due to greater detriments to subsequent performance, [29] for simplicity and ease of practitioner use, the present paper proposed equal weighting be given to both intensity and volumes. It would be preferable in future studies of this type if quantified measures of intensity and volume (and restrictions there-of) could be used (e.g., intensity linked to heart rate or Vo_2 max data; volume linked to GPS data) to provide more accurate values (although this may not be appropriate for some pure skill-based sports). An additional parameter, which measured the effectiveness of changes in training modality, such as replacing weight-bearing with nonweight-bearing activities, could also be added to provide more information in some studies.

5. Conclusion

Although training methods seek to improve athlete performance through the aggregation of marginal gains [42], the impact of injuries/illnesses on training is a key perspective, particularly in an elite sport setting. Where previously, time-loss has been used as a gross measure of the consequence of injuries/illnesses in sport, new discussions are emerging on the merits of alternate methods for quantifying levels of injury/illness-related athlete function and restriction in training. The current proposal to include an additional category of performance-restriction and pain scores, could provide greater detail in the understanding of the impact of injuries and illnesses on athlete availability and performance. With better understanding of this relationship, prevention initiatives can be better targeted to reduce the impact of athlete injuries and illnesses and improve athletic performance. The IIPP study continues into its fifth year of data collection in Great Britain Olympic athletes preparing for the Sochi 2014 and Rio 2016 Olympic Games.

Acknowledgments

The authors would like to thank the Sports' National Governing Body Medical, Strength and Conditioning, and Sport Science and coaching personnel, without whose input during data collection, this study would not have been possible.

References

[1] G. Langevoort, G. Myklebust, J. Dvorak, and A. Junge, "Handball injuries during major international tournaments," *Scandinavian Journal of Medicine and Science in Sports*, vol. 17, no. 4, pp. 400–407, 2007.

[2] J. M. Alonso, A. Junge, P. Renström, L. Engebretsen, M. Mountjoy, and J. Dvorak, "Sports injuries surveillance during the 2007 IAAF world athletics championships," *Clinical Journal of Sport Medicine*, vol. 19, no. 1, pp. 26–32, 2009.

[3] A. Junge, L. Engebretsen, M. L. Mountjoy et al., "Sports injuries during the Summer Olympic Games 2008," *American Journal of Sports Medicine*, vol. 37, no. 11, pp. 2165–2172, 2009.

[4] J.-M. Alonso, P. M. Tscholl, L. Engebretsen, M. Mountjoy, J. Dvorak, and A. Junge, "Occurrence of injuries and illnesses during the 2009 IAAF World Athletics Championships," *British Journal of Sports Medicine*, vol. 44, no. 15, pp. 1100–1105, 2010.

[5] M. Mountjoy, A. Junge, J. M. Alonso et al., "Sports injuries and illnesses in the 2009 FINA World Championships (aquatics)," *British Journal of Sports Medicine*, vol. 44, no. 7, pp. 522–527, 2010.

[6] J. Dvorak, A. Junge, W. Derman, and M. Schwellnus, "Injuries and illnesses of football players during the 2010 FIFA World Cup," *British Journal of Sports Medicine*, vol. 45, no. 8, pp. 626–630, 2011.

[7] L. Engebretsen, K. Steffen, J. M. Alonso et al., "Sports injuries and illnesses during the winter olympic games 2010," *British Journal of Sports Medicine*, vol. 44, no. 11, pp. 772–780, 2010.

[8] J.-M. Alonso, P. Edouard, G. Fischetto, B. Adams, F. Depiesse, and M. Mountjoy, "Determination of future prevention strategies in elite track and field: analysis of Daegu 2011 IAAF Championships injuries and illnesses surveillance," *British Journal of Sports Medicine*, vol. 46, no. 7, pp. 505–514, 2012.

[9] C. Fuller, K. Sheerin, and S. Targett, "Rugby world cup 2011: international rugby board injury surveillance study," *British Journal of Sports Medicine*, 2012.

[10] M. Schwellnus, W. Derman, T. Page et al., "Illness during the 2010 Super 14 Rugby Union tournament—a prospective study involving 22 676 player days," *British Journal of Sports Medicine*, vol. 46, no. 7, pp. 499–504, 2012.

[11] A. Ljungqvist, "Sports injury prevention: a key mandate for the IOC," *British Journal of Sports Medicine*, vol. 42, no. 6, p. 391, 2008.

[12] W. Van Mechelen, "The severity of sports injuries," *Sports Medicine*, vol. 24, no. 3, pp. 176–180, 1997.

[13] C. W. Fuller, J. Ekstrand, A. Junge et al., "Consensus statement on injury definitions and data collection procedures in studies of football (soccer) injuries," *British Journal of Sports Medicine*, vol. 40, no. 3, pp. 193–201, 2006.

[14] A. Junge, L. Engebretsen, J. M. Alonso et al., "Injury surveillance in multi-sport events: the International Olympic Committee approach," *British Journal of Sports Medicine*, vol. 42, no. 6, pp. 413–421, 2008.

[15] C. W. Fuller, M. G. Molloy, C. Bagate et al., "Consensus statement on injury definitions and data collection procedures for studies of injuries in rugby union," *Clinical Journal of Sport Medicine*, vol. 17, no. 3, pp. 177–181, 2007.

[16] J. W. Orchard, D. Newman, R. Stretch, W. Frost, A. Mansingh, and A. Leipus, "Methods for injury surveillance in international cricket," *British Journal of Sports Medicine*, vol. 39, no. 4, p. e22, 2005.

[17] B. M. Pluim, C. W. Fuller, M. E. Batt et al., "Consensus statement on epidemiological studies of medical conditions in tennis, April 2009," *British Journal of Sports Medicine*, vol. 43, no. 12, pp. 893–897, 2009.

[18] M. Turner, C. W. Fuller, D. Egan et al., "European consensus on epidemiological studies of injuries in the thoroughbred horse racing industry," *British Journal of Sports Medicine*, vol. 46, no. 10, pp. 704–708, 2012.

[19] C. W. Fuller, R. Bahr, R. W. Dick, and W. H. Meeuwisse, "A framework for recording recurrences, reinjuries, and exacerbations in injury surveillance," *Clinical Journal of Sport Medicine*, vol. 17, no. 3, pp. 197–200, 2007.

[20] R. Bahr, "No injuries, but plenty of pain? On the methodology for recording overuse symptoms in sports," *British Journal of Sports Medicine*, vol. 43, no. 13, pp. 966–972, 2009.

[21] D. W. Creighton, I. Shrier, R. Shultz, W. H. Meeuwisse, and G. O. Matheson, "Return-to-play in sport: a decision-based model," *Clinical Journal of Sport Medicine*, vol. 20, no. 5, pp. 379–385, 2010.

[22] D. Palmer-Green, G. Hunter, R. Jaques, C. Fuller, and C. Price, "Methods for epidemiological study of injury and illness in Great Britain Olympic sport: the injury/illness performance project," in *Proceedings of the IOC World Conference on Prevention of Injury & Illness in Sport*, Monte-Carlo, Monaco, April 2011, Abstract available at: *British Journal of Sports Medicine*, vol. 45, p. 367, 2011.

[23] B. Clarsen, G. Myklebust, and R. Bahr, "Development and validation of a new method for the registration of overuse injuries in sports injury epidemiology: the Oslo Sports Trauma Research Centre (OSTRC) overuse injury questionnaire," *British Journal of Sports Medicine*, vol. 47, pp. 495–502, 2013.

[24] J. Jacobsson, T. Timpka, J. Ekberg, J. Kowalski, S. Nilsson, and P. Renström, "Design of a protocol for large-scale epidemiological studies in individual sports: the Swedish Athletics injury study," *British Journal of Sports Medicine*, vol. 44, no. 15, pp. 1106–1111, 2010.

[25] J. Hawley and L. Burke, *Peak Performance. Training and Nutritional Strategies For Sport*, St. Leonards, Allen and Unwin, New South Wales, Australia, 1998.

[26] I. Mujika and S. Padilla, "Cardiorespiratory and metabolic characteristics of detraining in humans," *Medicine and Science in Sports and Exercise*, vol. 33, no. 3, pp. 413–421, 2001.

[27] I. Mujika and S. Padilla, "Muscular characteristics of detraining in humans," *Medicine and Science in Sports and Exercise*, vol. 33, no. 8, pp. 1297–1303, 2001.

[28] I. Mujika and S. Padilla, "Detraining: loss of training induced physiological and performance adaptation. Part I. Short term insufficient training stimulus," *Sports Medicine*, vol. 30, no. 2, pp. 79–87, 2000.

[29] I. Mujika and S. Padilla, "Detraining: loss of training-induced physiological and performance adaptations. Part II: long term insufficient training stimulus," *Sports Medicine*, vol. 30, no. 3, pp. 145–154, 2000.

[30] M. L. Harringe, S. Lindblad, and S. Werner, "Do team gymnasts compete in spite of symptoms from an injury?" *British Journal of Sports Medicine*, vol. 38, no. 4, pp. 398–401, 2004.

[31] L. J. Pen and C. A. Fisher, "Athletes and pain tolerance," *Sports Medicine*, vol. 18, no. 5, pp. 319–329, 1994.

[32] L. B. Cottler, A. Ben Abdallah, S. M. Cummings, J. Barr, R. Banks, and R. Forchheimer, "Injury, pain, and prescription opioid use among former National Football League (NFL) players," *Drug and Alcohol Dependence*, vol. 116, no. 1–3, pp. 188–194, 2011.

[33] P. M. Tscholl and J. Dvorak, "Abuse of medication during international football competition in 2010—lesson not learned," *British Journal of Sports Medicine*, vol. 46, no. 16, pp. 1140–1141, 2012.

[34] R. Bahr and J. C. Reeser, "Injuries among world-class professional beach volleyball players: the Fédération Internationale de Volleyball Beach Volleyball Injury Study," *American Journal of Sports Medicine*, vol. 31, no. 1, pp. 119–125, 2003.

[35] W. H. Meeuwisse and J. P. Wiley, "The sport medicine diagnostic coding system," *Clinical Journal of Sport Medicine*, vol. 17, no. 3, pp. 205–207, 2007.

[36] B. R. Kirkwood and J. A. C. Sterne, *Essential Medical Statistics*, Blackwell Scientific Publications, London, UK, 2nd edition, 2003.

[37] K. Steffen, T. Soligard, and L. Engebretsen, "Health protection of the Olympic athlete," *British Journal of Sports Medicine*, vol. 46, no. 7, pp. 466–470, 2012.

[38] B. Clarsen, O. Rønsen, M. Myklebust, T. W. Flørenes, and R. Bahr, "The Oslo Sports Trauma Research Center questionnaire on health problems: a new approach to prospective monitoring of illness and injury in elite athletes," *British Journal of Sports Medicine*, 2013.

[39] C. F. Finch, "No longer lost in translation: the art and science of sports injury prevention implementation research," *British Journal of Sports Medicine*, vol. 45, no. 16, pp. 1253–1257, 2011.

[40] J. H. M. Brooks and C. W. Fuller, "The influence of methodological issues on the results and conclusions from epidemiological studies of sports injuries: illustrative examples," *Sports Medicine*, vol. 36, no. 6, pp. 459–472, 2006.

[41] W. H. Meeuwisse, H. Tyreman, B. Hagel, and C. Emery, "A dynamic model of etiology in sport injury: the recursive nature of risk and causation," *Clinical Journal of Sport Medicine*, vol. 17, no. 3, pp. 215–219, 2007.

[42] The Independent, "'Head of Marginal Gains' helps GB gold machine stay in front," August 2012, http://www.independent.co.uk/sport/olympics/cycling/head-of-marginal-gains-helps-gb-gold-machine-stay-in-front-8010110.html.

16

The Incidence of Concussion in a Professional Australian Rugby League Team, 1998–2012

Jason Savage,[1] Chloe Hooke,[2] John Orchard,[3] and Richard Parkinson[4]

[1] *Monash Health, Department of Oral and Maxillofacial Surgery, Melbourne, VIC 3168, Australia*
[2] *Monash Health, Melbourne, VIC 3168, Australia*
[3] *School of Public Health, University of Sydney, Sydney, NSW 2006, Australia*
[4] *St Vincent's Hospital, Department of Neurosurgery, Sydney, NSW 2010, Australia*

Correspondence should be addressed to Jason Savage; jason.sav@hotmail.com

Academic Editor: Karim Chamari

Background. Rugby league is a physically demanding team sport and the National Rugby League is the highest-level competition of rugby league in Australia. Frequent tackles and collisions between players result in a high incidence of injury to players. Concussion injuries have been the source of much debate, with reporting varying greatly depending on the definition used. *Method.* Injury records of 239 players from one professional National Rugby League were analysed during a continuous period of 15 years, with particular interest in the incidence and recurrence of concussions and the change in incidence over time. *Result.* A total of 191 concussions were recorded, affecting 90 players. The incidence of concussion injuries was found to be 28.33 per 1000 player match hours, with an increase over time ($P = 0.0217$). Multiple concussions were recorded for 51 players. *Conclusion.* A statistically significant increase in the incidence of concussion injuries was found, without a concurrent increase in the number of head injuries or total injuries. New rules which mandate removal of players from the field may be beneficial for protection of players on the long term, although they risk being counterproductive, if they make players less likely to report their symptoms during matches.

1. Introduction

The National Rugby League (NRL) is the highest level of professional competition of rugby league in Australia. The playing season runs from March (autumn) to October (spring) each year. Rugby league is a full-body contact, physically demanding team sport consisting of 13 on field players: 6 forwards, 7 backs, and up to 4 interchange players [1–5]. Forwards are chosen for their size, strength, and tackling ability as they are involved in more body contact, whilst backs are often chosen for their speed and agility and are less involved in defensive physical contact [2, 3, 6, 7]. Compared to rugby union, contests for the ball in rugby league are decided in favour of the team in possession for up to 5 tackles with a handover occurring on the 6th tackle to the opposing team [1, 2, 4]. Player tackles and collisions make rugby league a popular spectator sport, but also one with a high reported incidence of injury [8]. Concussion is an injury with relatively low incidence if the injury definition requires players to miss a match, but higher incidence if "non-time-loss" injuries are taken into account [8–12].

2. Aims

A review of the literature regarding injuries occurring in rugby league revealed that previous studies have been of a short duration, and are not concussion injury specific or used a definition of injury that relied on the affected player being unavailable for the following match likely under reporting the true incidence of concussion injuries [8, 13, 14]. This study was conducted at a professional rugby league team where one of the authors (JO) has kept continuous injury records of injuries managed by the team medical officer since the inaugural season of the NRL, in 1998. The purpose of this study was to identify all presenting concussion injuries and their severity, during the 15-year recorded period for this professional rugby league team. Our aim was to describe the true concussion incidence and consider any changes over time. We hope this study will promote further research into the monitoring of concussion injuries and aid in awareness of the risks of multiple concussion injuries.

3. Method

Injury records for a cohort of professional rugby league players competing in the NRL, from 1998 until the conclusion of the 2012 season, were made available for retrospective analysis. During this period all injuries that occurred were recorded by the team's medical officer. This sports physician was employed for the duration of the study and was present at >95% of matches. Injuries were recorded in accordance with protocols described by Orchard using a modified Orchard sports injury Classification System [15].

Data was collected and managed in accordance with the Declaration of Helsinki for the Conduct of Clinical Research and Australian National Health and Medical Research Council guidelines [16, 17].

Injury data included details of the following:

(i) nature of the injury,

(ii) site of the injury,

(iii) time of injury onset,

(iv) team played for and against,

(v) time loss as a result of injury.

In the setting of multiple player injuries, all injuries were recorded.

An injury was defined in this study as "any physical or medical condition that required a player to receive medical attention" [18, 19].

In the context of this study, a concussion was defined as any neurological disturbance reported by the player to the team doctor, no matter how transient (and irrespective of whether the player had fully recovered by the time he was examined) [20–22]. A recurrent concussion injury was defined as "any subsequent concussion injury that occurred after a player had returned to full team participation from the index concussion," without necessarily being in the same season [23]. The definition of a concussion for this study differs from some recent interpretations of concussion guidelines, in which a borderline condition is recognised (i.e., transient headache ± dizziness which quickly resolves but does not involve unconsciousness, amnesia, or prolonged symptoms) [24, 25]. It is not clear whether these "mild" cases are necessarily concussions and whether they should be removed from the field, but for the purposes of this study they have been recorded [25, 26].

During the study, the number of players on the field remained constant at 13 per match, with 4 players on the interchange bench. All participants were male, aged 18 and over.

Statistical analysis consisted of the calculation of the injury incidence. The injury incidence is reported as the number of injuries per 1000 player match hours (1000 pmh), where

Incidence = 1000 ∗ (number of injuries per season)/1.33 (80 minute matches) ∗ (number of matches per season) ∗ 13 (on field players) [27].

A regression analysis of the incidence of concussion injury, head injury, and total number of injuries was performed using the R software package and the data was fitted using a linear model with hypothesis testing for a nonzero slope.

Additionally the incidence of injury between the playing positions of forward or back was compared as a difference between 2 proportions (of those playing hours where there was an injury).

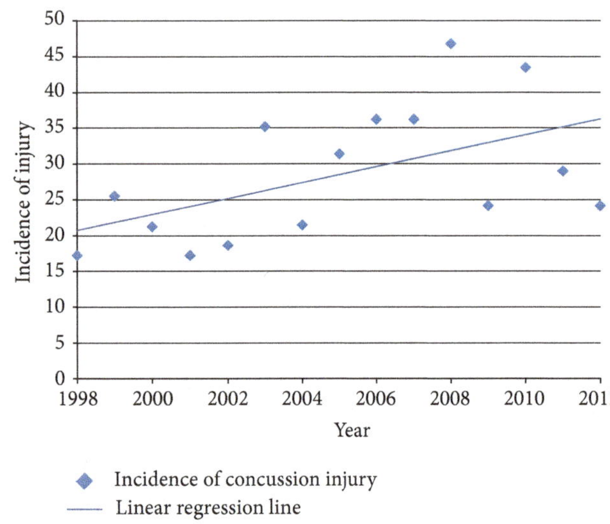

Figure 1: Incidence of concussion injuries. (Slope of regression line of the incidence of concussions = 1.11).

4. Results

The cohort consisted of 239 players, 99 that played a single NRL season and 140 that played multiple NRL seasons. During 15 consecutive professional NRL seasons a total of 191 concussions were recorded, affecting 90 players. 101 concussions were recurrent injuries according to our study definition (i.e., in the setting of a recorded previous concussion at this team at any time in the past). The exposure time of the study was calculated at 6743.1 hours of professional NRL competition, over 390 matches. The incidence of concussion injuries was calculated to be 28.33 per 1000 pmh. We found that the concussion incidence increased over time, with the linear regression slope found to be 1.11 ± 1.07 with 95% CI (hypothesis test passed: $P = 0.0217$) (Figure 1). The incidence of repeated concussion injuries was found to be 15.13 per 1000 pmh during the 15 consecutive seasons.

The total number of head injuries (excluding concussion) sustained during matches in the study period was 386. The total number of injuries sustained to players during the study period was 2352 (Table 1). The number of head injuries and the total number of injuries remained fairly constant over

Table 1: Concussion injuries and incidence.

	1998	1999	2000	2001	2002	2003	2004	2005	2006	2007	2008	2009	2010	2011	2012	Total	Average
Total concussion injuries (recurrent)	8 (0)	11 (2)	11 (7)	8 (4)	9 (5)	17 (6)	10 (9)	13 (8)	15 (10)	15 (9)	21 (12)	10 (8)	21 (11)	12 (9)	10 (2)	191 (102)	12.7
Head and neck injuries (excluding concussions)	24	18	37	30	33	29	18	22	18	31	20	23	30	29	24	386	25.7
Total number of injuries	190	142	203	138	166	125	120	143	146	163	156	149	235	167	111	2352	156.8
Number of matches played	27	25	30	27	28	28	27	24	24	24	26	24	28	24	24	390	26
Number of players monitored each season	43	41	43	46	48	49	39	38	38	41	30	27	30	30	31	239*	—
Concussion incidence (per 1000 player hours)	17.1	25.4	21.2	17.1	18.6	35.1	21.4	31.3	36.1	36.1	46.7	24.1	43.3	28.9	24.1	—	28.3
Recurrent concussion incidence (per 1000 player hours)	0	4.6	13.5	8.6	10.3	12.4	19.3	19.3	24.1	21.6	26.7	19.3	22.7	21.7	4.8	—	15.1

*The total number of players monitored over 15 seasons; 140 players were monitored over more than one season.

TABLE 2: Frequency of repeat concussions and timing of injury.

Number of concussions sustained	Number of players	Portion of players injured	Average duration between concussion injuries
1	39	16.3%	—
2	22	9.2%	583 days
3	17	7.1%	309 days
4	6	2.5%	491 days
5	4	1.7%	318 days
6	1	0.5%	587 days
7	1	0.5%	204 days
Total number of players with multiple concussions	**51**	**21.3%**	**381 days**

the study period, with no statistically significant increase in later seasons (head injury $P = 0.349$, total number of injuries $P = 0.319$).

Multiple concussions during the course of the study affected 51 players. Up to 7 concussions to the same player were recorded. Within the same season 27 players sustained a second concussion, 4 players sustained a third, and 2 players sustained a fourth (Table 2).

Players in a forward field position recorded a higher incidence of injury than those in a back, with an incidence of 32.1 compared with 25.1 injuries per 1000 pmh (Table 3). There are 6 forwards and 7 backs on the field. One would expect that as all positions on the field have equal exposure the result should be comparable. This was found to be clinically but not statistically significant ($P = 0.081$). The position of hooker sustained the highest incidence and recurrence of concussion injuries.

Concussion injuries caused a total of only 7 matches to be missed, with 2 matches missed by players due to multiple injuries including concussion. All other players who sustained a concussion were eligible to play the following match. In only one case did a player sustain a subsequent concussion in the following match, which constitutes a recurrence rate of <1% if only the return to play match is considered. Fitness to play in subsequent matches was allowed if

(1) the player no longer reported any symptoms of concussion,

(2) scores on neuropsychological testing had returned to baseline levels or above. Neuropsychological testing in the first ten years was performed with a DSST (Digit Symbol Substitution Test) and over the last five years with Cogsport, a reliable cognitive function test [28].

During the study period, no associated structural brain injury and fatal or nonfatal catastrophic injuries were reported. Although it was not specifically measured as part of the study, no player was forced into compulsory medical retirement from rugby league due to sequelae of concussion. However, the author who was the team doctor (JO) can recall 3 players who retired at a relatively young age (mid-20s) who cited multiple reasons for choosing early retirement. All three players sustained multiple concussions in a single season, not necessarily in their last season, and all three players were forwards. Two of the three players also played NRL at previous clubs. On the players request, a player can withhold the medical records at the time of club transfer. This can lead to an underestimation in the number of injuries the player may have sustained.

TABLE 3: Player position concussion incidence.

Player position (number of positions)	Total number of concussion injuries (recurrent injuries)	Incidence of concussion injuries (recurrent injuries)
Forwards	100 (50)	32.1 (16.1)
Prop (2)	25 (10)	24.1 (9.6)
Hooker	25 (16)	48.2 (30.8)
Second row (2)	44 (23)	42.4 (22.2)
Lock	6 (1)	11.6 (1.9)
Backs	91 (35)	25.1 (9.6)
Halfback	14 (8)	27.0 (15.4)
Five-eighth	10 (3)	19.3 (5.8)
Centre (2)	30 (15)	28.9 (14.5)
Wing (2)	14 (3)	13.5 (2.9)
Fullback	23 (6)	44.3 (11.6)

5. Discussion

This study found that 191 concussions occurred during the 15 seasons of the study. A statistically significant increase was found in the reported concussion incidence. A low of 17.1 concussions per 1000 pmh was found in 1998 and 2001, and a high of 46.7 concussions per 1000 pmh was found in 2008. In 2 of the last 5 years of the study the incidence rate was over 40 concussion injuries per 1000 pmh, whereas in the previous 10 years of the study, concussion injuries had never exceeded 36. There has been a statistically significant increase in concussion injuries, without a significant increase in the number of head injuries (excluding concussions), such as contusions, lacerations, facial and dentoalveolar injuries, or total injuries over the same period. A similar finding was made in amateur Rugby Union; Swain et al. found a significant increase in concussion incidence without an increase in head injuries [27].

The statistically significant increase in rate of reported concussions could be due to

(1) the increased degree of reporting to the club doctor. Over the years the "team doctor" position has gradually increased from a consultant position (attending games only and then otherwise seeing players at clinic) to a permanent part-time role (including regular clinics/sessions being conducted at the club training ground). Greater contact of the doctor with players may have increased the likelihood that players will report symptoms to the doctor. Greater player education about the potential long-term effects of concussion may have also increased likelihood of reporting symptoms to the doctor,

(2) a true increase in the actual rate of concussion,

(3) an increase in professionalism of clubs and athletes,

(4) the differences in the reporting of concussion, due to differences in definition and assessment.

The concussion incidence observed in this study (28.33 per 1000 pmh) is considerably high when compared to the incidence described by other studies. In professional Rugby League, the incidence of concussion has been reported as 8 to 8.1 per 1000 pmh [13]. In a professional AFL team, another prominent male contact sport in Australia, the incidence of concussion over a 10-year period was reported to be 16.7 per 1000 pmh when considering all presentations to medical staff [29], which is higher than rates reported when only injuries causing missed games are reported.

We found that 90 of the players monitored sustained a concussion, yet 191 concussions were recorded, 101 of these concussions were recurrent. Multiple concussions were sustained by 51 players, the majority sustaining a second (22) or third (17) concussion, with 6 a fourth, 4 a fifth, 2 a sixth, and 1 a seventh over the study. The average duration of time between the first and second and second and third concussions gradually reduced from 583 days to 309 days. Due to the small numbers of players who sustain a fourth or subsequent concussion, it is difficult to draw conclusions about the decreasing number of days between these concussion injuries.

Depending on the definition of recurrence chosen, concussion could be seen as an injury with a very low recurrence rate (<1%) the following week (if formal neuropsych testing is used to clear return to play) but a much higher recurrence rate over the course of a player's career (e.g., >50%). This is similar to another football code where in depth analysis has been conducted [30]. These divergent rates of recurrence are relevant to the two separate questions which are considered after every concussion—(1) is it safe for this player to return to play this week? (low recurrence rate if cleared by neuropsych tests) compared to (2) is it safe for this player's long-term health to continue playing a contact sport? (high recurrence rate considering career incidence).

The concussion incidence of the forwards was 32.1 per 1000 pmh compared with 25.1 per 100 pmh for backs;however, this was found not to be statistically significant. Findings were consistent with other studies that found that the incidence of injury was higher for forwards than for backs [7, 9, 31]. A contributing factor may be that certain positions on field attract players with specific physical characteristics, which may increase their risk of injury [3].

We found that the forward position of hooker was the player most at risk of sustaining a concussion injury, with an incidence of 48.2 per 1000 pmh. This was 4 times more likely than a player in the lock position, which sustained the lowest incidence of injury, with an incidence of 11.6 per 1000 pmh. Hookers have a heavy offensive and defensive role; they are positioned in the middle of the defensive ruck and are responsible for restarting offensive play, distributing the ball to support players after each "play the ball" stoppage [7]. Meir found that the hooker is the second lightest player on the field, while Gabbett found that they are the lightest and shortest of the 13 on-field player positions [3, 6]. The hooker has been found to have a significantly higher risk of injury from falling and stumbling injuries [7]. This may explain why the hooker has an increased risk of concussions, as they are constantly exposed to physical contact at head height by larger, heavier opponents. Gabbett believed that the hookers significant involvement in critical phases of play, both offensive and defensive, would result in a greater risk of injury to the player [7]. To rectify this, he suggested in 2005 that hookers could benefit from position-specific injury prevention programs, such as agility training to reduce the number of injuries from falling and stumbling [7].

Multiple concussions were sustained in the same season by 33 players. Of these players, 27 player sustained a second concussion, 4 players sustained a third concussion, and 2 players sustained four concussions within the same season. This finding was similar to what Gibbs had described, a high rate of concussion recurrence in AFL players who had sustained a previous concussion [29]. In his study over 10 years, 20 AFL players had a second concussion and 3 players a third concussion within the same season [29].

Recent changes made by the NRL will mean that "any player suspected of having a concussion must be removed from the game and be assessed by the first aider" and "a player who has suffered a concussion must not be allowed to return to play in the same game" [32]. However, clarification of this rule has indicated that it relates to clear-cut cases of concussion (e.g., unconscious, unsteady, or amnesic player) rather than the borderline symptoms (e.g., transient headache and dizziness which quickly resolves). The AFL advises that in the management of concussion injuries every case should be assessed by a medical doctor and that "if in doubt sit them out" as approach should be taken [33]. That is, "in general, the safest course of action is that the player not be allowed to return to play in the match or training session" [33].

This approach is supported by the "International Conference on Concussions in Sport," which suggests that a player diagnosed with a concussion should not be allowed to return to play in the current game [20, 21]. Similarly in the United States since May 2009, the Zachery Lystedt Law has legislated that youth athletes "shall be removed from competition" and "may not return to play until the athlete is evaluated by a licensed health care provider" [34]. Although these policies act to make sports safer by protecting concussed players from further injury, it has been suggested that these guidelines may lead to a change in the way that sports injuries are diagnosed on the pitch or sideline. There is concern that club doctors, whilst attempting to put player safety first, may feel pressure from the clubs that employ them to return injured players to the field as quickly as possible. The renaming of a "mild transient concussion" to "traumatic migraine" or delaying assessment of the player until the match is complete may assist this cause, meaning that a player could remain on the field for the match. Gibbs' study found that of AFL players who sustained a concussion injury only 26% were removed from the field and did not return to play in that match [29].

A concern with the more conservative concussion rule is that players may be less likely to report symptoms to the team medical staff (for an injury with no observed mechanism of head trauma from the sideline), if they personally feel safe to play and they expect to be taken off the field for reporting symptoms. In the case of professional athletes, there will always be an expectation to return to play as soon as possible [35]. We need to ensure that a return to play is not detrimental to the long-term health of the players.

The management of concussion injuries is guided by clinical assessment. Gibbs suggests that clinical assessment of signs and subjective symptoms is still the gold standard to assess if a player should return to play [29]. Computerised testing of cognitive function in players is now used as a reliable baseline and as an ongoing monitoring tool following a concussion, until symptoms are fully resolved [36].

The long-term risk to sports players of sustaining multiple concussions over their careers has been a well-publicised concern. Gronwall's study concluded that the effect of concussions has been shown to be cumulative [37]. In this context, consideration of the trends of concussion incidence and recurrent concussion frequency are immensely important. Further research into possible rule changes or new protective equipment is needed to identify opportunities to decrease the risk of concussions that face professional rugby league players.

Concussion as an injury is thought to be underreported as it often does not result in a missed game and is sometimes not even detected by the treating doctor [29]. Underestimation is expected to be a common error in studies of concussion. Within this study, there are several limitations to consider. For example, each player's first concussion during the study period was labelled as an "index"; however, this may in fact have been a recurrent concussion injury, where the true "index" concussion was sustained as a junior player, whilst playing for another club or prior to the study commencing. This may cause a skew in the data, where there are more "index" concussions in the early years of the study and more "recurrent" concussions later on in the study period. Also to be considered, the number of matches recorded within each season ranged from 24 to 30. Another source of variation was the squad size, which differed each season. This may be due to a change in the player substitution rule, where in 2001 the number of interchanges was limited to 12, from a pool of 4 players on the bench. However, since the calculated incidences in this paper are recorded in "1000 player match hours" these variations in number of matches and squad size should not cause error.

A significant limitation of this study was that the mechanism of injury was not recorded. It would have been of significant interest to identify the way in which concussions occurred in matches, particularly when considering ways to decrease the risk to players. There is also a risk of bias as the concussions were reported by an employee of the club. Baseline player neurological testing was not used over the entire study period and the diagnosis of a concussion was based on clinical judgement. However, by having just one person diagnosing the concussion injuries, the opportunity for measurement bias to occur is minimised.

It should be remembered that this study analysed players within one National Rugby League team and that concussions were recorded only when they occurred during matches. National Rugby League players change teams regularly. The majority has played ten or more years of junior rugby league and may play in other leagues such as state or national squads where they are also exposed to concussion injuries. The incidence of concussions reported to the doctor in National Rugby League matches has been recorded accurately in this study, but the true incidence of recurrent concussions is likely to be much higher. It would require accurate medical records to be maintained for each player at club, school, state, and national levels. We would suggest that until we have a national concussion database recording all concussion injuries (which exists in New Zealand), it will be difficult to fully identify the real risk that repeat concussions have on a player's life.

6. Conclusion

This study shows that there has been a statistically significant increase in the incidence of concussion injuries over 15 seasons in a professional rugby league team. Of note, there has not been a concurrent increase in the total number of injuries sustained to players. Multiple concussions, especially within the same season, are a cause for great concern, yet this study found that no recurrent concussions occurred within the same match and only one in the subsequent week. Whilst changes to the concussion laws of games, such as the NRL, are made in the best interests of players, these may be counterproductive, providing an incentive for players to avoid reporting symptoms. More research is required to identify the risk of repeat concussions in rugby league.

References

[1] W. Hoskins, H. Pollard, K. Hough, and C. Tully, "Injury in rugby league," *Journal of Science and Medicine in Sport*, vol. 9, no. 1-2, pp. 46–56, 2006.

[2] T. J. Gabbett, "Science of rugby league football: a review," *Journal of Sports Sciences*, vol. 23, no. 9, pp. 961–976, 2005.

[3] R. Meir, R. Newton, E. Curtis, M. Fardell, and B. Butler, "Physical fitness qualities of professional rugby league football players: determination of positional differences," *The Journal of Strength & Conditioning Research*, vol. 15, no. 4, pp. 450–458, 2001.

[4] T. Gabbett, T. King, and D. Jenkins, "Applied physiology of rugby league," *Sports Medicine*, vol. 38, no. 2, pp. 119–138, 2008.

[5] R. Meir, P. Colla, and C. Milligan, "Impact of the 10-meter rule change on professional rugby league: implications for training," *Strength & Conditioning Journal*, vol. 23, no. 6, pp. 42–46, 2001.

[6] T. J. Gabbett, "A comparison of physiological and anthropometric characteristics among playing positions in sub-elite rugby league players," *Journal of Sports Sciences*, vol. 24, no. 12, pp. 1273–1280, 2006.

[7] T. J. Gabbett, "Influence of playing position on the site, nature, and cause of rugby league injuries," *Journal of Strength and Conditioning Research*, vol. 19, no. 4, pp. 749–755, 2005.

[8] N. Gibbs, "Injuries in professional rugby league. A three-year prospective study of the South Sydney Professional Rugby League Football Club," *American Journal of Sports Medicine*, vol. 21, no. 5, pp. 696–700, 1993.

[9] T. J. Gabbett, "Incidence of injury in semi-professional rugby league players," *British Journal of Sports Medicine*, vol. 37, no. 1, pp. 36–43, 2003.

[10] J. H. M. Brooks, C. W. Fuller, S. P. T. Kemp, and D. B. Reddin, "A prospective study of injuries and training amongst the England 2003 Rugby World Cup squad," *British Journal of Sports Medicine*, vol. 39, no. 5, pp. 288–293, 2005.

[11] T. J. Gabbett, "Influence of injuries on team playing performance in Rugby League," *Journal of Science and Medicine in Sport*, vol. 7, no. 3, pp. 340–346, 2004.

[12] T. J. Gabbett, "Incidence, site, and nature of injuries in amateur rugby league over three consecutive seasons," *British Journal of Sports Medicine*, vol. 34, no. 2, pp. 98–103, 2000.

[13] C. Gissane, C. Gissane, and D. Jennings, "Injury in rugby league: a four year prospective survey," *British Journal of Sports Medicine*, vol. 30, no. 4, pp. 331–334, 1996.

[14] C. Gissane, D. Jennings, K. Kerr, and J. White, "Injury rates in rugby league football: impact of change in playing season," *American Journal of Sports Medicine*, vol. 31, no. 6, pp. 954–958, 2003.

[15] K. Rae and J. Orchard, "The orchard sports injury classification system (OSICS) version 10," *Clinical Journal of Sport Medicine*, vol. 17, no. 3, pp. 201–204, 2007.

[16] J. L. Hopper, "Australian NHMRC twin registry: a resource for pediatric research," *Pediatric Cardiology*, vol. 16, no. 2, p. 100, 1995.

[17] WMA. World Medical Association, *Declaration of Helsinki. Ethical Principles for Medical Research Involving Human Subjects*, 2008.

[18] H. Seward, J. Orchard, H. Hazard, and D. Collinson, "Football injuries in Australia at the elite level," *Medical Journal of Australia*, vol. 159, no. 5, pp. 298–301, 1993.

[19] D. A. King and T. J. Gabbett, "Training injuries in New Zealand amateur rugby league players," *Journal of Science and Medicine in Sport*, vol. 11, no. 6, pp. 562–565, 2008.

[20] P. McCrory, W. Meeuwisse, K. Johnston et al., "Consensus statement on concussion in sport—the 3rd International Conference on Concussion in Sport held in Zurich, November 2008," *PM and R*, vol. 1, no. 5, pp. 406–420, 2009.

[21] P. McCrory, K. Johnston, W. Meeuwisse et al., "Summary and agreement statement of the 2nd International Conference on Concussion in Sport, Prague 2004," *British Journal of Sports Medicine*, vol. 39, no. 4, pp. 196–204, 2005.

[22] M. Aubry, R. Cantu, J. Dvorak et al., "Summary and agreement statement of the first International Conference on Concussion in Sport, Vienna 2001. Recommendations for the improvement of safety and health of athletes who may suffer concussive injuries," *British Journal of Sports Medicine*, vol. 36, no. 1, pp. 6–10, 2002.

[23] C. W. Fuller, J. Ekstrand, A. Junge et al., "Consensus statement on injury definitions and data collection procedures in studies of football (soccer) injuries," *British Journal of Sports Medicine*, vol. 40, no. 3, pp. 193–201, 2006.

[24] C. C. Giza, J. S. Kutcher, S. Ashwal et al., "Summary of evidence-based guideline update: evaluation and management of concussion in sports: report of the Guideline Development Subcommittee of the American Academy of Neurology," *Neurology*, vol. 80, no. 24, pp. 2250–2257.

[25] K. G. Harmon, J. A. Drezner, M. Gammons et al., "American Medical Society for Sports Medicine position statement: concussion in sport," *British Journal of Sports Medicine*, vol. 47, no. 1, pp. 15–26, 2013.

[26] J. A. Langlois, W. Rutland-Brown, and M. M. Wald, "The epidemiology and impact of traumatic brain injury: a brief overview," *Journal of Head Trauma Rehabilitation*, vol. 21, no. 5, pp. 375–378, 2006.

[27] M. S. Swain, H. P. Pollard, and R. Bonello, "Incidence, severity, aetiology and type of neck injury in men's amateur rugby union: a prospective cohort study," *Chiropractic and Osteopathy*, vol. 18, article 18, 2010.

[28] A. Collie, P. Maruff, M. Makdissi, P. McCrory, M. McStephen, and D. Darby, "CogSport: reliability and correlation with conventional cognitive tests used in postconcussion medical evaluations," *Clinical Journal of Sport Medicine*, vol. 13, no. 1, pp. 28–32, 2003.

[29] N. Gibbs, "Concussion management in a professional senior AFL team over 10 years: returning to play guidelines assessing re-injury rate and performance level," in *Annual Scientific Conference of the Australian College of Sports Physicians*, Queensland, Australia, 2009.

[30] M. Makdissi, P. McCrory, A. Ugoni, D. Darby, and P. Brukner, "A prospective study of postconcussive outcomes after return to play in australian football," *American Journal of Sports Medicine*, vol. 37, no. 5, pp. 877–883, 2009.

[31] T. J. Gabbett, "Incidence of injury in amateur rugby league sevens," *British Journal of Sports Medicine*, vol. 36, no. 1, pp. 23–26, 2002.

[32] NRL, *Management of Concussion in Rugby League. Guidelines for Trainers, First-Aid Providers, Coaches and Parents*, NRL, 2012.

[33] M. Makdissi, *The Management of Concussion in Australian Football*, AFL, 2008.

[34] W. So, "Youth sports-head injury policies, Zackery Lystedt law," in *Engrossed House Bill 1824*, W. So, Ed., p. 3, 2009.

[35] A. S. McIntosh and P. McCrory, "Preventing head and neck injury," *British Journal of Sports Medicine*, vol. 39, no. 6, pp. 314–318, 2005.

[36] A. Collie, D. Darby, and P. Maruff, "Computerised cognitive assessment of athletes with sports related head injury," *British Journal of Sports Medicine*, vol. 35, no. 5, pp. 297–302, 2001.

[37] D. Gronwall and P. Wrightson, "Cumulative effect of concussion," *The Lancet*, vol. 2, no. 7943, pp. 995–997, 1975.

17

Quantifying the "Slosh Stomach": A Novel Tool for Assessment of Exercise-Associated Gastroparesis Symptoms in Endurance Athletes

Amy Sue Biondich and Jeremy D. Joslin

Department of Emergency Medicine, SUNY Upstate Medical University, Syracuse, NY, USA

Correspondence should be addressed to Jeremy D. Joslin; joslinj@upstate.edu

Academic Editor: Nancy J. Rehrer

Introduction. We describe a novel scale and its field use for evaluation of exercise-associated gastroparesis in the endurance athlete. *Methods.* A scale was created based on gastroparesis tools previously described in the medical literature. Surveys of the tool were administered to runners participating in a 210 km multiday foot race in Sri Lanka. *Results.* Use of this novel scale was demonstrated to be useful in assessing gastroparesis severity scores of athletes and how these symptoms affected their race performance. Of the 27 race participants who completed the survey, 27 felt that the tool adequately captured their symptoms. *Conclusions.* This novel survey tool was able to assess the presence and severity of exercise-associated gastroparesis symptoms in endurance racers in a remote location. This tool may be helpful with further research of the identification and management of gastroparesis and other gastrointestinal upset in the endurance race environment.

1. Introduction

Interest and participation in endurance events and ultramarathons has become increasingly popular [1, 2]. Attempts have been made to understand what factors not only impact athletic performance in these events but also ultimately delineate the finishers from the nonfinishers [3, 4]. The bulk of physiologic research concentrates on marathons and shorter running events. However, there has been an increasing body of work aimed solely at understanding medical issues specific to the endurance athlete during race day [5, 6]. These ultramarathons frequently occur in remote geography and often subject athletes to harsh environmental conditions.

Although the importance of physical activity to one's overall health cannot be overstated, it is well-known that strenuous exertion has a multitude of possibly detrimental effects on gastrointestinal function [7–10]. Several authors report data from endurance events describing gastrointestinal (GI) distress as a common and pervasive problem even if only temporary [4, 11–16].

The physiology behind the GI distress experienced by endurance events participants is not well-understood and is likely multifactorial [9]. Proposed mechanisms include the mechanical stress on the GI tract as a result of the repetitive pounding action of running [17, 18], reduced splanchnic blood flow as a product of changes of blood distribution during strenuous activity [10, 19], electrolyte disturbances (especially hyponatremia) from excessive fluid intake [20], or general malaise from dehydration [21–25].

An etiology of gastrointestinal distress that is gaining interest in the endurance foot-race industry is exercise-associated gastroparesis (EAG) which is colloquially known as "slosh stomach." Although gastroparesis is well reported in the gastroenterology literature, there is a paucity of published literature specific to endurance athletic events; and there is no objective tool to quantitatively measure the severity of these symptoms. There are several validated gastroparesis severity scales utilized by gastroenterologists [26, 27], which are not completely applicable to the endurance athlete. Utilizing previously well-validated scoring symptoms, a modified and novel scale to capture GI symptoms in endurance racers was created and subsequently tested in the field.

The purpose of this prospective study was to trial the field expediency of a quantitative measurement tool for the

TABLE 1: Percentage of patients reporting severity scores for each symptom before and after treatment. Scores that indicate improvement after treatment are shown in bold font.

	None (0)		Mild (1)		Moderate (2)		Severe (3)		Very severe (4)		Unbearable (5)	
	Initial	Follow-up	Initial	Follow-up	Initial	Follow-up	Initial	Follow-up	Initial	Follow-up	Initial	Follow-up
Nausea	0	22	26	44	48	**33**	19	**0**	7	**0**	0	0
Vomiting	70	96	26	**4**	4	**0**	0	0	0	0	0	0
Loss of appetite	11	41	44	**37**	22	**19**	19	**4**	4	**0**	0	0
Loss of desire to drink	22	59	41	**30**	30	**11**	4	**0**	4	**0**	0	0
Abdominal sloshing	67	96	11	**0**	22	**4**	0	0	0	0	0	0
Abdominal pain	78	85	22	**15**	0	0	0	0	0	0	0	0

common ailment of exercise-associated gastroparesis, as well as the satisfaction of the athlete and physician with its use.

2. Methods

Institutional Review Board approval was obtained (Upstate Medical University Proposal #722316) to survey consented athletes at the Wild Elephant Trail, a 6-day, multistage, remote ultramarathon that registered 52 runners (63% male and average age 48.9 years) and held its inaugural race in March 2015. The race covers 210 km through rural and remote Sri Lanka in the area between Yapahuwa Temple and Sigiriya Rock. Environmental conditions are typically tropical with average temperatures between 24°C and 32°C. Geography includes rolling hills, jungle climbs, and wet stretches of relatively flat paddy fields.

A convenience sample of athletes was surveyed by the event physician. Surveys were administered either when the athlete approached the medical team requesting medical care of gastrointestinal symptoms, or when the physician performed routine athlete health assessments and discovered a gastrointestinal complaint. Survey answers were collected just prior to any treatment or physician recommendations and then at time of reassessment. All medical management was based on current best practices and standard of care and was not altered for the purposes of the study. Surveys were made anonymous after posttreatment assessment was completed.

The survey instrument was adapted from previously published tools which have been used to measure symptom severity of gastroparesis in the context of chronic illness [26, 27]. From these previously described tools, we selected 6 symptoms which we felt were germane to the endurance athlete based on the collective authors' experience with hundreds of athletes over several years. Symptoms included in our tool were nausea, vomiting, loss of appetite, loss of desire to drink, abdominal "sloshing," and abdominal pain. Once in the field, the severity of these 6 symptoms of interest was recorded on a 0–5 (none to unbearable) Likert scale. The total scores of all 6 symptoms were summated to produce a gastroparesis severity score (GSS). Finally, our instrument consisted of the time of initial assessment and reassessment, along with treatment provided and the activity being performed by the athlete at the time of the complaint (rest, exertion, and meals).

At the same time, a separate question of our survey used a Visual Analog Scale (VAS) to assess the more generic question "how much are the symptoms affecting your race performance?" where one end was "no problems at all" and the other end was "I'm thinking of dropping out." The single mark on the VAS was measured in millimeters and converted to a percent.

After management of the symptoms by rest, medication, or watchful waiting, reassessment was performed using the same Likert scale for the same 6 symptoms of interest as well as the same VAS question and scale. The change in GSS was used to measure improvement in symptoms. The change in VAS was used to measure the athlete's perceived performance impact from these symptoms. Two new questions were also asked at this time. To the athlete, it was "Did you feel like this score adequately captured all of your symptoms as well as their severity?" and to the physician administering the survey it was "Did you feel like this score adequately captured the runner's symptoms?"

Survey results were analyzed descriptively with SPSS (version 22; SPSS Inc., Chicago, IL).

3. Results

A total of 27 surveys were obtained which included both the pretreatment and posttreatment assessments for athletes with gastroparesis symptoms. Surveys were administered to athletes either during exertion on the race course (16/27; 59%), during an attempt to take a meal (1/27; 4%), or after stage completion during recovery activities (10/27; 37%). No statistical differences were seen associating symptoms experienced with type of activity.

Summation of the severity scores (0–5 Likert scale) of all six symptoms was used to calculate a global gastroparesis severity score (GSS) of 0–30 for each athlete. The median pretreatment GSS was 6 (range: 2–16) with 23 athletes reporting improvement of their GSS and 4 athletes reporting no change or worsening of their symptoms. The median posttreatment GSS was 2 (range: 0–9). Table 1 describes the percent of athletes who experienced each symptom at initial evaluation (before treatment) and at follow-up (after treatment), stratified by symptom severity on the Likert scale (0–5).

Reassessments were done at the convenience of the athlete and without time constraints given. The median time between assessments was 1:05 hours (range 00:05 hours to

TABLE 2: Final exercise-associated gastroparesis severity score.

Symptom	None	Mild	Moderate	Severe	Very severe	Unbearable
Nausea	0	1	2	3	4	5
Vomiting	0	1	2	3	4	5
Loss of appetite	0	1	2	3	4	5
Loss of desire to drink	0	1	2	3	4	5
Abdominal sloshing	0	1	2	3	4	5
Abdominal pain	0	1	2	3	4	5

Gastroparesis severity score (GSS) = sum of all circled numbers.

9:55 hours; SD 2:33 hours). No statistical differences were seen associating GSS with time elapsed between assessments.

Medical management of athletes included anticipatory guidance (7/27; 26%), prescribed rest (13/27; 48%), or medication (7/27; 26%). Anticipatory guidance included suggestions for the athlete to shed their heat load by cooling themselves by rest or shade. Medications used included metoclopramide (1/27) and ondansetron (6/27). Median GSS decrease was 1 for anticipatory guidance, 2 for prescribed rest, and 5 for medication ($p = 0.446$).

Athletes with a GSS improvement of at least 3 points (top 50th percentile) had a median improvement in their VAS of 25.9% whereas athletes with a GSS improvement less than 3 points (lower 50th percentile) had a median improvement in their VAS of 7.14%.

Finally, all (100% of responses) athletes indicated that the survey instrument adequately captured their symptoms and severity. Similarly, the physician administering the surveys felt that, throughout the athlete encounters, the symptoms were adequately captured (100% of responses).

4. Discussion

Although this analysis does not specifically test sensitivity or specificity of the symptom domains, it does demonstrate that this tool can be used in the field to effectively capture the most common symptoms that occur with exercise-associated gastroparesis. The fact that athlete improvement in GSS was predictive of improvement of their VAS score suggests that the symptoms we chose were important to the athletes' race performance. Further psychometric validation would be needed to ascertain the strengths of each component, but because all of the athletes felt that their symptoms were captured, it is plausible that future analysis of this novel tool would demonstrate statistical sensitivity. Specificity of the symptoms would require a larger number of participants and a larger number of symptoms captured.

The severity of runner's symptoms was not associated with the activity that they were involved in at the time of questioning. The timing at which the runner was reassessed also did not have an association with the symptom score. Although this was not the primary objective of this study, it was noted that nausea and loss of appetite were associated most with the runner's overall attitude in their ability to complete the race. This finding may help guide future studies, including those that have to do with the treatment of EAG.

During this event, no athletes developed intractable symptoms that would prompt the race physician to consider other, more sinister, causes of nausea or fatigue. No athletes received intravenous fluids or required medical disqualification or evacuation. Information on "Did not finish" (DNF) status of athletes was not included in the data collected during this study. Though not statistically significant, there is a suggestion that medication may be more effective than simply rest alone.

Although EAG is a well-recognized and described syndrome in endurance medicine [10, 23–25], there has yet to be any symptom assessment instruments developed or any formal or extensive discussion of treatment published. Recent work has added greatly to our understanding of GI distress in the setting of endurance events by studying the incidence, severity, and timing of GI symptoms in finishers and nonfinishers of a 161 km race [16]; however a tool to discretely measure these symptoms in a race setting has yet to be developed. Although a formal validation study is still needed, results of our study suggest that our novel, field-expedient survey tool can be used to measure and assess the presence and severity of exercise-associated gastroparesis symptoms. The gastrointestinal symptoms chosen for our survey are widely considered to be common amongst endurance athletes.

Our novel EAG scale was developed by adapting other publications that have demonstrated the usefulness and validity of GI symptom severity scores [26, 27]. The symptoms chosen for inclusion in the survey were a result of previous gastroparesis research as well as the authors' experience with athletes in the race environment. Previous GI symptoms scores have included both discrete Likert-type questions for specific symptoms and a continuous VAS component attempting to capture more of a global understanding of the effects of the studied symptoms [26]. Though we utilized both elements to trial our tool, we have opted to only use the Likert questions in future iterations due to the ease of use. See Table 2 for a proposed EAG scale that does not include the VAS or other questions that were included for purposes of understanding the perception of this tool and its field expediency.

Limitations of this study involve those inherent in obtaining a convenience study sample. This limitation is difficult to control for in the remote, ultramarathon setting where athletes do not typically wish to participate in any kind of extraneous activities that may slow their competitive intents.

The race physician who was queried by the survey was also the treating physician, which may introduce some ascertainment bias. Finally, because no athletes had any serious illness we cannot assess the utility of this tool in more critically ill athletes; however, this was not our intent and should not be the proposed target of the use of this tool.

This novel EAG score was developed in an attempt to provide researchers and clinicians with a tool to quantify the severity of this illness and response to therapy. To our knowledge no clinical trials have been conducted assessing the several treatments available for EAG. Further study is needed to determine if this questionnaire is valid, but our development of a scoring system to quantify largely subjective symptoms in an austere environment is not without precedent. For example, the Lake Louise Criteria for Acute Mountain Sickness were developed by expert consensus [28] and then trialed in the field to validate [29–31]. Our hope is that this expert-derived scoring system could derive further validation from future field use. One such immediate use would be to quantify symptoms in order to assess the effectiveness of medication-based interventions during races.

5. Conclusions

A simple Likert scale of the severity of nausea and loss of appetite seems to provide a useful tool for measuring the severity of exercise-associated gastroparesis in endurance athletes. Further research efforts focusing on this clinical syndrome may benefit from a numeric scoring system as described in this novel exercise-associated gastroparesis severity scale.

Competing Interests

The authors declare that they have no competing interests.

References

[1] M. D. Hoffman, J. C. Ong, and G. Wang, "Historical analysis of participation in 161 km ultramarathons in North America," *International Journal of the History of Sport*, vol. 27, no. 11, pp. 1877–1891, 2010.

[2] B. Knechtle, P. Knechtle, and R. Lepers, "Participation and performance trends in ultra-triathlons from 1985 to 2009," *Scandinavian Journal of Medicine and Science in Sports*, vol. 21, no. 6, pp. e82–e90, 2011.

[3] J. Joslin, R. Worthing, T. Black, W. D. Grant, T. Kotlyar, and S. M. Wojcik, "Analysis of weight change and borg rating of perceived exertion as measurements of runner health and safety during a 6-day, multistage, remote ultramarathon," *Clinical Journal of Sport Medicine*, vol. 24, no. 3, pp. 245–250, 2014.

[4] M. D. Hoffman and K. Fogard, "Factors related to successful completion of a 161-km ultramarathon," *International Journal of Sports Physiology and Performance*, vol. 6, no. 1, pp. 25–37, 2011.

[5] M. D. Hoffman, K. Fogard, J. Winger, T. Hew-Butler, and K. J. Stuempfle, "Characteristics of 161-km ultramarathon finishers developing exercise-associated hyponatremia," *Research in Sports Medicine*, vol. 21, no. 2, pp. 164–175, 2013.

[6] M. D. Hoffman, I. R. Rogers, J. Joslin, C. A. Asplund, W. O. Roberts, and B. D. Levine, "Managing collapsed or seriously ill participants of ultra-endurance events in remote environments," *Sports Medicine*, vol. 45, no. 2, pp. 201–212, 2015.

[7] D. L. Costill and B. Saltin, "Factors limiting gastric emptying during rest and exercise," *Journal of Applied Physiology*, vol. 37, no. 5, pp. 679–683, 1974.

[8] H. P. F. Peters, W. R. De Vries, G. P. Vanberge-Henegouwen, and L. M. A. Akkermans, "Potential benefits and hazards of physical activity and exercise on the gastrointestinal tract," *Gut*, vol. 48, no. 3, pp. 435–439, 2001.

[9] H. Zoller, M. Creus, J. Roos, and W. Vogel, "Clinical investigation of athletes and gastrointestinal symptoms: where is the starting line?" *International SportMed Journal*, vol. 6, no. 3, pp. 141–150, 2005.

[10] E. P. de Oliveira and R. C. Burini, "Food-dependent, exercise-induced gastrointestinal distress," *Journal of the International Society of Sports Nutrition*, vol. 8, pp. 12–18, 2011.

[11] F. Brouns, "Etiology of gastrointestinal disturbances during endurance events," *Scandinavian Journal of Medicine and Science in Sports*, vol. 1, no. 2, pp. 66–77, 1991.

[12] K. J. Stuempfle, M. D. Hoffman, and T. Hew-Butler, "Association of gastrointestinal distress in ultramarathoners with race diet," *International Journal of Sport Nutrition and Exercise Metabolism*, vol. 23, no. 2, pp. 103–109, 2013.

[13] B. Glace, C. Murphy, and M. McHugh, "Food and fluid intake and disturbances in gastrointestinal and mental function during an ultramarathon," *International Journal of Sport Nutrition and Exercise Metabolism*, vol. 12, no. 4, pp. 414–427, 2002.

[14] H. P. F. Peters, M. Bos, L. Seebregts et al., "Gastrointestinal symptoms in long-distance runners, cyclists, and triathletes: prevalence, medication, and etiology," *American Journal of Gastroenterology*, vol. 94, no. 6, pp. 1570–1581, 1999.

[15] S. M. Simons and R. G. Kennedy, "Gastrointestinal problems in runners," *Current Sports Medicine Reports*, vol. 3, no. 2, pp. 112–116, 2004.

[16] K. J. Stuempfle and M. D. Hoffman, "Gastrointestinal distress is common during a 161-km ultramarathon," *Journal of Sports Sciences*, vol. 33, no. 17, pp. 1814–1821, 2015.

[17] N. J. Rehrer and G. A. Meijer, "Biomechanical vibration of the abdominal region during running and bicycling," *The Journal of Sports Medicine and Physical Fitness*, vol. 31, no. 2, pp. 231–234, 1991.

[18] S. N. Sullivan and C. Wong, "Runners' diarrhea: different patterns and associated factors," *Journal of Clinical Gastroenterology*, vol. 14, no. 2, pp. 101–104, 1992.

[19] M. I. Qamar and A. E. Read, "Effects of exercise on mesenteric blood flow in man," *Gut*, vol. 28, no. 5, pp. 583–587, 1987.

[20] T. Hew-Butler, M. H. Rosner, S. Fowkes-Godek et al., "Statement of the third international exercise-associated hyponatremia consensus development conference, New Carlsbad, California, 2015," *Clinical Journal of Sport Medicine*, vol. 25, no. 4, pp. 303–320, 2015.

[21] S. M. Gil, E. Yazaki, and D. F. Evans, "Aetiology of running-related gastrointestinal dysfunction: how far is the finishing line?" *Sports Medicine*, vol. 26, no. 6, pp. 365–378, 1998.

[22] N. J. Rehrer, G. M. E. Janssen, F. Brouns, and W. H. M. Saris, "Fluid intake and gastrointestinal problems in runners competing in a 25-km race and a marathon," *International Journal of Sports Medicine*, vol. 10, no. 1, pp. S22–S25, 1989.

[23] I. Carrió, M. Estorch, R. Serra-Grima et al., "Gastric emptying in marathon runners," *Gut*, vol. 30, no. 2, pp. 152–155, 1989.

[24] P. D. Neufer, A. J. Young, and M. N. Sawka, "Gastric emptying during exercise: effects of heat stress and hypohydration," *European Journal of Applied Physiology and Occupational Physiology*, vol. 58, no. 4, pp. 433–439, 1989.

[25] K. van Wijck, K. Lenaerts, J. Grootjans et al., "Physiology and pathophysiology of splanchnic hypoperfusion and intestinal injury during exercise: strategies for evaluation and prevention," *American Journal of Physiology—Gastrointestinal and Liver Physiology*, vol. 303, no. 2, pp. G155–G168, 2012.

[26] H. J. Bovenschen, M. J. R. Janssen, M. G. H. van Oijen, R. J. F. Laheij, L. G. M. van Rossum, and J. B. M. J. Jansen, "Evaluation of a gastrointestinal symptoms questionnaire," *Digestive Diseases and Sciences*, vol. 51, no. 9, pp. 1509–1515, 2006.

[27] D. A. Revicki, A. M. Rentz, D. Dubois et al., "Development and validation of a patient-assessed gastroparesis symptom severity measure: the Gastroparesis Cardinal Symptom Index," *Alimentary Pharmacology and Therapeutics*, vol. 18, no. 1, pp. 141–150, 2003.

[28] "The lake louise consensus on the definition and quantification of altitude illness," in *Hypoxia and Mountain Medicine*, J. R. Sutton, G. Coates, and C. S. Houston, Eds., Queen City Printers, Burlington, Vt, USA, 1992.

[29] G. Savourey, A. Guinet, Y. Besnard, N. Garcia, A.-M. Hanniquet, and J. Bittel, "Evaluation of the Lake Louise acute mountain sickness scoring system in a hypobaric chamber," *Aviation Space and Environmental Medicine*, vol. 66, no. 10, pp. 963–967, 1995.

[30] D. P. Hall, I. J. C. MacCormick, A. T. Phythian-Adams et al., "Network analysis reveals distinct clinical syndromes underlying acute mountain sickness," *PLoS ONE*, vol. 9, no. 1, Article ID e81229, 2014.

[31] M. J. MacInnis, S. C. Lanting, J. L. Rupert, and M. S. Koehle, "Is poor sleep quality at high altitude separate from acute mountain sickness? Factor structure and internal consistency of the Lake Louise Score Questionnaire," *High Altitude Medicine and Biology*, vol. 14, no. 4, pp. 334–337, 2013.

18

Examining Measures of Weight as Risk Factors for Sport-Related Injury in Adolescents

Sarah A. Richmond,[1,2,3] Alberto Nettel-Aguirre,[2,4,5] Patricia K. Doyle-Baker,[2] Alison Macpherson,[3] and Carolyn A. Emery[2,4]

[1]*Child Health Evaluative Sciences, Hospital for Sick Children, 555 University Avenue, Toronto, ON, Canada M5G 1X8*
[2]*Sport Injury Prevention Research Centre, Faculty of Kinesiology, University of Calgary, 2500 University Drive, Calgary, AB, Canada T2N 1N4*
[3]*School of Kinesiology and Health Science, York University, 4700 Keele Street, Toronto, ON, Canada M3J 1P3*
[4]*Alberta Children's Hospital, Institute for Child and Maternal Health, 2888 Shaganappi Trail NW, Calgary, AB, Canada T3B 6A8*
[5]*Departments of Pediatrics and Community Health Sciences, Cumming School of Medicine, University of Calgary, 2500 University Drive, Calgary, AB, Canada T2N 1N4*

Correspondence should be addressed to Sarah A. Richmond; sarah.a.richmond@gmail.com

Academic Editor: Michael Gaetz

Objectives. To examine body mass index (BMI) and waist circumference (WC) as risk factors for sport injury in adolescents. *Design.* A secondary analysis of prospectively collected data from a pilot cluster randomized controlled trial. *Methods.* Adolescents ($n = 1{,}040$) at the ages of 11–15 years from two Calgary junior high schools were included. BMI (kg/m^2) and WC (cm) were measured from direct measures at baseline assessment. Categories (overweight/obese) were created using validated international (BMI) and national (WC) cut-off points. A Poisson regression analysis controlling for relevant covariates (sex, previous injury, sport participation, intervention group, and aerobic fitness level) estimated the risk of sport injury [incidence rate ratios (IRR) with 95% confidence intervals (CI)]. *Results.* There was an increased risk of time loss injury (IRR = 2.82, 95% CI: 1.01–8.04) and knee injury (IRR = 2.07, 95% CI: 1.00–6.94) in adolescents that were overweight/obese; however, increases in injury risk for all injury and lower extremity injury were not statistically significant. Estimates suggested a greater risk of time loss injury [IRR = 1.63 (95% CI: 0.93–2.47)] in adolescents with high measures of WC. *Conclusions.* There is an increased risk of time loss injury and knee injury in overweight/obese adolescents. Sport injury prevention training programs should include strategies that target all known risk factors for injury.

1. Introduction

Sport injury is the leading cause of injury in Canadian youth [1]. In the 2009-2010 Canadian Community Health Survey, children over the age of 12 reported sport as the activity where their most serious injury occurred, a total of 1,470,000 injuries over a one-year period [2]. Sport injury represents a large burden on both direct and indirect health care costs, including rehabilitation for the injury itself, and the costs associated with children spending time away from school and subsequent sport and physical activity. Lifelong participation in sport and physical activity is particularly important, as overweight/obesity is an established epidemic [3]. Overweight/obesity in youth in Canada has increased in past decades; the prevalence of obesity in 2004 was 2.5 times higher than measures in the late 1970s [3]. Self-report body mass index (BMI) data collected in the 2013 Health Indicator Profile reported that 421,350 Canadian children at the ages of 12–17 years were overweight or obese [3].

As part of a public health approach to reducing an injury problem, understanding the risk factors that place a child at increased risk for sport injury is a key part of the prevention pathway. Pediatric sport injury literature has long established nonmodifiable risk factors for sport injury to include age, sex, and previous injury, and there is some evidence for modifiable risk factors including low fitness levels (e.g., poor aerobic fitness and lack of preseason training) [4]. What is lesser known is the association of measures of obesity as independent risk factors for increases in sport injury rates in youth. This is not due to the lack of investigation, but rather a lack of consensus between studies, most likely due to differing methods of assessment of body composition, populations (sport versus non-sport specific), injury definitions, and study design, reducing the ability to synthesize data across studies. There are studies that demonstrate that children with higher BMI measures are at increased risk of a sport-related injury including Nilstad et al. (2014) where multivariable analyses demonstrated that female soccer players with a higher BMI were associated with greater odds of lower extremity injury (OR = 1.51, 95% CI: 1.21–1.90) [5]. There are also studies that demonstrate a protective effect for injury in children with higher BMI measures including Ezzat et al. (2014) who demonstrate a statistically significant reduction in the odds of sport injury in obese adolescents compared to their healthy weight counterparts (OR = 0.72, 95% CI: 0.53–0.99) [6]. The mixed results demonstrated in these studies may be due to the inconsistent measure and categorization of healthy weight in children, in addition to the lack of prospective data collection and direct measures of weight and height.

The current study is a follow-up to a previously reported study examining BMI as a risk factor for sport injury in adolescent youth in Alberta, Canada [7]. This study found that there was an increased odds of sport injury in obese adolescents compared to healthy weight adolescents; however, recommendations for future research included using prospective study designs and direct measures of weight [7]. Therefore, the aim of this study was to examine direct measures of BMI in youth and the association of these measures with sport-related injury.

2. Materials and Methods

This was a secondary analysis of data collected from a prospective, pilot cluster randomized controlled trial (RCT) in Calgary, Alberta, Canada [8]. The pilot study examined the effectiveness of a sport injury prevention program in junior high youth, comparing an intervention program implemented in physical education classes in two junior high schools (one intervention school and one control school) [8]. The two junior high schools chosen for this study were selected from similar, socioeconomic demographics. Students and their parent/guardian signed the consent form, approved by the Office of Medical Bioethics, University of Calgary, and the Calgary Board of Education.

The main outcome measure in this study was sport injury, defined as any injury resulting from sporting activity that required medical attention, time loss, and/or removal of the participant from the sporting activity. Secondary injury definitions included lower extremity injury (injury of the hip, knee, ankle, lower leg, and foot), time loss injury (an injury that resulted in time away from sport, physical activity, or school, greater than 7 days), and knee and ankle injury. Students reported any injury sustained in a sporting activity to the physical education teacher who instructed and assisted the student in completing an injury report form. Injury report forms were initiated by the student and followed up by a study physiotherapist who assessed each reported injury. The injury report forms used in this study have been previously validated in a sporting youth population [9, 10].

A certified exercise physiologist collected all weight and fitness measures (BMI, waist circumference, aerobic fitness, and vertical jump) and reliability was demonstrated using a one-week test-retest protocol [8]. BMI (kg/m^2) was estimated from direct measures of height (cm) and weight (kg) and overweight and obese categories were created using validated age and sex specific, international cut-off points [11]. The overweight and obese categories were combined to create one variable in this study. Included in the healthy categorization were children with low BMI measures. The health effects of cut-off points corresponding to low BMI measures in children have not been validated as markers of disease risk, particularly with injury [11].

Waist circumference (WC) was collected at baseline and measured to the nearest 0.50 cm using anthropometric tape. The protocol for all physical measures was taken from the Canadian Physical Activity, Fitness and Lifestyle Appraisal [12]. Waist circumference was then categorized into a binary variable (healthy or unhealthy) using national reference data [13].

Participating students from both schools completed a baseline medical questionnaire (including questions about previous six-week and one-year injury history) and weekly sport participation journal (including the total sport participation hours over the study period). Previous one-year injury as a binary variable (yes, no) was included in the final model. Sport participation was collected prospectively from a weekly sport participation journal, completed in the student's health classes. The total number of hours of sport participation was used as the offset in a Poisson regression model, controlling for the amount of play between students. Indirect aerobic fitness was collected using the Leger 20-metre shuttle run and used as a covariate in the model [14]. The child's maximum stage recorded was converted into a VO_2 measure, represented as the volume of oxygen consumption in millimetres per kilogram of body weight per minute ($mL \cdot kg^{-1} \cdot min^{-1}$). Vertical jump was collected as the maximum jump height attained from three trial jumps. The students highest jump measure was recorded in cm from the difference in standing height and maximum jump height.

All data were analyzed using STATA statistical software, version 12.0. Poisson regression analyses controlled for relevant covariates (sex, previous injury, sport participation, intervention group, and aerobic fitness level) and clustering by class was used to estimate the risk of sport injury, across injury definitions, reported using incidence rate ratios (IRR) with 95% confidence intervals (CI). Injury definitions included all sport injury, lower extremity injury, time loss injury, and ankle and knee sprain injury. The covariates considered in the final model were those significant at the 5% level. Two-way interactions were examined for evidence of

TABLE 1: Baseline characteristics by sex.

	Boys	Girls
Frequency, %	427 (41.0)	613 (58.9)
Age (median, IQR)	13 (12-13)	13 (12-13)
BMI (mean, 95% CI)	19.5 (19.2–19.8)	19.3 (19.1–19.5)
Missing (n)	9	9
Unhealthy BMI (%, 95% CI)	15.3 (11.9–18.9)	9.0 (6.7–11.2)
WC (mean, 95% CI)	69.2 (68.4–70.1)	66.5 (66.0–67.1)
Missing (n)	7	9
Unhealthy WC (%, 95% CI)	24.8 (20.7–28.9)	22.7 (19.4–26.0)
Sport participation* (median, IQR)	52.0 (32.0–80.0)	52.0 (31.0–77.0)
Aerobic fitness** (mean, 95% CI)	42.6 (41.8–43.3)	36.8 (36.3–37.3)
Missing (n)	11	25
Vertical jump (cm)	36.9 (36.1–37.8)	31.2 (30.7–31.7)
Missing (n)	28	39
Previous injury† (%, 95% CI)	23.5 (19.5–27.6)	22.4 (19.1–25.8)
Missing (n)	6	7

BMI: body mass index (kg/m^2). WC: waist circumference (cm).
*Total sport participation over study period (hours). **Indirect measure of aerobic fitness. †Injury reported in the previous 12 months (frequency).

effect modification by sex, previous injury, and intervention group. In the case of no effect modification, variables were taken out of the model to asses the change in betas to assess for confounding.

3. Results

The cohort participants included 1,040 children at the ages of 11–15 years. The median age of participants was 13 years (IQR: 12–13). At baseline (Table 1), the proportion of overweight/obese boys (15.3%, 95% CI: 11.9–18.9) was higher compared to girls (9.0%, 95% CI: 6.7–11.2). In addition, boys had higher levels of aerobic fitness (VO_2 max estimates = 42.6 mL·kg^{-1}·min^{-1}, 95% CI: 41.8–43.3) compared to girls (VO_2 max estimates = 36.8 mL·kg^{-1}·min^{-1}, 95% CI: 36.3–37.3) in addition to measures of vertical jump (cm) and WC (cm) (Table 1).

When examining the differences in measures of lower extremity strength (vertical jump, measured as the maximum jump height in cm), overweight/obese students had significantly lower measures of vertical jump (29.7 cm, SD = 6.94) compared to healthy weight students [34.0 cm, SD = 7.78, $t(957) = 5.51$, and $p \leq 0.0001$]. For WC, vertical jump measures were also lower for those students with unhealthy WC (32.1 cm, SD = 7.91) compared to students with healthy measures [34.0 cm, SD = 7.73, $t(971) = 3.22$, and $p = 0.0013$].

There was no evidence of effect modification by sex, previous injury, or intervention type. There were a total of 109 injuries that occurred during the study period, which represents an overall cohort injury rate of 1.80 injuries/1000 total hours of sport participation. The rate of lower extremity injury was 1.27/1000 hours, time loss injury was 0.63/1000 hours, knee injury was 0.48/1000 hours, and ankle injury was 0.45/1000 hours. The Poisson regression model demonstrated an increased risk of time loss injury (IRR = 2.82, 95% CI: 1.01–8.04) and knee injury (IRR = 2.07, 95% CI: 1.00–6.94) in overweight/obese adolescents (Table 2). There were no significant increases in injury risk for all sport injury and lower extremity injury in overweight/obese adolescents. Point estimates suggest a greater risk of time loss injury [IRR = 1.63 (95% CI: 0.93–2.47)] and knee injury [IRR = 1.43 (95% CI: 0.60–3.47)] in adolescents with unhealthy measures of WC; however, these effects were not statistically significant.

4. Discussion

This study was a follow-up to previous research demonstrating that obese students were at a 34% increased risk for sport injury, compared to healthy weight students [7]. The results of this study show that overweight/obese children are at a higher risk of time loss injury and knee injury, compared to healthy weight students. Overweight/obese adolescents may be at increased risk for sport-related injury due to the forces being absorbed through soft tissue and joints. Literature in this area has long established that a lack of lower extremity strength and power increases the risk of knee and ankle related injury [15]. There is an increased risk of anterior cruciate ligament injury (greater in females) with greater hamstring : quadriceps ratios [15]. In this study, students with greater unhealthy mass have poorer lower extremity strength that may be related to the lack of exposure to the type of activities that would increase lower extremity strength.

There is a breadth of literature describing components of neuromuscular training programs that reduce the burden of pediatric sport injury in a sport-specific population [16–21]. Less information is known about the components of programs that can reduce injury in the general population (e.g., students) [8, 22]. It is important to consider all potentially modifiable risk factors for sport injury in the development of prevention programs. Including exercises that can reduce

Table 2: Incidence rates (IR, 95% CI) and incidence rate ratios (IRR, 95% CI) by risk factors, adjusted for previous injury, sex, aerobic fitness, intervention group, and sport participation.

	Number of injuries	All sport IR (n = 109)	Lower extremity IRR* (n = 77)	Time loss IRR* (n = 38)	Knee IRR* (n = 29)	Ankle IRR* (n = 27)
BMI (kg/m^2)						
Healthy**	94	1.00	1.00	1.00	1.00	1.00
Unhealthy**	11	1.28 (0.65–2.49)	1.14 (0.50–2.61)	2.82 (1.01–8.04)	2.07 (1.00–6.94)	0.44 (0.06–3.43)
WC (cm)						
Healthy***	84	1.00	1.00	1.00	1.00	1.00
Unhealthy***	25	1.26 (0.78–2.07)	1.14 (0.90–1.75)	1.63 (0.93–2.47)	1.43 (0.60–3.47)	0.59 (0.17–2.05)
Previous injury (yes/no)						
No	69	1.00	1.00	1.00	1.00	1.00
Yes	38	1.47 (1.00–2.15)	1.43 (0.83–2.59)	2.16 (1.06–4.42)	2.60 (1.00–6.76)	1.25 (0.55–2.85)
Sex (males/females)						
Females	59	1.00	1.00	1.00	1.00	1.00
Males	50	0.78 (0.54–1.12)	0.73 (0.46–1.16)	0.58 (0.26–1.30)	0.54 (0.19–1.52)	0.74 (0.33–1.68)
Intervention (yes/no)						
No	60	1.00	1.00	1.00	1.00	1.00
Yes	49	0.30 (0.18–0.51)	0.30 (0.18–0.52)	0.37 (0.17–0.81)	0.32 (0.11–0.93)	0.37 (0.18–0.77)

BMI: body mass index. WC: waist circumference. *Adjusted model. **Based on international cutoffs. ***Based on national reference data.

measures of BMI as a risk factor of injury and, at the same time, increasing lower extremity strength and balance will have the greatest impact. In addition, applying these programs to children outside of a sport-specific setting can have large public health impact.

Strengths of this study include the prospective collection of sport injury assessed weekly by a study physiotherapist and direct measures of weight and fitness level. This study also prospectively collected hours of sport participation, which was used as the offset to represent a rate of injury per hour of participation. An additional strength of this study includes the low drop-out rate (0.41%) and the potential for socioeconomic status as a confounder was eliminated due to the homogeneity between the two groups being compared. Limitations in this study include the relatively small proportion of the population categorized as being overweight/obese (11.6%, 95% CI: 9.6–13.5). The RCT that these data were initially collected from was powered on an expected difference in injury proportion between the two schools. The ability to evaluate numerous injury definitions across primary exposure variables of interest leads to wide confidence intervals and increased risk of type II error. In addition, it is impossible to consider sport type, mechanism of injury, and injury type in the modeling of these data due to the numerous sports, mechanisms, and injury types reported. This may lead to spurious conclusions of overweight/obesity as a risk factor for sport injury. Upon visual examination of these data, however, the proportion of overweight/obese students participating in contact sports did not appear to be different compared to those of healthy weight. Finally, these data were limited to two schools; therefore, the generalizability of these data to populations beyond those reported here is limited.

5. Conclusion

The results from this study suggest that there is an increased risk of sport-related injury in overweight/obese adolescents when considering exposure to participation. Specifically, adolescents with higher BMIs demonstrate an increased risk of more severe injury (time loss greater than seven days) and knee injuries. Sport injury prevention training programs should include strategies targeting both injury prevention and healthy body weight.

Competing Interests

The authors declare that they have no competing interests.

Acknowledgments

The authors acknowledge the support of the Calgary Board of Education and all participating schools, teachers, and students who made this research possible. The Sport Injury Prevention Research Centre is one of the International Research Centres for Prevention of Injury and Protection of Athlete

Health supported by the International Olympic Committee. Carolyn A. Emery is funded through the Alberta Children's Hospital Foundation (Chair in Pediatric Rehabilitation).

References

[1] W. Pickett, M. Molcho, K. Simpson et al., "Cross national study of injury and social determinants in adolescents," *Injury Prevention*, vol. 11, no. 4, pp. 213–218, 2005.

[2] Statistics Canada, *Injuries in Canada: Insights from the Canadian Community Health Survey*, 2013, http://www.statcan.gc.ca/pub/82-624-x/2011001/article/11506-eng.htm.

[3] Statistics Canada, Body mass index, overweight or obese, self-reported, youth, http://www.statcan.gc.ca/tables-tableaux/sum-som/l01/cst01/health84a-eng.htm?sdi=body mass index.

[4] C. A. Emery, "Risk factors for injury in child and adolescent sport: a systematic review of the literature," *Clinical Journal of Sport Medicine*, vol. 13, no. 4, pp. 256–268, 2003.

[5] A. Nilstad, T. E. Andersen, R. Bahr, I. Holme, and K. Steffen, "Risk factors for lower extremity injuries in elite female soccer players," *American Journal of Sports Medicine*, vol. 42, no. 4, pp. 940–948, 2014.

[6] A. Ezzat, A. Schneeberg, and M. Koehoorn, "Weighty problems: sport injuries in overweight or obese active canadian adolescents," *British Journal of Sports Medicine*, vol. 48, article 592, 2014.

[7] S. A. Richmond, J. Kang, and C. A. Emery, "Is body mass index a risk factor for sport injury in adolescents?" *Journal of Science and Medicine in Sport*, vol. 16, no. 5, pp. 401–405, 2013.

[8] S. A. Richmond, J. Kang, P. K. Doyle-Baker, A. Nettel-Aguirre, and C. A. Emery, "A school-based injury prevention program to reduce sport injury risk and improve healthy outcomes in youth," *Clinical Journal of Sport Medicine*, vol. 26, no. 4, pp. 291–298, 2016.

[9] C. A. Emery, W. H. Meeuwisse, and S. E. Hartmann, "Evaluation of risk factors for injury in adolescent soccer: implementation and validation of an injury surveillance system," *The American Journal of Sports Medicine*, vol. 33, no. 12, pp. 1882–1891, 2005.

[10] C. A. Emery and W. H. Meeuwisse, "Injury rates, risk factors, and mechanisms of injury in minor hockey," *American Journal of Sports Medicine*, vol. 34, no. 12, pp. 1960–1969, 2006.

[11] T. J. Cole, M. C. Bellizzi, K. M. Flegal, and W. H. Dietz, "Establishing a standard definition for child overweight and obesity worldwide: international survey," *The British Medical Journal*, vol. 320, no. 7244, pp. 1240–1243, 2000.

[12] Canadian Society for Exercise Physiology, *The Canadian Physical Activity, Fitness and Lifestyle Appraisal*, Canadian Society for Exercise Physiology, Ontario, Canada, 3rd edition, 2003.

[13] P. T. Katzmarzyk, "Waist circumference percentiles for Canadian youth 11–18y of age," *European Journal of Clinical Nutrition*, vol. 58, no. 7, pp. 1011–1015, 2004.

[14] L. A. Léger, D. Mercier, C. Gadoury, and J. Lambert, "The multistage 20 metre shuttle run test for aerobic fitness," *Journal of Sports Sciences*, vol. 6, no. 2, pp. 93–101, 1988.

[15] T. E. Hewett, T. N. Lindenfeld, J. V. Riccobene, and F. R. Noyes, "The effect of neuromuscular training on the incidence of knee injury in female athletes. A Prospective Study," *American Journal of Sports Medicine*, vol. 27, no. 6, pp. 699–706, 1999.

[16] C. A. Emery, M. S. Rose, J. R. McAllister, and W. H. Meeuwisse, "A prevention strategy to reduce the incidence of injury in high school basketball: a cluster randomized controlled trial," *Clinical Journal of Sport Medicine*, vol. 17, no. 1, pp. 17–24, 2007.

[17] C. A. Emery and W. H. Meeuwisse, "The effectiveness of a neuromuscular prevention strategy to reduce injuries in youth soccer: a cluster-randomised controlled trial," *British Journal of Sports Medicine*, vol. 44, no. 8, pp. 555–562, 2010.

[18] U. G. Longo, M. Loppini, A. Berton, A. Marinozzi, N. Maffulli, and V. Denaro, "The FIFA 11+ program is effective in preventing injuries in elite male basketball players: a cluster randomized controlled trial," *The American Journal of Sports Medicine*, vol. 40, no. 5, pp. 996–1005, 2012.

[19] G. Myklebust, L. Engebretsen, I. H. Braekken, A. Skjølberg, O.-E. Olsen, and R. Bahr, "Prevention of noncontact anterior cruciate ligament injuries in elite and adolescent female team handball athletes," *Instructional Course Lectures*, vol. 56, pp. 407–418, 2007.

[20] O.-E. E. Olsen, G. Myklebust, L. Engebretsen, I. Holme, and R. Bahr, "Exercises to prevent lower limb injuries in youth sports: cluster randomised controlled trial," *The British Medical Journal*, vol. 330, no. 7489, pp. 449–452, 2005.

[21] T. Soligard, G. Myklebust, K. Steffen et al., "F-MARC 11+: a complete warm-up programme to prevent injuries in youth female football," *British Journal of Sports Medicine*, vol. 42, article 496, 2008.

[22] D. C. M. Collard, M. J. M. Chinapaw, E. A. L. M. Verhagen, I. Bakker, and W. van Mechelen, "Effectiveness of a school-based physical activity-related injury prevention program on risk behavior and neuromotor fitness a cluster randomized controlled trial," *International Journal of Behavioral Nutrition and Physical Activity*, vol. 7, article 9, 2010.

19

Graded Exercise Testing Protocols for the Determination of VO_2max: Historical Perspectives, Progress, and Future Considerations

Nicholas M. Beltz,[1] Ann L. Gibson,[1] Jeffrey M. Janot,[2] Len Kravitz,[1] Christine M. Mermier,[1] and Lance C. Dalleck[3]

[1]*Health, Exercise & Sports Sciences Department, University of New Mexico, Albuquerque, NM, USA*
[2]*Department of Kinesiology, University of Wisconsin-Eau Claire, Eau Claire, WI, USA*
[3]*Recreation, Exercise & Sports Science Department, Western State Colorado University, Gunnison, CO, USA*

Correspondence should be addressed to Nicholas M. Beltz; nbeltz@unm.edu

Academic Editor: Andrew Bosch

Graded exercise testing (GXT) is the most widely used assessment to examine the dynamic relationship between exercise and integrated physiological systems. The information from GXT can be applied across the spectrum of sport performance, occupational safety screening, research, and clinical diagnostics. The suitability of GXT to determine a valid maximal oxygen consumption (VO_2max) has been under investigation for decades. Although a set of recommended criteria exists to verify attainment of VO_2max, the methods that originally established these criteria have been scrutinized. Many studies do not apply identical criteria or fail to consider individual variability in physiological responses. As an alternative to using traditional criteria, recent research efforts have been directed toward using a supramaximal verification protocol performed after a GXT to confirm attainment of VO_2max. Furthermore, the emergence of self-paced protocols has provided a simple, yet reliable approach to designing and administering GXT. In order to develop a standardized GXT protocol, additional research should further examine the utility of self-paced protocols used in conjunction with verification protocols to elicit and confirm attainment of VO_2max.

1. Brief History of Graded Exercise Testing

The examination of the dynamic human physiological responses during incremental exercise has been an ever-evolving task for nearly 200 years. Beginning as early as the 18th century and continuing through the 19th century, pioneering physiologists such as Antoine Lavoisier and Nathan Zuntz have been credited with the first scientific examinations involving exercising humans under normal and hypoxic conditions. In 1918, Lambert described the use of a series of exercise tests to examine the impact on blood pressure to establish a reliable index of myocardial efficiency [1]. Inspired by Lambert and the foundational works of Francis Benedict, Goran Liljestrand, and August Krogh, British physiologist Archibald Vivian (A. V.) Hill conducted a fundamental series of experiments that remain the genesis of exercise physiology as an academic discipline [2]. Using Douglas bags to collect expired air samples, Haldane gas analyzers to determine fractional concentrations of oxygen and carbon dioxide, and a Tissot gasometer to measure air volumes, Hill and colleagues [3–6] repeated running trials of increasing speeds to plot the relationship between intensity and oxygen uptake (VO_2). Interestingly, it was concluded that a “ceiling” or upper limit in the maximal uptake of oxygen (VO_2max) existed [7]. It must be appreciated that a difference exists between VO_2peak and VO_2max and that these terms are often used interchangeably in the literature. That is, VO_2peak is the highest value attained during exercise and represents an individual’s exercise tolerance while VO_2max represents the highest physiologically attainable value [8]. Interestingly, a VO_2max is always a peak but a VO_2peak is not always maximal. The difference between VO_2peak and VO_2max is often determined by the presence of a VO_2 "plateau," although the plateau depends on many protocol variables. This review will further expound on this point. Hill's experiments and a century of observations before him led to the discovery of graded exercise testing (GXT), the gold standard for quantifying cardiorespiratory fitness (CRF) and measuring VO_2 during incremental to maximal exercise.

2. Applications of GXT

Graded exercise testing is used to observe the dynamic relationship between exercise workload and the integrated cardiovascular, pulmonary, musculoskeletal, and neuropsychological systems [9]. Protocols require a systematic and linear increase in exercise intensity over time until the individual is unable to maintain or tolerate the workload. Selected cardiovascular, pulmonary, and metabolic variables are collected during the test to evaluate exercise tolerance and represent the efficiency in which the cardiovascular system is able to deliver oxygenated blood to working skeletal muscle and the ability of muscle to utilize oxygen. Due to the widespread use of GXT in healthy populations, normative criteria have been established to help practitioners identify metabolic and ventilatory patterns. Moreover, these metabolic and ventilatory patterns may even assist in categorizing cardiovascular disease (CVD) states and prognoses [9].

The assessment of exercise tolerance has been used to establish the relationship between CRF, CVD, and all-cause mortality [10]. An early investigation by Blair et al. [10] examined the relationship between fitness and mortality in 32,421 men and women (20–80 years old) encompassing 264,978 living-years and 690 deaths. Their results were in agreement with a previous investigation [11] that found substantial strength and independence of low CRF as a predictor for all-cause mortality and future CVD. Similarly, a meta-analysis by Kodama et al. [12] showed that a 1-MET ($3.5\ mL{\cdot}kg^{-1}{\cdot}min^{-1}$) increase in VO_2max was associated with a 13% and 15% reduction in risk of all-cause mortality and CVD, respectively. Furthermore, a threshold to classify a substantially higher risk for all-cause mortality and CVD was established as low CRF (<7.9 METS) [12]. The evidence clearly demonstrates the influence of low CRF as an independent precursor to mortality and underpins the application of standardized protocols to monitor VO_2max in specific populations. These studies highlight the importance of accurate and reliable GXT results for minimal exercise tolerance and clinical evaluation of health status [10–12]. Furthermore, valid GXT results are relevant when interpreting studies using repeated measurements of VO_2max (and not VO_2peak) to establish a training effect or design exercise prescription.

Accurately capturing the dynamic physiological responses during GXT is essential to establish a valid VO_2max and to quantify CRF responses throughout various training interventions. Many independent factors contribute to the varying opinions surrounding the appropriateness of current standardized GXT guidelines, thereby limiting the ability to compare results between tests and population or apply them. The modes for administering GXT are traditionally limited to cycle and treadmill, each resulting in unique physiological responses. Protocol design variables such as stage length, workload increment per stage, and total test duration may individually limit the accuracy of GXT. Furthermore, the criteria used to confirm attainment of VO_2 plateau are not consistent or universally applied among studies. This review will examine the limitations within the current recommendations for GXT and highlight the importance of the continuous search for identifying an optimal protocol.

3. Applications of the Fick Equation

The importance of seminal works by Hill et al. [4–6] is apparent considering that the fundamental basis for quantifying oxygen transport, utilization, and mitochondrial energy production remain the same today as they did nearly 100 years ago. The Fick equation states that VO_2 is equal to the product of cardiac output (Q) and the difference between arterial and venous oxygen content at the level of the capillary (a-vO_{2diff}).

$$VO_2\left(mL{\cdot}kg^{-1}{\cdot}min^{-1}\right) = Q\left(L{\cdot}min^{-1}\right) \times (\text{a-}vO_{2diff})\left(mL{\cdot}L^{-1}\right). \tag{1}$$

The equation can be expanded to represent Q as the product of heart rate (HR) and left ventricular (LV) stroke volume (SV), with SV being parsed into the difference between LV end-diastolic volume (EDV) and end-systolic volume (ESV).

$$VO_2\left(mL{\cdot}kg^{-1}{\cdot}min^{-1}\right) = HR\left(b{\cdot}min^{-1}\right) \cdot \left(EDV\left(mL{\cdot}b^{-1}\right) - ESV\left(mL{\cdot}b^{-1}\right)\right)(\text{a-}vO_{2diff}) \cdot \left(mL{\cdot}L^{-1}\right). \tag{2}$$

Altogether, the components of Fick represent individual central (Q) and peripheral (a-vO_{2diff}) factors. The central component consists of factors that impact the diffusion of O_2 from the external environment into the arterial blood supply and transport of oxygenated blood to working skeletal muscle tissue. The peripheral component comprises various cellular and molecular mechanisms at the skeletal muscle level to diffuse O_2 from arterial blood to the mitochondria for consumption in the process of ATP regeneration [13].

3.1. Q Implications of the VO_2max Protocol. It has been well established that Q increases at a linear rate similar to VO_2 upon the initiation of incremental to maximal exercise [14–18]. In response to metabolically induced peripheral vasodilation in working skeletal muscle, blood pressure is maintained by increases in HR and SV [16]. Central medullary control of baroreceptors, chemoreceptors, and vascular tone contributes to the withdrawal of parasympathetic activity coupled with an increase in sympathetic drive. The result is an overall increase in chronotropic and inotropic characteristics of the heart.

Generally, HR increases linearly during incremental to maximal exercise; however, a breaking point (i.e., HR threshold) is eventually obtained after which the slope may increase or decrease until maximal heart rate (HRmax). The HR threshold is an individual phenomenon that may indicate chronotropic insufficiency [19]. Moreover, the significance of the flattened HR response following HR threshold, in particular, may be associated with a downregulation in beta-1 adrenergic receptor activation during greater exercise intensities. For instance, a study by Knight-Maloney et al. [19] examined HR responses during incremental to maximal exercise in 14 healthy individuals and found that eight subjects demonstrated a decelerated post-HR threshold response while six subjects showed an accelerated post-HR threshold response. These findings are in agreement with previous research that demonstrated the intersubject variability in HR responses [20–24].

Alongside the increasing inotropic response, shifts in sympathetic nervous system dominance raise chronotropic activity and influence central mechanical changes during incremental to maximal exercise. Neural drive enhances myocardial contractility, reducing ESV. Additionally, the intramuscular oscillations during exercise promote an increase in venous return to the heart. The improved blood flow to the LV enhances preload and promotes LV myocardial stretch, increasing elastic potential energy for additional contractile force. This is known as the Frank-Starling mechanism [25]. The net effect is an increase in SV, contributing to an increase in Q during incremental to maximal exercise. Contrary to traditional thought, SV within a healthy population may exhibit individual linear or plateau responses that are dependent on many factors.

Pioneering work by Astrand et al. [26] evaluating the SV response to incremental to maximal exercise established the widely accepted observation that SV plateaus are at approximately 40–50% of VO_2max [27, 28]. This finding was primarily attributed to tachycardiac limitations on diastolic filling time, therefore reducing EDV and blunting SV response [29]. More recently, a review by Vella and Robergs [30] underscores that the potential determinants of the intersubject variability in SV are more complex than originally established. Factors such as age, fitness level, and sex contribute to four main SV responses: the classic plateau, plateau with subsequent drop, plateau with subsequent rise, and gradual increase. While some studies have reported linear SV responses during incremental to maximal exercise in older individuals [31, 32] other studies showed that SV exhibited either a plateau or a subsequent drop at nonspecific points during incremental to maximal exercise [18, 33–35]. Although it may be logical to suggest that age has a negative impact on the maintenance of SV near maximal exercise due to reductions in myocardial compliance, the overall relationship between age and SV response remains unclear. Similarly, individual fitness level does not reliably predict the trend in SV during exercise. Some investigations showed a constant increase in SV up to maximal [36–39] and near maximal intensities [40] in trained individuals while others reported a plateau in both trained and untrained subjects [32, 41] and progressive increases until maximal exercise in untrained subjects [42–44]. One could postulate that adaptations consequent to aerobic training enhance SV through combinations of the following: increased blood volume leading to greater EDV, increased LV chamber size, improved LV compliance, greater myocardial contractility, and reduced afterload may explain the individual ability to increase SV progressively through incremental to maximal exercise [30].

3.2. A-vO_{2diff} Implications of the VO_2max Protocol. It has also been accepted that an increase in Q was the sole component of maintaining VO_2 during the onset of exercise due to a potential lag between oxygen demand and venous return [45–47]. This was tested by Casaburi et al. [48], who found that pulmonary artery desaturation occurred as soon as four seconds after the onset of 150-Watt cycle exercise. The results reported by the Casaburi et al. [48] were questioned by De Cort et al. [45] and attributed to immobilized vena caval blood. Compared to Casaburi et al. [48], who measured a-vO_{2diff} upon exercise from rest, De Cort et al. [45] began measurements starting at the first increase in VO_2 after the abrupt increase in cycling intensity from a submaximal level. Although a-vO_{2diff} may improve with aerobic training [49, 50], the cellular mechanisms contributing to oxygen extraction within skeletal muscle also increase at a predictable rate during incremental to maximal exercise. Recent meta-analyses by Montero et al. [51] and Montero and Diaz-Canestro [52] examined the effects of aerobic training on a-vO_{2diff} in untrained or moderately trained healthy young (<40 years old), middle-aged, and/or older (≥40 years old) individuals. These studies concluded that the improvements in VO_2max from 5 to 52 weeks of endurance training were due to linear improvements in Q_{max} but not a-vO_{2diff}. Therefore, the peripheral mechanisms are viewed as a complement to the central mechanisms contributing to VO_2max.

4. VO_2max Protocol Critical Considerations

The foundational study by Taylor et al. [53] demonstrated that the sensitivity and reliability of physiological responses during GXT were limited by subject characteristics and GXT protocol design. In an attempt to investigate this issue, 115 healthy males (18–35 years) completed a wide range of GXT protocols under various conditions of physical stressors (caloric restriction, bed rest, temperature, and illness). It was the first comprehensive study to examine the sensitivity and reliability of VO_2max based on modality, fitness status, illness, environment, gas sampling rate, test duration, and speed/grade increments.

Since then, there has been a search for an optimal standardized protocol suitable for the entire spectrum of fitness abilities and testing goals. The two modalities commonly used in GXT are treadmill and cycle ergometry. While the treadmill appears to be the most widely used modality due to familiarity with upright locomotion and greater muscle mass utilization, cycling protocols present an opportunity to test individuals with coordination or orthopedic limitations. Furthermore, opting to use a cycle ergometer over treadmill may result in a more quantifiable workload (Watts) and provides an opportunity to use a progressive ramp protocol allowing for more reproducible outcomes [9]. However, VO_2max attained using treadmill protocols tend to produce up to 20%

greater VO_2max values when compared to cycle protocols [54, 55]. This difference is attributed to a larger recruitment of exercising skeletal muscle mass, *Q* and a-vO_{2diff}, vascular conductance, and a lower rate of carbohydrate oxidation leading to a less severe development of metabolic acidosis at submaximal intensities [15, 56–60].

Realizing the need to investigate physiological responses to the earliest standardized GXT protocols, Pollock et al. [61] compared cardiopulmonary responses between four widely used treadmill testing protocols in 51 men (22 active, 29 sedentary): Balke [62], Bruce [63], Ellestad [64], and modified Astrand [65]. Each test differed in the method of increasing work rate in a step fashion (either speed or grade). The Balke protocol maintains a constant speed (3.3 mph) but increases grade by 1% each minute. The Bruce protocol increases speed and grade every 3 min. The Ellestad protocol increases speed each stage until the 10th minute upon introduction of a single increase in grade (to 5%) followed by subsequent increases in speed. Finally, the Astrand protocol maintains a constant running speed with increase in grade (2.5%) every 2 min. Pollock et al. [61] observed a similar VO_2max achieved between Balke, Bruce, Ellestad, and Astrand protocols (39.4, 40.0, 40.7, and 41.8 $mL{\cdot}kg^{-1}{\cdot}min^{-1}$, resp.) despite the difference in VO_2 plateau attainment (69%, 69%, 59%, and 80% of participants, resp.). Interestingly, this shows that the individual characteristics of similar protocols do not impact VO_2max but show inconsistencies in plateau. Their finding was one of the first to demonstrate the impact of protocol design characteristics on the attainment of VO_2max and a VO_2 plateau.

Early investigations by Whipp et al. [47] and Davis et al. [66] popularized the use of ramp protocols on electronically braked cycle ergometers. It was proposed that ramp cycle protocols would improve an individual's ability to reach VO_2max because the ramp increased work in a much more continuous fashion when compared to step increases in work rate used in traditional treadmill protocols [67]. Since workload was deliverable in a linear fashion, attention turned to examining the slope of the VO_2-work rate ($\Delta VO_2/\Delta WR$) relationship. Buchfuhrer et al. [67] compared cycle tests of various changes in work rates (15 $W{\cdot}min^{-1}$, 30 $W{\cdot}min^{-1}$, and 60 $W{\cdot}min^{-1}$) and noted that ramping at an intermediate rate (30 $W{\cdot}min^{-1}$) produced the greatest VO_2max values; however, the work rate was dependent on fitness status. In a similar study, Zhang et al. [68] compared multiple work rates (15 $W{\cdot}min^{-1}$, 20 $W{\cdot}min^{-1}$, and 30 $W{\cdot}min^{-1}$) applied in continuous ramp versus step (1 min, 2 min, and 3 min) fashion. Interestingly, no differences were found in aerobic parameters (VO_2max, anaerobic threshold (AT), AT/VO_2max, and $\Delta VO_2/\Delta WR$) between any of the protocols. Furthermore, this study emphasized the importance of work rate increments independent of the stage length used. In contrast, Myers et al. [54] showed that ramp protocols (treadmill and cycle) represented a higher correlation between VO_2 and workload compared to step, thus reducing the error in predicting the metabolic cost at individual workloads. Muscat et al. [55] completed the most comprehensive investigation to date, comparing physiological responses (cardiometabolic function, gas exchange, breathing patterns, pulmonary function, and leg discomfort) between ramp treadmill and ramp cycle protocol matched for work increase (25 W/2 min) in 15 healthy young men. It was concluded that VO_2, VCO_2, respiratory exchange ratio (RER), HR, O_2 pulse, ventilation, and respiratory muscle effort (diaphragm) responses were greater at maximal and submaximal workloads for treadmill compared to cycle exercise; however, the responses in ventilatory equivalents and ventilatory thresholds were similar. Their results suggested that either mode may be applied for purposes of evaluating mode-specific fitness and determining optimal training prescriptions when work rate increases are applied in a ramp fashion.

Similar to protocol mode (cycle versus treadmill), stage length, and work rate increments (ramp versus step), GXT protocol duration should be considered when comparing results. Buchfuhrer et al. [67] utilized 1-minute stage protocols to examine the impact of protocol duration on the achievement of VO_2max. Since VO_2max values were greater in protocols lasting between 8 and 17 min compared to tests outside these limits, the current duration recommendation of 8–12 min was established [67]. More recently, Yoon et al. [69] suggested that the Buchfuhrer et al. [67] study lacked appropriate statistical power and commented that overall test duration (5–14 min) may depend on age and training status [70–72]. Yoon et al. [69] compared VO_2max and incidence of VO_2 plateau across four protocols of different durations (5, 8, 12, and 16 min) using a cycle ramp protocol in moderate-to-highly trained individuals. They found that VO_2max was higher in men for the 8-minute protocol compared to 5-, 12-, and 16-minute protocols, while there was no difference in VO_2max in women. Further statistical analysis attributed this sex difference to lower fitness levels and perhaps more importantly the lower muscle mass (~45 kg in women versus ~67 kg in men) in women participating in the study. The impact of fitness level on test duration suggests that the steeper $\Delta VO_2/\Delta WR$ slope in shorter protocols may be disadvantageous to individuals of lower fitness. This could be due to increased reliance on nonmitochondrial energy systems, thus causing premature fatigue, as well as eliciting central cardiovascular limitations.

5. VO_2max Protocol Paradigm Shift

For the past 60 years the push to standardize GXT procedures has been essential to progress understanding of the complex and sensitive interaction between exercise and the integrated human physiological responses. In spite of the advancements that have given test administrators the ability to control fixed increments of intensities in an open-loop fashion (constant administrator testing variable manipulation without a fixed termination time), recent research has introduced an alternative approach to exercise protocols that allow the subject to self-pace the protocol in an incremental format [73–75]. In effect, this type of protocol would not negate past research that emphasized the role of the heart, lungs, circulatory, and other integrated systems in a limiting capacity but rather challenge the role of the brain as a potential simultaneous regulator. Although not entirely self-paced, studies by Pollock et al. [61, 76] used a model where speed was adjusted to accommodate individual movement efficiency and workload was increased by adding treadmill grade. In an effort to appreciate the evolution of self-paced protocols, the Pollock et al. [61, 76] investigations underscore the importance of identifying movement speeds that engage the greatest amount of muscle mass. Hagerman [77] was the first to report the ability of an individual to reach a greater VO_2 by self-pacing during a simulated competitive time trial compared to laboratory-based testing methods. The finding suggested that an individual's ability to self-regulate muscular power output may serve as the ultimate variable in maximizing physiologic responses. Intrigued by this finding, Foster et al. [78] compared the physiological responses between a self-paced laboratory 5-km cycle time trial and a GXT using a cycle ergometer. They found that maximal VO_2, HR, ventilation, and blood lactate (BLa^-) levels were significantly greater in the 5-km time trial compared to the cycle ergometer GXT. These initial findings raised an important fundamental question regarding exercise testing protocols: if an individual possesses the ability to achieve a greater physiological ceiling when self-paced, does the search for achieving standardized protocol procedures serve a pragmatic purpose?

Eston and Thompson [73] used a closed-loop (no constant administrator manipulation and a fixed termination time) perceptually-regulated protocol guided by the 6–20 Rating of Perceived Exertion Scale (RPE) [79] to estimate maximal work rate in patients receiving β-blocker treatment. Using 4 × 3 min stages at an RPE of 9 ("very light"), 13 ("somewhat hard"), 15 ("hard"), and 17 ("very hard"), they reported that RPE could be used to predict maximal functional capacity. Similar RPE protocols using various stage lengths (2, 3, and 4 min) have been validated to accurately predict VO_2max [74, 80–83]. Using a similar perceptually regulated paradigm, Mauger and Sculthorpe [75] investigated a self-paced cycle exercise protocol in 16 untrained university students. The test design consisted of 5 × 2-minute stages, totaling 10 min, at incremental intensities utilizing Borg's Rating of Perceived Exertion (RPE_{6-20}) Scale [79]. The protocol was designed as follows: stage one was clamped at an RPE of 11 ("fairly light"), stage two clamped at an RPE of 13 ("somewhat hard"), stage three clamped at an RPE of 15 ("hard"), stage four clamped at an RPE of 17 ("very hard"), and the final stage clamped at an RPE of 20 ("maximal exertion"). The unique aspect of the protocol was the additional stage of "maximal exertion" (RPE 20) to the established series of 2 min RPE-clamped stages as applied previously [80] in order to directly measure VO_2max. The participants achieved a significantly greater VO_2max (40 ± 10 versus 37 ± 8 mL·kg^{-1}·min^{-1}) and peak power output (273 ± 58 versus 238 ± 55 Watts) in the self-paced protocol compared to a traditional GXT despite the absence of significant differences in HRmax, RERmax, VEmax, and mean power output. It is important to note that the results of Mauger and Sculthorpe [75] have received considerable criticism over methodology. Their results have been attributed to discrepancies in test duration between self-paced (10 ± 0 min) and traditional (13 ± 3 min) protocols and that direct GXT protocol comparison must require a match in total test duration [84, 85]. Interestingly, the closed-loop nature of the test elicited a motivation or "final push" during the final stage of the test similar to that expected toward the end of an athletic competition. Moreover, the results support the role of the brain during a closed-loop setting when the individual is able to vary work rate constantly, balancing discomfort with a maintainable power output and willingness to complete the test. The simplicity of the protocol design has produced many speculative explanations for the results. Mauger et al. [86] showed that a speed-based self-paced treadmill test elicited significantly greater VO_2max and HRmax values compared to those relative to a traditional test. This study also received criticisms over flawed methods and lack of control, attributing findings to using different modes (motorized versus nonmotorized treadmill) and neglect of measurement error to test their hypothesis [83, 87–89]. Follow-up studies have shown a higher VO_2max attainment during self-pacing using a cycle ramp protocol [90], similar VO_2max attainment using motorized treadmill [83, 91–93] and cycle protocols [84, 94], and a lower VO_2max attainment using an automated treadmill [89]. It is important to note that findings showing no difference between self-paced and traditional protocols demonstrate the potential utility for self-paced GXT protocols, particularly when considering protocol duration. While test duration is tightly controlled during self-paced testing and the incremental steps in oxygen cost between stages have been shown to fall within recommended guidelines (1-2 METS) [95], physiological measurements that may distinguish self-paced from traditional protocols have yet to be adequately examined. It is purported that underlying variables that comprise the Fick equation, namely, Q and a-vO_{2diff}, and the role of blood flow redistribution may underpin differences between self-paced and traditional protocols [92, 93]. More recently, Astorino et al. [90] showed that a self-paced cycle protocol elicited higher VO_2 compared to a ramp protocol (50.2 ± 9.6 versus 47.2 ± 10.2 mL·kg^{-1}·min^{-1}). Additionally, they were the first to compare central cardiovascular responses between protocols and showed a higher Q_{max} during self-paced compared to ramp (21.9 ± 3.7 versus 20.7 ± 3.4 L·min^{-1}). It should be noted that their average test duration was not tightly controlled to 10 min (9.6 ± 0.8 min); therefore pacing was not restricted throughout the final 2-minute stage. Although initial results are intriguing, the investigation into the efficacy and suitability of self-paced protocols is in its infancy. Therefore, future researchers could choose to design studies to expound on the intertrial reliability using self-pacing protocols. Additionally, studies should examine the interaction between central, peripheral, and central regulating responses during self-paced exercise.

6. VO_2max Attainment Criteria

In order to increase the reliability and validity of a test, an undefined combination of standardized criteria must be met during the GXT including the following: VO_2 plateau, estimated HRmax, RER, BLa^-, and RPE. This widely accepted set of characteristics, or VO_2max criteria, has become a controversial topic of debate in recent years due to the high intersubject variability in attaining the criteria [96–99]. Furthermore, the number and type of criteria used to determine VO_2max are often contingent on the preference of the researcher or clinician administering the test [96]. Along with protocol design, other factors such as metabolic data processing methods and participant effort make comparing the results for clinical or research purposes difficult [53, 99, 100].

7. Detection of a VO_2 Plateau

As with many of the principles used today in exercise physiology, the original reports of a slowing or "plateau" of oxygen consumption despite increasing muscular work can be attributed to Bassett Jr. and Howley [101]. Taylor et al. [53] later confirmed the existence of a VO_2 plateau in 9 of 13 men during a treadmill test of incremental speed (increasing 1 mph) and 108 of 115 (94%) men during treadmill tests of incremental grade (2.5%). Studies have since demonstrated that a VO_2 plateau can be detected in 17% to 100% of subjects tested, suggesting that its existence represents an inconsistent "phenomenon" [100]. Taylor et al. [53] were the first to apply the VO_2 plateau criterion of $\leq$150 mL·min^{-1}, defined by a change in VO_2 $\leq$150 mL·min^{-1} despite a continuous increase in workload. This value, alongside the wide range of other values used as plateau criteria ($\leq$50 mL·min^{-1}, $\leq$100 mL·min^{-1}, $\leq$200 mL·min^{-1}, and $\leq$280 mL·min^{-1}), should not be applied universally since the criteria must reflect the expected rate of VO_2 increase per unit time relative to the protocol design [102]. Among the most important factors impacting the incidence of a VO_2 plateau are age [103], testing modality [104], and data analyses methodology [99, 105]. Astorino et al. [103] showed that the strongest predictor of VO_2 plateau among 30 men and women consisting of groups of endurance-trained (n = 9), recreationally active (n = 11), and strength trained (n = 10) individuals was age, not training status, body composition, or training history. Gordon et al. [104] demonstrated that treadmill testing (58%) was superior to cycle ergometer testing (8%) at eliciting a plateau. The diminished plateau in cycling was attributed to the increased metabolic cost of the eccentric skeletal muscle activity in treadmill running compared to the concentrically dominant cycle exercise. Furthermore, Astorino [105] confirmed that gas sampling rate impacted the incidence of a plateau. In this study, 13 sedentary, 48 recreationally active, and 47 competitive athletes completed a GXT using treadmill and cycle protocols. The group found that the incidence of plateau was greater using breath-by-breath (81%), 15-sec (91%), and 30-sec (89%) averaging compared to a longer sampling rate of 60-sec (59%). Collectively, these findings suggest that sampling rate in conjunction with the plateau threshold criteria may explain much of the discrepancy in incidence of VO_2 plateau across studies.

7.1. Heart Rate Response to the VO_2max Protocol. Due to its noninvasive nature, simplicity, and fairly predictable response to incremental to maximal exercise, HR is often used as a secondary criterion to VO_2 plateau. Much like plateau and other secondary criteria, the criteria for HR are highly variable. Typically, the threshold is established at a specific percentage using an age-predicted HRmax equation. Surprisingly, Fox et al. [106] created the 220-age equation by drawing an arbitrary best fit line from the observation of 10 studies [106]. Robergs and Landwehr [107] evaluated the Fox equation [106] and highlighted the fact that there were no statistical methods used to establish the regression equation from their data set. Instead, Fox and colleagues [106] summarize their methods by stating that "no single line will adequately represent the data on the apparent decline of HRmax with age. The formula, 220-age, defines a line not far from many data points." Curious to investigate the mystery of 220-age, Robergs and Landwehr [107] replicated the data set presented by Fox et al. [106], applied linear regression analysis, and found the equation to be 215.4–0.9147 (age) with a ±21 bpm error. Tanaka et al. [108] cross-validated an age-predicted HRmax equation by combining 351 studies (18,712 subjects) and a laboratory investigation using 514 subjects (18–81 years old). Their regression analysis established a new equation (208 $-$ 0.7 $\times$ age) with a less, yet still substantial (±7–11 bpm), error range. It was concluded that the 220-age equation underestimates age-predicted HRmax in individuals over the age of 40 years. For these reasons, equations with less inherent error should be applied when using "±10 bpm of age-predicted HRmax" as a secondary VO_2max criterion.

7.2. RER Implication of the VO_2max Protocol. The RER is another secondary VO_2max criterion that is used to reflect the balance between bicarbonate buffering and hydrogen ion accumulation in the face of incremental exercise. Upon increasing metabolic acidosis, bicarbonate buffering leads to an increase in CO_2 production, increased ventilation, and a subsequent increase in RER. A series of studies by Issekutz et al. [109, 110] was the first to examine the relationship between RER and incremental exercise, VO_2max, and the metabolic state of the exercising human. Using a series of 4-5 min intermittent maximal exercise tests, they calculated the difference between CO_2 and the product of a metabolic respiratory quotient constant and VO_2 ($CO_2 - VO_2 \times 0.75$). This value was termed "excess CO_2" and used to reflect the change in substrate utilization and exercise intensity with the increase in VO_2 [109, 110]. Ultimately, they established the most widely used threshold for RER criteria ($\geq$1.15) today. Much like HR and VO_2plateau criteria, a standard RER threshold value is not consistently applied, using 1.0, 1.05, 1.08, 1.10, 1.12, 1.13, or 1.20 to verify VO_2max attainment [96, 97]. The high intersubject variability in RER responses due to inconsistent effort levels and training status makes higher RER values difficult to achieve for many individuals [97].

7.3. VO_2max and Blood Lactate Accumulation. Analysis of postexercise BLa^- compared to preexercise BLa^- has been used as a reliable marker to quantify exercise intensity. Hill et al. [4–6] were the first to establish a relationship between BLa^- and exercise intensity during vigorous to maximal exercise. Regardless of the debate for practical application or metabolic circumstances, it is agreed that BLa^- accumulation is related to an individual's ability to tolerate and sustain exercise; therefore, it is commonly used as a surrogate measure of the metabolic perturbations during maximal exercise and a secondary VO_2max criterion [111, 112]. The origins of the criterion date back to an investigation by Astrand [113] who used postexercise BLa^- concentrations to verify VO_2max in young (14–18 years) boys and girls. Despite the fact that only half of the subjects demonstrated a VO_2 plateau, it was noted that the individuals who exhibited a plateau had postexercise BLa^- concentrations between 7.9 and 8.4 mM (average ≥ 8 mM). It has since been determined that factors such as age, training status, sex, and overall effort may impact the level of BLa^-. This has led to the use of a ≥10 mM threshold or even a complete disregard for maximal BLa^- concentration due to the high intersubject variability (anywhere from 1.2 to 18 mM) in postexercise lactate [96, 98, 114].

7.4. RPE Assessment in a VO_2max Protocol. The simplest and most controversial measurement traditionally used as a VO_2max criterion was developed by Borg [79], known as Borg's Rating of Perceived Exertion (RPE) Scale_{6-20}. While RPE is not a direct measurement of physiological responses, the behavioral, motivational, and physical factors that an individual perceives during GXT contribute greatly to the overall validity of the test. Many studies have shown a strong relationship between RPE, HR, and VO_2 [82, 115–117]; however, others have demonstrated RPE to be less related to these variables in less active or sedentary individuals [118, 119]. Interestingly, Noakes [120] suggested that thresholds may not be as simple as limitations in central and peripheral components but rather controlled by a "central governor" that regulates self-pacing and overall effort throughout various points of a maximal exercise bout. Despite the relationship among RPE, HR, and BLa^-, inconsistencies in recent studies call to question the validity of RPE. Edvardsen et al. [114] examined the attainment of the commonly used RPE criterion of ≥17 in 840 individuals (20–85 years) and found that 84% of the subjects were able to achieve the criterion. Due to the variability and subjective nature of the criterion, Magnan et al. [121] examined the attainment of an RPE ≥18 in 240 inactive individuals (18–45 years) and found that 93.7% of the individuals reached the desired RPE threshold despite the fact that only 59% were demonstrating a VO_2 plateau. Overall, the assumptions in employing an RPE criterion depend on the subject's understanding of the scale and associated verbal descriptors, ability to differentiate between discomfort and physiological fatigue, and motivation.

8. Verification Protocols of VO_2max

Many of the current criteria used to determine VO_2max were established with technology that is no longer used today. Douglas bags and Tissot gasometers have been replaced by sophisticated metabolic analyzing systems and pneumotach and turbine flow measurement devices. Furthermore, the VO_2max criteria were developed using certain modalities (treadmill versus cycle) on relatively small samples of homogenous populations. These reasons and the overall variability of the criteria have resulted in some researchers rejecting secondary criteria altogether. Recent attempts have been made to establish new VO_2max attainment criteria through the introduction of a verification protocol [97, 122–126]. The origin of the verification protocol is believed to exist in a text by Thoden et al. [127], in which the first recommendation was made to include a bout of supramaximal exhaustive exercise (higher workload than achieved during GXT) following the completion of GXT. Since the inception of the verification protocol, there has been much effort to establish verification protocol intensity, duration, rest period after completing initial GXT, and the criteria used to verify VO_2max attainment. In follow-up guidelines, Thoden [128] recommended that the recovery phase between GXT and verification protocol should be between 5 and 15 minutes and a workload of one stage higher than the final completed stage during GXT should be used. Unfortunately, the recommendations by Thoden et al. [127, 128] were theoretical rather than research-based guidelines. The first study to directly examine the efficacy of a verification protocol was done by NiemelÄ et al. [129], who performed a verification protocol at a workload equal to the greatest workload achieved during initial GXT within a week of completing initial GXT. Using a ±5% repeatability range for VO_2max [130], they were able to confirm attainment in 8 of the 16 subjects. Day et al. [8] sought to observe the differences between cycle GXT and a subsequent verification test in 38 healthy individuals (19–61 years) and reported no difference in VO_2max using a workload of ~90% W_{peak}. Follow-up studies commonly used verification workloads between 95 and 130% of peak workload achieved during initial cycle GXT or 0.5–1.6 km·hr^{-1} higher than the peak velocity achieved during initial treadmill GXT. The recovery time between tests ranged from the same day [122, 126, 131–134], 1–10 min active rest [122, 132, 133, 135], and 5–60 min passive rest [125, 135], to separate day testing [8, 123, 126]. Furthermore, tests were done on endurance-trained runners [122, 123], male athletes [135], recreationally active men and women [122, 125, 126], sedentary men and women [105], and middle-aged men and women [131]. Studies commonly revealed a nonsignificant mean difference in VO_2max between GXT and verification protocols when analyzed on an individual, rather than group mean, basis within the ±5% measurement error (accuracy of metabolic system when properly calibrated according to manufacturer) associated with VO_2 measurement [136–138]. Most recently, a study by Nolan et al. [125] investigated the impact of two verification intensities and rest periods. After an initial treadmill test, 12 active males and females completed each of the following four verification conditions: 105% maximal GXT workload, 20 min rest; 105% maximal GXT workload, 60 min rest; 115% maximal GXT workload, 20 min rest; and 115% maximal GXT workload, 60 min rest. Their results demonstrated a 100% success rate in verifying attainment of VO_2max when using 105% maximal GXT workload, regardless of the rest period between tests, and highlighted the current recommendation for intensity and rest period optimization during verification tests [125].

9. Error in VO_2max Measurement

The sophisticated metabolic systems used to collect and analyze data during exercise testing represent the most sensitive and reliable means for laboratory-based research. In order to compare results between studies, the data must be validated. Even if metabolic systems are appropriately maintained and calibrated, measurement error of ±5% is commonly accepted [136–138]. A study by Yule et al. [139] reported a 15% difference in VO_2max between three identical systems in the same laboratory. Furthermore, differences attributed to measurement error between 10 and 22% have been reported when comparing identical testing protocols using different metabolic systems [137]. A meta-analysis by Vickers [140] examined the test-retest reliability in maximal exercise testing and found that the average standard measurement error was 2.58 $mL{\cdot}kg^{-1}{\cdot}min^{-1}$. To account for total error, however, a source of biovariation reflecting the inherent biological fluctuations within an individual must also be considered [141]. Knowing that the underlying assumption for comparing VO_2max between and within studies is that biological variability must account for a portion of total error, Katch et al. [141] designed a study in which five participants completed an average of 16 maximal exercise tests over the course of a 2–4-week period. They found that, within the total error of ±5.6%, biological variability accounted for ~93% of the error while measurement error accounted for only ~7%. Meanwhile, recommendations by Balady et al. [138] report that the biological component of variability intrinsic to GXT is commonly accepted within 3-4%. Due to the numerous factors that contribute to biological variability and subsequent total error, an argument can be made against studies that consider only manufacturers' guidelines of measurement error when comparing tests [142]. This can be represented by a scenario comparing VO_2 responses to various protocol designs, whereas an individual who falls within the accepted measurement error range between tests may have only done so based on the small contribution in variance from the system rather than the large contribution from biological variability due to heredity, homeostatic stress, training status, psychological stress, sleep, or nutrition [143]. For this reason, comparing attainment of VO_2max between protocols may be more reliable when considering total error (biological variability + measurement) rather than measurement error alone.

10. Conclusion

Due to the valuable information gathered and the wide spectrum of applications for the use of GXT, it has become an increasingly important objective to derive an optimal set of standardized procedures for the determination of VO_2max. Many years of observations examining the potential sources for individual variability in GXT responses are cited in the literature. Despite the pitfalls in physiological variability, standardized tests using traditional methods for VO_2max verification remain the most commonly employed. Furthermore, the methods in which these criteria have been previously established, as well as the comparison between studies evaluating the appropriateness of universal protocols, do not consider combined sources of inherent measurement and biological error. These reasons underpin the current suitability of more standardized GXT guidelines and subsequent methods for determining test validity. More recent approaches have highlighted alternative methods for measuring exercise capacity using a closed-loop, self-paced testing model. Future research directions should seek investigating perceptually regulated (RPE-clamped) protocols with verification protocols for the overall suitability and individualization of GXT.

Competing Interests

The authors declare that they have no competing interests.

References

[1] G. Lambert, "The exercise blood pressure test of myocardial efficiency," *BMJ*, vol. 2, no. 3014, pp. 366–368, 1918.

[2] C. M. Tipton, *History of Exercise Physiology*, Human Kinetics, 2014.

[3] A. V. Hill and H. Lupton, "The oxygen consumption during running," *The Journal of Physiology*, vol. 56, pp. 32–33, 1922.

[4] A. V. Hill, C. N. H. Long, and H. Lupton, "Muscular exercise, lactic acid, and the supply and utilisation of oxygen-parts i-iii," *Proceedings of the Royal Society of London B: Biological*, vol. 96, pp. 438–475, 1924.

[5] A. V. Hill, C. Long, and H. Lupton, "Muscular exercise, lactic acid and the supply and utilisation of oxygen—Parts VII-VIII," *Proceedings of the Royal Society of London B: Biological*, vol. 97, pp. 155–176, 1924.

[6] A. V. Hill, C. N. H. Long, and H. Lupton, "Muscular exercise, lactic acid, and the supply and utilisation of oxygen- parts iv-vi," *Proceedings of the Royal Society of London B: Biological*, vol. 97, pp. 84–138, 1924.

[7] D. R. Bassett Jr., "Scientific contributions of A. V. Hill: exercise physiology pioneer," *Journal of Applied Physiology*, vol. 93, no. 5, pp. 1567–1582, 2002.

[8] J. R. Day, H. B. Rossiter, E. M. Coats, A. Skasick, and B. J. Whipp, "The maximally attainable $\dot{V}o_2$ during exercise in humans: the peak vs. maximum issue," *Journal of Applied Physiology*, vol. 95, no. 5, pp. 1901–1907, 2003.

[9] K. Albouaini, M. Egred, A. Alahmar, and D. J. Wright, "Cardiopulmonary exercise testing and its application," *Postgraduate Medical Journal*, vol. 83, no. 985, pp. 675–682, 2007.

[10] S. N. Blair, J. B. Kampert, H. W. Kohl III et al., "Influences of cardiorespiratory fitness and other precursors on cardiovascular disease and all-cause mortality in men and women," *Journal of the American Medical Association*, vol. 276, no. 3, pp. 205–210, 1996.

[11] S. N. Blair, H. W. Kohl III, C. E. Barlow, R. S. Paffenbarger Jr., L. W. Gibbons, and C. A. Macera, "Changes in physical fitness and all-cause mortality: a prospective study of healthy and unhealthy men," *The Journal of the American Medical Association*, vol. 273, no. 14, pp. 1093–1098, 1995.

[12] S. Kodama, K. Saito, S. Tanaka et al., "Cardiorespiratory fitness as a quantitative predictor of all-cause mortality and cardiovascular events in healthy men and women: a meta-analysis," *Journal of the American Medical Association*, vol. 301, no. 19, pp. 2024–2035, 2009.

[13] B. D. Levine, "VO2max: what do we know, and what do we still need to know?" *The Journal of Physiology*, vol. 586, no. 1, pp. 25–34, 2008.

[14] A. Crisafulli, F. Melis, F. Tocco et al., "Anaerobic threshold and the oxygen consumption-cardiac output relationship during exercise," *Sport Sciences for Health*, vol. 1, no. 2, pp. 75–80, 2005.

[15] J. A. Faulkner, D. E. Roberts, R. L. Elk, and J. Conway, "Cardiovascular responses to submaximum and maximum effort cycling and running," *Journal of applied physiology*, vol. 30, no. 4, pp. 457–461, 1971.

[16] S. F. Lewis, W. F. Taylor, R. M. Graham, W. A. Pettinger, J. E. Schutte, and C. G. Blomqvist, "Cardiovascular responses to exercise as functions of absolute and relative work load," *Journal of Applied Physiology: Respiratory, Environmental and Exercise Physiology*, vol. 54, no. 5, pp. 1314–1323, 1983.

[17] W. W. Stringer, J. E. Hansen, and K. Wasserman, "Cardiac output estimated noninvasively from oxygen uptake during exercise," *Journal of Applied Physiology*, vol. 82, no. 3, pp. 908–912, 1997.

[18] D. N. Proctor, K. C. Beck, P. H. Shen, T. J. Eickhoff, and M. J. Halliwill Joyner Jr., "Influence of age and gender on cardiac output-VO2 relationships during submaximal cycle ergometry," *Journal of Applied Physiology*, vol. 84, no. 2, pp. 599–605, 1998.

[19] M. Knight-Maloney, R. A. Robergs, A. Gibson, and F. Ghiasvand, "Threshold changes in blood lactate, beat-to-cardiovascular function, and breath-by-breath VO2 during incremental exercise," *Journal of Exercise Physiology Online*, vol. 5, no. 3, pp. 39–53, 2002.

[20] V. Bunc, P. Hofmann, H. Leitner, and G. Gaisl, "Verification of the heart rate threshold," *European Journal of Applied Physiology and Occupational Physiology*, vol. 70, no. 3, pp. 263–269, 1995.

[21] F. Conconi, M. Ferrari, P. G. Ziglio, P. Droghetti, and L. Codeca, "Determination of the anaerobic threshold by a noninvasive field test in runners," *Journal of Applied Physiology Respiratory Environmental and Exercise Physiology*, vol. 52, no. 4, pp. 869–873, 1982.

[22] P. Hofmann, R. Pokan, K. Preidler et al., "Relationship between heart rate threshold, lactate turn point and myocardial function," *International Journal of Sports Medicine*, vol. 15, no. 5, pp. 232–237, 1994.

[23] P. Hofmann, R. Pokan, S. P. Von Duvillard, F. J. Seibert, R. Zweiker, and P. Schmid, "Heart rate performance curve during incremental cycle ergometer exercise in healthy young male subjects," *Medicine and Science in Sports and Exercise*, vol. 29, no. 6, pp. 762–768, 1997.

[24] A. M. Jones and J. H. Doust, "Lack of reliability in Conconi's heart rate deflection point," *International Journal of Sports Medicine*, vol. 16, no. 8, pp. 541–544, 1995.

[25] D. G. Allen and J. C. Kentish, "The cellular basis of the length-tension relation in cardiac muscle," *Journal of Molecular and Cellular Cardiology*, vol. 17, no. 9, pp. 821–840, 1985.

[26] P. O. Astrand, T. E. Cuddy, B. Saltin, and J. Stenberg, "Cardiac output during submaximal and maximal work," *Journal of Applied Physiology*, vol. 19, pp. 268–274, 1964.

[27] S. Bevegard, A. Holmgren, and B. Jonsson, "The effect of body position on the circulation at rest and during exercise, with special reference to the influence on the stroke volume," *Acta Physiologica Scandinavica*, vol. 49, pp. 279–298, 1960.

[28] G. Grimby, N. J. Nilsson, and B. Saltin, "Cardiac output during submaximal and maximal exercise in active middle-aged athletes," *Journal of Applied Physiology*, vol. 21, no. 4, pp. 1150–1156, 1966.

[29] D. E. R. Warburton, M. J. Haykowsky, H. A. Quinney, D. Blackmore, K. K. Teo, and D. P. Humen, "Myocardial response to incremental exercise in endurance-trained athletes: influence of heart rate, contractility and the Frank-Starling effect," *Experimental Physiology*, vol. 87, no. 5, pp. 613–622, 2002.

[30] C. A. Vella and R. A. Robergs, "A review of the stroke volume response to upright exercise in healthy subjects," *British Journal of Sports Medicine*, vol. 39, no. 4, pp. 190–195, 2005.

[31] C. G. Wiebe, N. Gledhill, V. K. Jamnik, and S. Ferguson, "Exercise cardiac function in young through elderly endurance trained women," *Medicine and Science in Sports and Exercise*, vol. 31, no. 5, pp. 684–691, 1999.

[32] A. M. Rivera, A. E. Pels III, S. P. Sady, M. A. Sady, E. M. Cullinane, and P. D. Thompson, "Physiological factors associated with the lower maximal oxygen consumption of master runners," *Journal of Applied Physiology*, vol. 66, no. 2, pp. 949–954, 1989.

[33] P. F. McLaren, Y. Nurhayati, and S. H. Boutcher, "Stroke volume response to cycle ergometry in trained and untrained older men," *European Journal of Applied Physiology and Occupational Physiology*, vol. 75, no. 6, pp. 537–542, 1997.

[34] T. Ogawa, R. J. Spina, W. H. Martin III et al., "Effects of aging, sex, and physical training on cardiovascular responses to exercise," *Circulation*, vol. 86, no. 2, pp. 494–503, 1992.

[35] S. D. McCole, M. D. Brown, G. E. Moore, J. M. Zmuda, J. D. Cwynar, and J. M. Hagberg, "Cardiovascular hemodynamics with increasing exercise intensities in postmenopausal women," *Journal of Applied Physiology*, vol. 87, no. 6, pp. 2334–2340, 1999.

[36] N. Gledhill, D. Cox, and R. Jamnik, "Endurance athletes' stroke volume does not plateau: major advantage is diastolic function," *Medicine and Science in Sports and Exercise*, vol. 26, no. 9, pp. 1116–1121, 1994.

[37] B. Zhou, R. K. Conlee, R. Jensen, G. W. Fellingham, J. D. George, and A. G. Fisher, "Stroke volume does not plateau during graded exercise in elite male distance runners," *Medicine and Science in Sports and Exercise*, vol. 33, no. 11, pp. 1849–1854, 2001.

[38] M. H. Crawford, M. A. Petru, and C. Rabinowitz, "Effect of isotonic exercise training on left ventricular volume during upright exercise," *Circulation*, vol. 72, no. 6, pp. 1237–1243, 1985.

[39] S. Ferguson, N. Gledhill, V. K. Jamnik, C. Wiebe, and N. Payne, "Cardiac performance in endurance-trained and moderately active young women," *Medicine and Science in Sports and Exercise*, vol. 33, no. 7, pp. 1114–1119, 2001.

[40] J. H. P. Vanfraechem, "Stroke volume and systolic time interval adjustments during bicycle exercise," *Journal of Applied Physiology Respiratory Environmental and Exercise Physiology*, vol. 46, no. 3, pp. 588–592, 1979.

[41] R. J. Spina, T. Ogawa, W. M. Kohrt, W. H. Martin III, J. O. Holloszy, and A. A. Ehsani, "Differences in cardiovascular adaptations to endurance exercise training between older men and women," *Journal of Applied Physiology*, vol. 75, no. 2, pp. 849–855, 1993.

[42] C. B. Chapman, J. N. Fisher, and B. J. Sproule, "Behavior of stroke volume at rest and during exercise in human beings," *The Journal of Clinical Investigation*, vol. 39, pp. 1208–1213, 1960.

[43] B. Krip, N. Gledhill, V. Jamnik, and D. Warburton, "Effect of alterations in blood volume on cardiac function during maximal exercise," *Medicine and Science in Sports and Exercise*, vol. 29, no. 11, pp. 1469–1476, 1997.

[44] M. Martino, N. Gledhill, and V. Jamnik, "High VO2max with no history of training is primarily due to high blood volume," *Medicine and Science in Sports and Exercise*, vol. 34, no. 6, pp. 966–971, 2002.

[45] S. C. De Cort, J. A. Innes, T. J. Barstow, and A. Guz, "Cardiac output, oxygen consumption and arteriovenous oxygen difference following a sudden rise in exercise level in humans," *The Journal of Physiology*, vol. 441, pp. 501–512, 1991.

[46] K. Wasserman, B. J. Whipp, and J. A. Davis, "Respiratory physiology of exercise: metabolism, gas exchange, and ventilatory control," *International Review of Physiology*, vol. 23, pp. 149–211, 1981.

[47] B. J. Whipp, J. A. Davis, F. Torres, and K. Wasserman, "A test to determine parameters of aerobic function during exercise," *Journal of Applied Physiology Respiratory Environmental and Exercise Physiology*, vol. 50, no. 1, pp. 217–221, 1981.

[48] R. Casaburi, J. Daly, J. E. Hansen, and R. M. Effros, "Abrupt changes in mixed venous blood gas composition after the onset of exercise," *Journal of Applied Physiology*, vol. 67, no. 3, pp. 1106–1112, 1989.

[49] C. G. Blomqvist and B. Saltin, "Cardiovascular adaptations to physical training," *Annual Review of Physiology*, vol. 45, pp. 169–189, 1983.

[50] B. Ekblom, P. O. Astrand, B. Saltin, J. Stenberg, and B. Wallström, "Effect of training on circulatory response to exercise," *Journal of Applied Physiology*, vol. 24, no. 4, pp. 518–528, 1968.

[51] D. Montero, C. Diaz-Canestro, and C. Lundby, "Endurance training and VO2max," *Medicine & Science in Sports & Exercise*, vol. 47, pp. 2024–2033, 2015.

[52] D. Montero and C. Diaz-Canestro, "Endurance training and maximal oxygen consumption with ageing: role of maximal cardiac output and oxygen extraction," *European Journal of Preventive Cardiology*, vol. 23, no. 7, pp. 733–743, 2016.

[53] H. L. Taylor, E. Buskirk, and A. Henschel, "Maximal oxygen intake as an objective measure of cardio-respiratory performance," *Journal of Applied Physiology*, vol. 8, pp. 73–80, 1955.

[54] J. Myers, N. Buchanan, D. Walsh et al., "Comparison of the ramp versus standard exercise protocols," *Journal of the American College of Cardiology*, vol. 17, no. 6, pp. 1334–1342, 1991.

[55] K. M. Muscat, H. G. Kotrach, C. A. Wilkinson-Maitland, M. R. Schaeffer, C. T. Mendonca, and D. Jensen, "Physiological and perceptual responses to incremental exercise testing in healthy men: effect of exercise test modality," *Applied Physiology, Nutrition and Metabolism*, vol. 40, no. 11, pp. 1199–1209, 2015.

[56] L. Hermansen, B. Ekblom, and B. Saltin, "Cardiac output during submaximal and maximal treadmill and bicycle exercise," *Journal of Applied Physiology*, vol. 29, no. 1, pp. 82–86, 1970.

[57] I. Jacobs and B. Sjödin, "Relationship of ergometer-specific VO2 max and muscle enzymes to blood lactate during submaximal exercise," *British Journal of Sports Medicine*, vol. 19, no. 2, pp. 77–80, 1985.

[58] K. Okita, H. Nishijima, K. Yonezawa et al., "Skeletal muscle metabolism in maximal bicycle and treadmill exercise distinguished by using in vivo metabolic freeze method and phosphorus-31 magnetic resonance spectroscopy in normal men," *American Journal of Cardiology*, vol. 81, no. 1, pp. 106–109, 1998.

[59] J. Porszasz, R. Casaburi, A. Somfay, L. J. Woodhouse, and B. J. Whipp, "A treadmill ramp protocol using simultaneous changes in speed and grade," *Medicine & Science in Sports & Exercise*, vol. 35, no. 9, pp. 1596–1603, 2003.

[60] D. A. Tanner, J. W. Duke, and J. M. Stager, "Ventilatory patterns differ between maximal running and cycling," *Respiratory Physiology and Neurobiology*, vol. 191, no. 1, pp. 9–16, 2014.

[61] M. L. Pollock, R. L. Bohannon, K. H. Cooper et al., "A comparative analysis of four protocols for maximal treadmill stress testing," *American Heart Journal*, vol. 92, no. 1, pp. 39–46, 1976.

[62] B. Balke and R. W. Ware, "An experimental study of physical fitness of Air Force personnel," *United States Armed Forces Medical Journal*, vol. 10, no. 6, pp. 675–688, 1959.

[63] R. A. Bruce, J. R. Blackmon, J. W. Jones, and G. Strait, "Exercising testing in adult normal subjects and cardiac patients," *Pediatrics*, vol. 32, pp. 742–756, 1963.

[64] M. H. Ellestad, W. Allen, M. C. Wan, and G. L. Kemp, "Maximal treadmill stress testing for cardiovascular evaluation," *Circulation*, vol. 39, no. 4, pp. 517–522, 1969.

[65] N. C. Dey, A. Samanta, and R. Saha, "The pulse rate and energy expenditure profile of underground coal miners in India," *Mining Technology*, vol. 113, no. 3, pp. 137–141, 2004.

[66] J. A. Davis, B. J. Whipp, N. Lamarra, D. J. Huntsman, M. H. Frank, and K. Wasserman, "Effect of ramp slope on determination of aerobic parameters from the ramp exercise test," *Medicine & Science in Sports & Exercise*, vol. 14, no. 5, pp. 339–343, 1982.

[67] M. J. Buchfuhrer, J. E. Hansen, T. E. Robinson, D. Y. Sue, K. Wasserman, and B. J. Whipp, "Optimizing the exercise protocol for cardiopulmonary assessment," *Journal of Applied Physiology Respiratory Environmental and Exercise Physiology*, vol. 55, no. 5, pp. 1558–1564, 1983.

[68] Y.-Y. Zhang, M. C. Johnson, N. Chow, and K. Wasserman, "Effect of exercise testing protocol on parameters of aerobic function," *Medicine & Science in Sports & Exercise*, vol. 23, no. 5, pp. 625–630, 1991.

[69] B. Yoon, L. Kravitz, and R. Robergs, "VO2max, protocol duration, and the VO2 plateau," *Medicine & Science in Sports & Exercise*, vol. 39, no. 7, pp. 1186–1192, 2007.

[70] T. A. Astorino, J. C. Rietschel, P. A. Tam et al., "Reinvestigation of optimal duration of VO_2max testing," *Journal of Exercise Physiology Online*, vol. 7, no. 6, pp. 1–8, 2004.

[71] P. M. Lepretre, J. P. Koralsztein, and V. L. Billat, "Effect of exercise intensity on relationship between $\dot{V}o_{2max}$ and cardiac output," *Medicine & Science in Sports & Exercise*, vol. 36, no. 8, pp. 1357–1363, 2004.

[72] S. D. McCole, A. M. Davis, and P. T. Fueger, "Is there a disassociation of maximal oxygen consumption and maximal cardiac output?" *Medicine & Science in Sports & Exercise*, vol. 33, no. 8, pp. 1265–1269, 2001.

[73] R. G. Eston and M. Thompson, "Use of ratings of perceived exertion for predicting maximal work rate and prescribing exercise intensity in patients taking atenolol," *British Journal of Sports Medicine*, vol. 31, no. 2, pp. 114–119, 1997.

[74] R. G. Eston, K. L. Lamb, G. Parfitt, and N. King, "The validity of predicting maximal oxygen uptake from a perceptually-regulated graded exercise test," *European Journal of Applied Physiology*, vol. 94, no. 3, pp. 221–227, 2005.

[75] A. R. Mauger and N. Sculthorpe, "A new VO_2max protocol allowing self-pacing in maximal incremental exercise," *British Journal of Sports Medicine*, vol. 46, no. 1, pp. 59–63, 2012.

[76] M. L. Pollock, C. Foster, D. Schmidt, C. Hellman, A. C. Linnerud, and A. Ward, "Comparative analysis of physiologic responses to three different maximal graded exercise test protocols in healthy women," *American Heart Journal*, vol. 103, no. 3, pp. 363–373, 1982.

[77] F. C. Hagerman, "Applied physiology of rowing," *Sports Medicine*, vol. 1, no. 4, pp. 303–326, 1984.

[78] C. Foster, M. A. Green, A. C. Snyder, and N. N. Thompson, "Physiological responses during simulated competition,"

Medicine & Science in Sports & Exercise, vol. 25, no. 7, pp. 877–882, 1993.

[79] G. A. V. Borg, "Psychophysical bases of perceived exertion," *Medicine and Science in Sports and Exercise*, vol. 14, no. 5, pp. 377–381, 1982.

[80] R. G. Eston, J. A. Faulkner, E. A. Mason, and G. Parfitt, "The validity of predicting maximal oxygen uptake from perceptually regulated graded exercise tests of different durations," *European Journal of Applied Physiology*, vol. 97, no. 5, pp. 535–541, 2006.

[81] M. Morris, K. Lamb, D. Cotterrell, and J. Buckley, "Predicting maximal oxygen uptake via a Perceptually Regulated Exercise Test (PRET)," *Journal of Exercise Science and Fitness*, vol. 7, no. 2, pp. 122–128, 2009.

[82] J. B. Coquart, M. Garcin, G. Parfitt, C. Tourny-Chollet, and R. G. Eston, "Prediction of maximal or peak oxygen uptake from ratings of perceived exertion," *Sports Medicine*, vol. 44, no. 5, pp. 563–578, 2014.

[83] N. J. Hanson, C. M. Scheadler, T. L. Lee, N. C. Neuenfeldt, T. J. Michael, and M. G. Miller, "Modality determines $VO_{2\max}$ achieved in self-paced exercise tests: validation with the Bruce protocol," *European Journal of Applied Physiology*, vol. 116, no. 7, pp. 1313–1319, 2016.

[84] W. Chidnok, F. J. DiMenna, S. J. Bailey et al., "VO2max is not altered by self-pacing during incremental exercise," *European Journal of Applied Physiology*, vol. 113, no. 2, pp. 529–539, 2013.

[85] R. Eston, "Use of ratings of perceived exertion in sports," *International Journal of Sports Physiology and Performance*, vol. 7, no. 2, pp. 175–182, 2012.

[86] A. R. Mauger, A. J. Metcalfe, L. Taylor, and P. C. Castle, "The efficacy of the self-paced $\dot{V}O_{2max}$ test to measure maximal oxygen uptake in treadmill running," *Applied Physiology, Nutrition, and Metabolism*, vol. 38, no. 12, pp. 1211–1216, 2013.

[87] R. G. Eston, A. Crockett, and A. M. Jones, "Discussion of 'the efficacy of the self-paced VO2 max test to measure maximal oxygen uptake in treadmill running'," *Applied Physiology, Nutrition and Metabolism*, vol. 39, no. 5, pp. 581–582, 2014.

[88] D. C. Poole, "Discussion: 'the efficacy of the self-paced $\mathring{V}$ $o_{2\max}$ test to measure maximal oxygen uptake in treadmill running'," *Applied Physiology Nutrition and Metabolism*, vol. 39, no. 5, pp. 581–582, 2014.

[89] C. M. Scheadler and S. T. Devor, "VO2max measured with a self-selected work rate protocol on an automated treadmill," *Medicine & Science in Sports & Exercise*, vol. 47, no. 10, pp. 2158–2165, 2015.

[90] T. A. Astorino, D. W. McMillan, R. M. Edmunds, and E. Sanchez, "Increased cardiac output elicits higher VO2max in response to self-paced exercise," *Applied Physiology, Nutrition and Metabolism*, vol. 40, no. 3, pp. 223–229, 2015.

[91] P. F. Sperlich, H.-C. Holmberg, J. L. Reed, C. Zinner, J. Mester, and B. Sperlich, "Individual versus standardized running protocols in the determination of VO_2max," *Journal of Sports Science and Medicine*, vol. 14, no. 2, pp. 386–393, 2015.

[92] J. Faulkner, A. R. Mauger, B. Woolley, and D. Lambrick, "The efficacy of a self-paced VO_{2max} test during motorized treadmill exercise," *International Journal of Sports Physiology and Performance*, vol. 10, no. 1, pp. 99–105, 2015.

[93] J. S. Hogg, J. G. Hopker, and A. R. Mauger, "The self-paced VO2max test to assess maximal oxygen uptake in highly trained runners," *International Journal of Sports Physiology and Performance*, vol. 10, no. 2, pp. 172–177, 2015.

[94] A. M. Straub, A. W. Midgley, G. S. Zavorsky, and A. R. Hillman, "Ramp-incremented and RPE-clamped test protocols elicit similar $VO_{2\max}$ values in trained cyclists," *European Journal of Applied Physiology*, vol. 114, no. 8, pp. 1581–1590, 2014.

[95] J. Faulkner, G. Parfitt, and R. Eston, "Prediction of maximal oxygen uptake from the ratings of perceived exertion and heart rate during a perceptually-regulated sub-maximal exercise test in active and sedentary participants," *European Journal of Applied Physiology*, vol. 101, no. 3, pp. 397–407, 2007.

[96] E. T. Howley, D. R. Bassett, and H. G. Welch, "Criteria for maximal oxygen uptake: review and commentary," *Medicine and Science in Sports and Exercise*, vol. 27, no. 9, pp. 1292–1301, 1995.

[97] A. W. Midgley, L. R. McNaughton, R. Polman, and D. Marchant, "Criteria for determination of maximal oxygen uptake: a brief critique and recommendations for future research," *Sports Medicine*, vol. 37, no. 12, pp. 1019–1028, 2007.

[98] A. W. Midgley, S. Carroll, D. Marchant, L. R. McNaughton, and J. Siegler, "Evaluation of true maximal oxygen uptake based on a novel set of standardized criteria," *Applied Physiology, Nutrition and Metabolism*, vol. 34, no. 2, pp. 115–123, 2009.

[99] R. A. Robergs, "An exercise physiologist's 'contemporary' interpretations of the 'ugly and creaking edifices' of the VO_2max concept," *Journal of Exercise Physiology Online*, vol. 4, no. 1, pp. 1–44, 2001.

[100] T. A. Astorino, R. A. Robergs, F. Ghiasvand, D. Marks, and S. Burns, "Incidence of the oxygen plateau at VO_{2max} during exercise testing to volitional fatigue," *Journal of Exercise Physiology Online*, vol. 3, no. 4, pp. 1–12, 2000.

[101] D. R. Bassett Jr. and E. T. Howley, "Limiting factors for maximum oxygen uptake and determinants of endurance performance," *Medicine & Science in Sports & Exercise*, vol. 32, no. 1, pp. 70–84, 2000.

[102] G. R. Cumming and W. Friesen, "Bicycle ergometer measurement of maximal oxygen uptake in children," *Canadian Journal of Physiology and Pharmacology*, vol. 45, no. 6, pp. 937–946, 1967.

[103] T. A. Astorino, J. Willey, J. Kinnahan, S. M. Larsson, H. Welch, and L. C. Dalleck, "Elucidating determinants of the plateau in oxygen consumption at VO_{2max}," *British Journal of Sports Medicine*, vol. 39, no. 9, pp. 655–660, 2005.

[104] D. Gordon, M. Mehter, M. Gernigon, O. Caddy, D. Keiller, and R. Barnes, "The effects of exercise modality on the incidence of plateau at VO_2max," *Clinical Physiology and Functional Imaging*, vol. 32, pp. 394–399, 2012.

[105] T. A. Astorino, "Alterations in VO_2max and the VO_2 plateau with manipulation of sampling interval," *Clinical Physiology and Functional Imaging*, vol. 29, no. 1, pp. 60–67, 2009.

[106] S. M. Fox, J. P. Naughton, and W. L. Haskell, "Physical activity and the prevention of coronary heart disease," *Annals of Clinical Research*, vol. 3, no. 6, pp. 404–432, 1971.

[107] R. A. Robergs and R. Landwehr, "The surprising history of the "HRmax=220-age" equation," *Journal of Exercise Physiology Online*, vol. 5, no. 2, pp. 1–10, 2002.

[108] H. Tanaka, K. D. Monahan, and D. R. Seals, "Age-predicted maximal heart rate revisited," *Journal of the American College of Cardiology*, vol. 37, no. 1, pp. 153–156, 2001.

[109] B. Issekutz and K. Rodahl, "Respiratory quotient during exercise," *Journal of Applied Physiology*, vol. 16, pp. 606–610, 1961.

[110] B. Issekutz, N. C. Birkhead, and K. Rodahl, "Use of respiratory quotients in assessment of aerobic work capacity," *Journal of Applied Physiology*, vol. 17, no. 1, pp. 47–50, 1962.

[111] G. A. Brooks, "Anaerobic threshold: review of the concept and directions for future research," *Medicine and Science in Sports and Exercise*, vol. 17, no. 1, pp. 22–31, 1985.

[112] P. J. Maud and C. Foster, *Physiological Assessment of Human Fitness*, Human Kinetics, 2006.

[113] P. O. Astrand, *Experimental Studies of Physical Working Capacity in Ventilation to Sex and Age*, Einar Munkagaard, Copenhagen, Denmark, 1952.

[114] E. Edvardsen, E. Hem, and S. A. Anderssen, "End criteria for reaching maximal oxygen uptake must be strict and adjusted to sex and age: a cross-sectional study," *PLoS ONE*, vol. 9, no. 1, Article ID e85276, 2014.

[115] B. E. Ainsworth, R. G. McMurray, and S. K. Veazey, "Prediction of peak oxygen uptake from submaximal exercise tests in older men and women," *Journal of Aging and Physical Activity*, vol. 5, no. 1, pp. 27–38, 1997.

[116] M. J. Chen, X. Fan, and S. T. Moe, "Criterion-related validity of the Borg ratings of perceived exertion scale in healthy individuals: a meta-analysis," *Journal of Sports Sciences*, vol. 20, no. 11, pp. 873–899, 2002.

[117] R. G. Eston, "Perceived exertion: recent advances and novel applications in children and adults," *Journal of Exercise Science and Fitness*, vol. 7, pp. S11–S17, 2009.

[118] A. R. Hoogeveen, C. Schep, and J. Hoogsteen, "The ventilatory threshold, heart rate, and endurance performance: relationships in elite cyclists," *International Journal of Sports Medicine*, vol. 20, no. 2, pp. 114–117, 1999.

[119] D. V. B. James and J. H. Doust, "Oxygen uptake during moderate intensity running: response following a single bout of interval training," *European Journal of Applied Physiology and Occupational Physiology*, vol. 77, no. 6, pp. 551–555, 1998.

[120] T. D. Noakes, "Testing for maximum oxygen consumption has produced a brainless model of human exercise performance," *British Journal of Sports Medicine*, vol. 42, no. 7, pp. 551–555, 2008.

[121] R. E. Magnan, B. M. Kwan, J. T. Ciccolo, B. Gurney, C. M. Mermier, and A. D. Bryan, "Aerobic capacity testing with inactive individuals: the role of subjective experience," *Journal of Physical Activity and Health*, vol. 10, no. 2, pp. 271–279, 2013.

[122] C. Foster, E. Kuffel, N. Bradley et al., "VO_{2max} during successive maximal efforts," *European Journal of Applied Physiology*, vol. 102, no. 1, pp. 67–72, 2007.

[123] M. N. Hawkins, P. B. Raven, P. G. Snell, J. Stray-Gundersen, and B. D. Levine, "Maximal oxygen uptake as a parametric measure of cardiorespiratory capacity," *Medicine & Science in Sports & Exercise*, vol. 39, pp. 103–107, 2007.

[124] C. M. Mier, R. P. Alexander, and A. L. Mageean, "Achievement of VO_2max criteria during a continuous graded exercise test and a verification stage performed by college athletes," *Journal of Strength and Conditioning Research*, vol. 26, no. 10, pp. 2648–2654, 2012.

[125] P. B. Nolan, M. L. Beaven, and L. Dalleck, "Comparison of intensities and rest periods for VO_2max verification testing procedures," *International Journal of Sports Medicine*, vol. 35, no. 12, pp. 1024–1029, 2014.

[126] D. C. Poole, D. P. Wilkerson, and A. M. Jones, "Validity of criteria for establishing maximal O_2 uptake during ramp exercise tests," *European Journal of Applied Physiology*, vol. 102, no. 4, pp. 403–410, 2008.

[127] J. S. Thoden, J. D. MacDougall, and B. A. Wilson, *Testing Aerobic Power*, Mouvement Publications Inc, 1982.

[128] J. S. Thoden, *Testing Aerobic Power*, Human Kinetics, 1991.

[129] K. NiemelÄ, I. Palatsi, M. Linnaluoto, and J. Takkunen, "Criteria for maximum oxygen uptake in progressive bicycle tests," *European Journal of Applied Physiology and Occupational Physiology*, vol. 44, no. 1, pp. 51–59, 1980.

[130] C. H. Wyndham, "Submaximal tests for estimating maximum oxygen intake," *Canadian Medical Association Journal*, vol. 96, no. 12, pp. 736–745, 1967.

[131] L. C. Dalleck, T. A. Astorino, R. M. Erickson, C. M. McCarthy, A. A. Beadell, and B. H. Botten, "Suitability of verification testing to confirm attainment of VO2max in middle-aged and older adults," *Research in Sports Medicine*, vol. 20, no. 2, pp. 118–128, 2012.

[132] A. W. Midgley, L. R. McNaughton, and S. Carroll, "Verification phase as a useful tool in the determination of the maximal oxygen uptake of distance runners," *Applied Physiology, Nutrition and Metabolism*, vol. 31, no. 5, pp. 541–548, 2006.

[133] H. B. Rossiter, J. M. Kowalchuk, and B. J. Whipp, "A test to establish maximum O_2 uptake despite no plateau in the O_2 uptake response to ramp incremental exercise," *Journal of Applied Physiology*, vol. 100, no. 3, pp. 764–770, 2006.

[134] R. M. Weatherwax, T. B. Richardson, N. M. Beltz, P. B. Nolan, and L. Dalleck, "Verification testing to confirm VO_2max in altitude-residing, endurance-trained runners," *International Journal of Sports Medicine*, vol. 37, no. 7, pp. 525–530, 2016.

[135] A. W. Midgley, L. R. McNaughton, and S. Carroll, "Time at $V{\bullet}O_{2\max}$ during intermittent treadmill running: test protocol dependent or methodological artefact?" *International Journal of Sports Medicine*, vol. 28, no. 11, pp. 934–939, 2007.

[136] American Thoracic Society and American College of Chest Physicians, "ATS/ACCP statement on cardiopulmonary exercise testing," *American Journal of Respiratory and Critical Care Medicine*, vol. 167, no. 2, pp. 211–277, 2003.

[137] C. Babineau, L. Léger, A. Long, and L. Bosquet, "Variability of maximum oxygen consumption measurement in various metabolic systems," *Journal of Strength and Conditioning Research*, vol. 13, no. 4, pp. 318–324, 1999.

[138] G. J. Balady, R. Arena, K. Sietsema et al., "Clinician's guide to cardiopulmonary exercise testing in adults: a scientific statement from the American heart association," *Circulation*, vol. 122, no. 2, pp. 191–225, 2010.

[139] E. Yule, L. A. Kaminsky, D. A. Sedlock, B. A. King, and M. H. Whaley, "Inter-laboratory reliability of VO_2max and submaximal measurements," *Medicine & Science in Sports & Exercise*, vol. 28, no. 5, p. S15, 1996.

[140] R. R. Vickers, *Measurement Error in Maximal Oxygen Uptake Tests*, Naval Health Research Center, 2003.

[141] V. L. Katch, S. S. Sady, and P. Freedson, "Biological variability in maximum aerobic power," *Medicine and Science in Sports and Exercise*, vol. 14, no. 1, pp. 21–25, 1982.

[142] A. W. Midgley and S. Carroll, "Emergence of the verification phase procedure for confirming 'true' VO_{2max}," *Scandinavian Journal of Medicine and Science in Sports*, vol. 19, no. 3, pp. 313–322, 2009.

[143] T. N. Mann, R. P. Lamberts, and M. I. Lambert, "High responders and low responders: factors associated with individual variation in response to standardized training," *Sports Medicine*, vol. 44, no. 8, pp. 1113–1124, 2014.

20

Efficiency of an Active Rehabilitation Intervention in a Slow-to-Recover Paediatric Population following Mild Traumatic Brain Injury

Sarah Imhoff,[1,2,3] Philippe Fait,[1,2,3,4] Frédérike Carrier-Toutant,[3,5] and Geneviève Boulard[3,5]

[1]*Department of Human Kinetics, Université du Québec à Trois-Rivières (UQTR), 3351 Boulevard des Forges, Trois-Rivières, QC, Canada G9A 5H7*
[2]*Research Group on Neuromusculoskeletal Dysfunctions (GRAN), UQTR, 3351 Boulevard des Forges, Trois-Rivières, QC, Canada G9A 5H7*
[3]*Cortex Médecine et Réadaptation Concussion Clinic, 205-1035 Avenue Wilfrid-Pelletier, Québec City, QC, Canada G1W 0C5*
[4]*Research Center in Neuropsychology and Cognition (CERNEC), Université de Montréal, 90 rue Vincent d'Indy, Montréal, QC, Canada H2V 2S9*
[5]*Clinique Neuropsychologique, 206-1379 Chemin Ste-Foy, Québec City, QC, Canada G1S 2N2*

Correspondence should be addressed to Philippe Fait; philippe.fait@uqtr.ca

Academic Editor: S. John Sullivan

Objective. The aim of this study was to identify whether the addition of an individualised Active Rehabilitation Intervention to standard care influences recovery of young patients who are slow-to-recover following a mTBI. *Methods.* Fifteen participants aged 15±2 years received standard care and an individualised Active Rehabilitation Intervention which included (1) low- to high-intensity aerobic training; (2) sport-specific coordination exercises; and (3) therapeutic balance exercises. The following criteria were used to measure the resolution of signs and symptoms of mTBI: (1) absence of postconcussion symptoms for more than 7 consecutive days; (2) cognitive function corresponding to normative data; and (3) absence of deficits in coordination and balance. *Results.* The Active Rehabilitation Intervention lasted 49 ± 17 days. The duration of the intervention was correlated with self-reported participation ($\overline{x}$ = 84.64 ± 19.63%, $r = -0.792$, $p < 0.001$). The average postconcussion symptom inventory (PCSI) score went from a total of 36.85 ± 23.21 points to 4.31 ± 5.04 points after the intervention ($Z = -3.18$, $p = 0.001$). *Conclusion.* A progressive submaximal Active Rehabilitation Intervention may represent an important asset in the recovery of young patients who are slow-to-recover following a mTBI.

1. Introduction

Mild traumatic brain injury (mTBI), or concussion, is an acute neurological disorder induced after a direct or indirect mechanical impact to the head (acceleration, deceleration, rotational force, etc.) [1]. MTBI is the most common type of brain injury, and it represents a major health problem in children and adolescents, as they are highly represented in sport-related head injury [2–5]. The annual incidence of mTBI in Canadians is estimated at 600 per 100,000 inhabitants [6, 7]. Although recovery following mTBI is usually a short-lived process (7–10 days), physical, cognitive, and emotional symptoms and sleep disorder may persist beyond the expected recovery period of one to three months in 10–30% of mTBI cases in youth [8–11]. Postconcussion syndrome (PCS) refers to persisting symptoms for more than 1 month following a mTBI, including headache, nausea, dizziness, fatigue, vision impairment, sensitivity to noise and/or light, balance impairment, difficulty concentrating, memory impairment, drowsiness, anxiety, irritability, and feeling "in a fog" (WHO ICD-10). Barlow et al. [8] found that 58.5% of children aged from 0 to 18 years who sustained a mTBI were still symptomatic 1 month following the incident. Whereas children and adolescents presenting postconcussion symptoms beyond 1 month following a mTBI are considered slow-to-recover, there is a need to develop feasible and valid interventions to improve recovery in the paediatric population who sustained a mTBI.

Little is known about the treatment of mTBI, especially when postconcussion symptoms persist beyond the normal expected period of convalescence. Up to now, rest has been considered as "the gold standard" after sustaining a mTBI. Thus, consensus statements either recommend that athletes should rest until they are asymptomatic before introducing physical activity [12–14] or do not state on how and when physical activity should be introduced when symptoms persist beyond the expected recovery period [1, 15]. It has been suggested that aerobic exercise could restore cerebrovascular function and autonomic balance following mTBI [16–24]. Recent reviews of the literature support the benefits of exercise as an active rehabilitation treatment when postconcussion symptoms persist beyond the expected recovery period after injury [20, 21, 25, 26]. Indeed, it has been postulated that the introduction of physical activity may have a positive impact on the chronic symptoms following mTBI [17, 24, 27–42]. Preliminary evidence demonstrated that exercise, when used as a treatment, reduces reported symptoms in adults [17, 18, 22, 43, 44] and in youth who are slow-to-recover after mTBI [9, 35, 45]. For the sake of improving knowledge about the care of youth with atypical recovery following a mTBI, we studied the effectiveness of the integration of an Active Rehabilitation Intervention coupled with standard care while participants were still experiencing postconcussion symptoms at rest. Considering the lack of available scientific literature on active rehabilitation, we adapted the paediatric active rehabilitation program described by Gagnon et al. [9]. Our Active Rehabilitation Intervention differed in training frequency (3 times a week versus daily) and intensity reached by the end of the treatment.

The aim of this study was to identify whether the addition of an individualised Active Rehabilitation Intervention to standard care influences recovery of young patients who are slow-to-recover following an mTBI and still symptomatic at rest.

2. Methods

2.1. Participants. Eighteen participants aged from 10 to 17 years who complained of postconcussion symptoms for more than 4 weeks following a mTBI were referred to the Active Rehabilitation Intervention study through the *Cortex Medicine and Rehabilitation Concussion Clinic (Québec city, Qc, Canada)*. Participants received an interdisciplinary intervention consisting of rest, general education, school adaptations, and putting a halt to participation in physical activities, as proposed by the Zurich Consensus [1]. The study was explained to the families by a registered neuropsychologist during an initial 1-hour meeting in which the interdisciplinary approach was presented and the patient interview was conducted. Written parental consent and participant assent were obtained if both indicated an interest in the study. The research project was approved by the Ethics Review Board of Université du Québec à Trois-Rivières (UQTR).

2.2. Study Design. Participants underwent a full assessment looking for symptoms and neurological, balance, and coordination impairments before and after the Active Rehabilitation Intervention. The initial evaluation was conducted 49 ± 17 days after mTBI. A standardized mTBI history questionnaire was administered by a trained neuropsychologist to obtain detailed information about the mTBI history, including the date of the injury, the mechanism of injury, the clinical symptoms (loss of consciousness, confusion, and amnesia), and the number of autoreported previous mTBI. Participation in the program and self-report symptoms were assessed during a weekly follow-up phone call. Final evaluation was conducted when the participants reported being asymptomatic for a minimum of seven days. The following criteria were used to determine the resolution of signs and symptoms of mTBI: (1) absence of postconcussive symptoms for more than seven consecutive days; (2) cognitive function corresponding to normative data when assessed by a neuropsychologist; and (3) absence of deficits in coordination and balance.

2.3. Active Rehabilitation Intervention. Since participants were still presenting postconcussion symptoms at rest, they could not perform the standard 6-step gradual return to physical activities as proposed by the 2013 Zurich Consensus [1]. They were asked to perform a personalized home-based active rehabilitation program which consisted of (1) progressive submaximal low- to high-intensity (based on perceived exertion) aerobic training for up to 20 min, (2) low-intensity sport-specific coordination exercises for up to 10 min, and (3) therapeutic balance exercises (Figure 1). The active rehabilitation program was initially performed in a clinic under the supervision of a licensed kinesiologist. Participants were asked to perform the active rehabilitation program 3 times a week at home, at school, at a sport facility, or at the clinic. The individualised home-based program was inspired from the Montréal Children's Hospital Trauma Centre Concussion Clinic/Mild Traumatic Brain Injury Program (MCH) [9, 45], but differed in the frequency of participation (3 times a week in the present study versus daily at the MCH) in order to facilitate treatment compliance and minimize the impact on participants' daily life. This also enabled a greater difference in daily participation in exercises, allowing better monitoring of symptoms that may have been created through exercise since symptoms can be compared between a day without physical activity and the day where the rehabilitation program was conducted. It allowed assurances that the intervention was not harmful to the participant. This training schedule also enables a day of rest between high-intensity training periods. This allowed the exercise session to be more difficult without risking overtiredness for the participant and creating an increase in symptoms. Our Active Rehabilitation Intervention also differed in the intensity and duration of aerobic exercise reached by the end of the program, which was similar to those of rehabilitation programs conducted in adults. The intensity reached by the end of the program was therefore closer to the one usually performed in organized sports. This may promote a better transition to the sport practised by the participant and could enable a more complete rehabilitation.

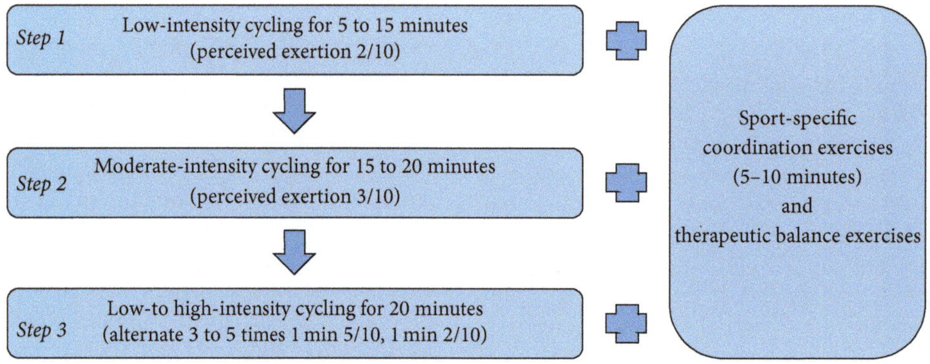

Figure 1: Active Rehabilitation Intervention.

Patients were requested to limit the duration and intensity of exercises to those prescribed according to their clinical evaluation. They were asked to perform their program even if they were symptomatic at rest but had to stop the exercise if any of the current symptoms increased by 1 point on a symptom intensity scale from 0 to 10 points or at any onset of a new symptom. Participants had to regress one stage in the program if symptoms were exacerbated after exercise participation.

2.3.1. Aerobic Training. Participants were asked to use an upright cycling ergometer to perform individualised progressive aerobic training program. Because of difficult access to a cycling ergometer, participant #7 used an elliptic. The level of perceived exertion was monitored using the 10-point Borg category-ratio scale (CR10), where effort is rated from none (0) to maximal (10) [46]. This scale was incorporated into the home program in order to help participants monitor exercise intensity. First, participants were asked to perform a symptom-dependent low-intensity supervised aerobic training session aiming to determine the volume at which they would initiate the aerobic training progression (between 5 and 15 min). In this protocol, participants evolved through three progressive stages in terms of volume and intensity, until symptom free: (1) 5 min progression every two sessions, from 5 to 15 min of low-intensity aerobic activity (perceived exertion of 2/10), (2) 5 min progression every two sessions, from 15 to 20 minutes of moderate-intensity aerobic activity (perceived exertion of 3/10), and (3) 5 min of low-intensity aerobic activity (perceived exertion of 2/10), followed by three-to-five low- to high-intensity intervals (alternate 1 min at high-intensity (perceived exertion of 5/10) and 1 min at low-intensity aerobic activity (perceived exertion of 2/10)), followed by 5 min low-intensity aerobic activity (perceived exertion of 2/10). The onset or increase of symptoms led to immediate termination of exercise for a minimum of 24 hours. Patients were asked to return to the previous stage if any of the symptoms increased by 1 point on a 10-point symptoms intensity scale during or after exercise. They had to progress through stages if they successfully completed a stage twice in a row. They were instructed not to exercise for two consecutive days.

2.3.2. Sport-Specific Coordination Exercises. Participants had to perform low-intensity (2/10) sport-specific coordination skills (shooting drills, dribbling drills, agility, etc.) for 5 to 10 min after every session of aerobic training. The activity had to be stopped if it generated any symptoms.

2.3.3. Therapeutic Balance Exercises. Participants were asked to perform three 30-seconds repetition of three therapeutic exercises consisting in balance exercises (standing on one foot with eyes closed, feet in tandem on an unstable surface, etc.) (Figure 3).

The home program included all three components of the Active Rehabilitation Intervention program and was provided to the families on paper. Progression was monitored through a weekly follow-up phone call. The participants and parents were asked to contact the study coordinator for any questions or if symptoms worsened or resolved. Follow-up was conducted until the participant reported being symptom-free for at least 7 days.

2.4. Participation in the Active Rehabilitation Intervention. Participation in the Active Rehabilitation Intervention was monitored through weekly follow-up phone calls and was determined by comparing a participant's report of exercises sessions performed with exercise sessions prescription (%). Correlation between the duration of the intervention and self-reported participation was calculated to evaluate the dose-response relationship.

2.5. Signs and Symptoms Assessment

2.5.1. Symptoms Assessment. Current postconcussion symptoms and preinjury symptoms severity were assessed by the Postconcussive Symptom Inventory scale (PCSI) [42]. The PCSI is a validated questionnaire of 21 items rated from 0 to 6 (0 = absence of symptom and 6 = severe problem) for youth of 13 to 18 years old who sustained a mTBI, where item 21 is a self-reported abnormality score rated from "0" indicating "No Difference" to "4" indicating "Very Different." The first 20 items' scores were added in order to create the PCSI score (0–120 points). The 18-item PCSI questionnaire form was used for participants under 13 years of age. Parents were asked to complete the PCSI parent version to rate their children's perceived symptom severity. Pre- and postintervention PCSI scores and self-reported abnormality scores were compared for each participant and parent and between the participant and their parent. The PCSI score results for participants #3 and #11 have not been considered in the statistical analysis due to the use of incompatible versions of the questionnaires.

2.5.2. Neuropsychological Assessment. A battery of neuropsychological tests was used to assess multiple aspects of cognitive functioning, including verbal memory (Rey Auditory Verbal Learning Test (RAVLT) [47]), verbal fluency (Delis-Kaplan executive function system (D-KEFS) [48]), working memory (Digit Span from the Weschler Adult Intelligent Scale (WAIS-IV) [49] or from the Weschler Intelligence Scale for Children (WISC-IV) [50]), information processing (Symbol Digit Modality Test (SDMT) [51]), and attention processes (Continuous Performance Test II (CPT-II) [52]). The tests were selected to evaluate the most affected cognitive functions following an mTBI as reported in the literature [53, 54]. This neuropsychological test battery was administered by a trained neuropsychologist. The test administration was standardized and uniform for all participants.

A psychological inventory (State-Trait Anxiety Inventory (STAI) [55]) was also administered to the participants' parents to measure their anxiety about their child's condition and their anxiety level as a personal characteristic [55].

2.5.3. Coordination and Balance. Coordination and balance were assessed by subtests from the Sport Concussion Assessment Tool v3 (SCAT3) Balance examination tests and coordination examination [1] through the Modified Balance Error Scoring System (BESS) testing, the tandem gait and the Finger-to-nose task. Participants performed the Modified Clinical Test of Sensory Interaction on Balance (m-CTSIB) [56], which measures static postural sway, and the Limit of Stability test (LOS), which measures dynamic postural control within a normalized sway envelope on a Biodex Biosway™ force platform (Biodex Medical Systems, Inc. Shirley, NY, USA) [57]. Finally, balance and coordination were also assessed by the Bruininks-Oseretsky Test of Motor Proficiency 2nd Edition (BOT-2) subtests of bilateral coordination, balance, and upper-limb coordination [58].

2.6. Statistical Analysis. Spearman correlation between the duration of the intervention and self-reported participation in the Active Rehabilitation Intervention and between Active Rehabilitation Intervention duration and time post mTBI preintervention were calculated. The Wilcoxon non parametric test for related samples was conducted on every other outcome measures. Outcome measures statistical analyses were conducted with the Statistical Package for the Social Sciences (SPSS) version 22 (SPSS. Inc., Chicago, Illinois, USA). BOT-2 subtests total point scores were converted to derived scores in order to have uniform meaning between subtests and participants. Normalized age and sex scale scores were used for statistical analysis.

3. Results

All participants were previously engaged in organized recreational to high performance sport groups for 6 ± 4 hours per week. Most sustained a sport-related mTBI in their principal competitive activity ($n = 14$) or in another recreational activity ($n = 2$). Two participants sustained a motor vehicle-related incident. From the previous 18 participants screened, 15 children and adolescents (9 females) aged 15.00 ± 1.69 years were included in this study. Three participants were excluded from the data analysis for the following reasons: one participant was not able to complete the final assessment because he suffered from a fractured toe and therefore decided to quit the rehabilitation program and two other participants returned to their sport without the consent of their treating clinicians, although they were still experiencing postconcussion symptoms. Participant characteristics are presented in Table 1. All participants had a normal academic progress and reported no cognitive, behavioural, neurological, or musculoskeletal impairments. Participant #4 was treated with carbamazepine (Mylan-Carbamazepine CR) for epilepsy. Participant #6 was diagnosed with influenza during the study and had flu symptoms for 10 days, after being asymptomatic for five days. Participant #7 suffered from iron deficiency anaemia and anxiety disorder, had a history of migraines and was treated with iron supplements, almotriptan (Axert®), and amitriptyline (Elavil®). No participants had sustained an mTBI in the previous 6 months before data collection. Seven participants reported amnesia of the event, three had lost consciousness, and five had sought medical attention at the emergency department. Participants #3 and #12 had an impact to the head during the study without convincing signs of mTBI. Screening and treatment for associated conditions of cervical ($n = 13$), oculomotor ($n = 10$), vestibular ($n = 5$), and temporomandibular ($n = 1$) dysfunctions were conducted by a registered physiotherapist.

3.1. Intervention Duration before Recovery. Participants were initially evaluated at 48 ± 88 days after mTBI. The intervention lasted 49 ± 17 days before recovery was attained. The final evaluation was conducted after 9 ± 2 days without symptoms (Table 1). Spearman correlation revealed no correlation between the Active Rehabilitation Intervention duration and the duration of postconcussion symptoms before the intervention ($r = -0.120$, $p = 0.671$).

3.2. Participation in the Active Rehabilitation Intervention. Participants completed on average $85 \pm 20\%$ of the Active Rehabilitation Intervention sessions prescribed. Duration of the intervention was correlated with self-reported participation score ($r = -0.796$, $p \leq 0.001$) (Figure 2). Three participants did the Active Rehabilitation Intervention program 3 to 4 times a week (every two days) which explained participation score higher than 100%.

3.3. Symptoms. Symptom frequency and severity decreased significantly after the intervention (see Table 2). Before the intervention, the participants reported an average of 8.9 ± 2.1 symptoms on the PCSI. The number of self-reported symptoms decreased significantly to 1.8 ± 1.4 following the intervention ($Z = -3.933$, $p \leq 0.001$). The most frequently symptoms from the pretest were fatigue ($n = 13$), difficulty concentrating ($n = 12$), headache ($n = 11$), and answering

TABLE 1: Participants characteristics.

Participants	Age (years)	Sex	Weight (kg)	Height (m)	Number of previous mTBIs	Amnesia	LOC	Sport	Duration of postconcussion symptoms before the intervention (days)	Active rehabilitation duration (days)	Time without symptoms after intervention (days)
01	15.0	F	46.8	1.60	1	Yes	No	Soccer	60	53	9
02	16.0	F	50.9	1.63	1	Yes	No	Basketball	86	44	10
03	12.3	M	38.6	1.56	2	No	No	Hockey*	30	27	13
04	13.6	F	47.7	1.58	0	Yes	Yes	Gymnastics	30	30	7
05	14.8	M	72.7	1.78	2	No	No	Hockey	48	49	9
06	15.0	M	75.9	1.73	1	No	No	Basketball	41	65	7
07	17.5	F	65.0	1.67	1	Yes	No	Synchronized swimming*	158	53	8
08	14.0	F	61.4	1.72	0	No	No	Soccer	373	63	9
09	15.8	M	92.3	1.83	2	Yes	Yes	Football**	120	14	10
10	15.3	F	66.4	1.71	0	Unclear	No	Basketball	60	24	14
11	11.3	M	36.4	1.39	2	No	No	Hockey	31	65	8
12	15.4	F	53.6	1.58	1	No	No	Soccer	30	56	9
13	17.1	M	70.5	1.66	0	Yes	Yes	Snowboarding	64	23	13
14	15.0	F	54.5	1.64	0	No	No	Soccer	36	48	10
15	16.8	F	81.8	1.67	0	Unclear	No	Cycling**	45	49	10

*Motor vehicle-related mTBI.
**Sport-related mTBI in another recreational sport.
LOC: loss of consciousness.

Table 2: Participants' postconcussion symptom inventory results.

	Before intervention	After intervention	Z	p
PCSI score (sum of 20 items)*	36.9 ± 23.2	4.3 ± 5.0	-3.180^b	0.001
Self-reported abnormality score*	2.0 ± 3.3	0.2 ± 0.4	-2.877^b	0.004

*Significant statistical difference.
[b]Based on positive ranks.

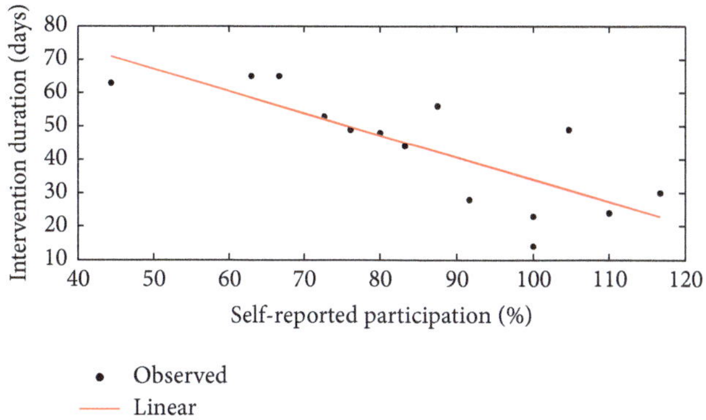

Figure 2: Correlation of duration of the intervention to self-reported participation.

questions more slowly than usual (n = 11). The PCSI score went from a total of 36.9 ± 23.2 points before the intervention to 4.3 ± 5.0 points after the intervention (Z = −3.18, p = 0.001). The self-reported abnormality score (PSCI item 21) decreased significantly from 2.0 ± 3.3 points to 0.2 ± 0.4 points (Z = −2.88, p = 0.004). Parents reported similar decrease in symptom perception of the PCSI score from 38.8 ± 20.3 to 12.8 ± 9.6 points (Z = −2.904, p = 0.004). They reported an abnormality score (item 21) of 2.1 ± 0.7 and 0.6 ± 0.5 points before and after the intervention, respectively (Z = −2.879, p = 0.004). Abnormality scores were similar between participants and their parents (Z = −1.342, p = 0.180).

3.4. Neuropsychological Results. The results of the neuropsychological test assessment are summarized in Table 3. Participants showed better performance in verbal episodic memory, both in total learning (Z = −2.843, p = 0.004) and in immediate recall (Z = −2.68, p = 0.001), in switching semantic verbal fluency (Z = −2.147, p = 0.032) and working memory (operational component (backward)) (Z = −2.54, p = 0.011) and they made less omission type errors in a task measuring different attention processes (Z = −2.386, p = 0.017) after the Active Rehabilitation Intervention. Other neuropsychological subtests did not differ when compared to the initial evaluation. No correlations were found between the Active Rehabilitation Intervention duration and the parental anxiety measured by the STAI for state anxiety (r = 0.112, p = 0.692) and trait anxiety (r = 0.042, p = 0.881).

3.5. Coordination and Balance. Coordination and balance results are presented in Table 4. Modified Balance Error Scoring System (BESS) on one leg (Z = −3.068, p = 0.002) and tandem (Z = −2.149, p = 0.032) stances, tandem gait (Z = −3.233, p = 0.001), and the Finger-to-nose (Z = −3.234, p = 0.001) scores improved after the intervention. Modified Clinical Test of Sensory Interaction on Balance (m-CTSIB) under the conditions: *Eyes opened, firm surface* (Z = −2.217, p = 0.027), *Eyes opened, foam surface* (Z = −2.309, p = 0.021) and *Eyes closed, foam surface* (Z = −3.068, p = 0.002) were significantly improved. Limit of Stability (LOS) improved from 56.6 ± 13.1% to 70.8 ± 9.9% (Z = −3.068, p = 0.002). Finally, the BOT-2 subtests of *bilateral coordination* (Z = −2.673, p = 0.008) and *upper-limb coordination* (Z = −3.121, p = 0.002) improved significantly after the intervention while the *balance* subtest remained unchanged (Z = −0.841, p = 0.400).

4. Discussion

The present study investigated the effects of an Active Rehabilitation Intervention integrated with standard care [1] on recovery, assessed by a postconcussion symptom inventory, cognitive function, and coordination and balance performance in a slow-to-recover paediatric population following a mTBI. All participants reported full recovery. The duration of the intervention was correlated with self-reported participation. The majority of coordination and balance assessment tests presented a significant improvement following the intervention.

Since postconcussion symptoms are not specific to mTBI, some patients may report symptoms on PCSI even if they report having recovered from their mTBI [42]. In this study, participant's self-reported abnormality score normalized after the Active Rehabilitation Intervention. Although there is a need to develop accessible and valid interventions to improve recovery in paediatric mTBI population, the literature supports the use of exercise as an Active Rehabilitation Intervention when symptoms persist beyond the expected recovery period after mTBI in adults [25, 26]. To date, only three similar studies conducted such interventions in youth [9, 35, 45]. Our intervention was inspired by the Montréal Children's Hospital Trauma Centre Mild Traumatic Brain Injury Program [9, 45]. Although our intervention differs in frequency of participation per week and in intensity/duration of aerobic exercise reached at the end of the program, the total duration of the Active Rehabilitation Intervention before recovery (49 ± 17 days) was similar to those observed by others [9, 45]. The Active Rehabilitation Intervention duration was not correlated with duration of autoreported postconcussion symptoms since the last mTBI (r = 0.205, p = 0.464). Considering that all participants reported a complete recovery from mTBI after the intervention, it is possible that physical activity had promoted recovery after mTBI, although recovery time overlaps this, as observed

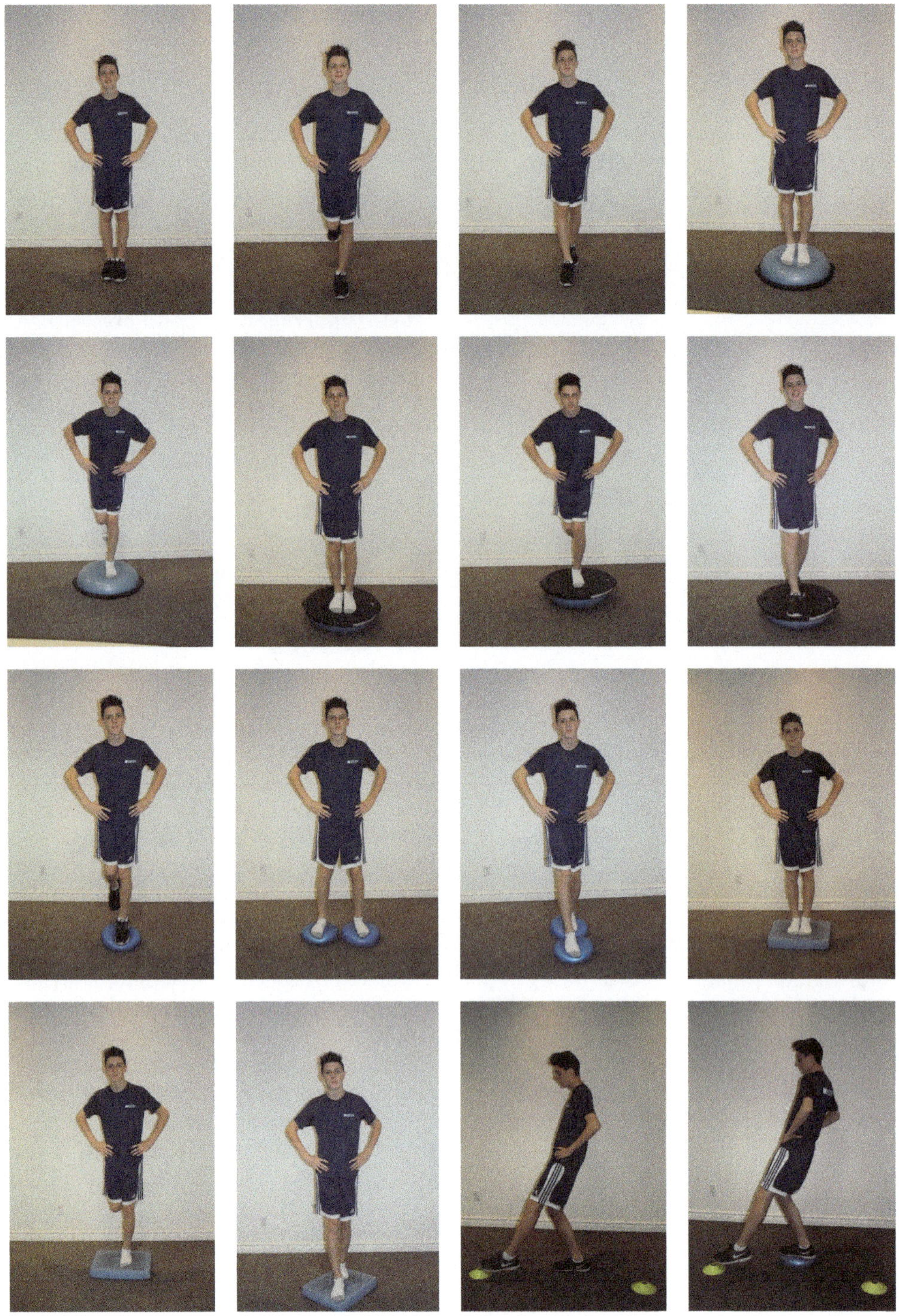

FIGURE 3: Therapeutic exercises.

by Barlow et al. [8]. Moreover, there is an apparent dose-response relationship between duration of the intervention and self-reported participation ($r = -0.792$, $p \leq 0.001$). This leaves us to believe in the effectiveness of exercise to decrease postconcussion symptoms. On the other hand, we cannot rule out the possibility of a bias created by the self-reported nature of the participation assessment.

Neuropsychological results suggest that athletes showed better performance in some verbal episodic memory, verbal fluency, working memory (operational component), and attention processes after the Active Rehabilitation Intervention. These results are consistent with the literature, indicating that episodic verbal memory, verbal fluency, working memory, and attention processes appear to be affected following a mTBI [53, 54]. Although there is a significant improvement in some parameters of cognitive functions, other parameters were not affected by the intervention (i.e., verbal memory (ListB, Delayed), verbal fluency (phoenemic,

Table 3: Neuropsychological results.

	Before intervention	After intervention	Z	p
RAVLT				
Trials 1 to 5 total*	47.46 ± 6.18	54.38 ± 7.34	−2.843[b]	0.004
List B interference	4.76 ±1.59	6.23 ± 1.36	−1.736[b]	0.083
Immediate recall*	9.77 ± 2.20	11.54 ± 1.90	−2.568[b]	0.001
Delayed recall	10.08 ± 2.66	11.15 ± 2.27	−1.724[b]	0.085
Verbal fluency (words)				
Phonemic	26.60 ± 7.23	29.60 ± 9.43	−1.449[b]	0.147
Semantic	37.64 ± 4.24	35.21 ± 4.81	−1.749[c]	0.080
Semantic switching (total responses)*	14.50 ± 2.21	11.93 ± 2.62	−2.147[c]	0.032
Semantic switching (total switching)	13.64 ± 2.37	11.36 ± 2.41	−1.891[c]	0.059
Digit span				
Forward	9.14 ± 1.70	9.29 ± 1.49	−0.426[b]	0.670
Backward*	7.43 ± 1.10	8.64 ± 1.91	−2.537[b]	0.011
SDMT				
Total	53.43 ± 7.59	56.86 ± 9.53	−1.857[b]	0.063
CPT II				
Omission*	4.33 ± 3.94	1.18 ± 1.17	−2.386[c]	0.017
Commission	23.92 ± 10.08	19.81 ± 7.08	−1.532[c]	0.126
Hit	380.80 ± 56.99	369.48 ± 35.67	−0.533[c]	0.594
Hit reaction time	6.10 ± 2.66	4.73 ± 1.24	−1.600[c]	0.110
Variability	10.04 ± 7.23	6.32 ± 1.61	−0.800[c]	0.424
Detectability	0.42 ± 0.585	0.52 ± 0.33	−1.512[c]	0.130

*Significant statistical difference.
Note: RAVLT, Rey auditory verbal learning test; SDMT, symbol-digit modalities test; CPT, Continuous Performance Task.
[b]Based on negative ranks.
[c]Based on positive ranks.

Table 4: Coordination and balance.

	Beforeintervention	After intervention	Z	p
SCAT3				
BESS double leg stance	0.07 ± 0.26	0.00 ± 0.00	−1.000[b]	0.317
BESS one leg stance*	5.20 ± 2.96	1.73 ± 2.63	−3.068[b]	0.002
BESS tandem stance*	2.80 ± 2.48	1.20 ± 2.01	−2.149[b]	0.032
Tandem gait*	17.93 ± 7.89	13.21 ± 4.08	−3.233[b]	0.001
Finger-to-nose*	3.54 ± 0.55	3.00 ± 0.48	−3.234[b]	0.001
Biosway				
mCTSIB eyes opened firm surface*	0.53 ± 0.27	0.39 ± 0.17	−2.217[b]	0.027
mCTSIB eyes closed firm surface	1.12 ± 0.88	0.69 ± 0.21	−1.874[b]	0.061
mCTSIB eyes opened foam surface*	0.78 ± 0.21	0.67 ± 0.19	−2.309[b]	0.021
mCTSIB eyes closed foam surface*	2.27 ± 0.60	1.87 ± 0.46	−1.960[b]	0.050
LOS*	56.6 ± 13.14	70.8 ± 9.92	−3.068[c]	0.002
BOT2				
Bilateral coordination*	12.33 ± 4.69	16.07 ± 4.03	−2.673[c]	0.008
Balance	12.07 ± 4.82	13.27 ± 4.43	−0.841[c]	0.400
Upper-limb coordination*	13.73 ± 4.08	18.33 ± 4.03	−3.121[c]	0.002

*Significant statistical difference.
[b]Based on positive ranks.
[c]Based on negative ranks.

semantic, semantic switching), working memory (forward), information processing, and attention processing (commission, hit, Hit reaction time, variability, and detectability)). This finding may be explained by the fact that athletes initially did not show any cognitive impairment. It may also relate to an incomplete recovery process, although participants report a subjective improvement in terms of number and intensity of autoreported symptoms. This is consistent with the literature indicating that although, in most cases, cognitive recovery largely overlaps with the time course of symptom recovery, it may occasionally follow clinical symptom resolution [1, 59, 60]. However, the limitations of the study, including the use of a small sample size and the use of alternative forms of neuropsychological tests, which could have induced a learning effect on the posttest measures, may have reduced the scope of this study. Participants demonstrated a significant improvement in coordination and balance following the intervention. These results are consistent with the literature indicating that coordination and balance are known to be altered after a mTBI in youth and young adults [53, 61–64]. The coordination and balance components of the Active Rehabilitation Intervention could impact the coordination and balance assessment results under the effect of practice. Therefore, the interpretation of the results must be made cautiously.

The lack of a control group and the limited number of participants do not allow us to draw conclusions about the effectiveness of this intervention. However, it is likely that maintaining physical rest is not optimal when the recovery process is longer than expected in youth. No participant reported having a deterioration of their condition following the Active Rehabilitation Intervention. Therefore, it is likely that the initiation of progressive low- to high-intensity physical activity, without risk of fall or impact, is safe in young athletes one month following mTBI. Physiotherapy treatments may also have had an impact on physical postconcussive symptoms.

5. Conclusion

A progressive submaximal Active Rehabilitation Intervention may be an important asset in the recovery in young patients who are slow-to-recover following a mTBI. The majority of coordination and balance assessment tests and some cognitive functions, such as working memory, verbal memory, verbal fluency, and attention processes, presented a significant improvement following the Active Rehabilitation Intervention. Symptoms resolved in every participant independently of the onset of the Active Rehabilitation Intervention in the recovery process. It is unclear how the Active Rehabilitation Intervention has influenced these results. This study is a step toward the integration of a multimodal rehabilitation intervention in patients who are slow-to-recover after a mTBI. Further studies including more participants and a control group are needed to validate this promising new approach. This study has the potential to influence traumatology practice and may promote sports therapy in mTBI rehabilitation, although additional research in this area is needed.

Competing Interests

The authors declare that there is no conflict of interests regarding the publication of this manuscript.

Acknowledgments

The authors' sincere thanks are due to the health care professionals from Cortex Médecine et Réadaptation Concussion Clinic who supported this research. This project was held in a Canadian collective effort to improve the care of children and adolescents with mTBI in collaboration with the paediatric mTBI Rehabilitation Intervention Study. This study was funded by Fonds de recherche du Québec-Santé (FRQ-S) and the Corporation des Thérapeutes du Sport du Québec research grant.

References

[1] P. McCrory, W. Meeuwisse, M. Aubry et al., "Consensus statement on concussion in sport—the 4th International conference on concussion in sport held in Zurich, November 2012," *Clinical Journal of Sport Medicine*, vol. 23, no. 2, pp. 89–117, 2013.

[2] Canadian Institute for Health Information, Head injuries in Canada: A Decade of Change (1994-1995 to 2003-2004), 2006, http://www.cihi.ca/.

[3] J. L. Guerrero, D. J. Thurman, and J. E. Sniezek, "Emergency department visits associated with traumatic brain injury: United States, 1995-1996," *Brain Injury*, vol. 14, no. 2, pp. 181–186, 2000.

[4] A. W. Selassie, D. A. Wilson, E. E. Pickelsimer, D. C. Voronca, N. R. Williams, and J. C. Edwards, "Incidence of sport-related traumatic brain injury and risk factors of severity: A Population-Based Epidemiologic Study," *Annals of Epidemiology*, vol. 23, no. 12, pp. 750–756, 2013.

[5] D. J. Thurman, "The epidemiology of traumatic brain injury in children and youths: a review of research since 1990," *Journal of Child Neurology*, vol. 31, no. 1, pp. 20–27, 2016.

[6] J. D. Cassidy, L. J. Carroll, P. M. Peloso et al., "Incidence, risk factors and prevention of mild traumatic brain injury: results of the WHO Collaborating Centre Task Force on Mild Traumatic Brain Injury," *Journal of Rehabilitation Medicine*, vol. 43, pp. 28–60, 2004.

[7] W. H. A. Ryu, A. Feinstein, A. Colantonio, D. L. Streiner, and D. R. Dawson, "Early identification and incidence of mild TBI in Ontario," *Canadian Journal of Neurological Sciences*, vol. 36, no. 4, pp. 429–435, 2009.

[8] K. M. Barlow, S. Crawford, A. Stevenson, S. S. Sandhu, F. Belanger, and D. Dewey, "Epidemiology of postconcussion syndrome in pediatric mild traumatic brain injury," *Pediatrics*, vol. 126, no. 2, pp. e374–e381, 2010.

[9] I. Gagnon, C. Galli, D. Friedman, L. Grilli, and G. L. Iverson, "Active rehabilitation for children who are slow to recover following sport-related concussion," *Brain Injury*, vol. 23, no. 12, pp. 956–964, 2009.

[10] J. Ponsford, C. Willmott, A. Rothwell et al., "Cognitive and behavioral outcome following mild traumatic head injury in children," *Journal of Head Trauma Rehabilitation*, vol. 14, no. 4, pp. 360–372, 1999.

[11] R. Zemek, N. Barrowman, S. B. Freedman et al., "Clinical risk score for persistent postconcussion symptoms among children

with acute concussion in the ED," *The Journal of the American Medical Association*, vol. 315, no. 10, pp. 1014–1025, 2016.

[12] C. C. Giza, J. S. Kutcher, S. Ashwal et al., "Summary of evidence-based guideline update: evaluation and management of concussion in sports: report of the Guideline Development Subcommittee of the American Academy of Neurology," *Neurology*, vol. 80, no. 24, pp. 2250–2257, 2013.

[13] M. E. Halstead and K. D. Walter, "American Academy of Pediatrics. Clinical report—sport-related concussion in children and adolescents," *Pediatrics*, vol. 126, no. 3, pp. 597–615, 2010.

[14] Ontario Neurotrauma Fondation, *Guidelines for Concussion/mTBI and Persistant Symptoms*, 2nd edition, 2013.

[15] R. Zemek, S. Duval, and C. Dematteo, *Guideline for Diagnosing and Managing Pediatric Concussion*, Neurotrauma Foundation, Ontario, Canada, 1st edition, 2014.

[16] W. E. Amonette and K. A. Mossberg, "Ventilatory anaerobic thresholds of individuals recovering from traumatic brain injury compared with noninjured controls," *Journal of Head Trauma Rehabilitation*, vol. 28, no. 5, pp. E13–E20, 2013.

[17] J. G. Baker, M. S. Freitas, J. J. Leddy, K. F. Kozlowski, and B. S. Willer, "Return to full functioning after graded exercise assessment and progressive exercise treatment of postconcussion syndrome," *Rehabilitation Research and Practice*, vol. 2012, Article ID 705309, 7 pages, 2012.

[18] M. Clausen, D. R. Pendergast, B. Willer, and J. Leddy, "Cerebral blood flow during treadmill exercise is a marker of physiological postconcussion syndrome in female athletes," *The Journal of Head Trauma Rehabilitation*, vol. 31, no. 3, pp. 215–224, 2016.

[19] R. L. Conder and A. A. Conder, "Heart rate variability interventions for concussion and rehabilitation," *Frontiers in Psychology*, vol. 5, article 890, 2014.

[20] J. Leddy, A. Hinds, D. Sirica, and B. Willer, "The role of controlled exercise in concussion management," *PM&R*, vol. 8, no. 3, supplement, pp. S91–S100, 2016.

[21] J. J. Leddy, J. G. Baker, and B. Willer, "Active rehabilitation of concussion and post-concussion syndrome," *Physical Medicine & Rehabilitation Clinics of North America*, vol. 27, no. 2, pp. 437–454, 2016.

[22] J. J. Leddy, K. Kozlowski, J. P. Donnelly, D. R. Pendergast, L. H. Epstein, and B. Willer, "A preliminary study of subsymptom threshold exercise training for refractory post-concussion syndrome," *Clinical Journal of Sport Medicine*, vol. 20, no. 1, pp. 21–27, 2010.

[23] J. J. Leddy, K. Kozlowski, M. Fung, D. R. Pendergast, and B. Willer, "Regulatory and autoregulatory physiological dysfunction as a primary characteristic of post concussion syndrome: implications for treatment," *NeuroRehabilitation*, vol. 22, no. 3, pp. 199–205, 2007.

[24] C. O. Tan, W. P. Meehan III, G. L. Iverson, and J. A. Taylor, "Cerebrovascular regulation, exercise, and mild traumatic brain injury," *Neurology*, vol. 83, no. 18, pp. 1665–1672, 2014.

[25] K. J. Schneider, G. L. Iverson, C. A. Emery, P. McCrory, S. A. Herring, and W. H. Meeuwisse, "The effects of rest and treatment following sport-related concussion: a systematic review of the literature," *British Journal of Sports Medicine*, vol. 47, no. 5, pp. 304–307, 2013.

[26] N. D. Silverberg and G. L. Iverson, "Is rest after concussion 'the best medicine?': recommendations for activity resumption following concussion in athletes, civilians, and military service members," *Journal of Head Trauma Rehabilitation*, vol. 28, no. 4, pp. 250–259, 2013.

[27] T. Archer, "Influence of physical exercise on traumatic brain injury deficits: scaffolding effect," *Neurotoxicity Research*, vol. 21, no. 4, pp. 418–434, 2012.

[28] T. Archer, K. Svensson, and M. Alricsson, "Physical exercise ameliorates deficits induced by traumatic brain injury," *Acta Neurologica Scandinavica*, vol. 125, no. 5, pp. 293–302, 2012.

[29] S. Brand, M. Gerber, J. Beck, M. Hatzinger, U. Pühse, and E. Holsboer-Trachsler, "High exercise levels are related to favorable sleep patterns and psychological functioning in adolescents: a comparison of athletes and controls," *Journal of Adolescent Health*, vol. 46, no. 2, pp. 133–141, 2010.

[30] C. De Matteo, K. A. Volterman, P. G. Breithaupt, E. A. Claridge, J. Adamich, and B. W. Timmons, "Exertion testing in youth with mild traumatic brain injury/concussion," *Medicine and Science in Sports and Exercise*, vol. 47, no. 11, pp. 2283–2290, 2015.

[31] I. Ensari, T. A. Greenlee, R. W. Motl, and S. J. Petruzzello, "Meta-analysis of acute exercise effects on state anxiety: an update of randomized controlled trials over the past 25 years," *Depression and Anxiety*, vol. 32, no. 8, pp. 624–634, 2015.

[32] G. S. Griesbach, F. Gomez-Pinilla, and D. A. Hovda, "The upregulation of plasticity-related proteins following TBI is disrupted with acute voluntary exercise," *Brain Research*, vol. 1016, no. 2, pp. 154–162, 2004.

[33] G. S. Griesbach, D. A. Hovda, R. Molteni, A. Wu, and F. Gomez-Pinilla, "Voluntary exercise following traumatic brain injury: brain-derived neurotrophic factor upregulation and recovery of function," *Neuroscience*, vol. 125, no. 1, pp. 129–139, 2004.

[34] K. Hotting and B. Roder, "Beneficial effects of physical exercise on neuroplasticity and cognition," *Neuroscience & Biobehavioral Reviews*, vol. 25, no. 13, pp. 00101–00102, 2013.

[35] B. G. Kurowski, J. Hugentobler, C. Quatman-Yates et al., "Aerobic exercise for adolescents with prolonged symptoms after mild traumatic brain injury: an exploratory randomized clinical trial," *The Journal of Head Trauma Rehabilitation*, In press.

[36] L. Larun, K. G. Brurberg, J. Odgaard-Jensen, and J. R. Price, "Exercise therapy for chronic fatigue syndrome," *The Cochrane Database of Systematic Reviews*, vol. 2, Article ID CD003200, 2015.

[37] J. J. Leddy, J. G. Baker, K. Kozlowski, L. Bisson, and B. Willer, "Reliability of a graded exercise test for assessing recovery from concussion," *Clinical Journal of Sport Medicine*, vol. 21, no. 2, pp. 89–94, 2011.

[38] C. W. Majerske, J. P. Mihalik, D. Ren et al., "Concussion in sports: postconcussive activity levels, symptoms, and neurocognitive performance," *Journal of Athletic Training*, vol. 43, no. 3, pp. 265–274, 2008.

[39] A. L. Rebar, R. Stanton, D. Geard, C. Short, M. J. Duncan, and C. Vandelanotte, "A meta-meta-analysis of the effect of physical activity on depression and anxiety in non-clinical adult populations," *Health Psychology Review*, vol. 9, no. 3, pp. 366–378, 2015.

[40] C. D. Rethorst, B. M. Wipfli, and D. M. Landers, "The antidepressive effects of exercise: a meta-analysis of randomized trials," *Sports Medicine*, vol. 39, no. 6, pp. 491–511, 2009.

[41] J. Rimer, K. Dwan, D. A. Lawlor et al., "Exercise for depression," *The Cochrane Database of Systematic Reviews*, vol. 7, Article ID CD004366, 2012.

[42] M. D. Sady, C. G. Vaughan, and G. A. Gioia, "Psychometric characteristics of the postconcussion symptom inventory in children and adolescents," *Archives of Clinical Neuropsychology*, vol. 29, no. 4, pp. 348–363, 2014.

[43] L. M. Chin, L. Chan, J. G. Woolstenhulme, E. J. Christensen, C. N. Shenouda, and R. E. Keyser, "Improved cardiorespiratory fitness with aerobic exercise training in individuals with traumatic brain injury," *The Journal of Head Trauma Rehabilitation*, vol. 30, no. 6, pp. 382–390, 2015.

[44] J. J. Leddy, J. L. Cox, J. G. Baker et al., "Exercise treatment for postconcussion syndrome: a pilot study of changes in functional magnetic resonance imaging activation, physiology, and symptoms," *Journal of Head Trauma Rehabilitation*, vol. 28, no. 4, pp. 241–249, 2013.

[45] I. Gagnon, L. Grilli, D. Friedman, and G. L. Iverson, "A pilot study of active rehabilitation for adolescents who are slow to recover from sport-related concussion," *Scandinavian Journal of Medicine and Science in Sports*, vol. 26, no. 3, pp. 299–306, 2016.

[46] G. A. V. Borg, "Psychophysical bases of perceived exertion," *Medicine and Science in Sports and Exercise*, vol. 14, no. 5, pp. 377–381, 1982.

[47] M. Schmidt, *Rey Auditory Verbal Learning Test*, Western Psycho-logical Services, Los Angeles, Calif, USA, 1996.

[48] D. C. Delis, E. Kaplan, and J. H. Kramer, *Kaplan Executive Function System (D-KEFS)*, Psychological Corporation, 2001.

[49] D. Wechsler, *Wechsler Adult Intelligence Scale*, NCS Pearson, San Antonio, Tex, USA, 4th edition, 2008.

[50] D. Wechsler, *Wechsler Intelligence Scale for Children-WISC-IV*, Pychological Corporation, 2003.

[51] A. Smith, *Symbol Digit Modalities Test (SDMT) Manual*, Western Psychological Services, Los Angeles, Calif, USA, 1982.

[52] C. K. Conners and M. H. S. Staff, *Conners' Continuous Performance Test II (CPT II V. 5)*, Multi-Health Systems, North Tonawanda, NY, USA, 2000.

[53] K. M. Guskiewicz, S. E. Ross, and S. W. Marshall, "Postural stability and neuropsychological deficits after concussion in collegiate athletes," *Journal of Athletic Training*, vol. 36, no. 3, pp. 263–273, 2001.

[54] A. Lundin, C. de Boussard, G. Edman, and J. Borg, "Symptoms and disability until 3 months after mild TBI," *Brain Injury*, vol. 20, no. 8, pp. 799–806, 2006.

[55] C. D. Spielberger, "State-Trait Anxiety Inventory," *Corsini Encyclopedia of Psychology. 1*, 2010.

[56] H. Cohen, C. A. Blatchly, and L. L. Gombash, "A study of the clinical test of sensory interaction and balance," *Physical Therapy*, vol. 73, no. 6, pp. 346–354, 1993.

[57] M. L. Pickerill and R. A. Harter, "Validity and reliability of limits-of-stability testing: a comparison of 2 postural stability evaluation devices," *Journal of Athletic Training*, vol. 46, no. 6, pp. 600–606, 2011.

[58] R. Bruininks and B. Bruininks, *Bruininks-Oseretsky Test of Motor Proficiency*, NCS Pearson, Minneapolis, Minn, USA, 2nd edition, 2005.

[59] J. Bleiberg, A. N. Cernich, K. Cameron et al., "Duration of cognitive impairment after sports concussion," *Neurosurgery*, vol. 54, no. 5, pp. 1073–1080, 2004.

[60] P. Fait, B. J. McFadyen, B. Swaine, and J. F. Cantin, "Alterations to locomotor navigation in a complex environment at 7 and 30 days following a concussion in an elite athlete," *Brain Injury*, vol. 23, no. 4, pp. 362–369, 2009.

[61] K. M. Guskiewicz, "Assessment of postural stability following sport-related concussion.," *Current Sports Medicine Reports*, vol. 2, no. 1, pp. 24–30, 2003.

[62] K. M. Guskiewicz and J. K. Register-Mihalik, "Postconcussive impairment differences across a multifaceted concussion assessment protocol," *PM&R*, vol. 3, no. 10, supplement 2, pp. S445–S451, 2011.

[63] L. A. King, F. B. Horak, M. Mancini et al., "Instrumenting the balance error scoring system for use with patients reporting persistent balance problems after mild traumatic brain injury," *Archives of Physical Medicine and Rehabilitation*, vol. 95, no. 2, pp. 353–359, 2014.

[64] A. G. Schneiders, S. J. Sullivan, A. R. Gray, G. D. Hammond-Tooke, and P. R. McCrory, "Normative values for three clinical measures of motor performance used in the neurological assessment of sports concussion," *Journal of Science and Medicine in Sport*, vol. 13, no. 2, pp. 196–201, 2010.

21

A Scoping Review of the Associations of Golf with Eye Injuries in Adults and Children

Evan Jenkins,[1] Roger Hawkes,[2] and Andrew Murray[1,2]

[1]*Sport and Exercise, the University of Edinburgh, St. Leonard's Land, Edinburgh EH8 8AQ, UK*
[2]*European Tour Performance Institute, Virginia Water GU25 4LX, UK*

Correspondence should be addressed to Andrew Murray; docandrewmurray@gmail.com

Academic Editor: Laura Guidetti

Introduction. Sport presents a risk of ocular trauma and accounts for a significant number of eye injuries that require hospital admission. The sport of golf presents a risk to eyesight from fast moving objects such as golf clubs and balls. This study aims to investigate the associations of golf with eye injuries and the reasons that these injuries occur. *Material/Methods.* A literature search was conducted using the databases MEDLINE, Web of Science, SPORTDiscus, and PsycINFO. Grey literature was searched using the WHO international clinical trials registry platform, Google Scholar, and ProQuest. Data was extracted using a standardised form and summarised into a report. *Results and Discussion.* Twenty-three studies were found relating to eye injuries in golf. Injuries appear to be rare, but more frequent in men and children. Injuries resulted in high rates of enucleation and visual impairment. Children sustained more injury from golf clubs whereas adults sustained more injuries from golf balls. *Conclusion.* Efforts are needed to encourage golf participants to understand the risks of ocular and indeed other head injuries. Initiatives to provide appropriate supervision and education on this topic are merited. Further research is needed to investigate the circumstances of eye injury in golf and assess the effects of interventions aimed at reducing risk of injury.

1. Introduction

Ocular injury is a recognised risk of taking part in sporting activity. Sport is estimated to be responsible for between 25 and 40% of all ocular injuries requiring hospital admission [1, 2]. Golf presents a risk to eye health from the swinging of golf clubs and golf balls in flight, both of which can transmit considerable force [3]. However, to our knowledge no review assessing ocular injuries in the sport of golf has been undertaken.

Golf is played by over 20 million participants in Europe alone and has seen a large increase in facilities worldwide [4]. Despite this, golf has one of the lowest rates of reported musculoskeletal injury of sports players [5], but eye and head injuries have been reported in the literature [6].

This review aimed to collate available evidence regarding ocular injuries in golf and assess the associations of golf with ocular injuries and any patterns in the occurrence of such incidents. This may alert golfers to possible risks, assist stakeholders attempting to improve health and safety for golf players, and highlight any gaps in the existing literature.

2. Materials and Methods

2.1. Databases. The following databases and search platforms were used to search for studies as part of a wider scoping review: MEDLINE, PsycINFO, SPORTDiscus, Web of Science, Google Scholar, WHO international clinical trials registry platform, and ProQuest.

2.2. Eligibility Criteria. The following inclusion and exclusion criteria were utilised:

Inclusion criteria are as follows.

(i) Research articles not limited by geographical location, language, or setting.

(ii) All age groups and both sexes of participants.

(iii) Research that looks at the general population, as well as specific population groups.

(iv) All forms of golf (including but not limited to 18 holes, 9 holes, driving range, and spectating).

(v) Research articles discussing ocular/eye injuries in the context of golf.

(vi) Sources of information including primary research studies, reviews (including but not limited to systematic reviews, scoping reviews, and meta-analyses), guidelines, and grey literature to include unpublished and on-going trials, annual reports, dissertations, and conference proceedings.

Explicit exclusion criteria identified are as follows.

(i) Opinion pieces/opinions, magazine and newspaper articles, case reports, and papers with no data.

2.3. Search Strategy. Using the keywords "golf" AND "health", a limited initial search for review articles was conducted using Google Advanced Search and SPORTDiscus. Fifty-six articles were retrieved from this search and were further analysed by the research team.

The team elected to maximise inclusivity by identifying "golf" as the primary search term. This term alone was used for the predominantly health related databases such as MEDLINE and PsycINFO. Secondary search terms were also included for Web of Science, Google Scholar, and SPORTDiscus, using the search terms "golf" AND "health OR illness OR injur* OR fitness OR mortality OR morbidity."

For grey literature searches, the term "golf" was used for the WHO international clinical trials registry platform. The search terms "golf AND health OR illness OR injur* OR fitness OR mortality OR morbidity" were also used when searching ProQuest database, the World Golf Foundation, the Royal and Ancient, the British Journal of Sports Medicine, the American College of Sports Medicine, and the Faculty of Sports and Exercise Medicine websites using the Google Advanced function. Grey literature studies were included if keywords appeared in the title.

All articles identified with keywords in the title were reviewed. This search strategy allowed the inclusion of articles relating to all aspects of golf and health. The results of databases and search platforms initially found 4041 articles, which were reduced to 3167 once duplicate articles were removed.

Following this, relevant articles were sought through the process outlined below:

(1) One reviewer (Andrew Murray) assessed all titles and abstracts applying the eligibility criteria. A second reviewer (Evan Jenkins) assessed 10% of these titles and abstracts, with excellent agreement. Following this, the full text of each remaining article was sourced and read, applying the same criteria by two reviewers (Andrew Murray and Evan Jenkins). Further articles were then identified from reading the reference lists of all relevant articles.

(2) Tables that are similar to those recommended for scoping reviews by the Joanna Briggs Institute [7] were used for data extraction of all remaining articles (see Table 1). Authors were contacted directly when further specific data was needed.

(3) Evidence extracted was collated and data synthesized relating to the number of cases, gender of participants, numbers needing surgery, and any serious visual impairment sustained.

3. Results and Discussion

3.1. Study Selection. The scoping review search yielded 3167 studies. Three hundred and fifty-six studies were read in full with 23 found to be directly relevant to eye injuries in golf.

3.2. Study Characteristics. Twenty-three studies were included in this review, after applying the eligibility criteria. These comprised 7 retrospective studies [6, 8–13], 2 prospective studies [14, 15], 2 patient case series [16, 17], 1 review of sports-related eye injuries [18], and ten [19–28] studies which described ocular injuries that resulted from exposure to the contents of liquid filled golf balls. These 10 studies included 4 histopathology investigations [19–22], 2 patient case series [23, 24], 3 case notes [25–27], and 1 commentary report [28]. Finally, a commentary review by Brunette [29] explored the link between golf and health.

3.3. Results. Data from all retrospective studies [6, 8–13], both prospective studies by Jones and Gregory [14, 15], and the review of sports-related eye injuries by Portis et al. [18] were deemed most relevant to current golf participants. These studies report 102 patients who presented to accident and emergency departments with golf-related ocular injuries, during the period of 1990–2007.

Using a large cohort of 309 patients, Fradkin et al. [6] demonstrated that ocular injuries were the second most common type of injury sustained from golf-related trauma, accounting for 8.1% of all injuries. Furthermore, Gregory [14] demonstrated that golf-related ocular injury (GROI) accounted for 2.2% of all sports-related ocular injuries that were admitted to the accident and emergency department of Sussex Hospital. This was similar to results from the study by Jones [15], where GROI accounted for 2.4% of all sports-related ocular injuries. After viewing records of golf-related ocular injuries at a pathology laboratory, Portis et al. [18] report that 14.0% of sports-related ocular injuries were from playing golf. However, each of these studies only presented data on the total number of GROI admitted to tertiary health centres. Therefore, these papers were not used for further analysis as none can contribute to results in other categories.

Ten studies [19–28] described injuries occurring from the expansion of liquid filled golf balls, which are no longer in popular use. Therefore, these studies are not relevant to modern golf participants. The review by Brunette [29] only made mention of an incidental case of GROI in a commentary. These 10 studies were not included in the synthesis of results. Data by Millar [16] and Takatama et al.

Table 1: Criteria used to extract data.

Author	Names of all authors involved in the study.
Article title	The full title of the study.
Year of publication	The year the study was published.
Type of publication	Which category of publication the study is in, for example, journal article, commentary, or letter.
Country	In which country was the study written?
Aims of the study	A description of questions the study is attempting to answer.
Population	How many people did the study discuss?
Methodology/methods	What methods did the study use to collect data?
Concept	What topic does the study investigate?
Context	In what setting does the study take place?
A priori themes: golf participation, physical activity and health, golf and physical activity, longevity, cardiorespiratory, metabolic, and musculoskeletal, accidents, illness, wellness, mental illness, special populations	Does the study discuss any of the outlined themes?
Any emergent themes not covered previously	Does the study note any points regarding themes not previously mentioned?

Table 2: Demographic information of patients who sustained golf-related ocular injuries.

Study	Number of cases	Patient group			Average age *(years)*
		Male	Female	Children *(<18 years)*	
Burnstine and Elner [8]	9	6	3	2	35.1
Fradkin et al.♦ [6]	16	—	—	16	—
Gregory♦ [14]	2	2	0	—	32.0
Hink et al. [9]	11	6	5	11	10.2
Jayasundera et al. [10]	11	8	3	4	26.3
Jones♦ [15]	2	—	—	—	—
Mieler et al. [11]	8	6	2	2	44.4
Millar♦ [16]	7	5	2	3	29.0
Park et al. [12]	22	16	6	0	48.5
Portis et al.♦ [18]	11	—	—	—	—
Takatama et al.♦ [17]	11	9	2	—	47.0
Townley et al.* [13]	10	8	1	4	29.0
Total	*120*	*66*	*23*	*42*	*33.5*

♦Not included in result synthesis.
*Case of a 1-year-old child where gender was not specified.

[17] are described separately as these case series cannot provide data on the incidence of injury.

In summary, 71 patients are reported to have suffered GROI. Fifty (70.4%) incidents occurred in males, 20 (28.2%) in females, and1 (1.4%) case of a 1-year-old where gender was not given (see Table 2). Twenty-one (29.6%) injuries were sustained from being hit by golf clubs and 50 (70.4%) from golf balls. Golf ball related trauma equated to 91.5% (43 cases) of all 47 adult injuries. Twenty-four (33.8%) injuries occurred in children of which 17 (70.8%) injuries were from being hit by golf clubs (children being defined here as aged 18 or under). Six injuries occurred in golf spectators, accounting for 8.5% of all cases (golf spectators were defined here as anyone not playing or practising golf).

As outlined in Table 3, the consequences of these injuries were often severe, with 55 (77.5%) injuries requiring surgery and 24 (33.8%) of these cases resulting in enucleation or evisceration of the eye. Blindness, in at least 1 eye, was reported in 27 (38.0%) patients of which 19 (70.4%) injuries were caused by impact from a golf ball and 8 (29.6%) from golf clubs. Furthermore, of the 6 studies which describe visual acuity, 34 (47.9%) out of the 71 patients had significant reductions in visual acuity below 20/40 Snellen, including those with no light perception [8–13]. As most studies reported visual acuity using the 20-foot US Snellen notation, this same notation was used for this review [8, 9, 11, 12]. For studies using the 6-meter UK based notation [10, 13], visual acuity changes below 6/12 were recorded and used to demonstrate impairment in visual acuity. This review regards any changes to visual acuity as a result of GROI as significant. Globe rupture was reported in 26 cases of which 22 (84.6%) were the result of impact from golf balls.Orbital fractures were reported in 5 studies

TABLE 3: Consequences of golf-related ocular injury.

Study	Cause of injury: Golf club (number of children injured)	Cause of injury: Golf ball (number of children injured)	Number needing surgery *(number of eyes)*	Number of globe ruptures *(number of eyes)*	Blindness in at least one eye *(number of eyes)*
Burnstine and Elner [8]	2 (2)	7 (0)	9	8	6
Fradkin et al.♦ [6]	—	—	—	—	—
Gregory♦ [14]	0 (—)	2 (—)	—	—	—
Hink et al. [9]	10 (10)	1 (1)	9	1	2
Jayasundera et al. [10]	4 (4)	7 (0)	7	5	2
Jones♦ [15]	—	—	—	—	—
Mieler et al. [11]	2 (0)	6 (2)	8	4	3
Millar♦+ [16]	4 (1)	3 (1)	2	2	2
Park et al. [12]	0 (0)	22 (0)	15	5	7
Portis et al.♦ [18]	8 (—)	3 (—)	11	—	11
Takatama et al.*♦ [17]	—	7 (—)	7	—	4
Townley et al. [13]	3 (1)	7 (3)	7	3	7
Total	*33 (18)*	*65 (7)*	*75*	*28*	*44*

♦Not included in synthesis of results.
+Incidence of child striking glass with a golf club resulting in a perforating injury.
*One incidence of ocular injury from a golf cart crash.

[8, 9, 11–13] and were present in 30 (50%) out of the 60 patients reported.

When collating these results with those of Millar [16] and Takatama et al. [17], a total of 89 ocular injuries were reported, with 64 (71.9%) cases occurring in males. Impact from golf balls resulted in 60 (67.4%) ocular injuries and 1 additional case describes injury from a golf cart crash. Numbers requiring surgery drop to 69.7% (62 cases) whilst rates of eye blindness remain relatively even at 33 (37.1%) cases.

Ten studies [19–28] discuss incidences of ocular injury from old style golf balls exploding and how the liquid centres commonly cause ocular injury in children. The studies commonly describe an "opaqueness" and corneal fibrosis that occur after contact with, what was found to be, inorganic crystalline material. The most recent report of this type of injury was from 1976 by Lucas et al. [20].

3.4. Discussion. Ocular injuries in the sport of golf are infrequent events which are associated with high rates of blindness and risk to sight. The setting of the included studies may partly explain the severity of the reported injuries, as each study took place in accident and emergency departments of either district hospitals or specialist eye hospitals [6, 8–13]. Further studies appraising eye injuries reported to golf course staff or primary care/family doctors may show a decreased severity of injury on average.

GROI occurs most often in males which may reflect the higher participation of men in golf [30]. It was also found that children sustained a greater number of injuries than adults; however, this may not be a fair estimate as 1 of the 6 studies used to collate results only collected data on children [10].

Children sustain more injuries from golf clubs through incidents that commonly occur away from golf courses and without adult supervision [10, 13]. This pattern highlights the need for adult supervision of children who use golf equipment. Adults must take such opportunities to teach children the correct golf etiquette and safety protocols, such as checking behind them before swinging a golf club.

Golf equipment should be kept safely out of reach of children to avoid the high number of injuries that occur outside of golf courses [9]. Townley et al. [13] suggest that large media campaigns and advertisements may assist in warning all owners of golf equipment about the dangers these items pose to children and of the need for supervision.

In contrast, adult injuries usually occur whilst playing golf and are often the result of impact from a golf ball. This suggests that further enforcement of golf health and safety protocols must be made clear to anyone present on a golf course [10]. This may be achieved through safety briefings, signs or posters situated around the golf course, or campaigns as described above. Jayasundera et al. [10] note that player experience had little to do with the risk of receiving ocular injury and therefore recommendations to lower the risk of injury must be accessible to players of all levels.

These measures should also be extended to golf spectators as there is some incidence of eye injury in this population. Safety should be considered in the layout of driving ranges. For example, play should not be in close proximity to walkways and protective measures such as signage and netting should be implemented [12]. When play is likely to occur in close proximity to crowds, such as driving ranges, it is possible for spectators to be injured by a golfer's backswing. Any danger of this can be addressed by implementing policies and safety measures to minimise danger from swinging golf clubs. This could include safety lines which spectators must stand behind during play.

As discussed by Jayasundera et al. [10], education of appropriate safety protocols is essential to preventing injury. For example, golfers who hit a wayward ball are expected to shout "fore" to warn passersby. If not appropriately informed, many golfers then choose to look up to see the approaching ball and increase injury risk. Therefore, all golfers must be taught to look down and shield their head to avoid such injury.

Finally, protective eye equipment is discussed by most studies and ultimately would guarantee some level of protection [12]. As mentioned by Townley et al. [13], fast moving golf balls can be difficult to avoid and such equipment would aid anyone unable to shield themselves. Mandatory use of these may be difficult to impose; however, such equipment may have a role when teaching children or introducing newcomers to the sport [12].

3.5. Strengths and Limitations. This review is limited by a relatively small patient population and having only 2 studies [13, 17] making comments on the specific circumstances that resulted in ocular injury. As a result, it is difficult to make recommendations regarding health and safety in golf. Additionally, 3 studies only collect information from specific patient populations or of certain modes of injury [6, 9, 12]. Therefore, evidence used to make recommendations is weak due to the limited availability of data. Furthermore, as the studies discussed use data from accident and emergency and trauma departments, they likely underreport less significant injuries that were not admitted to these departments. Therefore, this may reduce the amount of data regarding minor eye injuries in golf.

However, all retrospective studies [6, 8–13] collect data over at least 5 years, making these the best available evidence regarding the incidence of traumatic ocular injury in golf. All recommendations must be made from the best available evidence and modified as new evidence emerges. This review is the most current collection of evidences regarding eye injuries in golf.

The papers collected for this review have been peer-reviewed by 2 independent reviewers with experience working as physicians in primary and secondary care settings and experience working with golfing populations.

3.6. Recommendations for Future Research. Further cross-sectional studies are needed both to identify the cause of injury and to provide any comment regarding the circumstances surrounding each incident. Where practical, studies to assess the incidence of eye injuries would provide a better understanding of the frequency with which GROI occur. This may be achieved through large cohort studies of golfers and recording of all GROI. However, to most effectively quantify GROI, prospective studies taking place in well-circumscribed geographic areas are needed. Such studies should take place in both emergency and ophthalmology departments.

The overall results derived by this review are dependent on the reporting and publication of GROI, regardless of whether the studies provide data of GROI incidence. However, underreporting of these injuries is very likely as many clinicians will choose not to report GROI through published case series, such as that done by Takatama et al. [17]. Therefore, future studies may wish to use appropriate ICD-10 codes to help gather further data of eye injuries through billing and payer records.

Research is needed to assess golf players' knowledge of health and safety rules. This may include assessing the knowledge of golf players at all levels, regarding their understanding of golf safety, and then comparing this to knowledge held by the general public. This information may highlight areas of golf safety that are poorly understood and therefore need to be taught. It may also demonstrate gaps in public knowledge and help guide the health and safety information issued with golf equipment. Efforts must then be made to adapt these messages for children.

Future reviews may also wish to focus on all head and face injuries sustained in golf. These injuries are likely to occur under similar circumstances to eye injuries but will encompass a larger patient cohort. Alternately, collecting data through family doctors or general practitioners may also include a larger number of patients but with less severe injuries.

4. Conclusion

There is little published data regarding the incidence of GROI. Though GROI occurs relatively rarely, the severity of injury is high, with many cases resulting in loss of vision or enucleation [2]. Children sustain most of their ocular injuries from golf clubs, whilst adults are most frequently injured from golf balls. Children should have constant adult supervision whilst using golf equipment and be taught rules regarding safety. Anyone buying golf equipment should gain an understanding of these rules to minimise risk of injury.

The use of protective eye equipment should be considered and may be appropriate when teaching children. Considering the large population of golfers, targeted media campaigns may best inform players of how to avoid serious trauma [9]. Future studies should focus attention on all head injuries in golf and decide which aspects of health and safety are most important to advertise to players and the general public.

Competing Interests

The authors declare that there is no conflict of interests regarding the publication of this paper.

Acknowledgments

The authors would like to thank Luke Daines, Marshall Dozier, and colleagues from Sport and Exercise and the Physical Activity for Health Research Centre at the University of Edinburgh for their assistance in the preparation of this paper.

References

[1] A. Barr, P. S. Baines, P. Desai, and C. J. MacEwen, "Ocular sports injuries: the current picture," *British Journal of Sports Medicine*, vol. 34, no. 6, pp. 456–458, 2000.

[2] C. J. MacEwen and G. R. McLatchie, "Eye injuries in sport," *Scottish Medical Journal*, vol. 55, no. 2, pp. 22–24, 2010.

[3] M. R. Farrally, A. J. Cochran, D. J. Crews et al., "Golf science research at the beginning of the twenty-first century," *Journal of Sports Sciences*, vol. 21, no. 9, pp. 753–765, 2003.

[4] The R&A, Golf around the world 2015, http://www.randa.org/TheRandA/AboutTheRandA/DownloadsAndPublications.

[5] J. Arkkari, A. Natri, P. Kannus et al., "A controlled trial of the health benefits of regular walking on a golf course," *The American Journal of Medicine*, vol. 109, no. 2, pp. 102–108, 2000.

[6] A. J. Fradkin, P. A. Cameron, and B. J. Gabbe, "Children's misadventures with golfing equipment," *International Journal of Injury Control And Safety Promotion*, vol. 12, no. 3, pp. 201–203, 2005.

[7] M. Peters, C. Godfrey, P. McInerney, C. Soares, K. Hanan, and D. Parker, *The Joanna Briggs Institute Reviewers' Manual 2015: Methodology for JBI Scoping Reviews*, The Joanna Briggs Institute, Adelaide, Australia, 2015.

[8] M. A. Burnstine and V. M. Elner, "Golf-related ocular injuries," *American Journal of Ophthalmology*, vol. 121, no. 4, pp. 437–438, 1996.

[9] E. M. Hink, S. C. N. Oliver, A. V. Drack et al., "Pediatric golf-related ophthalmic injuries," *Archives of Ophthalmology*, vol. 126, no. 9, pp. 1252–1256, 2008.

[10] T. Jayasundera, B. Vote, and B. Joondeph, "Golf-related ocular injuries," *Clinical & Experimental Ophthalmology*, vol. 31, no. 2, pp. 110–113, 2003.

[11] W. F. Mieler, S. K. Nanda, M. D. Wolf, and J. Harman, "Golf-related ocular injuries," *Archives of Ophthalmology*, vol. 113, no. 11, pp. 1410–1413, 1995.

[12] S. J. Park, K. H. Park, J. W. Heo, and S. J. Woo, "Visual and anatomic outcomes of golf ball-related ocular injuries," *Eye*, vol. 28, no. 3, pp. 312–317, 2014.

[13] D. Townley, C. Kirwan, and M. O'Keefe, "Golf—recognising the risk of severe eye injury," *Irish Medical Journal*, vol. 101, no. 6, pp. 167–169, 2008.

[14] P. T. S. Gregory, "Sussex Eye Hospital sports injuries," *British Journal of Ophthalmology*, vol. 70, no. 10, pp. 748–750, 1986.

[15] N. P. Jones, "Eye injuries in sport: an increasing problem," *British Journal of Sports Medicine*, vol. 21, no. 4, pp. 168–170, 1987.

[16] G. T. Millar, "Golfing eye injuries," *The American Journal of Ophthalmology*, vol. 64, no. 4, pp. 741–742, 1967.

[17] A. Takatama, H. Saito, A. Noiri, H. Murakami, K. Sato, and K. Kawai, "Eleven cases of eye injury while playing golf," *Japanese Journal of Clinical Ophthalmology*, vol. 56, no. 4, pp. 567–570, 2002.

[18] J. M. Portis, S. A. Vassallo, and D. M. Albert, "Ocular sports injuries: a review of cases on file in the Massachusetts eye and ear infirmary pathology laboratory," *International Ophthalmology Clinics*, vol. 21, no. 4, pp. 1–19, 1981.

[19] F. B. Johnson and L. E. Zimmerman, "Barium sulfate and zinc sulfide deposits resulting from golf-ball injury to the conjunctiva and eyelid," *American Journal of Clinical Pathology*, vol. 44, no. 5, pp. 533–538, 1965.

[20] D. R. Lucas, A. C. Dunham, W. R. Lee, W. Weir, and F. C. F. Wilkinson, "Ocular injuries from liquid golf ball cores," *British Journal of Ophthalmology*, vol. 60, no. 11, pp. 740–747, 1976.

[21] R. O'Grady and D. Shoch, "Golf-ball granuloma of the eyelids and conjunctiva," *The American Journal of Ophthalmology*, vol. 76, no. 1, pp. 148–151, 1973.

[22] J. N. Taylor and C. H. Greer, "Ocular injuries by explosion of the liquid centres of golf balls," *The Medical Journal of Australia*, vol. 1, no. 12, pp. 632–633, 1969.

[23] R. Penner, "The liquid center golf ball: a potential ocular hazard," *Archives of Ophthalmology*, vol. 75, no. 1, pp. 68–71, 1966.

[24] M. M. Slusher, K. R. Jaegers, and W. H. Annesley Jr., "Liquid-center golf balls and ocular injury," *American Journal of Ophthalmology*, vol. 64, no. 4, pp. 736–740, 1967.

[25] L. W. Crigler, "Burn of eyeball due to caustic contents of golf-ball," *The Journal of the American Medical Association*, vol. 60, no. 17, article 1297, 1913.

[26] R. H. Elliot and W. S. Inman, "Serious injury to an eye from a bursting golf ball," *British Medical Journal*, vol. 1, no. 2829, pp. 501–502, 1915.

[27] H. E. Thomason, "Golf-ball burn of eye," *The Journal of the American Medical Association*, vol. 61, no. 12, article 965, 1913.

[28] H. Lowell, "Burn of eyes from contents of golf-ball core," *Journal of the American Medical Association*, vol. 61, no. 26, pp. 2302–2303, 1913.

[29] D. D. Brunette, "A good walk spoiled. Golf's links to medicine," *Minnesota Medicine*, vol. 80, no. 6, pp. 25–30, 1997.

[30] Golf Advisory Practice in EMEA, KPMG: Golf Participation for Europe 2016, http://golfbenchmark.com/article/golf_participation_report_for_europe_2016.

22

Muscle Activation Differs between Three Different Knee Joint-Angle Positions during a Maximal Isometric Back Squat Exercise

Paulo Henrique Marchetti,[1,2] Josinaldo Jarbas da Silva,[1] Brad Jon Schoenfeld,[3] Priscyla Silva Monteiro Nardi,[2] Silvio Luis Pecoraro,[1] Julia Maria D'Andréa Greve,[2] and Erin Hartigan[4]

[1]*Graduate Program in Science of Human Movement, College of Health Science (FACIS), Methodist University of Piracicaba, 13423-070 Piracicaba, SP, Brazil*
[2]*Institute of Orthopedics and Traumatology, School of Medicine, University of São Paulo, Laboratory of Kinesiology, 05403-000 São Paulo, SP, Brazil*
[3]*Department of Health Sciences, Program of Exercise Science, CUNY Lehman College, Bronx, NY 10468, USA*
[4]*Department of Physical Therapy, University of New England, Portland, ME 04103, USA*

Correspondence should be addressed to Paulo Henrique Marchetti; dr.pmarchetti@gmail.com

Academic Editor: Mark Willems

The purpose of this study was to compare muscle activation of the lower limb muscles when performing a maximal isometric back squat exercise over three different positions. Fifteen young, healthy, resistance-trained men performed an isometric back squat at three knee joint angles (20°, 90°, and 140°) in a randomized, counterbalanced fashion. Surface electromyography was used to measure muscle activation of the vastus lateralis (VL), vastus medialis (VM), rectus femoris (RF), biceps femoris (BF), semitendinosus (ST), and gluteus maximus (GM). In general, muscle activity was the highest at 90° for the three quadriceps muscles, yet differences in muscle activation between knee angles were muscle specific. Activity of the GM was significantly greater at 20° and 90° compared to 140°. The BF and ST displayed similar activation at all joint angles. In conclusion, knee position alters muscles activation of the quadriceps and gluteus maximus muscles. An isometric back squat at 90° generates the highest overall muscle activation, yet an isometric back squat at 140° generates the lowest overall muscle activation of the VL and GM only.

1. Introduction

The squat is one of the most frequently used exercises in the field of strength and conditioning. The squat is an exercise that increases hip and knee extensor muscle strength which then indirectly improves the quality of life in athletic and nonathletic populations [1]. The squat exercise utilizes muscles with different morphology (monoarticular and biarticular). Muscle forces also vary depending on joint positions (moment arm, length-tension relationship), whether the muscle acts as a prime mover or stabilizer, and whether the task is dynamic or static. Though evidence suggests that architecture, position, and function drive muscle performance during the squat, little is known about the neuromuscular changes that occur from a muscle activation standpoint. Elucidating how muscle activation patterns change in the monoarticular and biarticular knee and hip extensors during squatting at different knee angles would thus enhance our understanding of how one could capitalize on maximizing muscle activation and the best position to specific evaluations and sEMG normalization. This would be a first step to then apply the knowledge during exercise prescription that includes the squat.

Considering that the squat exercise is a multijoint task, a large number of muscle groups can be activated simultaneously in a more complex way. Several studies have shown that manipulating features of the squat exercise resulted in altered muscle activity. These manipulations include changes in foot position [2, 3], barbell position [4], stability of the surface on which the exercise is performed [5–9], different levels of intensity of load [10], range of motion [10–12], and different equipment [13].

As a multijoint exercise, the knee extensors (e.g., rectus femoris, RF; vastus lateralis, VL; and vastus medialis, VM) and hip extensors (e.g., gluteus maximus, GM; biceps femoris, BF; and semitendinosus, ST) are considered to be the prime movers during the squat exercise, with other muscles acting in a secondary capacity [1, 11, 14]. Caterisano et al. [11] measured the relative contributions of GM, BF, VM, and VL muscles of ten experienced lifters while performing dynamics squats at 3 depths (partial squat (the angle between the femur and the tibia was ~2.36 rad at the knee joint), parallel squat (the angle between the femur and the tibia was ~1.57 rad at the knee joint), and full-depth squat (the angle between the femur and the tibia was ~0.79 rad at the knee joint)), using 100–125% of body weight as resistance. The results suggested that the GM was most active, rather than the BF, the VM, or the VL, during a concentric contraction as squat depth increases. On the contrary, Robertson et al. [12] determined that the GM displayed a reduced activity level at maximum squat depth. Robertson et al. [12] also showed that the biarticular muscles functioned mainly as stabilizers of the ankle, knee, and hip joints by working eccentrically to control descent or transferring energy among the segments during ascent. Whether monoarticular and biarticular hip and knee extensors have different muscle activation during an isometric squat and whether activation changes during different knee angles are unclear. Consequently, the rationale of the present study was to evaluate, indirectly, the muscle activation in different mechanical positions related to differences in the joint-angle-torque diagram and the sticking region effect in all three joint angles (20°, 90°, and 140°).

Finally, differences in muscle activity during dynamic and isometric squat exercise have received less attention in the physical education and rehabilitation area. Others have shown the isometric squat (90° and 120° of knee join position) as a reliable test to provide an indicator of changes in dynamic strength (1-repetition maximum barbell back squat, 1RM) and power performance [15, 16]; however, whether muscle activity changes as an isometric squat is manipulated is unknown. Although motor units are recruited differently during dynamic movements, they generate the same relative force/torque during a static contraction [17]. Despite inherent neural and mechanical differences between isometric and dynamic contractions, the isometric squat exercise performed in different knee joint angles may be used to understand changes in muscle activation patterns without confounding any other external effects such as the stretch-shortening cycle from dynamic movements [18]. Therefore, the purpose of this study was to evaluate the maximal isometric muscle activation of the lower limbs during three different knee joint-angle positions in the back squat exercise.

2. Methods

2.1. Subjects. We collected the peak amplitude of the root mean square (RMS) from VL sEMG data during a pilot study to drive this power analysis. Based on a statistical power analysis derived from these data (RMS VL EMG), it was determined that twelve subjects would be necessary to achieve an alpha level of 0.05, effect size of 1.41, and a power $(1 - \beta)$ of 0.80 [19]. Therefore, we recruited fifteen young, healthy, resistance-trained men (age: 30 ± 7 years, height: 174 ± 6 cm, and total body mass: 76 ± 9 kg, with 5 ± 1 years of experience on the back squat exercise) to participate in this study. Subjects had no previous lower back injury, no surgery on the lower extremities, and no history of injury with residual symptoms (pain, "giving-away" sensations) in the lower limbs within the last year. This study was approved by the university research ethics committee and all subjects read and signed an informed consent document.

2.2. Procedures. Prior to data collection, subjects were asked to identify their preferred leg for kicking a ball, which was then considered their dominant leg [20]. All subjects were right-leg dominant. Volunteers attended one session in the laboratory, and they reported to have refrained from performing any lower body exercise other than activities of daily living for at least 48 hours prior to testing. Subjects performed a 5-minute cycle warm-up and a familiarization session with all isometric conditions. The familiarization session was performed in all joint angles used during the experimental procedure (20°, 90°, and 140°) for 1 set of 3 seconds each. After the warm-up and familiarization, all subjects performed three trials of 10-second maximal isometric contractions against a locked smith machine under three different knee joint-angle positions in a randomized, counterbalanced order: back squat at 20 degrees (20°); back squat at 90 degrees (90°); and back squat at 140 degrees (140°). The knee joint-angle positions were evaluated by a goniometer (Plastic 12″ Goniometer 360 Degree ISOM), and, for all angles, full knee extension was considered the "zero" position. The subjects' feet were always positioned at hip width and vertically aligned with the barbell position. The barbell was positioned on the shoulders (high-bar position) for all subjects and experimental conditions. A rest period of 15 minutes was provided between conditions with 3 minutes afforded between sets. All measures were performed at the same hour of the day, between 9 and 12 AM, and by the same researcher.

2.3. Measures

2.3.1. Surface Electromyography (sEMG). The subjects' hair was shaved at the site of electrode placement and the skin was cleaned with alcohol before the sEMG electrode was affixed. Bipolar active disposable dual Ag/AgCl snap electrodes were used which were 1 cm in diameter for each circular conductive area with 2 cm center-to-center spacing. Electrodes were placed on the dominant limb along the axes of the muscle fibers, according to the SENIAM/ISEKI protocol [21]: gluteus maximus (GM) at 50% of the distance between the sacral vertebrae and the greater trochanter; vastus lateralis (VL) at 2/3 of the distance between the anterior spine iliac and the superior aspect of the lateral side of the patella; rectus femoris (RF) at 50% on the line from the anterior spine iliac to the superior part of patella; vastus medialis (VM) at 80% on the line between the anterior spine iliac superior and the joint space in front of the anterior border of the medial ligament; biceps femoris (BF) at 50% on the line between the ischial tuberosity and the lateral epicondyle of the tibia; and semitendinosus (ST) at 50% on the line between the ischial tuberosity and the medial epicondyle of the tibia. The sEMG signals were recorded by an electromyographic acquisition system (EMG832C, EMG System do Brasil, São José dos Campos, Brazil) with a sampling rate of 2000 Hz using a commercially designed software program (EMG System do Brasil, São José dos Campos, Brazil). EMG activity was amplified (bipolar differential amplifier, input impedance = 2 MΩ, common mode rejection ratio > 100 dB min (60 Hz), gain × 20, noise > 5 μV) and converted from an analog to digital signal (12 bits). A ground electrode was placed on the right clavicle. EMG signals collected during all conditions were normalized to a maximum voluntary isometric contraction (MVIC) against fixed strap resistance. Then, two trials of five-second MVICs were performed for each muscle with one-minute rest between actions for the dominant leg. The first MVIC was performed to familiarize the participant with the procedure. For GM MVIC, subjects were in the prone position with their knee flexed at 90° and resistance placed on the distal region of the thigh with the pelvis stabilized. For VL, VM, and RF MVICs, subjects were seated with their knee flexed at 90° and resistance placed on the distal tibia. For BF and ST MVICs, subjects were seated with their knee flexed at 90° and resistance placed on the distal tibia. Verbal encouragement was given during all MVICs. The order of MVICs was counterbalanced to avoid any potential neuromuscular fatigue.

TABLE 1: Effect size (d) comparisons for iEMG between knee joint-angle positions.

Angle	VL	VM	RF	BF	ST	GM
20° × 90°	0.99	0.91	0.98	0.08	0.20	0.03
90° × 140°	1.87	0.87	0.65	0.27	0.05	1.81
20° × 140°	0.95	0.18	0.50	0.36	0.24	1.76

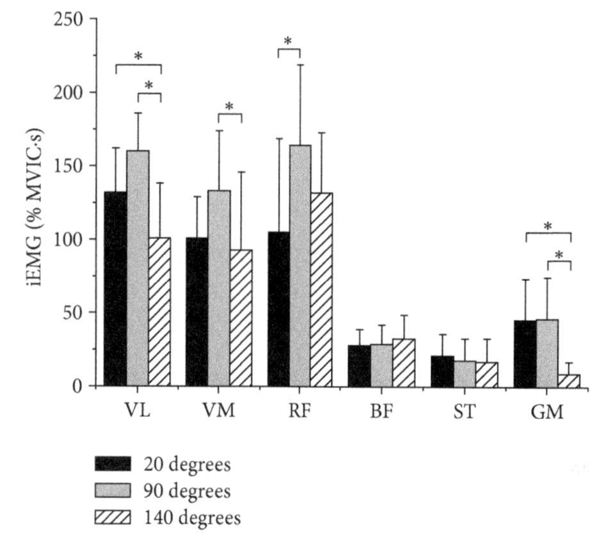

FIGURE 1: Mean and standard deviation of iEMG in three different knee joint-angle positions. *Significant differences, $P < 0.05$.

2.4. Data Analyses. All sEMG data were analyzed with customized Matlab routine (MathWorks Inc., USA). The digitized sEMG data were band-pass filtered at 20–400 Hz using a fourth-order Butterworth filter with zero lag. For muscle activation time domain analysis, RMS (150 ms moving window) was calculated during the MVIC. Isometric back squat data was then normalized to the RMS peak of the two peak MVICs, the first second was removed from RMS normalized, and the following 3 seconds of each trial were integrated (iEMG).

2.5. Statistical Analyses. The normality and homogeneity of variances within the data were confirmed with the Shapiro-Wilk and Levene's tests, respectively. To test differences for each muscle activity (iEMG), repeated measures ANOVAs were used. Post hoc comparisons were performed with the *Bonferroni* test. Cohen's formula for effect size (d) was calculated, and the results were based on the following criteria: <0.35 trivial effect; 0.35–0.80 small effect; 0.80–1.50 moderate effect; and >1.5 large effect, for recreationally trained subjects [22]. Interrater reliability was assessed for the researcher who positioned and evaluated iEMG tracings for all muscles and conditions. Reliability was operationalized using the following criteria: <0.4 poor; 0.4–<0.75 satisfactory; ≥0.75 excellent [23]. The ICCs ranged between 0.91 and 0.99 (excellent) for all iEMG data. An alpha of 5% was used to determine statistical significance.

3. Results

There was a significant main effect of VL ($P < 0.001$), VM ($P = 0.030$), RF ($P = 0.018$), and GM ($P < 0.001$) for muscle activity during three different knee joint-angle positions (20°, 90°, and 140°) in the isometric back squat.

The VL activity was significantly less in 140° than 20° ($P = 0.027$, Δ% = 24.4) and 90° ($P < 0.001$, Δ% = 37.5). The VM activity was significantly less in 140° than 90° ($P = 0.036$, Δ% = 30). The RF activity was significantly less in 20° than 90° ($P = 0.015$, Δ% = 36). The GM activity was significantly less in 140° than 90° ($P < 0.001$, Δ% = 80.4) and 20° ($P < 0.001$, Δ% = 80) (Table 1 and Figure 1).

4. Discussion

The purpose of this study was to evaluate the maximal isometric muscle activation of the lower limbs during three different knee joint-angle positions in the back squat exercise. The architecture, position, and function influence muscle forces during the squat; however, little is known about the neuromuscular changes that occur from a muscle activation standpoint. The primary finding of this investigation was that, during isometric squatting, a position of 90° of knee joint angle demonstrated the overall highest muscle activation of the quadriceps and gluteus maximus, whereas the 140° knee joint-angle position presented the lowest muscle activation values for almost all muscles that act as prime movers. Interestingly, the activation of the hamstring did not differ among knee joint-angle positions and the three quadriceps muscles responded differently as the knee went from a relatively extended position to a more flexed position.

Given the close chain nature of the squat, as the knee joint changes position, the hip joint angles also change positions. Consequently, the squat exercise simultaneously utilizes several muscles with different morphologies (monoarticular and biarticular) in a manner that produces "muscle coordination" [24]. A multijoint task to strengthen the knee and hip extensors is more complex for the neuromuscular system as two joints work in concert to achieve the task [12]. Also, since some muscles cross more than one joint, the complexity increases compared to open chain terminal knee extension or isolated hip extension exercise [12]. During the squat exercise, there are several biarticular muscles interacting including the hamstrings and RF [1]. Biarticular muscles such as RF, BF, and ST have intermediate activation when the muscles have agonistic action at one joint and antagonistic action at the other joint; this is in contrast with the high activation seen when a biarticular muscle works as an agonist for both joints simultaneously [24]. Lombard [25] suggested that biarticular muscles of the lower extremity act in a "paradoxical" fashion when the movement is constrained or controlled (named *Lombard's paradox*); it is observed when RF, BF, and ST contract concurrently when rising from a chair. The extension seen from both the hip and the knee is the result of the differential moment arms of the two muscles at each joint. The present results showed low muscle activation for BF and ST in all knee positions, probably because these muscles act more like a joint stabilizer at the knee and a prime mover at the hip. Both BF and ST have the longer moment arm at the hip thereby creating a hip extensor moment. Thus, the BF and ST muscles allow for the extension of both the knee and the hip [12]. Since the RF has a greater moment arm across the knee, due to the patella, it creates an extensor moment at the knee joint. Considering the present results, the RF showed higher muscle activation at 90° when compared to 20°; however, it was similar to 140° of knee angle. This may represent a higher effect on muscle activation during the initial phase of the squat movement (between 20° and 90°) than after 90° since the muscle activation did not change.

On the other hand, monoarticular muscles act on one specific joint. During the squat exercise, several monoarticular muscles contribute to movement including the soleus, vasti (lateralis, medialis, and intermedius), and GM [1]. The present results showed that muscle activation for all monoarticular muscles (e.g., VM, VL, and GM) did not differ between 20° and 90°. Additionally, the highest muscle activation was observed at 90° when compared to 20° and 140°; on the other hand, 140° presented the lowest activation for VL and GM muscles. Interestingly, the VM behaved differently from the other monoarticular muscles, even the VL, as the muscle activation of the VM did not differ between the 20- and 140-degree knee joint angles.

Usually, when monoarticular muscles perform as agonists, the activation increases as the joint moment increases [24]. Additionally, monoarticular muscles are affected by the sticking region which is considered a poor mechanical force position in which the mechanical advantage of the muscles involved is such that their capacity to exert force is reduced and where the lifter experiences difficulty in exerting force against the external load [26–30]. Cardinale et al. [31] displayed that the higher muscle activation during the squat exercise occurs at 90° of knee joint-angle position, which is considered the sticking region. The present results support this finding for all monoarticular muscles analyzed (VL, VM, and GM). Our findings support this theory as all monoarticular muscles presented lower values of activation at 140° of knee joint-angle position when compared to 90°. In this specific position (at 140°), it is feasible to speculate that changes in muscle length modify muscle contractile abilities and, in turn, modify sEMG-force and sEMG-moment relationships [18, 24]. Alternatively, afferent signals from muscles could decrease motoneuronal firing frequency (i.e., Golgi tendon reflex) during isometric contractions when the muscle fibers are in an elongated position [17].

Others have also investigated muscle activation during the squat by comparing different knee joint angles, yet previous studies compared knee positions during a dynamic squat, not an isometric squat. Caterisano et al. [11] measured the relative contributions of GM, BF, VM, and VL muscles of ten experienced lifters while performing dynamics squats at 3 depths (partial squat (the angle between the femur and the tibia was ~2.36 rad at the knee joint), parallel squat (the angle between the femur and the tibia was ~1.57 rad at the knee joint), and full-depth squat (the angle between the femur and the tibia was ~0.79 rad at the knee joint)), using 100–125% of body weight as resistance. Caterisano et al. [11] found that, during the concentric phase of the dynamic squat, the GM activation was higher during full-depth (35.4%) squat compared to the partial (16.9%) and parallel (28.0%) squat exercise and that the BF, the VM, and the VL did not change. The results suggested that the GM, rather than the BF, the VM, or the VL, becomes more active in concentric contraction as squat depth increases. Others have also shown superior muscular hypertrophy when squatting throughout a full versus a partial range of motion [32, 33]. Our findings of less muscle activation at 140° do not support Bloomquist and colleagues' findings. The greater cross-sectional area of the muscles found by Bloomquist et al. [32] may be more related to time under tension than the muscle activation. However, without muscle activation data, this remains speculative. In opposition, when our subjects performed an isometric squat in different positions, the GM activity was the highest in the 90-degree position, not the deeper knee flexion position. Perhaps the change in 100–125% body weight load during the dynamic trials and our maximum isometric load in all three conditions influence the lack of agreement between the studies. Similar to our results, Robertson et al. [12] reported that the GM muscle activity level was reduced at maximum full (deep-knee) squat depth. Robertson et al. [12] also concluded that the biarticular muscles (BF, ST, and RF) functioned mainly as stabilizers of the knee and hip joints during the eccentric and concentric phases of a dynamic squat. The authors presumed that the reduced GM activity level at maximum squat depth was because the GM was not needed to maintain stability or perhaps it permitted an extra degree of hip flexion that created a deeper countermovement immediately before the ascent phase. From an activation standpoint, our findings suggest a diminished benefit from squatting beyond 90°. The reason for these seemingly contradictory findings among studies remains to be elucidated. Investigations comparing muscle activity during isometric and dynamic squatting are needed.

A limitation of this study includes the use of healthy, well-trained men only, and, therefore, our findings are not generalizable to other conditions, populations, or women. We also have a small sample size; thus, this study may be underpowered to identify differences between knee joint positions. We did not control for hip angles to create a more realistic squat performance.

5. Conclusion

Knee position alters muscles activation of the quadriceps and gluteus maximus muscles. An isometric back squat at 90° generates the highest overall muscle activation, yet an isometric back squat at 140° generates the lowest overall muscle activation of the VL and GM only. Knee angle did not affect muscle activation of the hamstrings. Thus, we recommend performing an isometric squat at 90° to maximize neuromuscular recruitment of the knee and hip extensors.

Competing Interests

The authors declare that there are no competing interests regarding the publication of this paper.

References

[1] B. J. Schoenfeld, "Squatting kinematics and kinetics and their application to exercise performance," *Journal of Strength and Conditioning Research*, vol. 24, no. 12, pp. 3497–3506, 2010.

[2] S. T. McCaw and D. R. Melrose, "Stance width and bar load effects on leg muscle activity during the parallel squat," *Medicine & Science in Sports & Exercise*, vol. 31, no. 3, pp. 428–436, 1999.

[3] A. Paoli, G. Marcolin, and N. Petrone, "The effect of stance width on the electromyographical activity of eight superficial thigh muscles during back squat with different bar loads," *Journal of Strength and Conditioning Research*, vol. 23, no. 1, pp. 246–250, 2009.

[4] J. C. Gullett, M. D. Tillman, G. M. Gutierrez, and J. W. Chow, "A biomechanical comparison of back and front squats in healthy trained individuals," *Journal of Strength and Conditioning Research*, vol. 23, no. 1, pp. 284–292, 2009.

[5] K. Anderson and D. G. Behm, "Trunk muscle activity increases with unstable squat movements," *Canadian Journal of Applied Physiology*, vol. 30, no. 1, pp. 33–45, 2005.

[6] E. J. Drinkwater, E. J. Pritchett, and D. G. Behm, "Effect of instability and resistance on unintentional squat-lifting kinetics," *International Journal of Sports Physiology and Performance*, vol. 2, no. 4, pp. 400–413, 2007.

[7] J. M. Kohler, S. P. Flanagan, and W. C. Whiting, "Muscle activation patterns while lifting stable and unstable loads on stable and unstable surfaces," *Journal of Strength and Conditioning Research*, vol. 24, no. 2, pp. 313–321, 2010.

[8] J. M. McBride, P. Cormie, and J. R. Deane, "Isometric squat force output and muscle activity in stable and unstable conditions," *Journal of Strength and Conditioning Research*, vol. 20, no. 4, pp. 915–918, 2006.

[9] J. M. McBride, T. R. Larkin, A. M. Dayne, T. L. Haines, and T. J. Kirby, "Effect of absolute and relative loading on muscle activity during stable and unstable squatting," *International Journal of Sports Physiology and Performance*, vol. 5, no. 2, pp. 177–183, 2010.

[10] R. R. Aspe and P. A. Swinton, "Electromyographic and kinetic comparison of the back squat and overhead squat," *Journal of Strength and Conditioning Research*, vol. 28, no. 10, pp. 2827–2836, 2014.

[11] A. Caterisano, R. F. Moss, T. K. Pellinger et al., "The effect of back squat depth on the EMG activity of 4 superficial hip and thigh muscles," *Journal of Strength and Conditioning Research*, vol. 16, no. 3, pp. 428–432, 2002.

[12] D. G. E. Robertson, J.-M. J. Wilson, and T. A. St Pierre, "Lower extremity muscle functions during full squats," *Journal of Applied Biomechanics*, vol. 24, no. 4, pp. 333–339, 2008.

[13] A. H. Saeterbakken, V. Andersen, and R. van den Tillaar, "Comparison of kinematics and muscle activation in free-weight back squat with and without elastic bands," *Journal of Strength and Conditioning Research*, vol. 30, no. 4, pp. 945–952, 2016.

[14] P. H. Marchetti, W. A. Gomes, W. A. Da Luz Junior et al., "Aspectos neuromecânicos do exercício agachamento," *Revista Centro de Pesquisas Avançadas em Qualidade de Vida*, vol. 5, no. 2, pp. 1–16, 2013.

[15] A. J. Blazevich, N. Gill, and R. U. Newton, "Reliability and validity of two isometric squat tests," *Journal of Strength and Conditioning Research*, vol. 16, no. 2, pp. 298–304, 2002.

[16] S. Demura, K. Miyaguchi, S. Shin, and Y. Uchida, "Effectiveness of the 1RM estimation method based on isometric squat using a back-dynamometer," *Journal of Strength and Conditioning Research*, vol. 24, no. 10, pp. 2742–2748, 2010.

[17] P. F. Gardiner, *Advanced Neuromuscular Exercise Physiology*, Human Kinetics, Champaign, Ill, USA, 2011.

[18] T. W. Worrell, G. Karst, D. Adamczyk et al., "Influence of joint position on electromyographic and torque generation during maximal voluntary isometric contractions of the hamstrings and gluteus maximus muscles," *Journal of Orthopaedic and Sports Physical Therapy*, vol. 31, no. 12, pp. 730–740, 2001.

[19] J. Eng, "Sample size estimation: how many individuals should be studied?" *Radiology*, vol. 227, no. 2, pp. 309–313, 2003.

[20] P. Maulder and J. Cronin, "Horizontal and vertical jump assessment: reliability, symmetry, discriminative and predictive ability," *Physical Therapy in Sport*, vol. 6, no. 2, pp. 74–82, 2005.

[21] H. J. Hermens, B. Freriks, C. Disselhorst-Klug, and G. Rau, "Development of recommendations for SEMG sensors and sensor placement procedures," *Journal of Electromyography and Kinesiology*, vol. 10, no. 5, pp. 361–374, 2000.

[22] M. R. Rhea, "Determining the magnitude of treatment effects in strength training research through the use of the effect size," *Journal of Strength and Conditioning Research*, vol. 18, no. 4, pp. 918–920, 2004.

[23] B. Rosner, *Fundamentals of Biostatistics*, Cengage Learning, Boston, Mass, USA, 7th edition, 2010.

[24] B. I. Prilutsky, "Coordination of two- and one-joint muscles: functional consequences and implications for motor control," *Motor Control*, vol. 4, no. 1, pp. 1–44, 2000.

[25] W. P. Lombard, "The action of two-joint muscles," *American Journal of Physics Education*, vol. 9, pp. 141–145, 1903.

[26] B. C. Elliott, G. J. Wilson, and G. K. Kerr, "A biomechanical analysis of the sticking region in the bench press," *Medicine & Science in Sports & Exercise*, vol. 21, no. 4, pp. 450–462, 1989.

[27] R. van den Tillaar and A. H. Saeterbakken, "Fatigue effects upon sticking region and electromyography in a six-repetition maximum bench press," *Journal of Sports Sciences*, vol. 31, no. 16, pp. 1823–1830, 2013.

[28] R. van den Tillaar, "Kinematics and muscle activation around the sticking region in free weight barbell back squat," *Kinesiologia Slovenica*, vol. 21, no. 1, pp. 15–25, 2015.

[29] R. van den Tillaar, V. Andersen, and A. H. Saeterbakken, "The existence of a sticking region in free weight squats," *Journal of Human Kinetics*, vol. 42, no. 1, pp. 63–71, 2014.

[30] R. Van den Tillaar and A. Sæterbakken, "The sticking region in three chest-press exercises with increasing degrees of freedom," *Journal of Strength and Conditioning Research*, vol. 26, no. 11, pp. 2962–2969, 2012.

[31] M. Cardinale, R. Newton, and K. Nosaka, *Strength and Conditioning—Biological Principles and Practical Applications*, John Wiley & Sons, Chichester, UK, 2011.

[32] K. Bloomquist, H. Langberg, S. Karlsen, S. Madsgaard, M. Boesen, and T. Raastad, "Effect of range of motion in heavy load squatting on muscle and tendon adaptations," *European Journal of Applied Physiology*, vol. 113, no. 8, pp. 2133–2142, 2013.

[33] G. E. McMahon, C. I. Morse, A. Burden, K. Winwood, and G. L. Onambélé, "Impact of range of motion during ecologically valid resistance training protocols on muscle size, subcutaneous fat, and strength," *Journal of Strength and Conditioning Research*, vol. 28, no. 1, pp. 245–255, 2014.

23

Validity of a Smartphone-Based Application for Determining Sprinting Performance

Robert Stanton, Melanie Hayman, Nyree Humphris, Hanna Borgelt, Jordan Fox, Luke Del Vecchio, and Brendan Humphries

School of Medical and Applied Sciences, Central Queensland University, Bruce Highway, Rockhampton, QLD 4702, Australia

Correspondence should be addressed to Robert Stanton; r.stanton@cqu.edu.au

Academic Editor: António Ascensão

Recent innovations in smartphone technology have led to the development of a number of applications for the valid and reliable measurement of physical performance. Smartphone applications offer a number of advantages over laboratory based testing including cost, portability, and absence of postprocessing. However, smartphone applications for the measurement of running speed have not yet been validated. In the present study, the iOS smartphone application, *SpeedClock*, was compared to conventional timing lights during flying 10 m sprints in recreationally active women. Independent samples t-test showed no statistically significant difference between *SpeedClock* and timing lights ($t(190) = 1.83$, $p = 0.07$), while intraclass correlations showed excellent agreement between *SpeedClock* and timing lights (ICC (2,1) = 0.93, $p = 0.00$, 95% CI 0.64–0.97). Bland-Altman plots showed a small systematic bias (mean difference = 0.13 seconds) with *SpeedClock* giving slightly lower values compared to the timing lights. Our findings suggest *SpeedClock* for iOS devices is a low-cost, valid tool for the assessment of mean flying 10 m sprint velocity in recreationally active females. Systematic bias should be considered when interpreting the results from *SpeedClock*.

1. Introduction

The use of emerging technologies such as smartphones and tablets offers researchers and coaches opportunities to undertake physical performance assessments in the field, rather than the sports science laboratory. Current smartphone technology includes advanced computing capacity, inertial sensors, a global positioning system, and high speed video capacity [1]. Recently developed smartphone applications (APPs) for sport have capitalised on these advances and are shown to be valid and reliable tools to assess lower limb functional performance during countermovement jump [2, 3], drop jump [3], balance [4, 5], and maximal strength [6] tests. However, while the assessments of jumping performance and muscular strength are important characteristics of human performance, sprint speed is critical for success in a range of activities including football [7] and netball [8]. Yet unlike other physical performance characteristics, the assessment of sprinting capacity has received relatively less attention in the peer-reviewed literature [9].

Although fully automated timing systems using pressure sensitive starting blocks or photo finish recording systems remain the gold standard for the assessment of sprint running performance, such systems are rarely found outside athletic venues. They lack portability and are cost prohibitive to many teams, coaches, and athletes. Dual beam photocell systems are increasingly used due to their lower cost, portability, and capability to wirelessly send data to a handheld receiver. Dual beam systems exhibit greater accuracy compared to single-beam systems and have been recommended over single-beam systems [10]. Recent developments in error detection algorithms to address some of the shortcomings associated with single-beam systems have shown promising results. For example, the SmartSpeed (Fusion Sport, Coopers Plains, Australia), single-beam system with error detection, has been shown to comply with Australia's National Sport Science Quality Assurance standards, which require sprint testing systems to achieve a maximal typical error of 0.05 seconds over 30 m. D'Auria and colleagues [11] showed that the SmartSpeed system achieved a typical error of ≤0.03 seconds at distances of 5, 10, and 20 m.

Studies also show that video analysis of running performance has been shown to closely match fully automated timing systems [12] and dual beam photocell systems [13], even when recorded at 50 or 100 Hz. Therefore, even low-speed video capture may represent a low-cost and portable option to assess running performance. Recent innovations in smartphone technology have seen video capture speeds up to 240 Hz on iPhone 6. Coupled with improved image detection algorithms and computing power, smartphone APPs have been developed to allow coaches and researchers to determine running speed using these popular and low-cost tools. One such APP is *SpeedClock* (http://appmaker.se/?m=5&s=0). *SpeedClock* uses the iOS device camera to detect and record motion and, with the user input of a reference distance, calculates speed. *SpeedClock* can be used on a single standalone device, with the reference frame defined by the edges of the image detection field, or connected via Bluetooth with a second iOS device to record time over longer distances.

Although APPs such as *SpeedClock* are purported to accurately record sprint performance, to the best of our knowledge, there are currently no studies which demonstrate the validity of *SpeedClock*. Such studies are important in confirming the usefulness of emerging technologies and are of great interest to athletes, coaches, and researchers. Therefore, the purpose of the present study is to examine the validity of the *SpeedClock* APP using timing lights as a reference.

2. Methods

2.1. Participants. Participants were a convenience sample of 24 recreationally active females (>18 years) recruited via personal discussion with investigators. An information sheet outlining the purpose, risks, and benefits of participation was provided to all potential participants. Prior to inclusion in the study, participants were screened for musculoskeletal, neurological, or cardiorespiratory concerns which would contraindicate the performance of maximal sprinting, using stage one of the Adult Preexercise Screening System [14]. Written informed consent was obtained from all participants prior to the commencement of data collection. This study was approved by the institutional human research ethics committee.

2.2. Protocols. Participants stature was measured using a Seca 213 portable stadiometer (Seca GMBH, Hamburg) and weight determined using a Seca robusta 813 portable scale (Seca GMBH, Hamburg). All measures were performed according to standardised protocols [15]. All participants underwent a standardised warm-up comprising five minutes of light jogging, static and dynamic stretching, and a series of submaximal sprints. Participants then performed four maximal effort 20 m sprints, separated by five minutes of passive rest. Participants started on a line between the first set of timing lights and commenced the sprint in their own time. Standardised instructions were provided regarding maximal effort and to decelerate only when past the final set of timing lights. All sprints were performed in an indoor sports stadium (~26°C, 50% RH) on a suspended timber floor. Participants wore their usual running shoes and apparel.

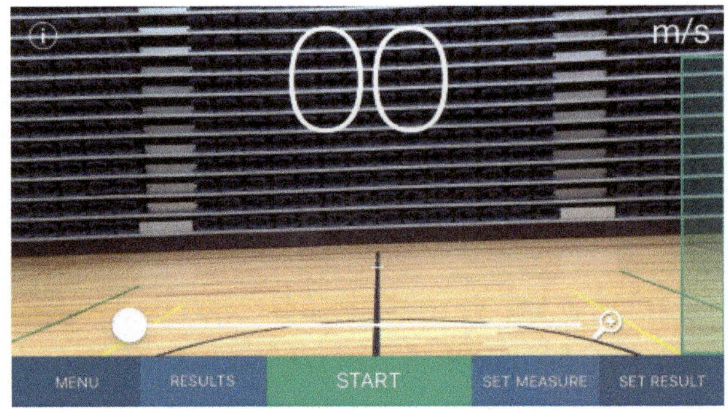

FIGURE 1: Screenshot of iPhone 5c showing motion detection zones at each edge of the field of view.

2.3. Instruments. Sprint times were recorded using SmartSpeed Pro timing lights (Fusion Sport, Coopers Plains, Australia), with gates at zero, 10, and 20 metres. This system uses a single-beam design to improve battery life and ease of setup, however, incorporates novel error detection algorithms to reduce false triggers. In the event of multiple triggers, the algorithm interprets the longest trigger as the true start time. Gates were set at a height of 1.0 m from the floor. Sprint times were converted to mean sprint velocity (m/s) for 0–10 m, 10–20 m, and 0–20 m using a standard linear motion equation ($v = d/t$). To examine the validity of the *SpeedClock* iOS application, the APP was installed on an iPhone 5c running iOS Version 9.2.1 (Apple Corporation, Cupertino, CA), which records video at 60 frames per second. In SpeedM (Motion) mode, the APP incorporates motion detection zones at each edge of the image which trigger and terminate data collection (Figure 1). For the present study, to ensure repeatability of the method and to minimise movement of the device, iPhone was mounted in a plastic tripod mount on a Velbon EX 330 tripod (Velbon Corporation, Tokyo, Japan), with the camera lens 1.0 m from the ground. The tripod was positioned 10.5 m perpendicular to the midpoint between the timing lights at 10 and 20 m, such that the motion detection zones of the application were aligned with the 10 and 20 m timing lights. The tracking sensitivity on the APP was set to 0.92 (arbitrary units) to avoid false triggers from background movement. In this manner, as the participant ran through the timing lights at 10 m, motion detection triggered data acquisition. Similarly, as the participant ran through the timing lights at 20 m, motion detection terminated data acquisition. Figure 2 shows the positioning of the timing lights and iOS device. Mean velocity (m/s) for the flying 10 m sprint was displayed on-screen and manually recorded for later analysis.

2.4. Statistical Analysis. Descriptive statistics were calculated for participant data. All four flying 10 m sprints recorded simultaneously using timing lights and the *SpeedClock* application were used for analysis. Independent sample t-tests

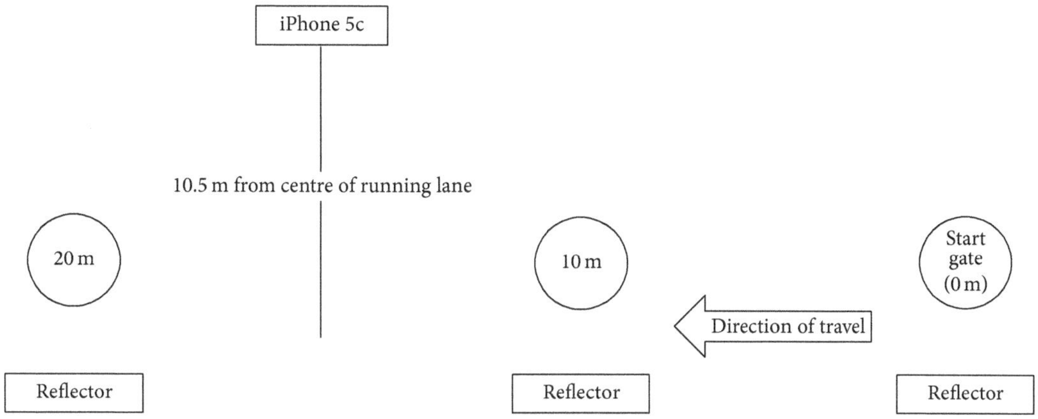

FIGURE 2: Positioning of the timing lights and iOS device.

TABLE 1: Mean flying 10 m sprint times for timing lights and *SpeedClock* APP.

Timing lights	*SpeedClock* APP
6.48 ± 0.49	6.31 ± 0.48

(two-tailed) were used to identify differences in average velocity obtained from the timing lights and *SpeedClock* APP. Between-device agreement was examined using intraclass correlation coefficients (ICC 2,1) with 95% confidence intervals (95% CI) and interpreted according to Munro [16]. Bland-Altman plots were then constructed using Microsoft Excel (Microsoft Corporation, Redmond, USA) to visualise the level of agreement between average velocity obtained from the timing lights and the *SpeedClock* APP. With the exception of Bland-Altman plots, all statistical analyses were performed using Statistical Package for the Social Sciences (SPSS), Version 22 (IBM Corporation, Chicago, Ill). Statistical significance was accepted at an alpha level of $p < 0.05$.

3. Results

Twenty-four recreationally active females (mean age 26.6 ± 5.4 years, mean body mass index 25.0 ± 3.1 kg·m^{-2}) provided informed consent and participated in the study. No adverse events were reported. Results for mean flying 10 m sprint times are shown in Table 1. Independent samples t-test showed no statistically significant difference in mean flying 10 m sprint velocity between data from the timing lights (6.47 ± 0.49 sec) and the *SpeedClock* APP (6.31 ± 0.48 sec) ($t(190) = 1.83$, $p = 0.07$). Intraclass correlations (ICC 2,1) showed excellent agreement in mean flying 10 m sprint velocity between data from the timing lights and the *SpeedClock* APP (ICC (2,1) = 0.93, $p = 0.00$, 95% CI 0.64–0.97). Bland-Altman plots to visualise the difference between mean flying 10 m sprint velocity determined by timing lights and *SpeedClock* APP are shown in Figure 3. A small systematic bias (mean difference = 0.13 seconds) shows the APP consistently gave slightly lower values compared to the timing lights.

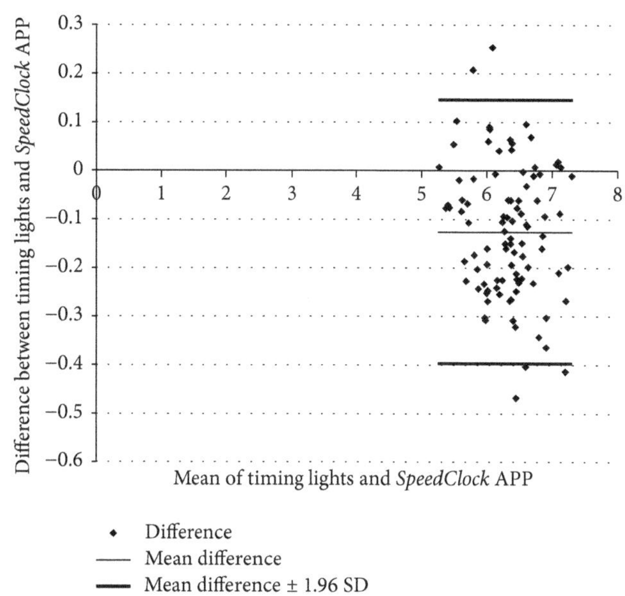

FIGURE 3: Bland-Altman plot depicting the level of agreement between timing lights and *SpeedClock* application for 10 m sprinting.

4. Discussion

To the best of our knowledge, no other studies comparing APP-based measures of sprint running speed have been published in the peer-reviewed literature. As such this study makes an important contribution to the exercise and sports science domain. The findings from the present study suggest that the *SpeedClock* APP installed on an iPhone 5c recording video at 60 frames per second is a valid measure of average flying 10 m sprint velocity in recreationally active females.

A number of other studies have examined the use of video technology in determining sprint running performance. For example, Haugen and colleagues [12] reported no systematic variation between Brower dual beam infrared timing and Dartfish-based video analysis of 40 m sprint times in national level male and female track athletes. In another study, Harrison and colleagues [13] reported the validity of video recorded at 50 Hz and at 100 Hz, to determine mean sprint velocity over 3 m. No statistically significant differences and excellent ICCs were observed between a laser sports measurement system and video recorded at either frame rate. However, at medium to fast sprinting velocities, video recorded at 100 Hz compared more favorably with laser-derived measures than video recorded at 50 Hz, due to the higher sampling rate. In the present study, mean flying 10 m sprit velocity recorded using the *SpeedClock* APP was not significantly different to that recorded using dual beam timing lights. Moreover, ICCs showed excellent agreement with Bland-Altman plots indicating only a small degree of systematic bias, with a mean difference of −0.13 seconds (1.97%). Although this level of mean difference may be significant with respect to changes in sprint performance over time, these values are likely within expected test-retest reliability of sprinting performance, and researchers should examine the smallest worthwhile change in performance to determine if a real change has occurred.

One notable difference between the timing lights and the *SpeedClock* APP is that the timing lights report data to three decimal places, while the *SpeedClock* APP reports data to two decimal places. Therefore, we reran our ICC analysis using velocities based on timing light data under similar conditions, firstly truncated and then rounded to two decimal places. The resultant analyses were not substantially different from our initial findings (ICC (2,1) = 0.92, p = 0.00, 95% CI 0.68–0.97, and 0.93, p = 0.00, 95% CI 0.64–0.97, resp.) and do not change our interpretation of the validity of this APP.

Emerging technologies such as the use of smartphone applications in sport have the potential to provide athletes, coaches, and researchers with additional data not otherwise available with a single laboratory based system. For example, when using *SpeedClock*, an image of the participant can be captured midway through the image capture field. This may provide valuable data to assess running technique, and, since the image is stamped with the mean velocity, it serves as a permanent record of the attempt. Unlike GPS-based system, *SpeedClock* is video-based and therefore can be used indoors. Finally, unlike manual stopwatch timing, the data is not affected by parallax error when standing at the start or finish line, and in the case of *SpeedClock*, two devices can be used together in a manner not unlike timing gates. In general, smartphone-based APPs for sprint performance assessment offer low-cost, portability, and ease of use, not otherwise available with laboratory based systems, and their widespread applicability to training, rehabilitation, and research warrants further investigation.

A strength of the present study is the use of Bland-Altman plots to examine systematic bias between methods used to determine sprint velocity. However, a potential limitation is the use of the iPhone 5c, which records video at 60 frames per second. Future studies should examine the use of high speed video on newer iOS devices as the increased resolution afforded by the higher frame rate may improve accuracy and reduce systematic bias. Future studies should also examine other speed recording APPs on Android operating systems, since, at the present time, *SpeedClock* is only available on iOS and, although iOS devices are widely utilised, they are not the sole software platform. Finally, future studies should examine the validity of the *SpeedClock* or similar APPs over shorter and longer distances and in clinical populations.

5. Conclusions

SpeedClock for iOS devices is a low-cost, valid tool for the assessment of mean flying 10 m sprint velocity in recreationally active females. Further studies are required in different populations and settings to generalise the findings from the present study.

Competing Interests

There is no conflict of interests to declare.

References

[1] M. B. del Rosario, S. J. Redmond, and N. H. Lovell, "Tracking the evolution of smartphone sensing for monitoring human movement," *Sensors*, vol. 15, no. 8, pp. 18901–18933, 2015.

[2] C. Balsalobre-Fernández, M. Glaister, and R. A. Lockey, "The validity and reliability of an iPhone app for measuring vertical jump performance," *Journal of Sports Sciences*, vol. 33, no. 15, pp. 1574–1579, 2015.

[3] F. Gallardo-Fuentes, J. Gallardo-Fuentes, R. Ramírez-Campillo et al., "Inter and intra-session reliability and validity of the My Jump app for measuring different jump actions in trained male and female athletes," *The Journal of Strength and Conditioning Research*, vol. 30, no. 7, pp. 2049–2056, 2016.

[4] R. Z. Amick, A. Chaparro, and J. A. Patterson, "Test-retest reliability of the sway balance mobile application," *Journal of Mobile Technology in Medicine*, vol. 4, no. 2, pp. 40–47, 2015.

[5] J. A. Patterson, R. Z. Amick, T. Thummar et al., "Validation of measures from the smartphone SWAY balance application: a pilot study," *International Journal of Sports Physical Therapy*, vol. 9, no. 2, pp. 135–139, 2014.

[6] C. Balsalobre-Fernández, M. Kuzdub, P. Poveda-Ortiz, and J. D. Campo-Vecino, "Validity and reliability of the push wearable device to measure movement velocity during the back squat exercise," *The Journal of Strength & Conditioning Research*, vol. 30, no. 7, pp. 1968–1974, 2016.

[7] O. Faude, T. Koch, and T. Meyer, "Straight sprinting is the most frequent action in goal situations in professional football," *Journal of Sports Sciences*, vol. 30, no. 7, pp. 625–631, 2012.

[8] J. K. Hewit, J. B. Cronin, and P. A. Hume, "Kinematic factors affecting fast and slow straight and change-of-direction acceleration times," *The Journal of Strength & Conditioning Research*, vol. 27, no. 1, pp. 69–75, 2013.

[9] T. Haugen and M. Buchheit, "Sprint running performance monitoring: methodological and practical considerations," *Sports Medicine*, vol. 46, no. 5, pp. 641–656, 2016.

[10] T. A. Haugen, E. Tønnessen, I. S. Svendsen, and S. Seiler, "Sprint time differences between single- and dual-beam timing systems," *The Journal of Strength & Conditioning Research*, vol. 28, no. 8, pp. 2376–2379, 2014.

[11] S. D'Auria, R. Tanner, J. Sheppard et al., "Evaluation of various methodologies used to assess sprint performance," in *Proceedings of the Australian Institute of Sport Applied Physiology Conference*, ACT, Canberra, Australia, 2006.

[12] T. A. Haugen, E. Tønnessen, and S. K. Seiler, "The difference is in the start: Impact of timing and start procedure on sprint running performance," *The Journal of Strength and Conditioning Research*, vol. 26, no. 2, pp. 473–479, 2012.

[13] A. J. Harrison, R. L. Jensen, and O. Donoghue, "A comparison of laser and video techniques for determining displacement and velocity during running," *Measurement in Physical Education and Exercise Science*, vol. 9, no. 4, pp. 219–231, 2005.

[14] ESSA, *Adult Pre-Exercise Screening System*, Exercise and Sports Science, Brisbane, Australia, 2011.

[15] K. Norton and T. Olds, *Anthropometrica*, UNSW Press, Sydney, Australia, 1996.

[16] B. Munro, *Statistical Methods for Health Care Research*, J. B. Lippincott, Philadelphia, Pa, USA, 1997.

24

Plasma Cytokine Profiles in Long-Term Strenuous Exercise

Hilde G. Nielsen,[1] Olav Øktedalen,[2] Per-Kristian Opstad,[3,4] and Torstein Lyberg[5]

[1] *Division for Society and Health, Department of Health, The Research Council of Norway, P.O. Box 564, 1327 Lysaker, Norway*
[2] *Department of Infectious Medicine, Oslo University Hospital, Ullevål, 0407 Oslo, Norway*
[3] *Norwegian Research Defence Establishment, P.O. Box 25, 2027 Kjeller, Norway*
[4] *Norwegian Military Academy, 0593 Oslo, Norway*
[5] *Department of Medical Biochemistry, Oslo University Hospital, Ullevål, P.O. Box 4956, Nydalen, 0424 Oslo, Norway*

Correspondence should be addressed to Hilde G. Nielsen; hildegrindvik.nielsen@hotmail.com

Academic Editor: Daniel A. Galvao

The open window theory indicates altered immunity 3 to 72 hours after exercise. The J-curve describes the risk of illness in response to exercise. The aim of this study was to examine the secretion of proinflammatory and anti-inflammatory cytokines before and after long-term strenuous exercise. Fourteen marathon and 16 half-marathon runners and 10 military cadets participating in a military ranger-training course were recruited to this study. Within-subject design was used measuring levels of plasma cytokines before, during, and after exercise. Plasma cytokines were measured using Luminex multiplex technology and ELISA. Comparing pre/post plasma levels both the marathon- and the half-marathon runners showed heavily increased levels of IL-6, IL-10, and IL-8 ($P < 0.001$). LPS stimulation among the half-marathon runners decreased the postrace levels of IL-6, IL-1b, and TNFα by 45%, 24%, and 43%, respectively ($P < 0.01$). During the ranger training course the spontaneous and LPS-stimulated levels of IL-6, IL-8, IL-10, IL-1b, and TNFα changed in a similar fashion as in the half-marathon runners although the fluctuations were smaller. Our study supports the open window and the J-curve theory; the immune system is more activated and the subjects are more threatened to infectious pathogens after intensive physical activity and in the period after exercise.

1. Introduction

The open window theory implies that there is altered immunity following an acute bout of exercise, which lasts from three to 72 hours after exercise depending on the parameter measured [1]. According to the theory, there is an increased risk of contracting infectious diseases after physical exercise [2]. The J-curve describes the risk of illness in response to exercise. The "J" means that individuals engaged in moderate physical activity are at lower risk compared with sedentary individuals [3]. On the other side, excessive volumes of strenuous endurance exercise may suppress immune function and thereby enhance the risk of illness [2].

Inflammation is a complex series of events, involving many cell types. It is evident that great numbers of molecules encompass the term "proinflammatory cytokines." These cytokines are produced very early in the response to multiple stresses and are important by being involved in both innate and acquired immunity. They function as intercellular signals that regulate local and systemic responses. Cytokines are characterised as being inducible and belong to different families, including proinflammatory cytokines (IL-1β, IL-2, IL-4, IL-6, IL-8, and TNFα), which are cytokines that promote systemic inflammation, and anti-inflammatory cytokines (IL-5, IL-6, and IL-10), which refer to the property of a substance that reduces and protects against inflammation. Inflammation in excess is detrimental and excessive production and release of TNFα and IL-1β may lead to pathology [4].

Vascular endothelial growth factor (VEGF) is a signal protein produced by cells that stimulates vasculogenesis and angiogenesis. VEGF participates in restoring oxygen supply to tissues when blood circulation is insufficient. Proinflammatory cytokines like IL-1β, IL-6, IL-8, TGF-β, and TNF-α variably increase VEGF expression, depending upon the dose, cell, or tissue type. When VEGF is overexpressed, it can contribute to disease [5].

Regular exercise and its effects may be a prototype of physical stress [6]. Surgery, trauma, burn, and sepsis induce a pattern of hormonal and immunological responses with the same response profile as that of exercise [7]. Earlier studies regarding exercise and effects on immunological parameters indicate that the profiles of proinflammatory and anti-inflammatory cytokine levels are stimulated based on the intensity and duration of the physical exercise [8, 9]. Long-distance runners, for example, marathon runners, have shown high postexercise levels of IL-1β, IL-6, and IL-8 after six hours' endurance exercise [9–11], while there were no changes observed in plasma cytokine levels after a 5-kilometre run [12]. Measurements from cycle ergometer and treadmill running show no response of short-term exercise with high and moderate intensity, an increase in IL-6 after one-hour cycling at 75% of maximal oxygen consumption (VO_2max) and three-hours alternating cycling and treadmill running at 60–65% of VO_2max showed high postexercise values of IL-6, IL-1β, and TNFα [13–15]. Other studies indicate that long-term sleep and energy deficiency lead to immune depression [16, 17].

Microsphere-based multiplexing bioassay system has, during the last few years, become an important tool in cytokine detection. The assay is performed with great speed and accuracy by making use of hundreds of specially prepared magnetic beads, or microspheres, and is reporting on the contents of the sample. This is in contrast to the classical analysis of cytokine expression patterns, which has been performed by enzyme-linked immunosorbent assays (ELISA) for each separate analysis. Very few studies within the field of exercise immunology have so far used the multiplex technology in cytokine detection in relation to exercise or physical activity executed by healthy people.

According to prior reports, we expect in our study that the marathon/half-marathon race and the ranger-training course will lead to immunological responses in the subjects as seen in surgery and sepsis patients.

The aim of this study was to examine the secretion of the cytokines IL-1β, IL-2, IL-4, IL-5, IL-6, IL-8, IL-10, IL-12, TNFα, IFN$_\gamma$, GM-CSF, and VEGF before and after three different trials of physical exercise: the Oslo marathon/half-marathon and a military training course of eight days continuous exercise combined with sleep and energy deprivation. Both the spontaneous secretion of the cytokines and the lipopolysaccharide- (LPS-) induced whole blood stimulation of cytokines were examined.

2. Material and Methods

2.1. Oslo Marathon/Half-Marathon and Norwegian Military Ranger-Training Course. Fourteen men participating in Oslo marathon race (mean age 40; range 29–56), eight women (mean age 36; range 27–39) and eight men (mean age 34; range 30–45) participating in Oslo half-marathon race, and ten physically well-trained male cadets from the Norwegian Military Academy in the age between 21 and 28 years were recruited to this study. The marathon runners were selected based on the previous year's result list with the criterion that the expected running time should be 3 h 30 min; the corresponding criterion for the half-marathon runners was 1 h 30 min for men and 1 h 45 min for women. The runners were on average fit and practiced running as an interest. The race was conducted in cloudy weather with a temperature of about 20°C. The ranger-training course took place in the eastern part of Norway, in a forest area at 500 m altitude. The temperature during the eight days of the course was between 18 and 30°C during daytime and between 5 and 15°C at night. The ranger-training course consisted of military duties during daytime and nighttime [16]. The cadets were provided nearly no food during the course and approximately 3 hours/8 d sleep was allowed [16]. In the restitution period (day 9 through day 11), the cadets followed regular sleeping and eating habits as before the course. The subjects were informed about the study and gave their written informed consent for participation. The Regional Committee for Medical Ethics had approved the test protocols.

2.2. Blood Sampling Protocols. For the marathon runners and the half-marathon runners, blood samples were collected shortly before the race and immediately after the race. For the military cadets, blood samples were collected at the start of the ranger-training course, after 2, 4, and 8 days (end of the ranger-training course), and after one (day 9) and three (day 11) days' recovery. The blood samples from the cadets were taken between 6 and 8 a.m. For all groups, venous blood was sampled into either EDTA-, Na-citrate-, or heparin-anticoagulated vacuum tubes (Becton Dickinson, Plymouth, UK). The blood samples from the ranger-training course were collected in the field, kept on ice, and transported within 60 minutes to the nearest military training camp, Terningmoen, where a temporary laboratory was established. The blood samples from the marathon and the half-marathon runners where collected in the start area of the race, kept on ice, and transported within 30 minutes to Ullevål university hospital. Plasma was separated at 2500 ×g for 10 minutes and samples were stored at −80°C until analysis. To compare the cytokine production capacities of leukocytes, one set of experiments was performed with heparinized whole blood from the half-marathon runners and the ranger-training cadets. The blood samples were stimulated *ex vivo* with the potent cytokine inducer lipopolysaccharide (LPS), 1 μg/mL (*working solution*) (from *Escherichia coli* 026: B6, Sigma St. Louis, Mo, USA) for 6 h at 37°C, before storing plasma samples at −80°C until analysis.

2.3. Haematological Analyses. White blood cell (WBC), platelet and erythrocyte counts, haemoglobin, and haematocrit were assessed in EDTA blood using the Technicon H2•™ System (Bayer Corporation, Tarrytown, NY, USA) at the Department of Medical Biochemistry, Oslo University Hospital, Ullevål.

2.4. Cytokine Analyses

2.4.1. Individual Cytokine Assays. Plasma levels of individual cytokines (IL-1β, IL-6, IL-8, IL-10, and TNFα) were measured using the Quantikine colorimetric sandwich enzyme-linked immunosorbent assays (ELISA) from R&D, Abingdon, UK, according to the manufacturer's instructions.

2.4.2. Multiplex Cytokine Assays. We used the multiplex bead-based sandwich immunoassay technology (Luminex, Austin, TX, USA) and a human cytokine 12-plex kit (R&D), strictly following the manufacturer's instructions, to measure the concentration of the following cytokines before and after the marathon race: IL-1β, IL-2, IL-4, IL-5, IL-6, IL-8, IL-10, IL-12, TNFα, IFN$_\gamma$, GM-CSF, and VEGF.

Unfortunately, we only had the multiplex bead-based sandwich immunoassay technology (Luminex) available for the study with the marathon runners. The levels of cytokine release in the half-marathon runners and the cadets from the ranger-training course were therefore measured using the Quantikine colorimetric sandwich enzyme-linked immunosorbent assays (ELISA).

2.5. Statistical Analyses. Results are given as means and standard errors of the mean (mean, SEM). Data were analysed using one-way ANOVA with Student's t-test. Corrections for multiple uses of the tests were performed *ad modum* Bonferroni. P values of less than 0.05 were considered statistically significant. Difference within groups (marathon and half-marathon) was analysed using two-tailed paired sample t-test. Independent sample t-test was used in order to compare men and women within the half-marathon group. Since we did not observe any statistically significant differences between the women and men, we have chosen to present the results from the half-marathon runners as one group. Paired sample t-test was used to compare results from day 0 to results after 2, 4, and 8 days during the ranger-training course, and after day 1 and 3 days recovery. In the ranger-training course the repeated and longitudinal values obtained before, during, and after the period of exercise which made the subjects being their own controls.

3. Results

3.1. Haematology. The total leukocyte counts (WBC) (10^9/L) increased by 3.2-fold (values before: 5.1, values after: 16.4, $P < 0.01$) after the marathon race, 2.4-fold (values before: 6.3, values after: 15.2, $P < 0.01$) after the half-marathon race, and 1.5-fold (values before: 6.3, values after: 9.5, $P < 0.01$) at the end of the ranger-training course (day 8). After the ranger-training course, WBC were back to normal values after one-day (day 9) recovery. The increase in WBC was mainly due to a significant increase in neutrophils after both of the marathon races and after the ranger-training course, but monocyte counts were also consistently increased in all three experimental settings.

The platelet counts (10^9/L) increased significantly after both the marathon race (values before: 194, values after: 243, $P < 0.01$) and the half-marathon race (values before: 255, values after: 313, $P < 0.05$) and after eight days at the ranger-training course (values before: 214, values after: 265, $P < 0.05$). Baseline platelets values were observed after three days' recovery (day 11).

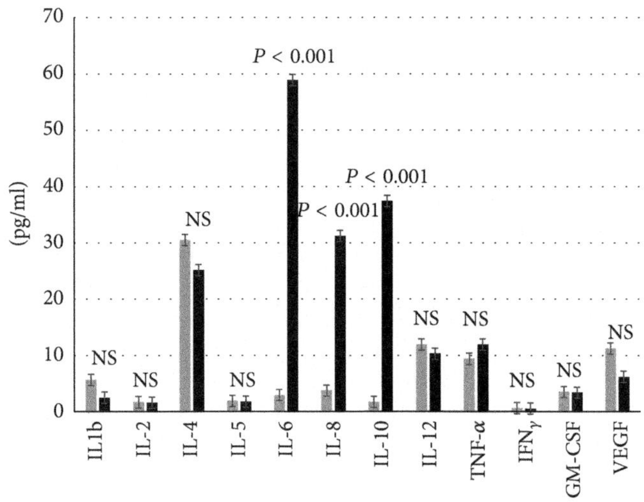

FIGURE 1: Multiplex cytokine analyses (pg/mL) before (grey colour) and after marathon race (black colour). $n = 14$. Data are expressed as mean and standard error of the mean. NS: nonsignificance.

We observed no changes in haemoglobin values after the marathon and the half-marathon races. A slight decrease in haemoglobin values was observed after eight days in the military training course ($P < 0.05$), maintained during the whole recovery period. The haematocrit values remained unchanged after the running races, whereas the values were reduced during days 4–8 of the ranger-training course as well as during the recovery phase.

3.2. Cytokine Profiles

Marathon (Figure 1). We performed a plain analysis of plasma levels of 12 cytokines in 14 individuals before and after a marathon race. Three of these cytokines were heavily increased when comparing pre/post plasma levels: IL-6 (26-fold increase, $P < 0.001$), IL-10 (28-fold increase, $P < 0.000$), and IL-8 (11-fold increase, $P < 0.001$). The other measured cytokines, IL-1β, IL-2, IL-4, IL-5, IL-12, TNFα, IFN$_\gamma$, GM-CSF, and VEGF, did not change significantly after the marathon race.

Half-Marathon (Table 1). In the half-marathon race we demonstrated significantly increased plasma levels of IL-6 (40-fold increase, $P < 0.001$), IL-10 (10-fold increase, $P < 0.001$), and IL-8 (14-fold increase, $P < 0.001$), whereas IL-1β and TNFα were unchanged after the race. When examining LPS-stimulated cytokine levels, IL-6, IL-1β, and TNFα were reduced after the race (IL-6 45% reduced, $P < 0.001$; IL-1β 24% reduced, $P < 0.05$; and TNFα 43% reduced, $P < 0.001$). On the contrary, IL-10 and IL-8 were further increased when LPS stimulation was superposed; IL-10 225% increased, $P < 0.01$, and IL-8 242% increased, $P < 0.001$.

Ranger-Training Course (Tables 2 and 3). The subjects of the ranger-training course showed smaller increase than in the half-marathon race with surprisingly highest levels in the postrace recovery period (Table 2). IL-1β, IL-6, IL-8,

TABLE 1: Individual cytokine analyses before and after half-marathon race. $n = 16$.

Cytokine	Unstimulated samples (pg/mL)			LPS-stimulated samples (ng/mL)		
	Pre	Post	P value	Pre	Post	P value
IL-1β	0.40 ± 0.02	0.5 ± 0.13	NS	72.7 ± 8.1	56 ± 8.0	0.05
IL-6	1.1 ± 0.2	36 ± 6	0.001	74 ± 5	45.4 ± 6.2	0.001
IL-8	1.7 ± 0.1	15.5 ± 1.1	0.01	4.4 ± 0.5	9.5 ± 1.30	0.001
IL-10 (pg/mL)	8.0 ± 0.2	71.8 ± 11.1	0.001	165 ± 28	275 ± 32	0.01
TNF-α	7 ± 3	5.3 ± 0.1	NS	53 ± 6	28.9 ± 4.5	0.001

Data are expressed as mean and standard error of the mean. NS: nonsignificance.

TABLE 2: Individual cytokine analyses (pg/mL) before, during, and after the ranger-training course. Unstimulated samples. $n = 10$.

Cytokines	Unstimulated samples					
	Day 0	Day 2	Day 4	Day 8	Day 9	Day 11
IL-1β	0.23 ± 0.04	0.4 ± 0.1	0.7 ± 0.2*	0.4 ± 0.1*	0.6 ± 0.1$^\$$	1.2 ± 0.2$^\#$
IL-6	2.2 ± 0.3	4.9 ± 1.8	4.3 ± 1.4	4.50 ± 1.02	6.6 ± 1.3*	6.1 ± 2.2
IL-8	1.1 ± 0.1	0.7 ± 0.1	2.0 ± 0.2*	1.5 ± 0.1	3.3 ± 0.3*	1.5 ± 0.1
IL-10	20.8 ± 5.4	28.1 ± 6.1	21.1 ± 2.5	27.2 ± 2.8	36 ± 3*	43.3 ± 1.5$^\#$
TNF-α	1.6 ± 0.1	1.5 ± 0.2	1.4 ± 0.2	1.5 ± 0.2	2.04 ± 0.24*	2.1 ± 0.2$^\$$

Data are expressed as mean and standard error of the mean. $^*P < 0.05$, $^\$P < 0.01$, and $^\#P < 0.001$.

TABLE 3: Individual cytokine analyses (ng/mL) before, during, and after the ranger-training course. LPS-stimulated samples. $n = 10$.

Cytokines	LPS-stimulated samples					
	Day 0	Day 2	Day 4	Day 8	Day 9	Day 11
IL-1β	119.6 ± 21.5	42.7 ± 4.6$^\$$	61.2 ± 7.4*	50.4 ± 6.2*	126.2 ± 22.6	67.4 ± 12.8$^\#$
IL-6	72 ± 4.5	41.1 ± 3.9$^\#$	52.5 ± 4.5$^\#$	41.9 ± 3.6$^\#$	68.1 ± 6.7	52.4 ± 4.6$^\#$
IL-8	11.1 ± 1.5	11.1 ± 1.4	17.4 ± 1.9*	13.1 ± 1.7	10.4 ± 1.2	9.7 ± 0.7
IL-10 (pg/mL)	90 ± 15	170.1 ± 30.5*	485.9 ± 85.5$^\#$	350 ± 90$^\$$	156.8 ± 41.4	90.9 ± 25.1
TNF-α	64.9 ± 8.2	53.2 ± 6.7	62.2 ± 7.8	60.9 ± 8.8	38.5 ± 3.6*	53.3 ± 4.7

Data are expressed as mean and standard error of the mean. $^*P < 0.05$, $^\$P < 0.01$, and $^\#P < 0.001$.

IL-10, and TNFα were all significantly increased at some stage during the course. Additional investigations including LPS stimulation of whole blood showed reduced production capacity for IL-1β, IL-6, and TNFα, whereas the IL-8 and IL-10 levels were further increased in a similar manner as after the half-marathon (Table 3).

4. Discussion

Several studies have observed leukocytosis after physical exercise [2, 18, 19]. Physical exercise leads to an excessive increase in total number of neutrophils immediately and is followed by a slightly smaller increase a few hours after the exercise [20]. In our study, the blood samples were taken immediately after the exercise and only the initial increase in leukocytes was measured. We observed a 3.2-fold and a 2.4-fold increase in leukocytes after the marathon race and the half-marathon race, respectively. At the end of the ranger-training course (day 8), the levels of leukocytes had increased by 1.5-fold. In agreement with former studies we found that the increase in leukocyte counts is primarily due to increase in neutrophils, although monocytes and lymphocytes were increased as well [21]. The first increase in neutrophils is mainly due to release of marginated cells caused by mechanical shear stress and catecholamines [22]. The reason for the different levels of leukocytes in the three exercise trials is probably due to the type and the duration of the activity [21], and this corresponds to earlier studies [23, 24].

Altered levels of cytokines are not only seen in inflammatory diseases. Acute exercise in healthy individuals has an effect on cytokines and the inflammatory response as well [9]. The intensity, duration, and type of physical exercise can all influence proinflammatory and anti-inflammatory cytokines and thereby influence the susceptibility to inflammatory diseases [19]. Ostrowski et al. [4, 25] reported a 2-fold increase in TNFα and IL-1β after a marathon race, in addition to a nearly 100-fold increase in IL-6 values. Exercise studies of three hours' duration performed in laboratories have shown increase in the same parameters [9].

We observed after the marathon and the half-marathon races a 26-fold and a 40-fold increase in IL-6. The magnitude of increase in IL-6 is closely related to the duration of the activity [26], the age of the athlete, the body mass index (BMI), and the physical condition of the person [13, 14]. The participants in our trials were moderate to well-trained individuals executing physical exercise of long duration. The half-marathon runners were on average 5 years younger compared to the marathon runners, they run half the distance of a marathon race, and they probably ran the half-marathon race with higher heart rate compared to the level of intensity of the marathon runners. Our study did not separately measure the effect of running intensity and running duration on the plasma cytokine levels after marathon and half-marathon running.

For the marathon runners we observed 11-fold and 28-fold increase in IL-8 and IL-10, respectively, but no change in TNFα and IL-1β. In the half-marathon runners, we observed a 10-fold increase in IL-10 and 14-fold increase in IL-8, but as for the marathon race, no changes in IL-1β and TNFα values were recorded. It seems that TNFα and IL-1β do not increase exponentially during exercise, which is different when compared to infections [27]. It could be hypothesized that the high levels of the anti-inflammatory cytokines IL-6 and IL-10 in our study might prevent the production of TNF-α and IL-1β after the races.

IL-6 is called an inflammatory responding cytokine described as a proinflammatory cytokine but can also stimulate anti-inflammatory cytokines. IL-6 is highly increased during strenuous physical exercise and thus takes part in the control of the inflammatory response to strenuous physical exercise [25, 28]. The proinflammatory TNFα is known to be inhibited by IL-10 [29] and induced by different stressors [30, 31]. The values obtained after physical exercise are inconstant related to the variations in duration and intensity of the exercise tasks [32].

In the ranger-training course, there was no increase in IL-6 or IL-10 during the period of activity, but, surprisingly, a small increase in the recovery phase (days 9 and 11). IL-1β and IL-8 showed a small increase during the course and in the recovery period. Both IL-1β and TNFα showed elevated values in the postexercise period.

The boosting of cytokine responses in peripheral blood leukocytes by LPS in many ways mimics the initial innate immune response to bacterial infection, LPS stimulation showed that the plasma levels of both IL-6, IL-1β, and TNFα were significantly reduced after the half-marathon race as well as during and after the ranger-training course. This corresponds to the observation made by Abbasi et al. [33] who have observed reduced IL-6, IL-1β, and TNFα- levels in LPS-stimulated samples 30 min and 3 h after exercise in half-marathon runners.

The observed reduction after the half-marathon race and the ranger-training course may be due to either actually reduced production capacity as a result of exercise or at least a temporary change in the regulatory pathways leading to altered cytokine synthesis and release. In contrast, IL-8 and IL-10 were boosted both by the exercise itself and after additional LPS stimulation. It seems that the anti-inflammatory IL-10 production is more triggered in the long-lasting marathon race (28-fold increase) compared with the shorter workload of the half-marathon race (10-fold increase). Furthermore, the IL-6 release was more pronounced in the more work-intensive half-marathon than the longer-lasting but less intensive marathon race (40-fold versus 26-fold increase), possibly being mainly due to a larger release from the muscle mass of the lower extremities [34]. Although a similar cytokine profile was registered in the ranger-training course, the magnitude of cytokine increases was not as impressive as for the corresponding marathon races, again possible due to a lesser work load per time unit as well as the lower work intensity. Regardless, we have in all three experimental settings demonstrated an increase of proinflammatory and anti-inflammatory cytokines, which in many ways are similar to the cytokine profile, which characterises inflammatory and infectious diseases [8, 27]. The balance between proinflammatory and anti-inflammatory cytokines during exercise may lay the ground for potentiation of the inflammatory status by introducing additional coincidental pathogens of both Gram-negative and Gram-positive origin, which thereby can tilt the balance into overt disease. Both LPS of Gram-negative bacteria and lipoteichoic acid (LTA), peptidoglycan, and purified protein derivative (PPD) of Gram-positive bacteria all have a number of biological activities, including also being potent cytokine inducers [35, 36].

Most of the studies do only look at the direct immunological responses occurring immediately after different types of physical activity. The very new part in our study is the three days follow-up after the end of the ranger-training course. The participants responded to a phone questionnaire one to two weeks after the course. None of the respondents reported upper respiratory tract infections or other infectious diseases. It may, however, be noted that the training course was performed at a season of the year where the general burden of common cold or influenza-like disease is at a minimum.

5. Conclusion

In conclusion, our study of long-term physical exercise performed in three different trials showed a significant increase in plasma levels of the cytokines IL-6, IL-8, and IL-10, whereas TNFα and IL-1β levels were unchanged or reduced. Our study supports the open window theory by an "open window" of altered immunity after long-term physical exercise and which lasts for at least 72 hours after the exercise. The results support the J-curve theory; athletes are more sensitive to pathogens in the immediate period after intensive physical exercise, probably due to the exercise-induced inflammatory state that can exaggerate the response to coincidentally occurring pathogens.

Disclosure

Present address of Hilde G. Nielsen is the following: The Research Council of Norway, P.O. Box 564, 1327 Lysaker, Norway.

Competing Interests

The authors wish to declare no conflict of interests that is relevant to the content of this paper.

Acknowledgments

The authors would like to thank the marathon and the half-marathon runners who voluntarily participated in this project and the Norwegian Defence Research Establishment (FFI) for cooperation. Special thanks are due to MLT Lisbeth Saetre for excellent technical and practical assistance and the Foundation ALMUS for economical support.

References

[1] B. K. Pedersen and H. Ullum, "NK cell response to physical activity: possible mechanisms of action," *Medicine and Science in Sports and Exercise*, vol. 26, no. 2, pp. 140–146, 1994.

[2] D. C. Nieman and B. K. Pedersen, "Exercise and immune function. Recent developments," *Sports Medicine*, vol. 27, no. 2, pp. 73–80, 1999.

[3] D. C. Nieman, "Exercise, upper respiratory tract infection, and the immune system," *Medicine and Science in Sports and Exercise*, vol. 26, no. 2, pp. 128–139, 1994.

[4] K. Ostrowski, T. Rohde, M. Zacho, S. Asp, and B. K. Pedersen, "Evidence that interleukin-6 is produced in human skeletal muscle during prolonged running," *The Journal of Physiology*, vol. 508, no. 3, pp. 949–953, 1998.

[5] M. Scianna and L. Preziosi, *Cellular Potts Models: Multiscale Extensions and Biological Applications*, Mathematical and Computational Biology Series, Chapman & Hall/CRC, Taylor & Francis Group, 2013.

[6] B. K. Pedersen, T. Rohde, and M. Zacho, "Immunity in athletes," *Journal of Sports Medicine and Physical Fitness*, vol. 36, no. 4, pp. 236–245, 1996.

[7] G. Camus, G. Deby-Dupont, J. Duchateau, C. Deby, J. Pincemail, and M. Lamy, "Are similar inflammatory factors involved in strenuous exercise and sepsis?" *Intensive Care Medicine*, vol. 20, no. 8, pp. 602–610, 1994.

[8] B. K. Pedersen and A. D. Toft, "Effects of exercise on lymphocytes and cytokines," *British Journal of Sports Medicine*, vol. 34, no. 4, pp. 246–251, 2000.

[9] B. K. Pedersen, "Exercise and cytokines," *Immunology and Cell Biology*, vol. 78, no. 5, pp. 532–535, 2000.

[10] J. P. H. Drenth, S. H. M. Van Uum, M. Van Deuren, G. J. Pesman, J. Van Der Ven- Jongekrijg, and J. W. M. Van Der Meer, "Endurance run increases circulating IL-6 and IL-1ra but downregulates ex vivo TNF-α and IL-1β production," *Journal of Applied Physiology*, vol. 79, no. 5, pp. 1497–1503, 1995.

[11] K. Suzuki, M. Yamada, S. Kurakake et al., "Circulating cytokines and hormones with immunosuppressive but neutrophil-priming potentials rise after endurance exercise in humans," *European Journal of Applied Physiology*, vol. 81, no. 4, pp. 281–287, 2000.

[12] J. P. H. Drenth, R. J. M. Krebbers, J. Bijzet, and J. W. M. Van der Meer, "Increased circulating cytokine receptors and ex vivo interleukin-1 receptor antagonist and interleukin-1β production but decreased tumour necrosis factor-α production after a 5-km run," *European Journal of Clinical Investigation*, vol. 28, no. 10, pp. 866–872, 1998.

[13] H. Ullum, P. M. Haahr, M. Diamant, J. Palmo, J. Halkjaer-Kristensen, and B. K. Pedersen, "Bicycle exercise enhances plasma IL-6 but does not change IL-1α, IL-1β, IL-6, or TNF-α pre-mRNA in BMNC," *Journal of Applied Physiology*, vol. 77, no. 1, pp. 93–97, 1994.

[14] J. A. Smith, R. D. Telford, M. S. Baker, A. J. Hapel, and M. J. Weidemann, "Cytokine immunoreactivity in plasma does not change after moderate endurance exercise," *Journal of Applied Physiology*, vol. 73, no. 4, pp. 1396–1401, 1992.

[15] A. I. Moldoveanu, R. J. Shephard, and P. N. Shek, "Exercise elevates plasma levels but not gene expression of IL-1β, IL-6, and TNF-α in blood mononuclear cells," *Journal of Applied Physiology*, vol. 89, no. 4, pp. 1499–1504, 2000.

[16] P. K. Opstad, "Medical consequences in young men of prolonged physical stress with sleep and energy deficiency," Tech. Rep. 5-89, Norwegian Defence Research Establishment, 1995.

[17] Y. Gundersen, P. K. Opstad, T. Reistad, I. Thrane, and P. Vaagenes, "Seven days' around the clock exhaustive physical exertion combined with energy depletion and sleep deprivation primes circulating leukocytes," *European Journal of Applied Physiology*, vol. 97, no. 2, pp. 151–157, 2006.

[18] R. J. Shephard and P. N. Shek, "Impact of physical activity and sport on the immune system," *Reviews on Environmental Health*, vol. 11, no. 3, pp. 133–147, 1996.

[19] B. K. Pedersen, "Special feature for the Olympics: effects of exercise on the immune system: exercise and cytokines," *Immunology & Cell Biology*, vol. 78, pp. 532–535, 2000.

[20] D. A. McCarthy and M. M. Dale, "The leucocytosis of exercise. A review and model," *Sports Medicine*, vol. 6, no. 6, pp. 333–363, 1988.

[21] H. G. Nielsen, I. A. Hagberg, and T. Lyberg, "Marathon running leads to partial exhaustion of ROS-generating capacity in leukocytes," *Medicine and Science in Sports and Exercise*, vol. 36, no. 1, pp. 68–73, 2004.

[22] A. Bøyum, P. Wiik, E. Gustavsson et al., "The effect of strenuous exercise, calorie deficiency and sleep deprivation on white blood cells, plasma immunoglobulins and cytokines," *Scandinavian Journal of Immunology*, vol. 43, no. 2, pp. 228–235, 1996.

[23] P. J. Robson, A. K. Blannin, N. P. Walsh, L. M. Castell, and M. Gleeson, "Effects of exercise intensity, duration and recovery on in vitro neutrophil function in male athletes," *International Journal of Sports Medicine*, vol. 20, no. 2, pp. 128–135, 1999.

[24] J. M. Peake, "Exercise-induced alterations in neutrophil degranulation and respiratory burst activity: possible mechanisms of action," *Exercise Immunology Review*, vol. 8, pp. 49–100, 2002.

[25] K. Ostrowski, T. Rohde, S. Asp, P. Schjerling, and B. K. Pedersen, "Pro- and anti-inflammatory cytokine balance in strenuous exercise in humans," *The Journal of Physiology*, vol. 515, no. 1, pp. 287–291, 1999.

[26] K. Ostrowski, C. Hermann, A. Bangash, P. Schjerling, J. N. Nielsen, and B. K. Pedersen, "A trauma-like elevation of plasma cytokines in humans in response to treadmill running," *The Journal of Physiology*, vol. 513, no. 3, pp. 889–894, 1998.

[27] A. M. W. Petersen and B. K. Pedersen, "The anti-inflammatory effect of exercise," *Journal of Applied Physiology*, vol. 98, no. 4, pp. 1154–1162, 2005.

[28] D. C. Nieman, C. L. Dumke, D. A. Henson, S. R. McAnulty, S. J. Gross, and R. H. Lind, "Muscle damage is linked to cytokine changes following a 160-km race," *Brain, Behavior, and Immunity*, vol. 19, no. 5, pp. 398–403, 2005.

[29] C. Gérard, C. Bruyns, A. Marchant et al., "Interleukin 10 reduces the release of tumor necrosis factor and prevents lethality in experimental endotoxemia," *The Journal of Experimental Medicine*, vol. 177, no. 2, pp. 547–550, 1993.

[30] J. C. Meltzer, B. J. MacNeil, V. Sanders et al., "Stress-induced suppression of in vivo splenic cytokine production in the rat

by neural and hormonal mechanisms," *Brain, Behavior, and Immunity*, vol. 18, no. 3, pp. 262–273, 2004.

[31] J. D. Johnson, K. A. O'Connor, M. K. Hansen, L. R. Watkins, and S. F. Maier, "Effects of prior stress on LPS-induced cytokine and sickness responses," *American Journal of Physiology—Regulatory Integrative and Comparative Physiology*, vol. 284, no. 2, pp. R422–R432, 2003.

[32] C. Weinstock, D. König, R. Harnischmacher, J. Keul, A. Berg, and H. Northoff, "Effect of exhaustive exercise stress on the cytokine response," *Medicine and Science in Sports and Exercise*, vol. 29, no. 3, pp. 345–354, 1997.

[33] A. Abbasi, E. Fehrenbach, M. Hauth et al., "Changes in spontaneous and LPS-induced ex vivo cytokine production and mRNA expression in male and female athletes following prolonged exhaustive exercise," *Exercise Immunology Review*, vol. 19, pp. 8–28, 2013.

[34] K. Ostrowski, P. Schjerling, and B. K. Pedersen, "Physical activity and plasma interleukin-6 in humans—effect of intensity of exercise," *European Journal of Applied Physiology*, vol. 83, no. 6, pp. 512–515, 2000.

[35] T. Saetre, H. Kähler, S. J. Foster, and T. Lyberg, "Aminoethyl-isothiourea inhibits leukocyte production of reactive oxygen species and proinflammatory cytokines induced by streptococcal cell wall components in human whole blood," *Shock*, vol. 15, no. 6, pp. 455–460, 2001.

[36] I. J. S. Blix, K. Helgeland, E. Hvattum, and T. Lyberg, "Lipopolysaccharide from Actinobacillus actinomycetemcomitans stimulates production of interleukin-1β, tumor necrosis factor-α, interleukin-6 and interleukin-1 receptor antagonist in human whole blood," *Journal of Periodontal Research*, vol. 34, no. 1, pp. 34–40, 1999.

25

The Influence of Methylsulfonylmethane on Inflammation-Associated Cytokine Release before and following Strenuous Exercise

Mariè van der Merwe and Richard J. Bloomer

School of Health Studies, The University of Memphis, Memphis, TN, USA

Correspondence should be addressed to Mariè van der Merwe; mvndrmrw@memphis.edu

Academic Editor: Ian L. Swaine

Background. Inflammation is associated with strenuous exercise and methylsulfonylmethane (MSM) has been shown to have anti-inflammatory properties. *Methods.* Physically active men were supplemented with either placebo or MSM (3 grams per day) for 28 days before performing 100 repetitions of eccentric knee extension exercise. *Ex vivo* and *in vitro* testing consisted of evaluating cytokine production in blood (whole blood and isolated peripheral blood mononuclear cells (PBMCs)) exposed to lipopolysaccharide (LPS), before and through 72 hours after exercise, while *in vivo* testing included the evaluation of cytokines before and through 72 hours after exercise. *Results.* LPS stimulation of whole blood after MSM supplementation resulted in decreased induction of IL-1β, with no effect on IL-6, TNF-α, or IL-8. After exercise, there was a reduced response to LPS in the placebo, but MSM resulted in robust release of IL-6 and TNF-α. A small decrease in resting levels of proinflammatory cytokines was noted with MSM, while an acute postexercise increase in IL-10 was observed with MSM. *Conclusion.* Strenuous exercise causes a robust inflammatory reaction that precludes the cells from efficiently responding to additional stimuli. MSM appears to dampen the release of inflammatory molecules in response to exercise, resulting in a less incendiary environment, allowing cells to still have the capacity to mount an appropriate response to an additional stimulus after exercise.

1. Introduction

Inflammation is a normal biological response to harmful stimuli, including pathogens and sterile tissue damage. The response originates with innate immune cells that sense danger through pattern recognition receptors (PRR) such as Toll-like receptor 4 (TLR4) and respond by producing molecules to initiate the inflammatory cascade that eventually leads to pathogen clearance and tissue repair [1]. This cascade of events is tightly controlled, as chronic inflammation has deleterious consequences and is associated with a plethora of diseases, including cardiovascular disease [2] and rheumatoid arthritis [3].

Methylsulfonylmethane (MSM) is an organosulfur compound that is widely used as a dietary supplement for inflammatory conditions such as osteoarthritis [4] and allergic rhinitis [5]. *In vitro* studies indicate that the anti-inflammatory activity of this compound is mediated by the inhibition of the proinflammatory nuclear factor kappa beta (NF-$\kappa\beta$) signaling pathway and attenuation of the NLR family pyrin domain containing 3 (NLRP3) inflammasome activation, resulting in decreased release of the proinflammatory cytokines such as interleukins IL-1β, IL-6, and IL-8 [6–8]. In addition to pathological conditions, MSM supplementation also alleviates markers of oxidative stress and muscle damage following acute bouts of exercise in a healthy population [9–12]. However, as strenuous exercise also induces an inflammatory response, it is not known what effect MSM has on the inflammatory cytokine production.

Considering the available evidence, we hypothesized that supplementation with MSM would reduce *in vivo* inflammatory cytokine production induced by a single bout of strenuous eccentric exercise—exercise which is known to induce an acute inflammatory response [13, 14]. In order

Table 1: Descriptive characteristics of 40 men assigned to either placebo or MSM.

Variable	Placebo $n = 20$	MSM $n = 20$
Age (yrs)	25.5 ± 1.2	25.1 ± 1.6
Height (cm)	178.8 ± 1.5	176.5 ± 1.4
Weight (kg)	83.6 ± 2.4	84.6 ± 1.5
BMI (kg·m^{-2})	26.1 ± 0.6	27.2 ± 0.5
Knee extensor 1RM (kg)	147.2 ± 4.1	151.9 ± 5.6
Compliance to capsule intake (%)	96.2 ± 1.4	96.6 ± 1.0

Data are mean ± SEM.
No statistically significant differences noted ($p > 0.05$).

to test this hypothesis, we analyzed human blood samples for cytokine production. Specifically, blood from healthy exercise-trained men was collected before and through 72 hours following the completion of an acute bout of strenuous eccentric exercise. In addition to *in vivo* cytokine analysis, blood samples were also stimulated *ex vivo* and *in vitro* with lipopolysaccharide (LPS) to determine changes in cytokine production induced by a Toll-like receptor 4 (TLR4) agonist.

2. Methods

2.1. Subjects. A total of 40 men began the study and completed testing. Subjects were healthy, physically active, and nonsmokers and did not have any cardiovascular or metabolic disorders. All subjects were required to have been performing resistance exercise for a minimum of six months prior to beginning the study, with at least one day per week of lower body resistance exercise. They were not using nutritional supplements or medications that may have impacted inflammatory status. If subjects were noted upon screening to be using supplements or medications thought to impact outcome measures, they were required to cease use for at least three weeks prior to the start of the study. Subject characteristics are provided in Table 1. As can be seen, the mean body mass index is greater than 25 kg/m^2. However, due to the exercise training status of subjects, many were muscular and carried more body mass because of this. By no means were these subjects carrying a significant amount of body fat. Subjects were informed of all procedures, potential risks, and benefits associated with the study, the procedures were approved by the University Institutional Review Board for Human Subjects Research, and subjects provided written informed consent.

2.2. Supplementation. This study involved a double-blind, placebo-controlled design in which a total of 40 subjects completed testing (*in vivo* portion only). Subjects were assigned to MSM ($n = 20$; 3 grams per day; OptiMSM®, Bergstrom Nutrition, Vancouver, WA) or placebo ($n = 20$; rice flour) capsules to ingest daily for four weeks, in addition to the three days following the exercise bout. The rice flour placebo has been used in many prior studies and noted to be inert. Compliance to intake was determined by counting capsules upon bottle return. Subjects assigned to each condition were matched based on age and body mass in an effort to retain similarity between the MSM and placebo groups.

2.3. Exercise Bout and Collection of Blood Samples. Subjects performed 10 sets of 10 repetitions (or repetitions to failure) of eccentric knee extension using roughly 100% of concentric one-repetition maximum, with a 2-minute rest period between sets. During the exercise, the weight on the apparatus was raised by the investigators to a level where the knees were fully extended. The subject then lowered the weight under control on a 4-second count (using a metronome) to the ending position. If the subject was unable to lower the weight over a 4-second count, the weight was reduced by approximately 10% for the remaining sets to maintain the repetitions at 10 per set. Several days prior to performing the actual exercise protocol, subjects were familiarized with the knee extension apparatus and performed dynamic repetitions in an attempt to prepare for the actual test session.

Before (Baseline 1) and following the 4-week supplementation period (Baseline 2), as well as at 0, 24, 48, and 72 hours after exercise, a venous blood sample was obtained from a forearm vein. Whole blood collected into ethylenediaminetetraacetic acid (EDTA) tubes was removed and treated accordingly for *ex vivo* and *in vitro* analysis ($n = 2$, placebo; $n = 3$, MSM). Blood collected into tubes containing no additive was allowed to clot at room temperature for 30 minutes and was then centrifuged to obtain serum and stored at −70°C until analyzed for cytokines.

2.4. Ex Vivo Analysis. As a pilot experiment and using a sample of only 5 of the 40 subjects, blood was collected and analyzed. For whole blood LPS stimulation, 250 μL of whole blood was incubated in a 96-well U-bottom plate with 50 μL culture media (RPMI 1640, Pen/Strep, and 10% fetal bovine serum (FBS)) containing LPS to a final concentration of 0.2 μg/mL. For unstimulated control samples, 50 μL of culture media was added to 250 μL of whole blood. All samples were incubated at 37°C for 24 h in a humidified environment containing 5% CO_2. After incubation, supernatants were collected after centrifugation and stored at −70°C.

Cytokine concentrations were measured using a Millipore multiplex magnetic bead system and a MAGPIX® analyzer. Antibodies for the following analytes were used: IL-1β, IL-17a, TNF-α, IL-8, IFN-γ, IL-10, IL-6, and MCP-1.

2.5. In Vitro Analysis. Peripheral blood mononuclear cells (PBMCs) were isolated using Ficoll (Ficoll-Paque PLUS, GE Healthcare Life Sciences) according to manufacturer's instructions. Cell number was determined and cells were diluted in culture media (RPMI 1640, Pen/Strep, and 10% FBS). 300,000 cells were plated per well in a 96-well U-bottom plate. LPS was added to a final concentration of 0.2 μg/mL. As an unstimulated control, cells were also incubated in culture media in the absence of LPS. Cells were incubated at 37°C for 24 h in a humidified environment containing 5% CO_2. After incubation, the supernatant was collected and stored at −70°C.

Cytokine concentrations were measured using a Millipore multiplex magnetic bead system and a MAGPIX analyzer. Antibodies for the following analytes were used: IL-1β, IL-17a, TNF-α, IL-8, IFN-γ, IL-10, IL-6, and MCP-1.

2.6. In Vivo Analysis. Whole blood was analyzed for cytokines using a MILLIPLEX MAP human custom cytokine magnetic bead panel including analytes for the following cytokines: IL-10, IL-17a, IL-1β, Il-6, IL-8, and TNF-α (EMD Millipore; HCYTOMAG-60K). Serum was used without dilution according to the manufacturer's instructions and analytes were quantified using MAGPIX and xPONENT software. All assays were performed in duplicate on the first thaw.

2.7. Statistical Analysis. For *in vivo* testing, cytokines were analyzed using repeated measures analysis of variance (RMANOVA), using data obtained from preexercise (Baseline 2 only) and all postexercise times. Tukey *post hoc* tests were used as needed. Baseline 1 and Baseline 2 values were compared using analysis of variance. Statistical significance for all tests was set at $p \leq 0.05$.

For *ex vivo* and *in vitro* analysis, statistical significance was not determined, as there were only $n = 2$ (placebo) and $n = 3$ (MSM). Mean ± SEM was calculated using GraphPad Prism 6.

3. Results

3.1. Ex Vivo. Exercise is a physiological stress that results in systemic alterations in hormones and cytokines and also affects leukocyte functionality and survival [15]. To determine the role of MSM in exercise-induced changes in leukocytes response, whole blood cultures (where blood was collected before and after exercise) were incubated with or without LPS and secreted cytokine levels determined. In the absence of MSM and LPS, exercise induced an acute increase in IL-1β and IL-6, with maximum response immediately after exercise (time = 0) and a return to baseline at 24 h. However, in the presence of MSM, this exercise-induced response is dampened immediately after exercise but appears to increase at later time points (24 h and 48 h after exercise) (Figures 1(a) and 1(b)). In addition, TNF-α and IL-8 appear to have a delayed cytokine response with maximum production at 48 h after exercise (Figures 1(c) and 1(d)).

In these experiments, LPS is used as a stimulus for *ex vivo* whole blood cultures to determine responsiveness of leukocytes present in the blood before and after exercise in the presence or absence of MSM. As whole blood is used for this experiment, MSM would be present in the soluble fraction. Incubation of whole blood (collected before exercise, baseline) with LPS induced robust release of IL-1β, IL-6, TNF-α, and IL-8 (Figures 2(a)-2(b)). This is consistent with LPS being a TLR4 agonist and inducing inflammatory cytokine synthesis and release. To normalize for cytokine levels present in blood plasma without LPS addition, fold changes in cytokine levels were calculated. MSM supplementation very efficiently suppressed IL-1β induction but was unable to suppress IL-6, TNF-α, and IL-8 to the same extent (Figure 2(b)).

We next determined the effect of MSM supplementation on LPS-induced cytokine levels after exercise from whole blood collected immediately after (time 0) and 24 h, 48 h, and 72 h hours after exercise (Figure 3). In the placebo group, there was a dramatic reduction in LPS-induced IL-1β and IL-6 secretion immediately after exercise (Figures 3(a) and 3(b)). Surprisingly, MSM appears to protect against this loss with IL-1β levels comparable to baseline and an increase in IL-6 secretion immediately after exercise in the MSM supplemented group (MSM *versus* placebo; 3104.233 pg/mL ± 1036.124 *versus* 1334.280 pg/mL ± 926.401). Neither exercise nor MSM appeared to influence the levels of LPS-induced TNF-α and IL-8 (Figures 3(c) and 3(d)).

To determine whether this induction is specific to IL-1β and IL-6, we also determined the effect of LPS on additional cytokines associated with tissue damage and inflammation. LPS did not induce the secretion of IL-17α, IFN-γ, and MCP-1 (data not shown).

IL-10 is a cytokine that can repress proinflammatory responses and limit unnecessary tissue damage. In whole blood samples incubated for 24 h in the absence of LPS, IL-10 levels were very low/undetectable (Figure 4). Similar to what was seen for IL-6, the placebo group had an increase in IL-10 immediately after exercise as seen in samples not stimulated by LPS (Figure 4 (−LPS)). This is consistent with the fact that both pro- and anti-inflammatory molecules are released in response to exercise with the goal of inducing and then resolving inflammation. With LPS stimulation of these samples, IL-10 is induced to the same extent for both groups, with a greater absolute increase in the MSM supplemented group at 24 hours after exercise (Figure 4, MSM (+LPS)).

3.2. In Vitro. To control for confounding factors present in the soluble fraction of blood and also to normalize for cell numbers, PBMCs were isolated from blood collected at time points mentioned earlier. *In vitro* cultures of PBMCs were corrected for cell number and incubated in tissue culture media in the presence or absence of LPS for 24 h. In addition to the loss of soluble factors, MSM would also not be present in these cultures. In cultures of PBMCs isolated from blood collected before exercise, LPS efficiently induced the secretion of IL-1β, IL-6, and TNF-α as seen in Figures 5(a)–5(c). Contradictory to the results from the *ex vivo* cultures, LPS-induced IL-1β secretion in preexercise cultures is more similar between the placebo and the MSM groups (Figure 5(a)), suggesting that there is a loss of the anti-inflammatory capability when culturing in tissue culture media. This result further implies that MSM present in the soluble fraction is responsible for inhibition of LPS-induced IL-1β secretion. In addition, cultured isolated PBMCs did not have the dramatic loss of LPS-induced cytokines immediately after exercise (Figures 5(a) and 5(b)), suggesting that, rather than loss of function, there is loss of leukocytes with exercise resulting in reduced cytokine release. Interestingly, IL-6 levels were still robustly induced with LPS in the MSM supplemented group immediately after exercise (Figure 5(b)). This is consistent with what is seen in the whole blood incubation, with IL-6 secretion not being suppressed by MSM but rather augmented by exercise. There was no difference between

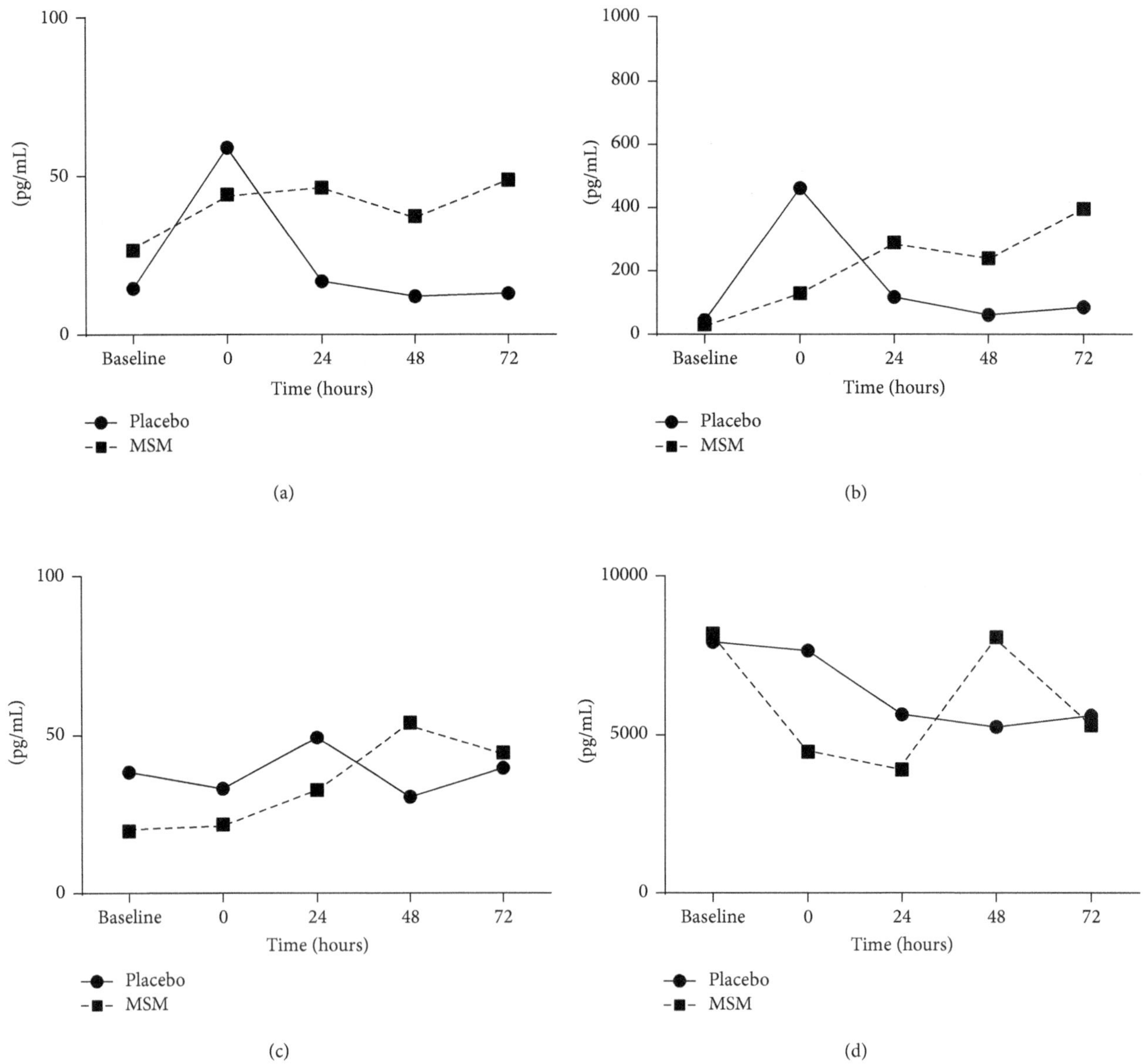

FIGURE 1: Reduced induction of inflammatory cytokines with MSM supplementation immediately after exercise. IL-β (a), IL-6 (b), TNF-α (c), and IL-8 (d) concentrations (pg/mL) were determined in whole blood *ex vivo* cultures from blood collected at baseline (24 h before exercise), immediately after exercise (Time 0), and then at 24 h, 48 h, and 72 h after exercise. Results represent mean ($n = 2$, placebo; $n = 3$, MSM).

the placebo and MSM supplemented groups for TNF-α (Figure 5(c)), IL-8 (data not shown), and IL-10 (Figure 5(d)).

3.3. In Vivo. For the *in vivo* testing, the following was noted: no condition ($p = 0.42$), time ($p = 0.99$), or interaction ($p = 0.91$) effect was noted for IL-6. No condition ($p = 0.19$), time ($p = 0.71$), or interaction ($p = 0.97$) effect was noted for IL-8. A condition effect was noted for IL-10 ($p = 0.001$), with values higher for MSM compared to placebo. No time effect ($p = 0.96$) or interaction effect ($p = 0.95$) was noted. A condition effect was noted for IL-17 ($p = 0.0005$), with values lower for MSM compared to placebo. No time effect ($p = 0.64$) or interaction effect ($p = 0.77$) was noted. A condition effect was noted for IL-1β ($p = 0.0003$), with values higher for MSM compared to placebo. No time effect ($p = 0.92$) or interaction effect ($p = 0.91$) was noted. A condition effect was noted for TNF-α ($p < 0.0001$), with values higher for MSM compared to placebo. A trend for a time effect was noted ($p = 0.08$). No interaction effect was noted ($p = 0.95$). Data are presented in Table 2.

4. Discussion

In the current study, we determined the effect of MSM supplementation on cytokine release in response to exercise and how it alters the response of leukocytes to an additional stimulus in the form of LPS. Blood was collected from healthy subjects before and after exercise. Cytokine release

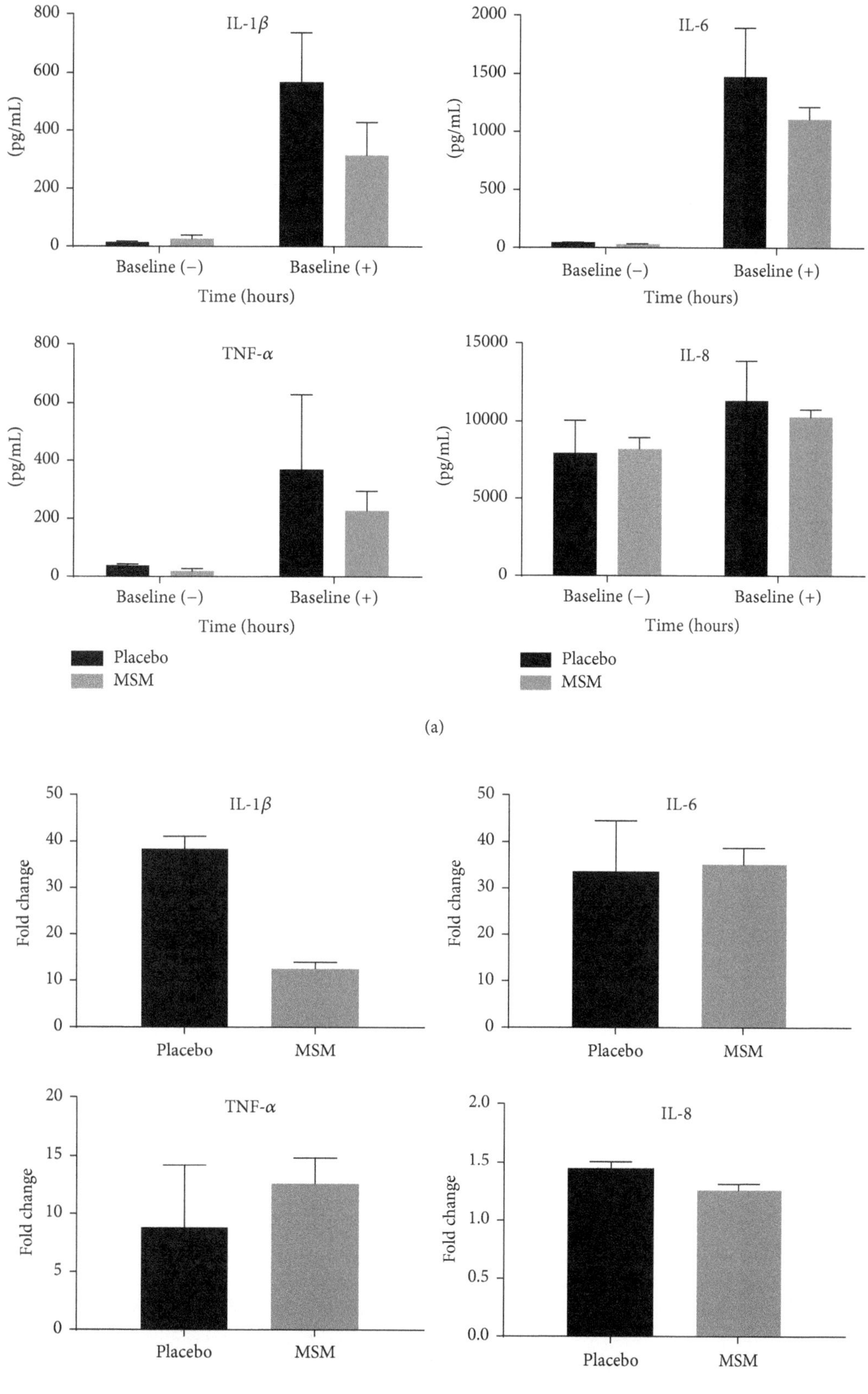

Figure 2: MSM reduces LPS-induced IL-1β secretion. Cytokine secretion was determined after LPS stimulation of *ex vivo* whole blood cultures and measured by Luminex multiplex bead assay. (a) In the absence of exercise, LPS induces robust release of IL-1β, IL-6, TNF-α, and IL-8. (b) Data from (a) are expressed as fold change from unstimulated samples. Results represent mean ± SEM (n = 2, placebo; n = 3, MSM).

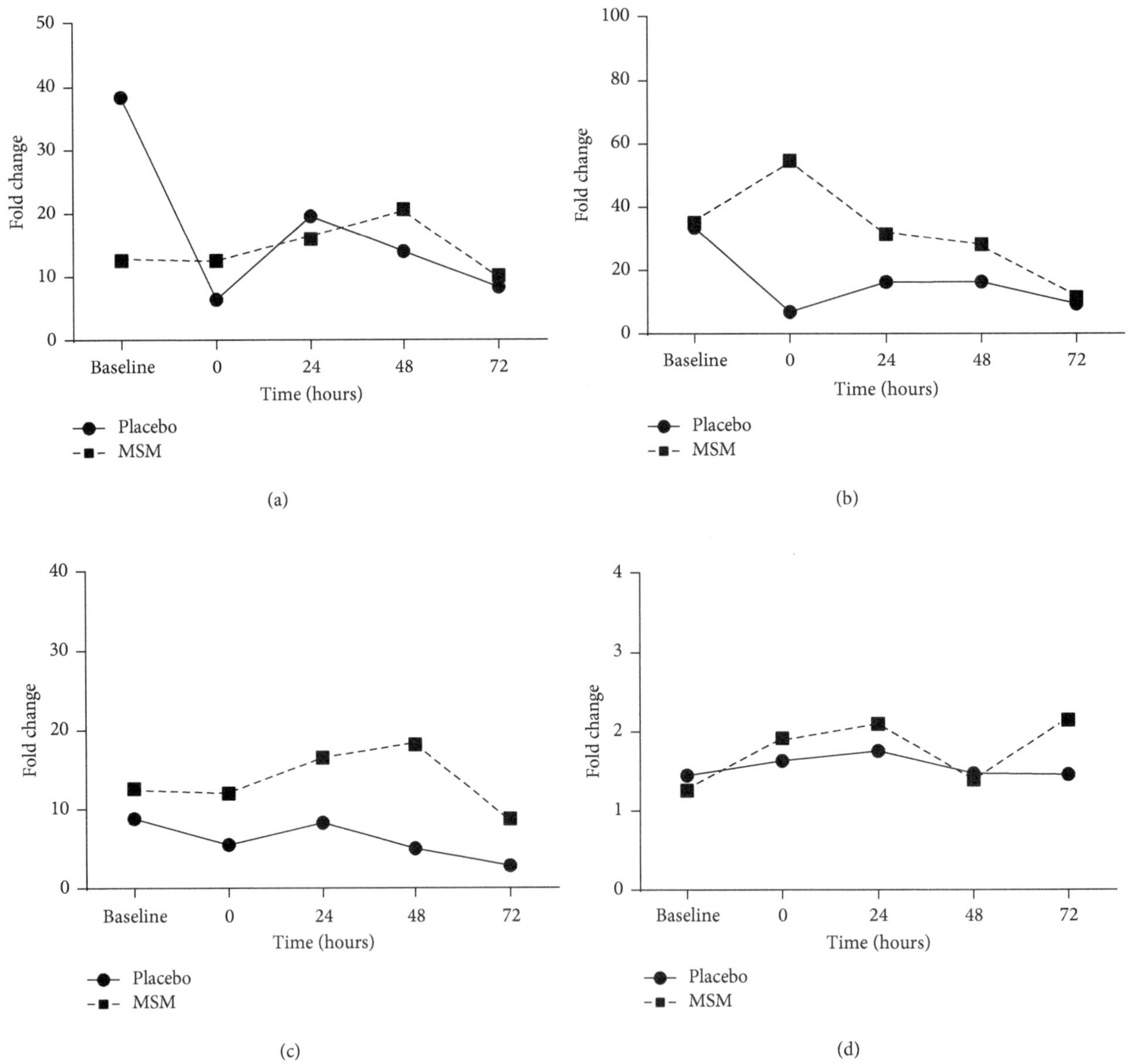

FIGURE 3: Exercise alters cytokine response to LPS. IL-1β (a), IL-6 (b), TNF-α (c), and IL-8 (d) induced by LPS, with MSM supplementation allowing for more efficient release of IL-6 and TNF-α after exercise. Data are represented as fold change from unstimulated samples. Results represent mean ± SEM ($n = 2$, placebo; $n = 3$, MSM).

was determined *ex vivo*, where whole blood was exposed to LPS; *in vitro*, isolated PBMCs exposed to LPS; and *in vivo*, where systemic cytokine levels were determined for each subject at different time points after exercise.

Consistent with previous data suggesting that MSM acts as an antioxidant [9–11], MSM was able to dampen the acute induction of IL-1β and IL-6 to an intense bout of exercise. Using LPS as a second stimulus, whole blood collected before exercise was stimulated and could very efficiently induce IL-1β, IL-6, TNF-α, and IL-8. However, MSM supplementation specifically inhibited the secretion of IL-1β and possibly IL-6 and TNF-α, but to a lesser extent. This reduction is also consistent with previous *in vitro* results demonstrating that MSM blocked IL-1β secretion from LPS-primed bone marrow-derived macrophages [6].

To determine the effect of MSM on exercise-induced changes in leukocytes, blood was also collected after exercise and stimulated with LPS to determine whether MSM supplementation alters the immune cell response after a stressor such as exercise. The acute bout of exercise resulted in a dramatic reduction in LPS-induced IL-1β, IL-6, and TNF-α after exercise in the placebo group. Interestingly, MSM supplementation protected against this loss and the LPS-induced response was similar to baseline levels for the MSM group. This immunosuppressed phenotype can be a consequence of changes in the soluble fraction of the blood, including differences in hormones or additional cytokine that was not measured. Intense bouts of exercise can also cause a decrease in TLR4 expression, decreasing response potential of the leukocytes [16]. In addition, it might also result from changes

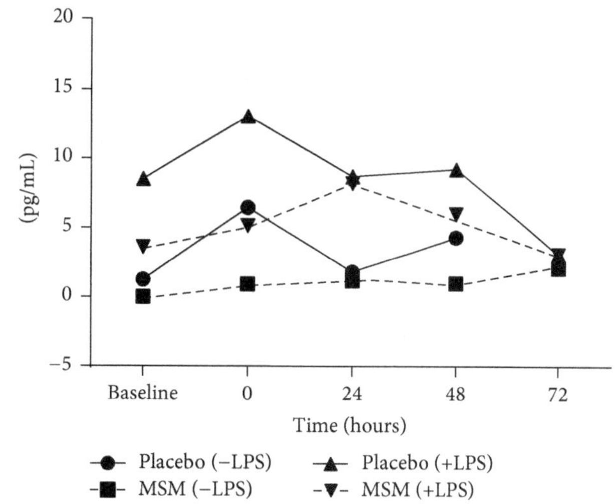

FIGURE 4: Induction of IL-10 by exercise and LPS in *ex vivo* cultures. Results represent mean ± SEM ($n = 2$, placebo; $n = 3$, MSM).

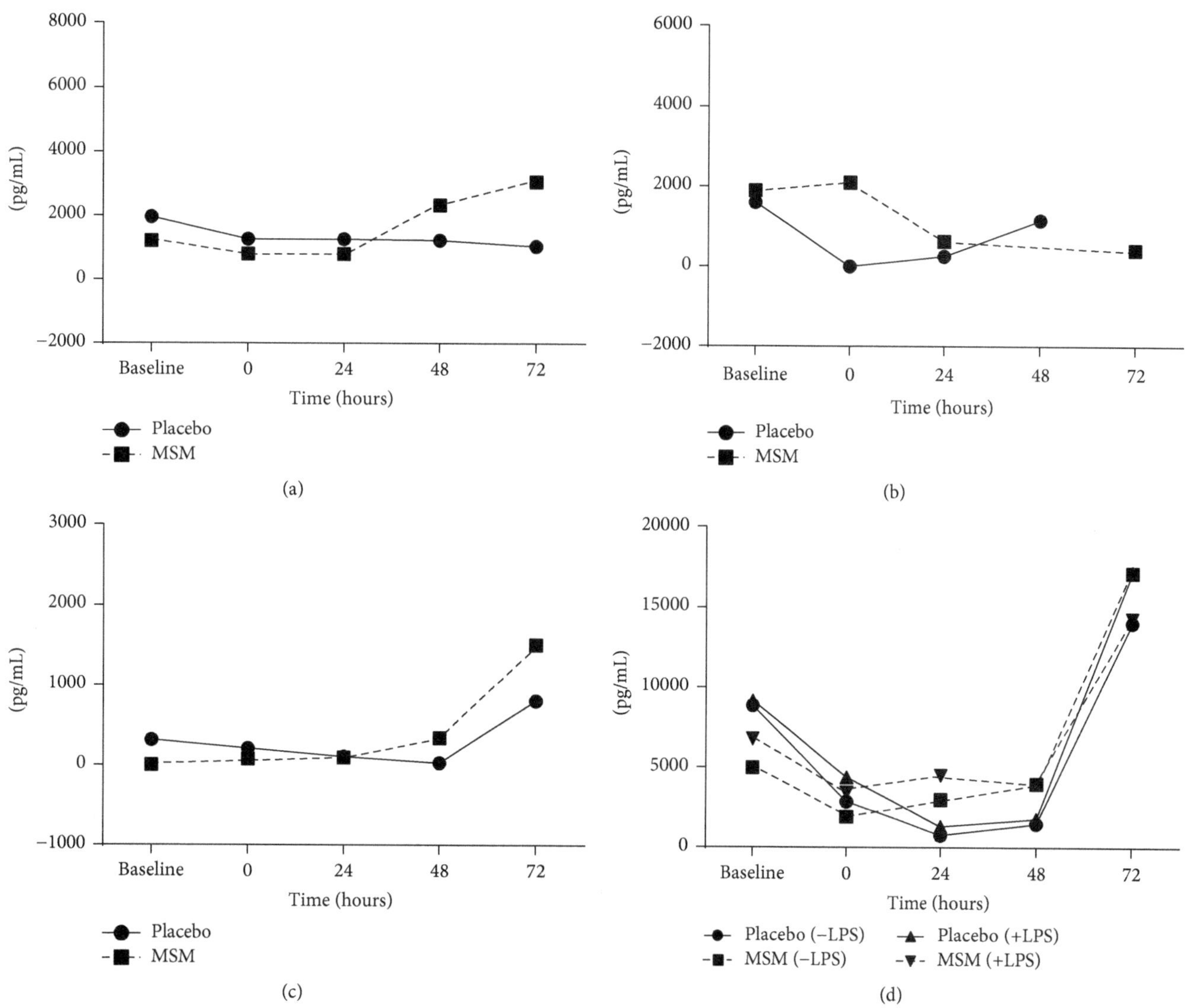

FIGURE 5: IL-1β (a), IL-6 (b), TNF-α (c), and IL-10 (d) release from *in vitro* LPS-stimulated PBMCs isolated from blood collected before (baseline) or after (0 h, 24 h, 48 h, and 72 h) exercise. Results represent mean ± SEM ($n = 2$, placebo; $n = 3$, MSM).

Table 2: Blood cytokine data of 40 men assigned to either placebo or MSM for four weeks.

	Baseline 1	Baseline 2	At 0 hrs	After 24 hrs	After 48 hrs	After 72 hrs
IL-6 ($pg{\cdot}mL^{-1}$) *Placebo*	10.3 ± 5.0	18.3 ± 7.2	16.8 ± 6.9	15.4 ± 6.3	19.1 ± 9.5	17.6 ± 11.2
IL-6 ($pg{\cdot}mL^{-1}$) *MSM*	14.4 ± 4.4	11.6 ± 2.9	16.0 ± 3.1	17.9 ± 4.5	13.7 ± 3.5	13.9 ± 3.5
IL-8 ($pg{\cdot}mL^{-1}$) *Placebo*	32.8 ± 10.0	39.7 ± 14.6	46.4 ± 15.9	30.7 ± 12.3	31.2 ± 13.7	41.3 ± 14.9
IL-8 ($pg{\cdot}mL^{-1}$) *MSM*	28.3 ± 6.1	24.0 ± 5.4	37.6 ± 8.3	30.2 ± 5.6	24.5 ± 4.4	29.6 ± 7.2
IL-10 ($pg{\cdot}mL^{-1}$)* *Placebo*	6.1 ± 1.6	6.5 ± 1.7	5.7 ± 1.2	6.2 ± 1.5	4.8 ± 1.1	6.0 ± 1.5
IL-10 ($pg{\cdot}mL^{-1}$) *MSM*	22.6 ± 8.1	17.7 ± 6.6	26.8 ± 9.4	19.3 ± 6.8	18.4 ± 7.0	18.1 ± 6.9
IL-17 ($pg{\cdot}mL^{-1}$)* *Placebo*	54.3 ± 15.3	65.7 ± 22.2	72.9 ± 26.3	42.6 ± 13.6	47.2 ± 16.8	69.5 ± 25.1
IL-17 ($pg{\cdot}mL^{-1}$) *MSM*	27.3 ± 8.4	24.4 ± 7.2	33.5 ± 8.2	30.1 ± 7.7	22.8 ± 5.0	28.5 ± 6.9
IL-1β ($pg{\cdot}mL^{-1}$)* *Placebo*	3.7 ± 1.1	2.7 ± 0.8	2.8 ± 0.8	2.8 ± 0.7	3.3 ± 1.1	3.3 ± 1.0
IL-1β ($pg{\cdot}mL^{-1}$) *MSM*	10.8 ± 3.2	10.4 ± 3.2	15.5 ± 4.6	18.7 ± 7.6	15.8 ± 5.8	12.0 ± 3.4
TNF-α ($pg{\cdot}mL^{-1}$)* *Placebo*	3.3 ± 0.8	2.1 ± 0.4	3.4 ± 0.6	2.3 ± 0.7	2.3 ± 0.6	2.7 ± 0.8
TNF-α ($pg{\cdot}mL^{-1}$) *MSM*	4.8 ± 0.6	3.8 ± 0.5	5.9 ± 0.6	4.7 ± 0.7	4.1 ± 0.5	4.6 ± 0.7

Values are mean ± SEM.
*Condition effect for IL-10 ($p = 0.001$), IL-17 ($p = 0.0005$), IL-1β ($p = 0.0003$), and TNF-α ($p < 0.0001$).
No other statistically significant effects noted ($p > 0.05$).

in leukocyte number due to redistribution or apoptosis, as previous studies [17] have shown that intense exercise leads to leukopenia, depending on exercise and intensity.

As we did not determine leukocyte number in the *ex vivo* cultures, PBMCs were isolated and equal cell numbers stimulated with LPS to see whether the results mimic the *ex vivo* cultures. These cultures were incubated in tissue culture media thereby removing any incongruent factors that might be present in the soluble fraction of the whole blood culture. IL-1β was again very efficiently induced by LPS in the PBMC cultures. Contradictory to the *ex vivo* cultures, cells from the MSM group responded similarly to the placebo group. As MSM is not present in the PBMC cultures (still present in the plasma in the *ex vivo* cultures), our data suggests that MSM is responsible for the inhibitory effect on IL-1β. However, we cannot rule out the fact that there are additional molecules in the soluble fraction that might influence the IL-1β release.

Of great importance is the fact that the PBMC cultures did not have a significant difference between the placebo and MSM group immediately after exercise, as seen with the *ex vivo* cultures, where there was a dramatic loss of responsiveness to LPS in the placebo group. This suggests that the decrease in LPS-induced cytokines in the placebo group reflects reduction in cell number. As there is no decrease from baseline to time 0 for the MSM group in *ex vivo* cultures, our data also suggests that MSM is protecting against exercise-induced leukopenia. Interestingly, LPS-induced IL-6 induction was as efficiently induced in *ex vivo* cultures as isolated PBMCs, indicating that the leukocytes have been primed previously to release IL-6 by the exercise-induced environment and that MSM does not inhibit this release of IL-6. IL-6 can act as a myokine and a proinflammatory cytokine and might be beneficial when released after a bout of tissue damaging exercise.

In vivo inflammatory markers were not different between MSM and placebo, with a great deal of variability across subjects in most measures (Table 2). While not statistically significant, MSM treatment tended to reduce resting proinflammatory cytokines (e.g., IL-6, IL-8, and IL-17) when viewing the change from Baseline 1 to Baseline 2, while these values increased with placebo treatment. In response to exercise, proinflammatory cytokines increased and gradually decreased from Baseline 2 through the postexercise period with a similar pattern in both groups. An anti-inflammatory cytokine (IL-10) increased immediately after eccentric exercise in the MSM group (51%) and decreased slightly in the placebo group. It was reported that IL-10 is increased in response to exercise which induces muscle damage [18] and this can act as an anti-inflammatory mediator by downregulating proinflammatory cytokines such as IL-1β and TNF-α [19]. The present study noted that IL-10 levels were correspondingly elevated after exercise, possibly to compensate for damage-induced increase in proinflammatory cytokines. This trend occurred only in the MSM group but not in the placebo group. Based on our observation, while only speculative, MSM supplementation may improve resting systemic inflammatory status while simultaneously sensitizing the acute anti-inflammatory response to eccentric exercise.

It should be noted that inflammation was only analyzed in blood samples. It is possible that inflammation may have been elevated in skeletal muscle. Our failure to include skeletal muscle samples for analysis may be considered a limitation of this work.

5. Conclusions

Taken together, these data suggest that an intense bout of exercise causes muscle damage that induces a robust inflammatory reaction that results in exercise-induced leukocyte death and temporary immunosuppression. MSM, acting as an antioxidant, is able to blunt tissue damage and the resulting inflammation and, as a consequence, prevent leukocyte apoptosis. As inflammation induced by exercise may cause prolonged muscle soreness, these data are in agreement with the results noting a reduction in muscle soreness after exercise with MSM supplementation [11]. Based on these results, we speculate that MSM taken during intense bouts of exercise would reduce postexercise immunosuppression.

Competing Interests

The authors declare that they have no competing interests.

Acknowledgments

This work was partially funded by Bergstrom Nutrition and the University of Memphis. Appreciation is extended to Matt Butawan for assistance in manuscript preparation.

References

[1] A. Mantovani, A. Sica, and M. Locati, "Macrophage polarization comes of age," *Immunity*, vol. 23, no. 4, pp. 344–346, 2005.

[2] E. Golia, G. Limongelli, F. Natale et al., "Inflammation and cardiovascular disease: from pathogenesis to therapeutic target," *Current Atherosclerosis Reports*, vol. 16, no. 9, article 435, 7 pages, 2014.

[3] R. Holmdahl, V. Malmström, and H. Burkhardt, "Autoimmune priming, tissue attack and chronic inflammation—the three stages of rheumatoid arthritis," *European Journal of Immunology*, vol. 44, no. 6, pp. 1593–1599, 2014.

[4] P. R. Usha and M. U. R. Naidu, "Randomised, double-blind, parallel, placebo-controlled study of oral glucosamine, methylsulfonylmethane and their combination in osteoarthritis," *Clinical Drug Investigation*, vol. 24, no. 6, pp. 353–363, 2004.

[5] E. Barrager and A. G. Schauss, "Methylsulfonylmethane as a treatment for seasonal allergic rhinitis: additional data on pollen counts and symptom questionnaire," *The Journal of Alternative and Complementary Medicine*, vol. 9, no. 1, pp. 15–16, 2003.

[6] H. Ahn, J. Kim, M.-J. Lee, Y. J. Kim, Y.-W. Cho, and G.-S. Lee, "Methylsulfonylmethane inhibits NLRP3 inflammasome activation," *Cytokine*, vol. 71, no. 2, pp. 223–231, 2015.

[7] Y. H. Kim, D. H. Kim, H. Lim, D.-Y. Baek, H.-K. Shin, and J.-K. Kim, "The anti-inflammatory effects of methylsulfonylmethane on lipopolysaccharide-induced inflammatory responses in murine macrophages," *Biological and Pharmaceutical Bulletin*, vol. 32, no. 4, pp. 651–656, 2009.

[8] B. Kloesch, M. Liszt, J. Broell, and G. Steiner, "Dimethyl sulphoxide and dimethyl sulphone are potent inhibitors of IL-6 and IL-8 expression in the human chondrocyte cell line C-28/I2," *Life Sciences*, vol. 89, no. 13-14, pp. 473–478, 2011.

[9] S. Barmaki, S. Bohlooli, F. Khoshkhahesh, and B. Nakhostin-Roohi, "Effect of methylsulfonylmethane supplementation on exercise—induced muscle damage and total antioxidant capacity," *Journal of Sports Medicine and Physical Fitness*, vol. 52, no. 2, pp. 170–174, 2012.

[10] B. Nakhostin-Roohi, S. Barmaki, F. Khoshkhahesh, and S. Bohlooli, "Effect of chronic supplementation with methylsulfonylmethane on oxidative stress following acute exercise in untrained healthy men," *Journal of Pharmacy and Pharmacology*, vol. 63, no. 10, pp. 1290–1294, 2011.

[11] D. S. Kalman, S. Feldman, A. R. Scheinberg, D. R. Krieger, and R. J. Bloomer, "Influence of methylsulfonylmethane on markers of exercise recovery and performance in healthy men: a pilot study," *Journal of the International Society of Sports Nutrition*, vol. 9, no. 1, article 46, 2012.

[12] K. Ostrowski, T. Rohde, S. Asp, P. Schjerling, and B. K. Pedersen, "Pro- and anti-inflammatory cytokine balance in strenuous exercise in humans," *The Journal of Physiology*, vol. 515, no. 1, pp. 287–291, 1999.

[13] L. Hirose, K. Nosaka, M. Newton et al., "Changes in inflammatory mediators following eccentric exercise of the elbow flexors," *Exercise Immunology Review*, vol. 10, pp. 75–90, 2004.

[14] F. M. DiLorenzo, C. J. Drager, and J. W. Rankin, "Docosahexaenoic acid affects markers of inflammation and muscle damage after eccentric exercise," *The Journal of Strength & Conditioning Research*, vol. 28, no. 10, pp. 2768–2774, 2014.

[15] K. Krüger and F. C. Mooren, "Exercise-induced leukocyte apoptosis," *Exercise Immunology Review*, vol. 20, pp. 117–134, 2014.

[16] M. Gleeson, B. McFarlin, and M. Flynn, "Exercise and toll-like receptors," *Exercise Immunology Review*, vol. 12, no. 1, pp. 34–53, 2006.

[17] D. C. Nieman, D. A. Henson, C. S. Sampson et al., "The acute immune response to exhaustive resistance exercise," *International Journal of Sports Medicine*, vol. 16, no. 5, pp. 322–328, 1995.

[18] B. K. Pedersen, "Muscles and their myokines," *Journal of Experimental Biology*, vol. 214, part 2, pp. 337–346, 2011.

[19] A. M. W. Petersen and B. K. Pedersen, "The anti-inflammatory effect of exercise," *Journal of Applied Physiology*, vol. 98, no. 4, pp. 1154–1162, 2005.

26

Comparison of Muscle Onset Activation Sequences between a Golf or Tennis Swing and Common Training Exercises Using Surface Electromyography

John M. Vasudevan,[1] Andrew Logan,[2] Rebecca Shultz,[2,3] Jeffrey J. Koval,[2] Eugene Y. Roh,[3] and Michael Fredericson[3]

[1]*Department of Physical Medicine & Rehabilitation, University of Pennsylvania, 1800 Lombard Street, Philadelphia, PA 19146, USA*
[2]*Human Performance Lab, Sports Medicine Center, Department of Orthopaedic Surgery, Stanford University, 341 Galvez Street, Lower Level, Stanford, CA 94305, USA*
[3]*Division of Sports Medicine, Department of Orthopaedic Surgery, Stanford University, 450 Broadway Street, Redwood City, CA 94063, USA*

Correspondence should be addressed to John M. Vasudevan; john.vasudevan@uphs.upenn.edu

Academic Editor: S. John Sullivan

Aim. The purpose of this pilot study is to use surface electromyography to determine an individual athlete's typical muscle onset activation sequence when performing a golf or tennis forward swing and to use the method to assess to what degree the sequence is reproduced with common conditioning exercises and a machine designed for this purpose. *Methods.* Data for 18 healthy male subjects were collected for 15 muscles of the trunk and lower extremities. Data were filtered and processed to determine the average onset of muscle activation for each motion. A Spearman correlation estimated congruence of activation order between the swing and each exercise. Correlations of each group were pooled with 95% confidence intervals using a random effects meta-analytic strategy. *Results.* The averaged sequences differed among each athlete tested, but pooled correlations demonstrated a positive association between each exercise and the participants' natural muscle onset activation sequence. *Conclusion.* The selected training exercises and Turning Point™ device all partially reproduced our athletes' averaged muscle onset activation sequences for both sports. The results support consideration of a larger, adequately powered study using this method to quantify to what degree each of the selected exercises is appropriate for use in both golf and tennis.

1. Introduction

Golf and tennis are popular sports for athletes of all ages and ability levels. There are over 30 million golfers and 28 million active tennis players in the United States and over 50 million golfers worldwide [1–4]. Both sports are associated with overuse injuries, as they rely on transferring the momentum from a club or a racquet to a ball for maximum velocity and accuracy [5].

The modern golf swing is characterized by increased shoulder rotation with restricted hip turning to maximize hip-shoulder separation. This technique may produce increased ball velocity and distance but comes at a cost of increased risk of musculoskeletal injury [5–10]. The modern golf swing has been shown to place nearly as much stress upon the spine as forces measured in college football linemen hitting a blocking sled [11]. Several biomechanical studies have assessed not only the golf swing, but also the role of axial rotation on loading and injury of the thoracolumbar spine, in which a supramaximal angle (termed the "dynamic X-factor") takes the player beyond a safe limit of flexibility [8–14]. Control of the dynamic X-factor requires conditioning not only spinal stabilizing muscles, but all limb and trunk muscles required of the swing.

The golf swing motion is separated into several phases: backswing, forward swing, acceleration, early follow through, and late follow through. The primary lower limb and trunk muscles involved in these phases have been described [2, 5]. Although EMG studies have identified muscles active in each phase, few studies have detailed the precise order of activation in an individual athlete or have only measured a limited set of muscles (i.e., lower limb or trunk, but rarely are both regions studied at once) [8, 9, 15].

As with golf, tennis has evolved over the years to become a more aggressive sport, requiring increasing loads to maximize power. This, in turn, increases the risk of injury across all skill levels [16]. There are no longitudinal cohort studies to identify risk factors and no randomized controlled trials designed to determine methods of injury prevention.

The tennis forehand stroke is divided into the backswing and forward swing. Power in the tennis forward swing is derived from sequential contractions in the lower limbs, axial torque through the pelvis and trunk in the transverse plane, and sequential rotation through the kinetic chain to the shoulder girdle and upper limb [17, 18]. As with the golf swing, this also requires hip-shoulder separation during backswing to increase potential energy and power from the stroke. Studies sequencing muscle activation in tennis are few in number, and most focus on the serve rather than forward swing [17]. Studies comparing athletes of varying skill levels have found that appropriate timing and velocity of pelvis and trunk rotation are critical to performance in athletes of all levels [19]. However, there is little information regarding typical muscle activation patterns of the trunk and pelvis in the tennis forward swing.

Conditioning exercises specific to the golf and tennis swing have been described to maximize efficiency of movement through the kinetic chain [2, 4, 17]. Although precise reproduction of sport-specific movement may not be necessary to condition or rehabilitate athletes, exercises are often tailored to athletes to accommodate for the complex movement patterns required of their sport. The purpose of this pilot study is to use surface electromyography to determine an individual athlete's typical muscle onset activation sequence from the limbs through the trunk, with a goal of determining how well the sequence is reproduced with common conditioning exercises (wood chop cable pull, medicine ball wall throw, or the novel Turning Point 4.0 Rotational Training Platform). We sought to determine whether this electromyographic measurement method used is appropriate to analyze motions used in both golf and tennis. Understanding how well an exercise simulates an athlete's swing may provide insight into the development of an optimal and individualized exercise regimen.

2. Materials and Methods

2.1. Participants. Informed consent for participation in study was obtained from 18 healthy male subjects (9 golfers and 9 tennis players). The number of participants was kept low for the pragmatic purpose of generating and analyzing pilot data. The participants ranged from 20 to 33 (mean = 22.2) years of age. The 9 golfers ranged from 20 to 33 (22.3) years of age. All golfers had been playing regularly for 1–14 (7) years and 2 of the participants played on an intercollegiate club golf team. The 9 tennis players were between the ages of 19 and 26 (22.4). Participants for tennis had been playing tennis ranging from 6 to 15 (9.9) years. Of the 9 tennis players, 2 had played with high school varsity, 2 are currently at the division III collegiate level and 3 at the club level, and the remaining 2 participants play recreationally. In an effort to minimize variability in the swing, only male university students without acute or chronic injuries of the spine or limbs (that could interfere with club or racquet swing capability) were recruited. All subjects primarily play one of the two sports. The study protocol was approved by the Stanford University Institutional Review Board.

2.2. Procedures. For this study, we chose the wood chop cable pull (WC) and medicine ball wall throw (MB) exercises because strength and conditioning coaches commonly use these exercises to train and rehabilitate athletes in these sports. These two exercises in isolation are by no means comprehensive in the training of the core musculature and proper motion through the kinetic chain. Rather, they are representative of many exercises used to train rotational movement and chosen based upon the advice of the strength and conditioning coaches at our university. The Turning Point 4.0 Rotational Training Platform (Turning Point Biotechnology, Toledo, Ohio; http://www.turningpointbiotech.com/index_draft.php) (TP) was included in this study because it was not only designed specifically for training of rotational strength, but also intended to provide more consistent and measurable movement due to its adjustable settings and computerized motion analysis [20, 21].

Prior to testing, participants were given five minutes to warm up with low-intensity cardiovascular exercise (e.g., treadmill walking) or stretching to their preference. Once ready, participants had the muscles of interest prepared for EMG electrode placement by gentle abrasion of the skin and treatment with alcohol to clean the area and provide an accurate reading. Ultrasound gel was also used to ensure that a clean EMG signal was recorded for all 15 channels used in this study. Location of electrode placement on each muscle was determined according to *Cram's Introduction to Surface Electromyography* [22].

Once all EMG electrodes were properly placed, participants completed four motions, performing 5 repetitions of each—a golf or tennis forward swing with ball contact, a wood chop cable pull (Figure 1), an 8-pound medicine ball wall throw in a perpendicular stance to a wall (Figure 2), and the Turning Point 4.0 Rotational Platform (Figure 3). We chose five repetitions for each motion to sample enough data while reducing any adverse effects of fatigue as each athlete progressed through the motions. The wood chop cable pull exercise is a dynamic, functional exercise that employs the lower limbs, trunk, and upper limbs in a natural motion. The person performing the exercise moves a bar or ball in diagonal fashion (e.g., from lower right to upper left in a right-handed golfer) in a controlled, spiral movement while keeping the torso as still as possible by coactivation of abdominals and paraspinals. A medicine ball wall throw

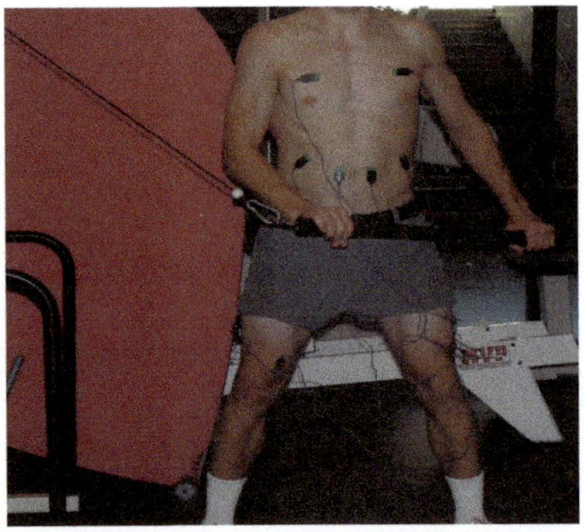

Figure 1: Surface EMG setup for wood chop cable pull exercise.

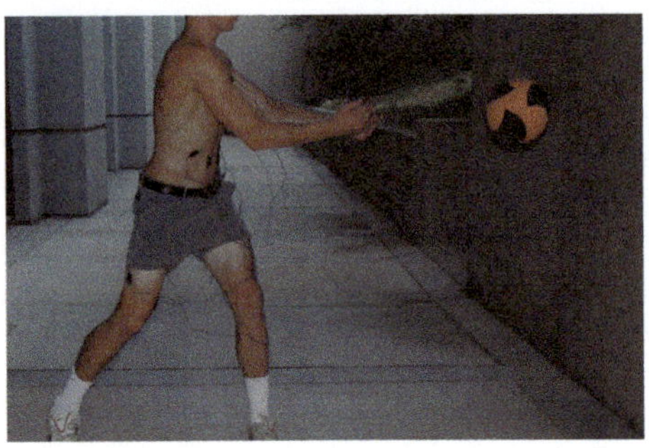

Figure 2: Surface EMG setup for medicine ball wall throw exercise.

exercise can be used in similar fashion to the wood chop but allows for a more natural take away (simulating backswing) and release of the ball toward a wall (simulating follow through), since the athlete is not tethered to a machine. The Turning Point 4.0 Rotational Training Platform places the user in a standing position and allows for shoulder-hip separation required of rotational movements as used in golf and tennis.

These exercises were performed in a randomized order for each participant. Randomization was done by use of a randomized number sheet. Participants were told to complete all motions at a self-selected comfortable pace. Resistance for the WC exercise was standardized to equal the torque created by an 8-pound medicine ball. Because settings on the TP platform were not directly comparable to the other exercises, resistance on the platform for each subject was set according to an equal level of self-perceived exertion when compared to the WC and MB exercises. All exercises were performed in the individual's self-selected natural swing stance. Each participant was given up to 5 minutes to practice the motions for each exercise and the Turning Point machine, followed by 5 minutes of rest prior to recorded trials. Five minutes of rest were given between each of the four motions to control for effects of fatigue.

2.3. Measuring Methods. Electromyographic (EMG) data were recorded (1200 Hz) from lower limb and trunk muscles (Bagnoli Desktop, Delsys Inc., Boston. MA, USA) using

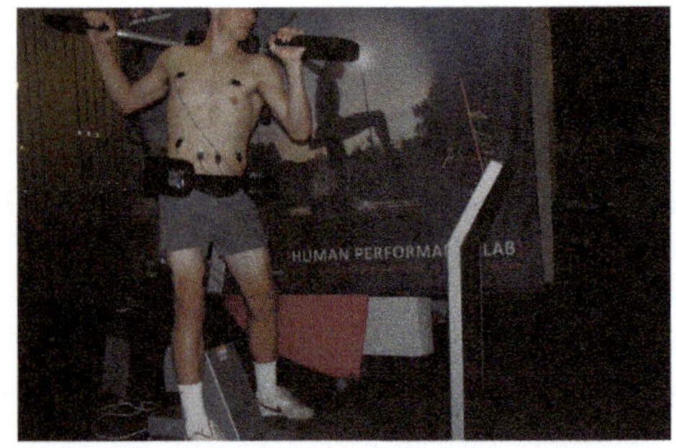

Figure 3: Surface EMG setup for Turning Point 4.0 Rotational Platform.

preamplified single differential, rectangular Ag electrodes with 10 mm interelectrode distance (DE-2.1, Delsys, Inc., Boston, MA, USA). The 15 specific muscles were bilateral erector spinae, pectoralis major, external oblique, rectus abdominis, internal oblique, vastus lateralis, gluteus maximus, and unilateral vastus medialis of each participant's trailing leg.

EMG data were bandpass filtered at 30–500 Hz, rectified, and low-pass filtered at 30 Hz. The evaluation of EMG onset was determined with computer analysis (MATLAB version 7.10.0. Natick, Massachusetts: The MathWorks Inc., 2010). The algorithm involved identification of the time point when the mean of a specified number of surrounding time samples exceeded the mean level by a predetermined number of standard deviations. This time point is considered the onset of activation for each muscle studied. The baseline mean level was averaged for 50 ms prior to signal to perform the activity. Following this, EMG activity was averaged over a sliding time window of 25 ms. If the average of the time window did not exceed the baseline by 3 standard deviations, the sliding time window was advanced one sample at a time until the onset was found. The algorithm and parameters used have previously been demonstrated to reduce observer bias and increase reliability [23].

The muscles studied in each subject were ranked in order of activation as described above from 1 to 15. For example, if the external oblique was the first to activate, it was ranked 1, and the last muscle to activate was ranked 15. In order to account for variability among swings in each individual, this activation order was averaged across the natural swing for each subject to determine his own "gold standard." We anticipated this variability based on a study by Meister et al. that demonstrated decreased consistency of the golf swing as handicap increases [6]. The muscle activation sequences for the wood chop cable pull (WC), medicine ball wall throw (MB), and Turning Point (TP) exercises were measured in similar fashion for comparison to each subject's natural swing.

2.4. Statistical Analyses. For each athlete, a Spearman correlation was calculated to estimate the congruence of muscle onset activation order between golf swing and the other exercises (i.e., WC, MB, and TP). For each exercise pair (e.g., golf swing versus WC) the correlations of each group

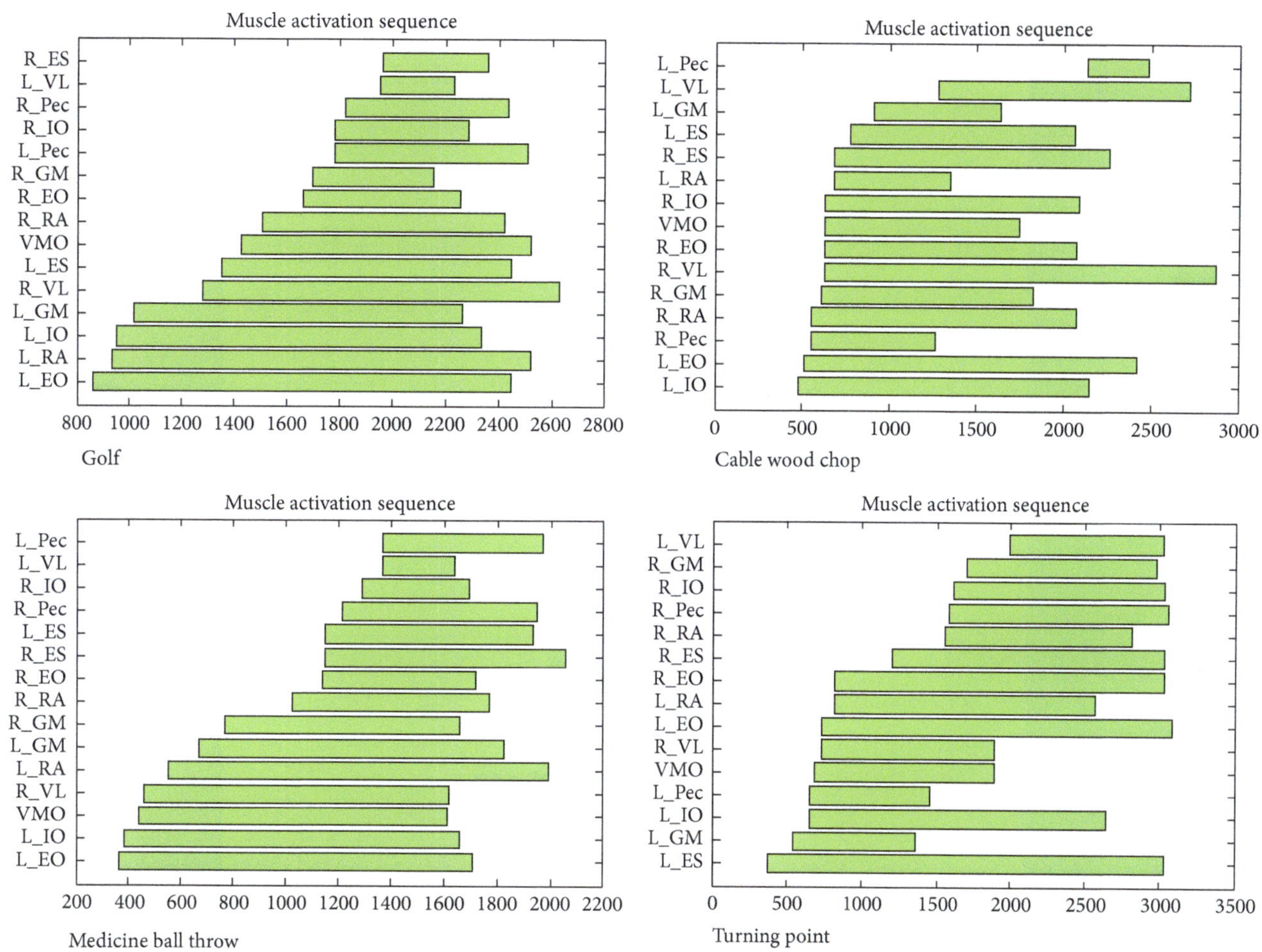

FIGURE 4: Example of one golf athlete's averaged muscle onset activation sequence for the forward golf swing, wood chop cable pull, medicine ball wall throw, and Turning Point 4.0 Rotational Platform. Each bar represents the average onset and duration of each subject's individual muscle activation. (x-axis: time (msec)). y-axis: muscles (e.g., L_EO = left external oblique).

of 9 athletes were pooled into overall estimates with 95% confidence intervals using a random effects meta-analytic strategy, implemented in the Metafor Package of the R statistical program. Meta-analysis is a statistical strategy to average or pool independent statistical results (in this case, player-specific Spearman's correlations) in a manner that retains information regarding within-player variability and number of observations [24]. Differences between the pooled correlations (e.g., golf swing versus WC compared to golf swing versus TP) were evaluated by inspecting the overlap between the 95% confidence intervals for the pooled correlations. The same method was used to estimate the congruence of muscle activation order between tennis swing and WC, MB, and TP exercises.

3. Results

3.1. Golf. Averaging of the 5 motions for each athlete determined the natural forehand swing for that athlete. An example of an individual athlete's muscle activation sequence for the golf swing and the three exercises studied is shown in Figure 4. There were differences in correlation (ranging from negative to positive) between the forward swing and each exercise among the 9 golf athletes, but these differences were within the range of the 95% confidence intervals. This is displayed along the x-axis in Figures 5(a)–5(c).

The majority of all athletes demonstrated a positive correlation between all exercises and the natural swing. For the minority of athletes in which there was a negative correlation, all confidence intervals crossed into the positive range (Figure 5, top 9 lines). When averaged among all athletes tested, the coefficients of correlation (with 95% confidence interval) between the WC, MB, and TP movements to the golf forward swing were 0.16 (95% CI: −0.01 to 0.32), 0.26 (95% CI: −0.01 to 0.52), and 0.23 (95% CI: 0.02 to 0.45), respectively (Figure 5, bottom line). The confidence intervals of these correlations overlap, indicating a nonsignificant difference among the exercises.

3.2. Tennis. An example of an individual athlete's muscle activation sequence for the tennis swing and the three exercises studied is shown in Figure 6, using the same methodology as with the golf athletes. Again, there were

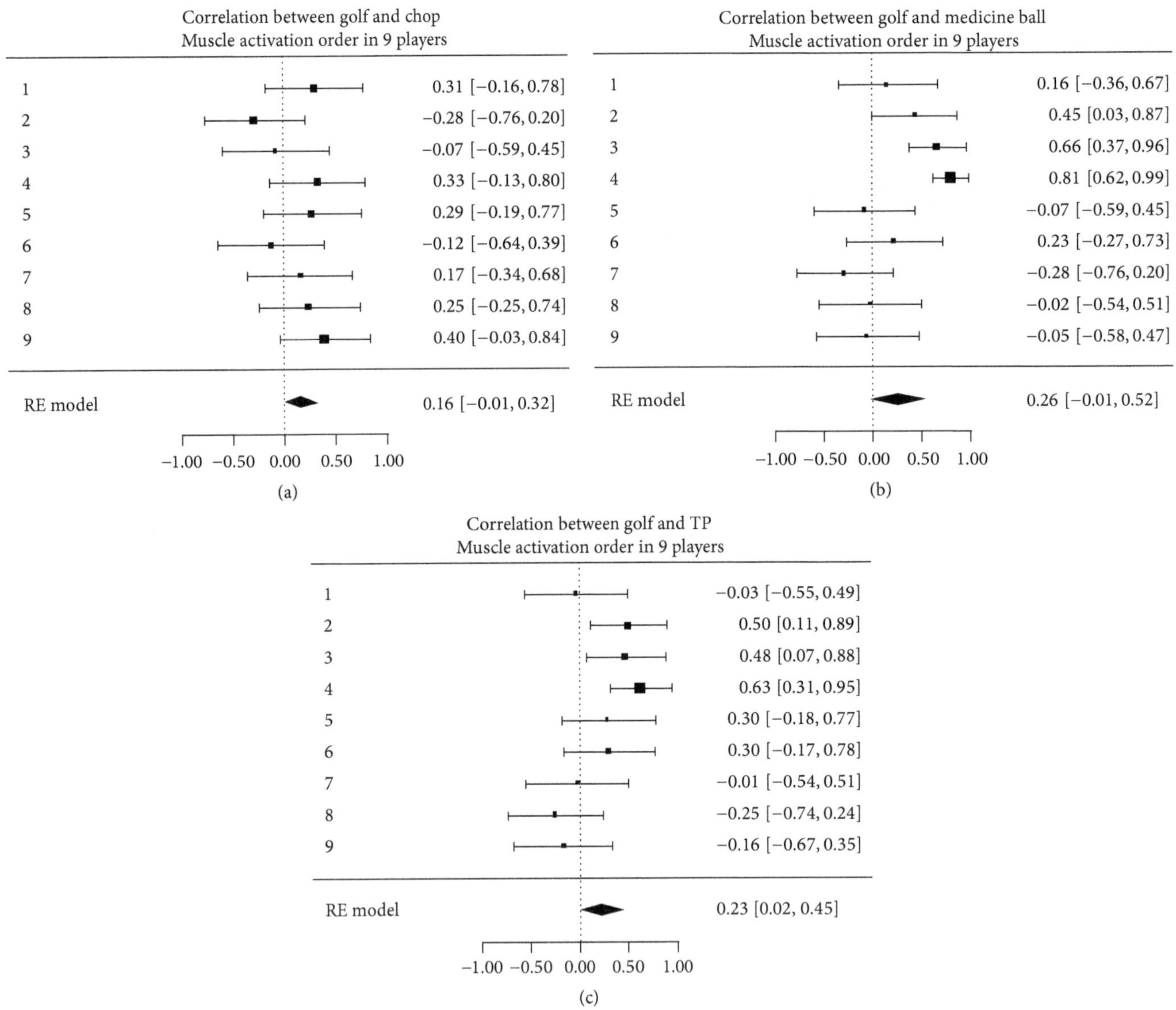

FIGURE 5: Correlation of muscle onset activation sequences between golf swing and the wood chop cable pull, medicine ball wall throw, and Turning Point 4.0 Rotational Platform. The top nine bars indicate each subject's individual correlation (with 95% confidence interval), and the bottom bar indicates the correlation averaged across all subjects tested (with 95% confidence interval).

differences in correlation (ranging from negative to positive) between the forward swing and each exercise among the 9 tennis athletes, with these differences within the range of the 95% confidence intervals. This is displayed along the x-axis in Figures 7(a)–7(c). This particular group studied exhibited less inconsistency than the golf athletes.

As with the golf cohort, the majority of all athletes demonstrated a positive correlation between all exercises and the natural swing. For the minority of athletes, in which there was a negative correlation, confidence intervals crossed into the positive range (Figure 7, top 9 lines). When averaged across all participants, the coefficients for WC, MB, and TP to the tennis forward swing were 0.16 (−0.02–0.34), 0.36 (0.16–0.56), and 0.42 (0.26–0.58), respectively (Figure 7, bottom line). The confidence intervals of these correlations overlap, indicating a nonsignificant difference among the exercises.

4. Discussion

This study utilized surface electromyography to observe the muscle activation sequences among recreational and club-level golf and tennis athletes. Seminal studies by Perry and colleagues, such as the ones by Pink et al. in 1990 and 1993 and Watkins et al. in 1996, helped establish the use of electromyography to evaluate muscle activation in the golf swing [25–27]. Because most of the available data is focused on trunk and shoulder musculature, recent reviews of electromyography variables related to the golf swing have identified a gap in the knowledge of lower limb muscle activation [28]. Based on what was already known (and yet unknown), the purpose of this pilot study was to not only define a method to readily identify the precise onset sequence of the lower limb through the trunk muscles in an athlete

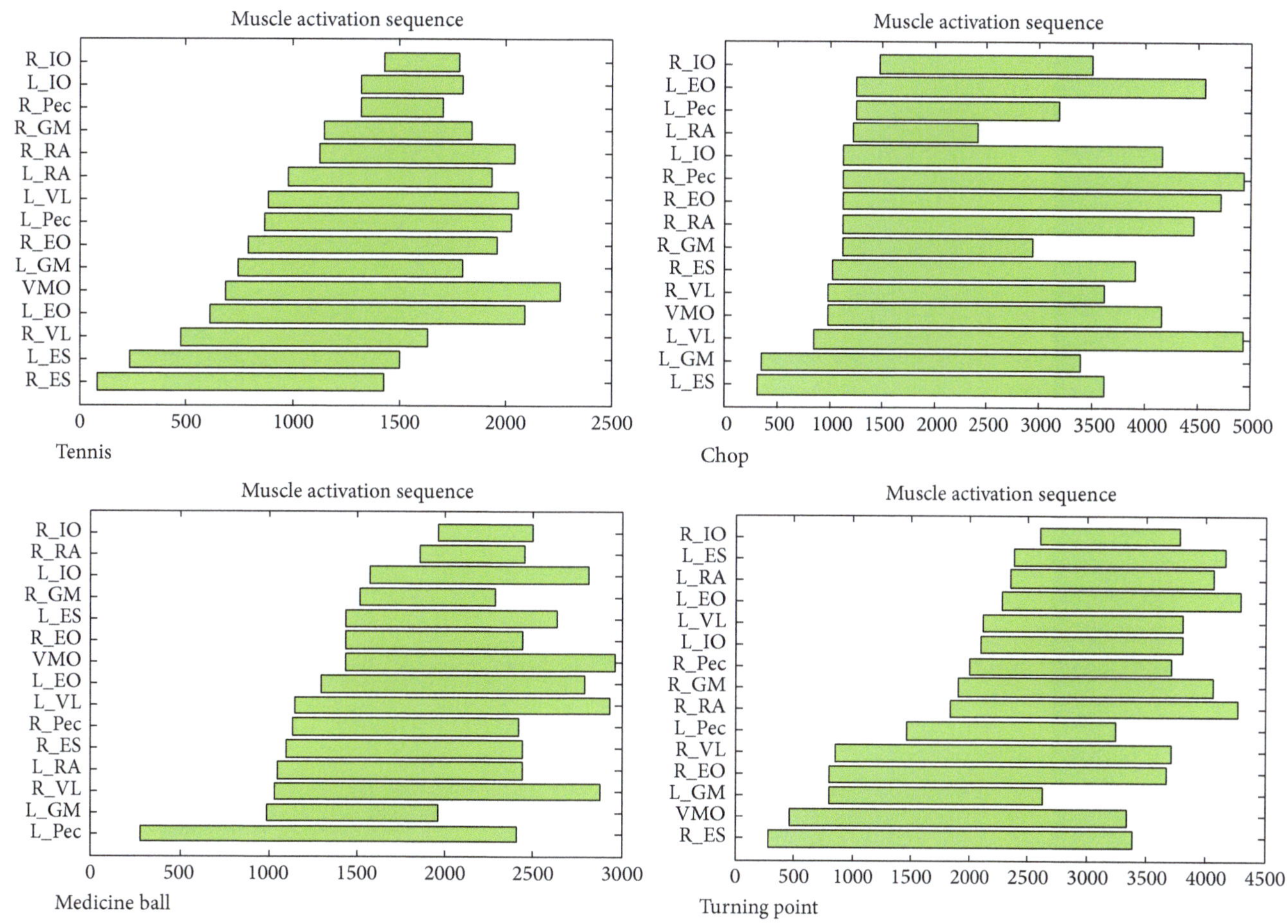

Figure 6: Example of one tennis athlete's averaged muscle onset activation sequence for the forehand tennis swing, wood chop cable pull, medicine ball wall throw, and Turning Point 4.0 Rotational Platform. Each bar represents the average onset and duration of each subject's individual muscle activation. (x-axis: time (msec)). y-axis: muscles (e.g., L_EO = left external oblique).

of any level, but also apply the method across multiple sport motions (e.g., golf and tennis forward swing).

Conclusions from the study data are limited by small sample size but suggest that the selected exercises may be appropriate for both golf and tennis. A larger, adequately-powered study would generate sufficient data to quantify the value of these exercises with greater certainty. The results of this study indicate that, when results are averaged across all athletes studied, there are positive correlations between the selected exercises and the natural forward golf and tennis swing in the population studied. The TP more closely correlates to the tennis swing than golf swing in the subjects tested, but not to a significant degree when compared to the other exercises studied. We suspect that the TP may have an advantage in tennis as the sport features more rotation in the transverse plane, of which the majority of the TP device's motion pertains. The golf swing not only employs transverse trunk motion, but also employs dynamic lateral trunk bending. While the TP device allows the user to set the trunk angle, this angle remains static throughout the motion of the device. Conversely, the tennis forward swing (as opposed to the overhead swing or serve) requires less dynamic change in trunk angle. These conclusions are made with caution, however, due to the small sample size. Because the confidence intervals overlapped among all motions tested, there was no demonstrable advantage to any one exercise.

A question for future study is to determine what degree of inconsistency or variability in sport motion is acceptable in order to achieve the desired performance outcome. Fleisig et al. studied the variability of pitching biomechanics from amateur to elite levels, and while professional athletes demonstrated less variability in their motions than their amateur counterparts, differences in temporal and kinetic variation were nonsignificant [29]. Wagner et al. found similar decreases in variability in certain motions in more highly skilled team handball players, but also they observed that athletes had an ability to maintain accuracy despite increases in movement variability required by the circumstances of the game [30]. The implication of these studies, as well as similar observations by Bartlett et al., is that a certain amount of variability may be desirable and functional without adversely affecting the sport task outcome or injury risk [31].

The most significant limitation of this study is the small sample size. However, the intention was to use a convenience sample size to develop pilot data that would promote use of this method in future studies. Another limitation is our

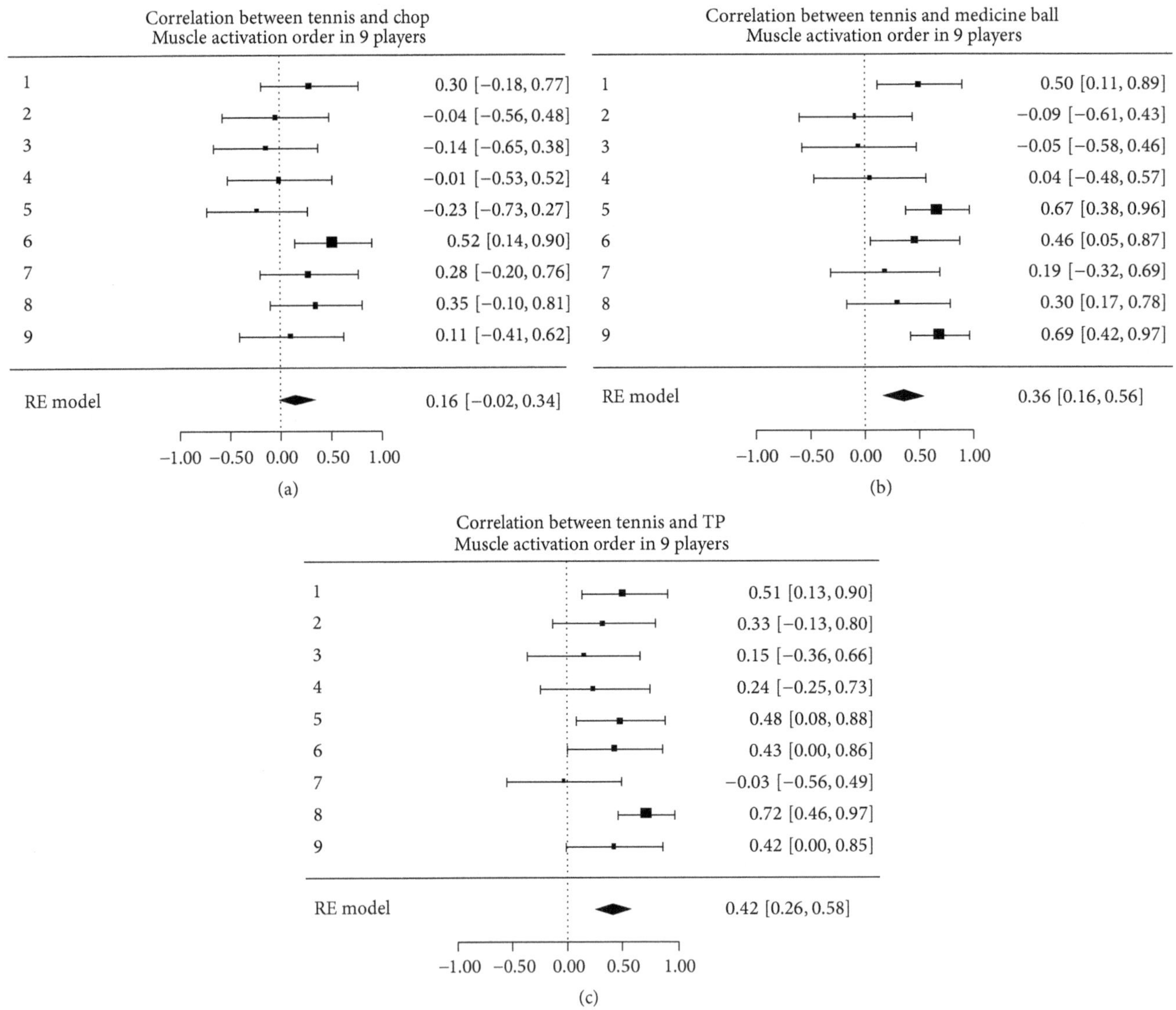

FIGURE 7: Correlation of muscle onset activation sequences between tennis swing and the wood chop cable pull, medicine ball wall throw, and Turning Point 4.0 Rotational Platform. The top nine bars indicate each subject's individual correlation (with 95% confidence interval), and the bottom bar indicates the correlation averaged across all subjects tested (with 95% confidence interval).

a priori assertion that the selected exercises are effective at reproducing a typical muscle activation sequence. No single exercise will perfectly simulate the natural swing, and a larger combination of exercises (whether they are intended to mimic the sport motion or not) is necessary to improve performance.

Movement patterns will vary not only by sport, but also by variations in the competitive environment [32]. Furthermore, muscle activation may vary in the context of recent injury [33]. Electromyographic methods have been used to measure the activation sequences in sport, but this is the first to our knowledge specifically studying the average muscle onset sequence from the lower limb through the trunk (distal-to-proximal kinetic chain) in the golf and tennis forward swing. The method used in this study has the potential for use in future studies to measure the precise timing of muscle onset activation in other sports and contexts (e.g., after injury) as well. The use of this method in future studies will allow for more significant conclusions to be drawn when examining the relationship of one exercise compared to another for the purposes of training and, eventually, determining benchmarks for return-to-play during injury rehabilitation.

5. Conclusions

Using surface electromyography to record the average onset muscle activation sequence of lower limb and trunk muscles in recreational and club-level golf and tennis athletes, there was a positive average correlation of the cable pull wood chop, medicine ball wall throw, and Turning Point 4.0 Rotational Platform to the natural golf and tennis forward swing in the amateur athlete population studied. Our pilot data suggest that a larger study using this method may effectively quantify to what degree these and other exercises are appropriate for golf and tennis athletes.

Disclosure

The Turning Point 4.0 Rotational Training Platform was donated as a gift from an alumnus of the University to the Human Performance Lab. There was no direct funding of this research study from Turning Point Biotechnology.

Competing Interests

Michael Fredericson was briefly a member of the Scientific Advisory Board for Turning Point Biotechnology, but not at the time of the study.

References

[1] J. F. Beditz and J. R. Kass, *Golf Participation in America, 2010–2020*, National Golf Foundation, Jupiter, Fla, USA, 2010, http://www.ngf.org/pages/future-of-golf-participation-us/.

[2] B. Brandon and P. Z. Pearce, "Training to prevent golf injury," *Current Sports Medicine Reports*, vol. 8, no. 3, pp. 142–146, 2009.

[3] United States Tennis Association, 2012 Year in Review: By The Numbers, http://www.usta.com/2012_year_in_review_by_the_numbers/.

[4] M. Reid and K. Schneiker, "Strength and conditioning in tennis: current research and practice," *Journal of Science and Medicine in Sport*, vol. 11, no. 3, pp. 248–256, 2008.

[5] E. Y. Roh, M. C. Geraci, and M. Smuck, "Preseason training for golfers with low back pain," *SpineLine*, vol. 1, pp. 17–21, 2012.

[6] D. W. Meister, A. L. Ladd, E. E. Butler et al., "Rotational biomechanics of the elite golf swing: benchmarks for amateurs," *Journal of Applied Biomechanics*, vol. 27, no. 3, pp. 242–251, 2011.

[7] J. Myers, S. Lephart, Y. S. Tsai, T. Sell, J. Smoliga, and J. Jolly, "The role of upper torso and pelvis rotation in driving performance during the golf swing," *Journal of Sports Sciences*, vol. 26, no. 2, pp. 181–188, 2008.

[8] A. McHardy and H. Pollard, "Muscle activity during the golf swing," *British Journal of Sports Medicine*, vol. 39, no. 11, pp. 799–804, 2005.

[9] M. H. Cole and P. N. Grimshaw, "Electromyography of the trunk and abdominal muscles in golfers with and without low back pain," *Journal of Science and Medicine in Sport*, vol. 11, no. 2, pp. 174–181, 2008.

[10] M. H. Cole and P. N. Grimshaw, "Trunk muscle onset and cessation in golfers with and without low back pain," *Journal of Biomechanics*, vol. 41, no. 13, pp. 2829–2833, 2008.

[11] G. S. Gluck, J. A. Bendo, and J. M. Spivak, "The lumbar spine and low back pain in golf: a literature review of swing biomechanics and injury prevention," *The Spine Journal*, vol. 8, no. 5, pp. 778–788, 2008.

[12] W. S. Marras and K. P. Granata, "A biomechanical assessment and model of axial twisting in the thoracolumbar spine," *Spine*, vol. 20, no. 13, pp. 1440–1451, 1995.

[13] S. H. M. Brown and S. M. McGill, "Co-activation alters the linear versus non-linear impression of the EMG-torque relationship of trunk muscles," *Journal of Biomechanics*, vol. 41, no. 3, pp. 491–497, 2008.

[14] S. Kumar, Y. Narayan, and D. Garand, "An electromyographic study of isokinetic axial rotation in young adults," *Spine Journal*, vol. 3, no. 1, pp. 46–54, 2003.

[15] J. F. Horton, D. M. Lindsay, and B. R. MacIntosh, "Abdominal muscle activation of elite male golfers with chronic low back pain," *Medicine and Science in Sports and Exercise*, vol. 33, no. 10, pp. 1647–1654, 2001.

[16] B. M. Pluim, J. B. Staal, G. E. Windler, and N. Jayanthi, "fTennis injuries: occurrence, aetiology, and prevention," *British Journal of Sports Medicine*, vol. 40, no. 5, pp. 415–423, 2006.

[17] E. P. Roetert, M. Kovacs, D. Knudson, and J. L. Groppel, "Biomechanics of the tennis groundstrokes: implications for strength training," *Strength & Conditioning Journal*, vol. 31, no. 4, pp. 41–49, 2009.

[18] B. Elliott, "Biomechanics and tennis," *British Journal of Sports Medicine*, vol. 40, no. 5, pp. 392–396, 2006.

[19] J. Landlinger, S. Lindinger, T. Stöggl, H. Wagner, and E. Müller, "Key factors and timing patterns in the tennis forehand of different skill levels," *Journal of Sports Science and Medicine*, vol. 9, no. 4, pp. 643–651, 2010.

[20] K. Marbaugh, V. K. Goel, D. Dick, and D. M. Pincivero, "Trunk and leg muscle EMG and perceived exertion during resisted trunk rotation exercise," in *Proceedings of the Annual Meeting of the American Society of Biomechanics*, State College, Pa, USA, August 2009, http://www.asbweb.org/conferences/2009/1065.pdf.

[21] B. J. AlSarraf, J. Brown, M. A. Waller, P. Esenman, and C. Hicks-Little, "Reliability of the turning point core trainer as a measure of peak upper torso rotational velocity, peak pelvic rotational velocity, and peak pelvic torso separation angle," in *Proceedings of the National Strength and Conditioning Associated National Conference*, Las Vegas, Nev, USA, July 2013, http://www.nsca.com/uploadedFiles/NSCA/Inactive_Content/Program_Books/Abstracts%20Inclusive.pdf.

[22] E. Criswell, *Cram's Introduction to Surface Electromyography*, Jones & Bartlett Publishers, Sudbury, Mass, USA, 2nd edition, 2011.

[23] P. W. Hodges and B. H. Bui, "A comparison of computer-based methods for the determination of onset of muscle contraction using electromyography," *Electroencephalography and Clinical Neurophysiology—Electromyography and Motor Control*, vol. 101, no. 6, pp. 511–519, 1996.

[24] L. V. Hedges and I. Olkin, *Statistical Methods for Meta-Analysis*, Academic Press, Cambridge, Mass, USA, 2014.

[25] M. Pink, F. W. Jobe, and J. Perry, "Electromyographic analysis of the shoulder during the golf swing," *American Journal of Sports Medicine*, vol. 18, no. 2, pp. 137–140, 1990.

[26] M. Pink, J. Perry, and F. W. Jobe, "Electromyographic analysis of the trunk in golfers," *American Journal of Sports Medicine*, vol. 21, no. 3, pp. 385–388, 1993.

[27] R. G. Watkins, G. S. Uppal, J. Perry, M. Pink, and J. M. Dinsay, "Dynamic electromyographic analysis of trunk musculature in professional golfers," *The American Journal of Sports Medicine*, vol. 24, no. 4, pp. 535–538, 1996.

[28] S. Marta, L. Silva, M. A. Castro, P. Pezarat-Correia, and J. Cabri, "Electromyography variables during the golf swing: a literature review," *Journal of Electromyography and Kinesiology*, vol. 22, no. 6, pp. 803–813, 2012.

[29] G. Fleisig, Y. Chu, A. Weber, and J. Andrews, "Variability in baseball pitching biomechanics among various levels of competition," *Sports Biomechanics*, vol. 8, no. 1, pp. 10–21, 2009.

[30] H. Wagner, J. Pfusterschmied, M. Klous, S. P. von Duvillard, and E. Müller, "Movement variability and skill level of various throwing techniques," *Human Movement Science*, vol. 31, no. 1, pp. 78–90, 2012.

[31] R. Bartlett, J. Wheat, and M. Robins, "Is movement variability important for sports biomechanists?" *Sports Biomechanics*, vol. 6, no. 2, pp. 224–243, 2007.

[32] H. Wagner, J. Pfusterschmied, M. Tilp, J. Landlinger, S. P. Von Duvillard, and E. Müller, "Upper-body kinematics in team-handball throw, tennis serve, and volleyball spike," *Scandinavian Journal of Medicine & Science in Sports*, vol. 24, no. 2, pp. 345–354, 2014.

[33] G. Sole, S. Milosavljevic, H. Nicholson, and S. J. Sullivan, "Altered muscle activation following hamstring injuries," *British Journal of Sports Medicine*, vol. 46, no. 2, pp. 118–123, 2012.

27

Cervical Spine Involvement in Mild Traumatic Brain Injury

Michael Morin,[1,2] Pierre Langevin,[3,4] and Philippe Fait[1,2,3,5]

[1]*Department of Human Kinetics, Université du Québec à Trois-Rivières (UQTR), Trois-Rivières, QC, Canada G9A 5H7*
[2]*Research Group on Neuromusculoskeletal Dysfunctions (GRAN), UQTR, Trois-Rivières, QC, Canada G9A 5H7*
[3]*Cortex Médecine et Réadaptation Concussion Clinic, Quebec City, QC, Canada G1W 0C5*
[4]*Department of Rehabilitation, Faculty of Medicine, Laval University, Quebec City, QC, Canada G1V 0A6*
[5]*Research Center in Neuropsychology and Cognition (CERNEC), Montreal, QC, Canada H3C 3J7*

Correspondence should be addressed to Philippe Fait; philippe.fait@uqtr.ca

Academic Editor: S. John Sullivan

Background. There is a lack of scientific evidence in the literature on the involvement of the cervical spine in mTBI; however, its involvement is clinically accepted. *Objective.* This paper reviews evidence for the involvement of the cervical spine in mTBI symptoms, the mechanisms of injury, and the efficacy of therapy for cervical spine with concussion-related symptoms. *Methods.* A keyword search was conducted on PubMed, ICL, SportDiscus, PEDro, CINAHL, and Cochrane Library databases for articles published since 1990. The reference lists of articles meeting the criteria (original data articles, literature reviews, and clinical guidelines) were also searched in the same databases. *Results.* 4,854 records were screened and 43 articles were retained. Those articles were used to describe different subjects such as mTBI's signs and symptoms, mechanisms of injury, and treatments of the cervical spine. *Conclusions.* The hypothesis of cervical spine involvement in post-mTBI symptoms and in PCS (postconcussion syndrome) is supported by increasing evidence and is widely accepted clinically. For the management and treatment of mTBIs, few articles were available in the literature, and relevant studies showed interesting results about manual therapy and exercises as efficient tools for health care practitioners.

1. Introduction

Mild traumatic brain injury (mTBI) is commonly known as concussion [1]. In a recent study, Statistics Canada estimated mTBI annual incidence to be 600 per 100,000 people [1]. The pediatric TBI population is the patients' subgroup who consulted the most often in the emergency room [1]. An estimated 1.6 to 3.8 million sport and recreation-related brain injuries occur in the United States annually, and up to 75% of them are classified as mild [2]. About 70 to 90 percent of all TBI cases are thought to be of mild severity, and the related symptoms usually resolve within 7 to 10 days [3, 4]. However, as many as 50% of concussions may go unreported [5]. In an epidemiologic study, Tator et al. (2007) reported that the highest incidence for TBI is in the age group under 18 years, with almost 45%. Additionally, approximately one-quarter of all patients with TBI are aged between 19 and 29 years [1]. The Centers for Disease Control and Prevention (CDC) describes mTBI as a silent epidemic [2].

Concussion in sports was defined in 2012 at the international consensus on concussion in sport held in Zurich as

> *a brain injury and is defined as a complex pathophysiological process affecting the brain, induced by biomechanical forces. Several common features that incorporate clinical, pathologic and biomechanical injury constructs may be utilized in defining the nature of a concussive head injury. This is caused by a direct blow to the head, face, neck or elsewhere on the body with an "impulsive" force transmitted to the head. [4]*

The number of reported concussions has increased in recent years for multiple reasons. Recent studies identified an increased awareness of the potential complications following concussion and repeated head trauma in the population [6] and higher involvement of health professionals in sports and in concussions recognition and follow-up [7]. Even though it is believed that most concussions usually resolve in between 7 and 10 days [3, 4], the symptoms may persist longer for up to 33 percent of cases [8]. Symptoms persisting for a few weeks to more than six months are defined in the literature as postconcussion syndrome (PCS) [8].

PCS is a complex medical subject that few articles and studies in the scientific literature explore concretely [4]. Considering that mTBI is a multifaceted injury, many signs and symptoms complicate its diagnosis [3]. Multiple impairments linked to this condition such as cognitive, vestibular, cervical, physical, and psychological dysfunctions [3, 4]. Therefore, with a multitude of clinical theories in the literature, it is difficult to determine clinical guidelines for PCS [3]. Current consensus identifies that a multidisciplinary approach is essential to the progress of the patient suffering from PCS [4].

One of the major challenges in the medical management of concussion is that there is no "gold standard" for assessing and diagnosing the injury [9]. It has been shown by Schneider et al. (2014) that a combination of cervical and vestibular physiotherapy decreased time to medical clearance for the return to sport in a cohort of 31 patients (12–30 years old) with persistent symptoms of dizziness, neck pain, and/or headaches following a sport-related concussion [10]. However, little research has been published on this very specific topic.

2. Problem

The problem targeted by this review of literature is the lack of data regarding the association between mTBI and cervicogenic impairment. The majority of scientific publications focus on diagnosing mTBI, and there is little evidence on the possible involvement of the cervical region [4]. Cervical spine examination after a cranial trauma is essential, but the association between symptoms and mTBIs is poorly described in the literature. A literature review will improve the medical knowledge of all medical professionals and help the diagnosis and treatment of mTBI.

3. Goals

The aim of this review was to target scientific articles describing mTBI and those involving cervicogenic headache (CGH) cases in order to look at the connections and similarities between these two types of injuries. The specific goals of this paper are (1) to determine the common signs and symptoms of mTBI (including PCS) and cervical dysfunctions, (2) to describe the mechanism of cranial trauma injury and link it with the impact on the cervical spine, and (3) to give an update on the various types of effective treatments for these conditions.

4. Methods

The following electronic resources were searched from January 1, 1990, to May 19, 2015: *PubMed, Index to Chiropractic Literature (ICL), SportDiscus, Physiotherapy Evidence Database (PEDro), Cumulative Index to Nursing and Allied Health Literature (CINAHL)*, and *Cochrane Library databases*. The following keywords were used in different combinations: *concussion, neck, TBI, mTBI, cervical, physiotherapy, physical therapy, athletic training, treatment, chiropractic, manipulation, manual therapy,* and *guideline*. For the complete list of combinations, see Table 1. Three data collections were carried out at different dates: February 16, 2014, May 15, 2014, and May 19, 2015. Reference lists of articles meeting the selection criteria were also collected. All abstracts in English and French dealing with concussion involving the neck were selected for a full reading of the article. A total of 4,854 abstracts were found on search engines. Following this search, the articles were selected according to three main streams:

(1) mTBI's and PCS symptoms related to the cervical spine.
(2) Mechanism of injury.
(3) Therapies of the cervical spine with symptoms related to mTBI.

Inclusion criteria, based on the precited keywords, were original data articles, literature reviews, and clinical recommendations, available in English and/or French, based on the objectives of this research. Exclusion criteria were foreign language papers other than English or French, case studies, magazine articles, and expert and editorial comments. The selection of articles is shown in Figure 1, and combinations are explained in Table 1.

5. Results

After a careful screening of 4,854 data entries, 82 abstracts met the inclusion criteria of our research and were reviewed. All these articles were read and analyzed. Thirty-eight articles were excluded because the main topic did not match the three topics of this study (n = 34) or were case studies (n = 2), magazine articles (n = 2), and expert commentary (n = 1). Finally, 43 papers were included in this literature review. Each selected article is described in Table 2 (see Appendix). These articles were analyzed and assigned to the different categories of topics discussed: (1) the association between cervical spine sprain and mTBI signs and symptoms, (2) mechanism of injury, and (3) treatments. Results are represented in Figure 1 and Table 1.

6. Discussion

6.1. The Association between Cervical Spine Sprain and mTBI Signs and Symptoms. The 2012 Zurich consensus on concussion in sports led by McCrory et al. (2013) defined a list of 22 common symptoms of mTBI divided into 4 main categories, as described in Table 3 [4, 6, 11–13]. The majority of mTBIs (80–90%) are resolved in 7 to 10 days [4, 14, 15]. However, in the remaining 10 to 20%, symptoms may persist for more than 10–14 days, and even for several months after trauma [4, 16]. This clinical picture is diagnosed as PCS and the etiology for PCS is not well defined in the literature [11, 14, 17].

As mentioned previously, the most common symptom in subjects after mTBI is posttraumatic headache (PTH) [18, 19].

TABLE 1: Preliminary search of literature (total results/abstracts (Abs) selection/articles (Art) for review).

	Date	January 1, 1990, to February 16, 2014			February 16, 2014, to May 15, 2014			May 15, 2014, to May 19, 2015		
Resources	Keywords	Total	Abs	Art	Total	Abs	Art	Total	Abs	Art
PubMed	Concussion, Neck	180	12	8	10	0	0	21	5	1
PubMed	TBI, Neck, Treatment	56	0	0	0	0	0	7	2	1
PubMed	TBI, Cervical	83	0	0	33	0	0	17	0	0
PubMed	Concussion, Chiropractic	12	4	1	2	0	0	2	0	0
PubMed	Concussion, Physiotherapy	53	3	2	3	0	0	12	2	1
PubMed	Concussion, Physical Therapy	—	—	—	138	4	1	38	6	1
PubMed	Concussion, Athletic Training, Cervical	30	2	2	0	0	0	6	1	0
ICL	Concussion	32	2	2	0	0	0	4	1	1
SportDiscus	Concussion, Neck	144	0	0	7	0	0	10	4	1
SportDiscus	TBI, Neck, Treatment	5	0	0	0	0	0	0	0	0
SportDiscus	Concussion, Neck, Treatment	15	1	1	4	1	0	3	1	1
SportDiscus	Concussion, Cervical	65	1	1	3	0	0	3	2	1
SportDiscus	Concussion, Chiropractic	9	2	0	0	0	0	2	0	0
SportDiscus	Concussion, Physiotherapy	34	2	2	0	0	0	7	2	1
SportDiscus	Concussion, Athletic Training, Cervical	13	1	1	0	0	0	1	1	1
CINAHL	Concussion, Manipulation	3	3	2	0	0	0	2	1	1
CINAHL	Concussion, Guideline	19	0	0	1	0	0	7	0	0
Cochrane	Concussion	4	1	1	0	0	0	1	1	0
PEDro	Concussion, Physical Therapy	2285	11	5	0	0	0	0	0	0
PEDro	mTBI, Physical Therapy	215	1	1	0	0	0	0	0	0
PEDro	mTBI, Manual Therapy	99	0	0	0	0	0	0	0	0
PEDro	Concussion, Manual Therapy	1132	2	2	0	0	0	0	0	0
PEDro	Concussion, Chiropractic	22	0	0	0	0	0	0	0	0
Total		4510	48	31	201	5	1	143	29	11

The incidence of PTH varies between 5 and 90% [16, 20]. Their prevalence in children with mTBI is from 73 to 93% [19]. The diagnosis of PTH can be difficult to address in subjects with a history of preexisting headaches. However, PTH syndrome diagnosis is considered when the intensity or frequency of headaches increases after trauma [19]. PTH is defined as a headache that occurs within 1 week after regaining consciousness or within 1 week following head trauma [17]. The majority of PTH resolve within 6 to 12 months, and it is caused by cervical muscle tension and posture impairment [17]. Because headache is one of the major causes of morbidity in mTBI subjects, health care professionals should manage this symptom with a high level of priority [17].

Biologically, concussions usually resolve 7 to 10 days after trauma in adults [4, 21]. PCS related symptoms are nonspecific. Professionals must consider other pathologies as alternative explanations to persistent symptoms [4, 17]. Meanwhile, a recent study suggests that even at 1 month or more after concussion, the cerebral blood flow is decreased in 36% of 11- to 15-year-old subjects who suffered mTBI compared to a nonconcussed control group [22]. Further studies are needed to clarify this phenomenon.

Rather than a structural problem, PCS would be related to a brain dysfunction problem [15]. This would explain the negative results on most of the medical imaging prescribed in emergencies [15]. In addition, a prospective Norwegian study of 348 participants identified through a questionnaire that headaches persisting for more than 3 months after trauma and diagnosed as PCS are often related to a musculoskeletal pathology. In other words, the head or brain injury does not cause the persistent symptoms [23]. These results show the importance of potential cervical impairment in patients with mTBI [4, 14, 16, 17].

6.2. Mechanism of Injury. Recent studies correlated mTBI with whiplash occurrence [12, 16, 24, 25]. Furthermore, Schneider et al. (2013) demonstrated in a prospective study with 3,832 male ice hockey players (11–14 years old) that

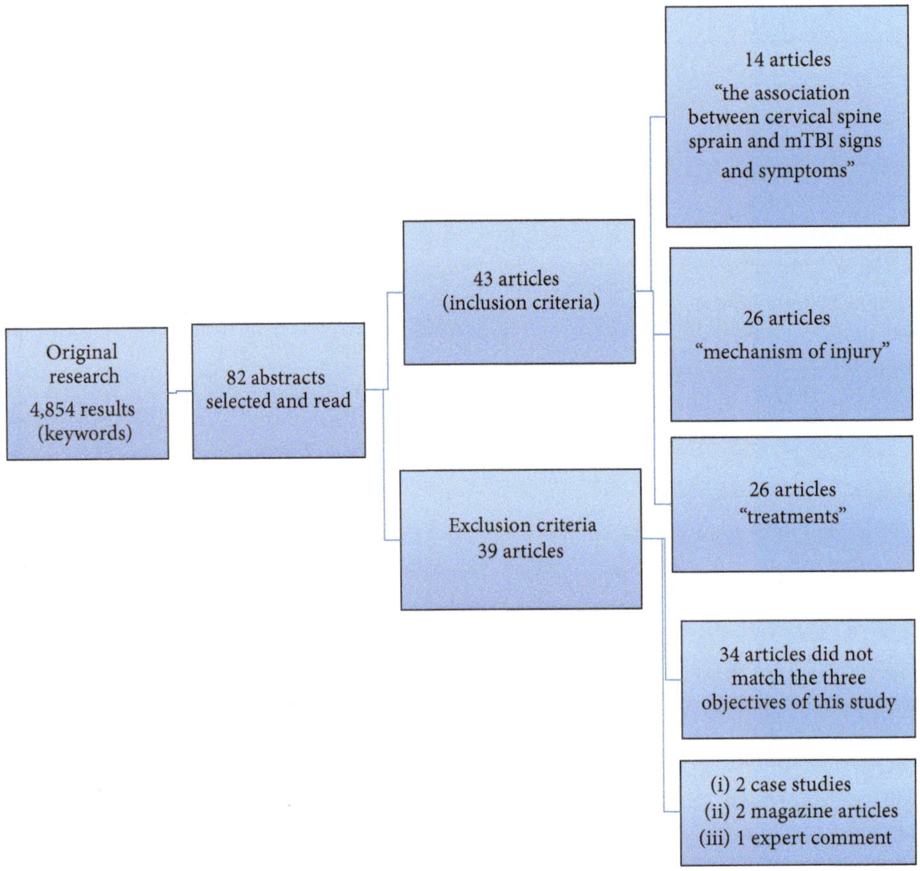

FIGURE 1: Research method for this review.

the presence of headache and neck pain in a preseason evaluation increases the risk of concussions during the season [26]. Consequently, a neck examination should be part of the postconcussion follow-up in addition to the neurological screening examination [6].

Whiplash is defined as a mechanism of acceleration-deceleration transferred to the cervical spine [6, 20, 27, 28] (see Table 4). With its large range of motion, the upper cervical spine is the most mobile part of the spine. During a whiplash, cervical structures are stressed at their end ranges of motion which can lead to neck injuries [29]. The impact generates stresses and injuries in the bones and soft tissues of the cervical spine, causing clinical manifestations [24]. Among those, whiplash symptoms include neck pain, cervicogenic headaches, chest pain, memory and concentration disturbances, muscle tension, sleep disturbances, dizziness, fatigue, cervical range of motion restrictions, irritability, tinnitus, and visual disturbances [12, 17, 20, 24, 25]. A preliminary study has demonstrated that low velocity impacts between 4 and 12 km/h can provoke neck and head injuries causing dysfunctions and pain [12]. These symptoms are often similar to those listed for mTBI, which leads to confusion for the medical community [12, 14, 16, 25].

The pathophysiology related to the patient's symptoms originates from one or several structures of the cervical spine. After a trauma involving the cervical region, the involvement of muscles, ligaments, arteries, nerves, the esophagus, the temporomandibular joint, intervertebral discs, zygapophysial joints, vertebrae, and the atlantooccipital joint creates a complex challenge for clinicians [16, 17, 20].

One of the hypotheses raised in the literature for the origin of neck pain is the involvement of the cervical zygapophysial joints [30]. Zygapophysial joints have been shown to be the source of neck pain, headaches, visual disturbances, tinnitus, and dizziness in patients who have sustained whiplash [14, 24, 25]. In this following order, the C1-C2, C2-C3, C0-C1, and C3-C4 levels are the most often described in association with cervical symptoms following mTBI [16, 24, 26, 31]. More specifically, cervical zygapophysial joint pain is expressed by a hypersensitivity and hyperexcitability of the spinal cord reflexes, causing an increase of nociceptive processes in the central nervous system [32]. The cross-sectional study of Smith et al. (2013) recruited 58 adults (18–52 years old) with chronic whiplash disorder and provided a facet joint block to all participants [32]. They analyzed characteristics of responders and nonresponders to facet joint block and concluded that patients with chronic Whiplash-Associated Disorder (WAD) show similar sensory disturbances, motor dysfunction, and psychological distress [32]. Another study published by Treleaven et al. (1994) supports the implication

Table 2: Included studies description.

Authors/sections	Study objective	Population	Methods	Main outcomes/findings
Becker [34]	This review was developed as part of a debate and takes the "pro" stance that abnormalities of structures in the neck can be a significant source of headache	Adult	Literature review	(i) Clinical treatment trials involving patients with proven painful disorders of upper cervical zygapophysial joints have shown significant headache relief with treatment directed at cervical pain generators (ii) Headaches related to cervical spine disorders (cervicogenic headache and chronic headache attributed to whiplash injury) remain one of the most controversial areas of headache medicine (iii) Diagnostic criteria for cervicogenic headache have been developed by the CHISG
Bogduk [30]	To summarize the evidence that implicates the cervical zygapophysial joints as the leading source of chronic neck pain after whiplash	Adult	Narrative review Data were retrieved from studies that addressed the postmortem features and biomechanics of injury to the cervical zygapophysial joints and from clinical studies	(i) Clinical studies have shown that zygapophysial joint pain is very common among patients with chronic neck pain after whiplash (ii) The fact that multiple lines of evidence, using independent techniques, consistently implicate the cervical zygapophysial joints as a site of injury and source of pain strongly implicates injury to these joints as a common basis for chronic neck pain after whiplash
Bonk et al. [38]	To evaluate the effectiveness of conservative management for acute Whiplash-Associated Disorder	Adult	Systematic review and meta-analysis of randomized controlled trials	Improvement of cervical movement in the horizontal plane short term could be promoted by the use of a conservative intervention. The use of a behavioral intervention (e.g., act-as-usual, education, and self-care including regular exercise) may be an effective treatment in reducing pain and improving cervical mobility in patients with acute WADII in the short-medium term
Borich et al. [2]	In this special interest article, we discuss the definition and risk factors associated with concussion, summarize and highlight some of the most widely used assessment tools, and critique the evidence for current principles of concussion management	Adult	Literature review	(i) Disease Control and Prevention describes *mild traumatic brain injury* (mTBI which includes concussion) as a silent epidemic (ii) An estimated 1.6 million to 3.8 million sport- and recreation-related brain injuries occur in the United States annually, and up to 75% are classified as mild (iii) "Rest" in the form of delaying return to competitive sports may be better served by a universal period of 7 to 10 days than by symptom monitoring, primarily to prevent the potential for reinjury

Table 2: Continued.

Authors/sections	Study objective	Population	Methods	Main outcomes/findings
Brolinson [7]	To systematically review the evidence for rest, treatment, and rehabilitation after sport-related concussion	Sports Adult Pediatric	Systematic review	(i) From 749 articles evaluating rest and 1,175 evaluating treatment, 2 studies met criteria for the effect of rest and 10 abstracts met criteria for treatment. Three further treatment articles were identified by the authors (ii) Health professionals are more involved in sports and in the concussions follow-up (iii) Interventions included manual spinal therapy, physiotherapy, and neuromotor and sensorimotor retraining compared with rest and graduated exercise, for up to 8 weeks
Collins et al. [43]	To develop and validate a cost-effective tool to measure neck strength in a high school setting and to determine if anthropometric measurements captured by ATs can predict concussion risk	6,704 high school athletes in boys' and girls' soccer, basketball, and lacrosse	Feasibility study Pilot study	(i) Differences in overall neck strength may be useful in developing a screening tool to determine which high school athletes are at higher risk of concussion. Once identified, these athletes could be targeted for concussion prevention programs
Eckner et al. [40]	The purpose of this study was to determine the influence of neck strength and muscle activation status on resultant head kinematics after impulsive loading	46 contact sport athletes 24 males; 22 females aged 8 to 30 years	Descriptive laboratory study	(i) Neck strength and impact anticipation are 2 potentially modifiable risk factors for concussion (ii) The results of this study suggest that greater neck strength attenuates the head's dynamic response to external forces
Fernández De Las Peñas et al. [24]	The aims of the present paper are to detail a manual approach developed by our research group, to help in future studies of the management of the sequels to whiplash injury, and to suggest explanations for the mechanisms of this protocol	Adult	Literature review	(i) The clinical syndrome of whiplash injury includes neck pain, upper thoracic pain, cervicogenic headache, tightness, dizziness, restriction of cervical range of motion, tinnitus, and blurred vision (ii) Spinal manipulation/mobilization and soft tissue mobilization techniques are manual therapies commonly used in the management of neck disorders

TABLE 2: Continued.

Authors/sections	Study objective	Population	Methods	Main outcomes/findings
Kennedy [14]	This document is intended to provide the user with instruction and direction in the rehabilitation of PCS	Ontario Hospital Canada Adult	PCS and treatment guidelines (i) Cervicogenic (ii) Autonomic (iii) Vestibular (iv) Vision (v) Education	(i) Anatomically, the cervical spine is closely linked to structures that can cause many of the same symptoms as concussion (ii) PCS treatment has traditionally consisted of rest, education, neurocognitive rehabilitation, and antidepressants with limited effectiveness (iii) Balance deficits and postural instability are commonly reported after concussion
Gravel et al. [36]	This systematic review investigated the effectiveness of interventions initiated in acute settings for patients who experience mTBI	Adult	Systematic review Cochrane's risk of bias assessment tool	(i) According to the published literature, no intervention initiated acutely has been clearly associated with a positive outcome for patients who sustain mTBI, and there is little evidence suggesting that follow-up interventions may be associated with a better outcome (ii) There is a paucity of well-designed clinical studies for patients who sustain mTBI. The large variability in outcomes measured in studies limits comparison between them
Guskiewicz et al. [9]	To review the current literature to identify the most sensitive and reliable concussion assessment components for inclusion in the revised version: the SCAT3	Adult	Literature review	(i) One of the major challenges in the medical management of concussion is that there is no single "gold standard" for assessing and diagnosing the injury (ii) Balance deficits or instability are often observable in patients following concussion and the presence of these deficits may be an indicator of vestibular disruption
Hanson et al. [6]	The purpose of this article is to review the current literature in the management and prevention of concussion	Pediatrics	Review	(i) The rise in the number of concussion diagnoses may be due, in part, to increased awareness regarding the potential for complications of concussions and sequelae of multiple concussions, as opposed to an actual increase in the incidence of concussion alone (ii) Typical signs and symptoms of concussion

Table 2: Continued.

Authors/sections	Study objective	Population	Methods	Main outcomes/findings
Harmon et al. [5]	To provide an evidence-based, best practices summary to assist physicians with the evaluation and management of sports concussion	Adult Children	Statement of the American Medical Society for Sport Medicine Review	(i) However, as many as 50% of the concussions may go unreported (ii) Headache is the most commonly reported symptom with dizziness the second most common
Headache Classification Committee of the International Headache Society (IHS) [33]	The International Classification of Headache Disorder may be reproduced freely for scientific, educational, or clinical uses by institutions, societies, or individuals	Adult Children	Review guideline	(i) Cervicogenic headache from (1) migraine and (2) tension-type headache includes side-locked pain, provocation of typical headache by digital pressure on neck muscles and by head movement, and posterior-to-anterior radiation of pain (ii) Diagnostic criteria
Hecht [16]	This article reviews the literature on management of posttraumatic headaches, presents an approach to the assessment and treatment of individuals with headaches following TBI that appear to be cervicogenic, focuses specifically on identifying occipital neuralgia, and discusses the technique of occipital nerve blocks	7 males (18–42 yo) 3 females (22–64 yo)	Retrospective review & Report of ten patients	(i) While there are a variety of different posttraumatic headaches, clinicians must be aware of all potential presentations including those emanating from the cervical spine and its affiliated structures (e.g., cervicogenic) (ii) Injury to these structures (innervated by afferent fibres of the 3 sup. cervical roots) (iii) These include but are not limited to muscles, ligaments, vessels, somatic and sympathetic nerves, esophagus, temporomandibular joint, discs, zygapophyseal joints, cervical vertebrae, and the atlantoaxial complex (iv) Whiplash syndrome may be the primary factor in many postconcussive headaches
Hynes and Dickey [12]	To examine the relationship between the occurrence of Whiplash-Associated Disorders and concussion symptoms in hockey players	High school, college/university, Ontario Hockey League, and men's recreational teams (15–35 yo) 20 teams	Prospective study	(i) 183 players were registered for this study; 13 received either a mechanical whiplash injury or a concussion injury (ii) There is a strong association between whiplash-induced neck injuries and the symptoms of concussion in hockey injuries (iii) Acceleration and deceleration of the head and neck complex occurs in sports and can potentially create injuries similar to those incurred in low velocity motor vehicle accidents, as stated in a recent literature review focused on Whiplash-Associated Disorders

Table 2: Continued.

Authors/sections	Study objective	Population	Methods	Main outcomes/findings
King et al. [35]	The objective was to determine the sensitivity, specificity, and likelihood ratio of manual examination for the diagnosis of cervical zygapophyseal joint pain	173 patients with neck pain in whom cervical zygapophyseal joint pain was suspected	Retrospective study	(i) Manual examination had a high sensitivity for cervical zygapophyseal joint pain, at the segmental levels commonly symptomatic, but its specificity was poor (ii) The present study found manual examination of the cervical spine to lack validity for the diagnosis of cervical zygapophyseal joint pain
Kozlowski et al. [3]	To assess exercise intolerance in male and female patients with PCS	34 patients (PCS) 17 males, 17 females Age = 25.9 ± 10.9 22 uninjured individuals	Cross-sectional study	(i) Symptoms from concussion typically resolve within 7 to 10 days (ii) The definition of PCS given by the World Health Organization includes a history of traumatic brain injury and 3 or more symptoms (iii) No cognitive testing, exclusion of other disorders, or symptom threshold exists for the diagnosis of PCS (iv) Patients with PCS had a symptom-limited response to exercise, and the treadmill test was a potentially useful tool to monitor the recovery from PCS
Kristjansson and Treleaven [29]	The purpose is to review dizziness in neck pain: implications for assessment and management	Adult	Review	(i) Disturbances to the afferent input from the cervical region in those with neck pain may be a possible cause of symptoms such as dizziness, unsteadiness, and visual disturbances, as well as signs of altered postural stability, cervical proprioception, and head and eye movement control
Leddy et al. [27]	The objective was to compare symptoms in patients with physiologic postconcussion disorder (PCD) versus cervicogenic/vestibular PCD	128 adults	Retrospective review Questionnaire	(i) Clinicians should consider specific testing of exercise tolerance and perform a physical examination of the cervical spine and the vestibular/ocular systems to determine the etiology of postconcussion symptoms (ii) Concomitant injury to the cervical spine resembling whiplash may occur as a result of the acceleration, deceleration forces sustained in concussive trauma (iii) Structural and functional injury to the cervical spine can be associated with prolonged symptoms such as headache, dizziness, blurred vision, and vertigo

Table 2: Continued.

Authors/sections	Study objective	Population	Methods	Main outcomes/findings
Leddy et al. [44]	This review focuses on rehabilitation of concussion and postconcussion syndrome	Adult Children	Review	(i) Early education, cognitive behavioral therapy, and aerobic exercise therapy have shown efficacy in certain patients but have limitations of study design
Leslie and Craton [25]	Based on the current medical evidence, we would suggest that the constellation of symptoms presently defined as concussion does not have to involve the brain	Adult	Editorial comment	(i) Concussion symptoms can emanate from the cervical spine (ii) Whiplash mechanisms of injury are identical to the "impulsive forces" described in concussive injuries (iii) Notably, symptoms such as headache, neck pain, disturbance of concentration or memory, dizziness, irritability, sleep disturbance, and fatigue have been described in both concussion and whiplash patients (iv) Cervical zygapophysial joints have been implicated as generators of headache and dizziness (v) The overlap with neck/whiplash injuries is evident
Lucas [19]	This article reviews the literature on headache management in concussion and mTBI	Adult Pediatric United States	Literature review	(i) Reports of headache after concussion or mTBI in children ranged from 72% to 93% (ii) Headache is one of the most common symptoms after TBI and PTH may be part of a constellation of symptoms that is seen in the postconcussive syndrome
Makdissi et al. [8]	The objectives of the current paper are to review the literature regarding difficult concussion and to provide recommendations for an approach to the investigation and management of patients with persistent symptoms	Adult Sport	Qualitative review	(i) Cases of concussion in sport where clinical recovery falls outside the expected window (i.e., 10 days) should be managed in a multidisciplinary manner by health care providers with experience in sports-related concussion
Marshall [11]	This paper is a review of recent literature on the topic of concussion, consisting of biomechanics, pathophysiology, diagnosis, and sideline management	Athletes United States	Narrative review	(i) The cervical spine not only is a potential source of injury that we must be aware of but also is implicated as a factor in the concussion itself (ii) Signs and symptoms of concussion from the Association of Sport College of Medicine (ACSM) updated consensus statement
Maugans et al. [22]	The goal of this investigation was to explore cerebral blood flow fluctuation after pediatric sport-related concussion	Twelve children Ages 11 to 15 years Control group	Clinical study	(i) Statistically significant alterations in cerebral blood flow were documented in the sport-related concussion group, with reduction in cerebral blood flow predominating. Improvement toward control values occurred in only 27% of the participants at 14 days and 64% at >30 days after sport-related concussion

TABLE 2: Continued.

Authors/sections	Study objective	Population	Methods	Main outcomes/findings
McCrory et al. [4]	The new 2012 Zurich Consensus statement is designed to build on the principles outlined in the previous documents and to develop further conceptual understanding of this problem using a formal consensus-based approach	International consensus (i) Adults (ii) Pediatric	International consensus Sport concussion	(i) An initial period of rest may be of benefit (ii) Multimodal physiotherapy treatment for individuals with clinical evidence of cervical spine and/or vestibular dysfunction may be of benefit (iii) Persistent symptoms (>10 days) are generally reported in 10–15% of concussions. In general, symptoms are not specific to concussion and it is important to consider other pathologies (iv) PCS should be managed in a multidisciplinary manner by health care providers with experience in sports concussion
Mihalik et al. [39]	The objective was to evaluate the effect of cervical muscle strength on head impact biomechanics	37 volunteer ice hockey players Age = 15.0 ± 1.0 years	Prospective cohort study	(i) The hypothesis that players with greater static neck strength would experience lower resultant head accelerations was not supported (ii) There is still nonempirical support for the role neck musculature may play in reducing the risk of mild TBI that is worthy of investigation in a young at-risk sample
Moser et al. [21]	The objective of this article is to evaluate the efficacy of cognitive and physical rest for the treatment of concussion	High school and collegiate athletes ($N = 49$) Range = 14–23 yo Mean = 15.0 yo 67% male 33% female	Retrospective analysis	(i) Participants showed significantly improved performance on Immediate Post-Concussion Assessment and Cognitive Testing and decreased symptom reporting following prescribed cognitive and physical rest (ii) These preliminary data suggest that a period of cognitive and physical rest may be a useful means of treating concussion-related symptoms, whether applied soon after a concussion or weeks to months later
Pelletier [18]	The purpose of this paper is to present a review of the diagnosis and treatment of the potentially catastrophic neck and head injuries caused by spearing in Canadian amateur football	Amateur football United States and Canada	Literature review	(i) Associated cervical trauma with concussion may include one or several of neck pain, reduced cervical range of movement, cervicogenic headache, cervicogenic vertigo, and occipital neuralgia (ii) Several manual techniques for the treatment of posttraumatic concussion syndrome have been described as either "direct" or "indirect"
Reid et al. [37]	This study aimed to determine the efficacy of sustained natural apophyseal glides (SNAGs) in the treatment of this condition	34 adults 17 SNAGs 17 Placebo	Double-blind randomized controlled clinical trial	(i) The SNAG treatment had an immediate clinically and statistically significant sustained effect in reducing dizziness, cervical pain, and disability caused by cervical dysfunction

Table 2: Continued.

Authors/sections	Study objective	Population	Methods	Main outcomes/findings
Schmidt et al. [42]	The purpose of this study was to compare the odds of sustaining higher magnitude in-season head impacts between athletes with higher and lower preseason performance on cervical muscle characteristics	49 high school and collegiate American football players	Cohort study	(i) The study findings showed that greater cervical stiffness and less angular displacement after perturbation reduced the odds of sustaining higher magnitude head impacts; however, the findings did not show that players with stronger and larger neck muscles mitigate head impact severity (ii) Male athletes also exhibit greater stiffness and capacity to store elastic energy compared with female athletes
Schneider et al. [26]	The objective of this study was to determine the risk of concussion in youth male hockey players with preseason reports of neck pain, headaches, and/or dizziness	3832 males Ice hockey players (11–14 yo) 280 teams	Prospective study	(i) Preseason reports of neck pain and headache were risk factors for concussion (ii) Dizziness was a risk factor for concussion in the Pee Wee nonbody checking (iii) A combination of any 2 symptoms was a risk factor in the Pee Wee nonbody checking cohort and the Bantam cohort (iv) Neck pain is the third most commonly reported baseline symptom in varsity athletes
Schneider et al. [10]	The objective of this study was to determine if a combination of vestibular rehabilitation and cervical spine physiotherapy decreased the time until medical clearance in individuals with prolonged postconcussion symptoms	18 males 13 females 12–30 years	Randomized controlled trial	(i) A combination of cervical and vestibular physiotherapy decreased time to medical clearance to return to sport in youth and young adults with persistent symptoms of dizziness, neck pain, and/or headaches following a sport-related concussion (ii) The cervical spine is cited as a source of pain in individuals with whiplash (iii) The upper cervical spine can cause cervicogenic headaches (iv) A combination of manual therapy and exercise has been shown to be more effective than passive treatment modalities in individuals with neck pain
Scorza et al. [13]	Current concepts in concussion	Children adolescents	Literature review	(i) Initial evaluation involves eliminating cervical spine injury and serious traumatic brain injury (ii) Selected symptoms of concussion

Table 2: Continued.

Authors/sections	Study objective	Population	Methods	Main outcomes/findings
Signoretti et al. [15]	The following review represents the authors' effort to piece together the current concepts and the most recent findings about the complex basic physiology underlying the injury processes of this particular type of brain trauma and to emphasize the nuances involved in conducting research in this area	European countries United States Adult	Literature review	(i) Postconcussive symptoms may be prolonged in a small percentage of cases, but the acute clinical symptoms largely reflect a functional disturbance rather than a structural injury, which usually is confirmed by the absence of abnormalities on standard neuroimaging studies (ii) The symptoms of concussion reflected a functional disturbance rather than a structural damage such as contusion, hemorrhage, or laceration of the brain
Smith et al. [32]	This preliminary study examined a sample of individuals who did and did not respond to facet block as well as healthy controls to determine whether there were differences in their physical and psychological features once the effects of the blocks had abated and symptoms had returned	58 adults (18–65 yo) Calgary, Canada	Cross-sectional study	(i) Following FB procedures, both WAD groups demonstrated generalized hypersensitivity to all sensory tests, decreased neck ROM, and increased superficial muscle activity with the CCFT compared to controls (ii) Both WAD groups demonstrated psychological distress (iii) Chronic WAD responders and nonresponders to feedback (FB) procedures demonstrate a similar presentation of sensory disturbance, motor dysfunction, and psychological distress. Higher levels of pain catastrophization and greater medication intake were the only factors found to differentiate these groups
Spitzer et al. [28]	The purpose was to expose the clinical classification of Whiplash-Associated Disorders	Adult	Guideline	(i) Grades 0 to 4 (clinical presentation)
Stovner et al. [23]	A main objective of this study was to assess the validity of this diagnosis by studying the headache pattern of concussed patients that participated in one historic (n = 131) and one prospective cohort (n = 217) study	200 patients (18–67 yo) Trauma involving LOC of < 15 min. Kaunas, Lithuania	Questionnaires study (after 3 months & 1 year)	(i) Existence of pretraumatic headache was a predictor of posttraumatic headache, although pretraumatic headache seems to have been underreported among the concussed patients (ii) This is negative correlation, and the lack of specificity indicates that headache occurring 3 months or more after concussion is not caused by the head or brain injury (iii) Rather it may represent an episode of one of the primary headaches, possibly induced by the stress of the situation

Table 2: Continued.

Authors/sections	Study objective	Population	Methods	Main outcomes/findings
Tator et al. [1]	This report is intended to improve understanding of the epidemiology of neurological conditions and the economic impact on the Canadian health care system and society	Adult Children Canada	Statistical report	(i) Cerebral concussions are commonly known as mild traumatic brain injury (mTBI) (ii) By contrast, Statistics Canada estimated in recent studies that the annual incidence for mTBI is 600 per 100,000 persons and 11.4 per 100,000 inhabitants for a traumatic brain injury (TBI) (iii) However, the highest age group incidence is between 19 and 29 years, representing approximately one-quarter of patients with cranial trauma (iv) Children (18 years and younger) represented almost 45% of the patients with head injury
Tierney et al. [41]	The purpose was to determine whether gender differences existed in head-neck segment kinematic and neuromuscular control variables responses to an external force application with and without neck muscle preactivation	20 females 20 males Adult	Cohort study	(i) Gender differences existed in head-neck segment dynamic stabilization during head angular acceleration (ii) Females exhibited significantly greater head-neck segment peak angular acceleration and displacement than males despite initiating muscle activity earlier (SCM only) and using a greater percentage of their maximum head-neck segment muscle activity
Treleaven et al. [31]	This study measured aspects of cervical musculoskeletal function in a group of patients (12) with postconcussional headache (PCH) and in a normal control group	8 males (15–48 yo) 4 females (20–44 yo)	Retrospective study	(i) Twelve of the 15 eligible patients consented to enter the study (ii) The most frequent major symptomatic segments were C1-C2, C2-C3, C0-C1, and C3-C4. Signs of cervical articular and muscular dysfunction distinguished the PCH group from the control group (iii) As upper cervical joint dysfunction is a feature of cervicogenic causes of headache, the results of this study support the inclusion of a precise physical examination of the cervical region in differential diagnosis of patients suffering persistent headache following concussion

Table 2: Continued.

Authors/sections	Study objective	Population	Methods	Main outcomes/findings
Watanabe et al. [20]	The specific goals of this review include (1) determination of effective interventions for PTH (2) development of treatment recommendations (3) identification of gaps in the current medical literature regarding PTHA treatment (4) suggestions for future directions in research to improve outcome for persons with PTHA	Adult Child	Literature review The level of evidence: American Academy of Neurology criteria	(i) Head pain may be related to direct damage to the skull or brain tissue; muscular, tendinous, and/or ligamentous injury to the cervical spine; and injuries to peripheral nerves. Other nervous system injuries, such as visual and vestibular system damage, also may contribute to headache syndromes (ii) Biologically based interventions included a variety of biofeedback mechanisms, physical therapy and manual therapy, immobilization devices, ice, and injections
Weightman et al. [17]	The purpose of this article is to provide a summary of the development process and to share specific recommendations for PT practice with service members who sustain MTBI	Military and civilian populations	Literature review MTBI-related, evidence-based reviews and guidelines	(i) Determine the disability and its severity related to the neck, jaw, and headaches (ii) Physical therapy interventions with the strongest evidence in the treatment of PTH include a multimodal approach of specific training in exercise and postural retraining, stretching and ergonomic education, and manipulation and/or mobilization in combination with exercise

TABLE 3: Most common symptoms of mTBI according to their categories [4, 6, 11–13].

References	Cognitive	Somatic physical	Affective emotional	Sleep disturbance
Marshall, 2012 [11] Hanson et al., 2014 [6] Hynes and Dickey, 2006 [12] Scorza et al., 2012 [13] McCrory et al., 2013 [4]	(i) Confusion (ii) Retrograde amnesia (iii) Anterograde amnesia (iv) Loss of consciousness (v) Disorientation (vi) Feeling foggy (in a fog) (vii) Vacant stare (viii) Inability to focus (ix) Delayed verbal responses (x) Delayed motor responses (xi) Slurred (xii) Incoherent speech (slurred) (xiii) Excessive drowsiness	(i) Headache (ii) Dizziness (iii) Balance disruption (iv) Nausea (v) Vomiting (vi) Visual disturbances (vii) Phonophobia	(i) Emotional liability (ii) Irritability (iii) Fatigue (iv) Anxiety (v) Sadness	(i) Trouble falling asleep (ii) Decreased sleep (iii) Increased sleep
Hanson et al., 2014 [6]	(i) Feeling slowed down (ii) Difficulty concentrating (iii) Difficulty remembering (iv) Forgetting of recent information (v) Confused about recent events (vi) Answers questions slowly (vii) Repeats questions	(i) Balance problems (ii) Visual problems (iii) Fatigue (iv) Sensitivity to light (v) Sensitivity to noise (vi) Dazed (vii) Stunned	(i) Nervousness	(i) Drowsiness
Hynes and Dickey, 2006 [12]	(i) Dysphagia (ii) Seeing stars	(i) Deafness (ii) Ringing in the ears (iii) Temporomandibular		
Scorza et al., 2012 [13]	(i) Disorientation (ii) Stunned (iii) Vacant stare	(i) Blurred vision (ii) Convulsions (iii) Light-headedness (iv) Numbness (v) Tingling (vi) Tinnitus	(i) Clinginess (ii) Depression (iii) Personality changes	

TABLE 4: Summary table of the Whiplash-Associated Disorder (WAD) classifications and concussion symptoms that can manifest themselves in any grade of WAD [6, 20, 27, 28].

WAD classification	Symptoms
0	No neck complaints
I	Complaint of neck pain, stiffness, or tenderness
II	Neck complaint with musculoskeletal signs
III	Neck complaint, musculoskeletal signs, and neurological signs
IV	Fracture and/or dislocation

of the cervical region by a precise physical examination in differential diagnosis of 12 patients suffering of persistent postconcussion headache [31].

Following a whiplash, the cervical spine is often the source of a patient's pain [4, 10]. The neck received the transmitted force of the impact and the same acceleration-deceleration mechanism that produces mTBI [28]. During the whiplash, the cause of cervicogenic and brain induced symptoms could be caused by either the mTBI or the cervical spine involvement or both at the same time [10]. There are similarities between the symptoms of neck disorders and the symptoms of mTBI [19]. The most common posttraumatic symptom is headache [4]. Cervicogenic headache and post-traumatic headache are well-known conditions [4, 13, 19, 33]. In fact, those upper cervical impairments, if not diagnosed and treated, can lead to chronicity of postconcussion headaches [10].

Cervicogenic headaches are common after a whiplash injury [16, 34]. Different studies showed that 3 to 4.6% of patients will develop chronic daily headaches after whiplash and 2% will be permanently disabled [34]. Upper cervical spine pain can arise from various anatomical structures such as muscles, joints, ligaments, and nerves [34]. Tensions in cervical muscles (trigger points) are the most common diagnosed type of headache [16, 23]. Becker (2010) explained that headaches related to cervical spine disorders (CGH) remain one of the most controversial areas of headache medicine [34]. Dysfunctions of the craniocervical zygapophysial (C0 to C4) joints can also cause headaches [16, 30]. In patients with headaches following a whiplash injury, dysfunctions of the C2-C3 zygapophysial joint are highly prevalent, particularly if there is tenderness over the C2-C3 facet joint [34]. Cervicogenic headaches may be unilateral or bilateral with the dominance depending on one or more of the structures that are affected [16]. Pain location usually begins in the occipital region of the neck [34]. After a whiplash injury, zygapophysial joints are clinically identified as the single most common source of pain in at least 50% of neck pain. Furthermore, facet joints appear to be the most common source of pain in the neck, with or without headache [34]. King et al. (2007) showed in their retrospective study, which included 173 patients, that manual examination had a high degree of sensitivity during zygapophysial joint pain evaluation [35]. Tension in the cervical muscles has the potential effect of reducing neck movement and generating local pain [16, 18]. A bad posture or sleeping position as well as physical activity performed with a faulty motor strategy can lead to neck pain and pain irradiating to the head [19]. In 2013, the Cervicogenic Headache International Study Group (CHISG) developed the diagnostic criteria for CGH [33] (see the following).

Summary of the Cervicogenic Headache (CGH) Diagnostic Criteria [33]

Unilaterality of pain, although it is recognized that bilateral cervicogenic headache may occur.

Restriction in range of motion in the neck.

Provocation of usual head pain by neck movement or sustained awkward neck positions.

Provocation of usual head pain with external pressure over the upper cervical or occipital region on the symptomatic side.

Ipsilateral neck, shoulder, or arm pain, usually of a vague nonradicular nature, occasionally radicular.

Posttraumatic headaches are a serious contributor to disability following cranial, cerebral, and cervical injury. Therefore, evaluating the cervical region after a head trauma is recommended [4]. This recommendation will highly contribute to limiting morbidity of mTBI and, furthermore, to help clinicians identify the International Headache Society (IHS) cervicogenic characteristics on mTBI patients. One of the improvements of SCAT3 and Child-SCAT3 compared to the SCAT2 is the introduction of the cervical assessment in posttrauma evaluation [4]. Knowing that the mechanism of mTBI is an external force transmitting energy to the head, it is possible that the neck, supporting the head, can also be injured during such an external force [11, 12, 16]. The Zurich consensus for concussion in sports (2012) recommended a multidisciplinary approach for patients who suffer PCS symptoms, such as headaches lasting longer than 6 weeks [4].

6.3. Treatments. The majority of articles in the literature currently focus on the diagnosis of mTBI, but few are dedicated to its management and treatments [7]. The 2012 Zurich consensus on concussion in sport suggested physical and cognitive rest until the end of the acute symptoms after trauma and a multidisciplinary approach involving experienced health care professionals when treating mTBI [4]. In their retrospective analysis, Moser et al. (2012) analyzed 49 high school and collegiate athletes (mean = 15.0 years old) and suggested that a period of cognitive and physical rest may be a useful mean of treating concussion-related symptoms [21]. This recovery time allows for a period of 7 to 10 days before the athlete returns to competition [2]. During this period, the symptoms should be evaluated daily and all activities that increase these symptoms should be stopped [4]. A Cochrane study mentioned that, based on present literature, no acutely initiated intervention has been clearly associated with a positive outcome for patients who sustain mTBI [36].

Return-to-play is allowed when athletes are symptom-free at rest, are able to do a full practice with contact without symptoms, no longer take any medications, and have returned to their baseline levels of cognitive functioning and postural stability [6].

The evaluation of the cervical region has been included as a new part of the SCAT3/Child-SCAT3, and a full clearance is essential before return-to-play [4]. According to some authors, post-mTBI subjects must have no pain in the neck, full mobility, and an adequate bilateral general strength to restart their sporting activities [12].

Treatments such as vertebral manual therapy, cervical tractions, manipulations, and exercises can relieve neck pain [16]. Brolinson (2014) has demonstrated that interventions of spinal manual therapy, physiotherapy, and neuromotor/sensorimotor training are more effective for mTBI recovery compared to a program of rest and exercises [7]. Another study demonstrated that the physical status of individuals with neck pain is improved with an exercise program combining manipulation, proprioceptive neuromuscular facilitation, acupressure on trigger points, and range of motion exercises, along with proprioceptive exercises compared to a neck pain control group of similar patients treated with information and advice [29]. Treatment of the cervical spine (sustained natural apophyseal glides) has been shown to be effective in 17 individuals with suspected cervicogenic dizziness compared to a control group (17 adults) [37]. Schneider et al. (2014) established that a significantly higher proportion of post-mTBI individuals (more than 3 weeks after trauma) were medically cleared to return to sport within 8 weeks of initiating treatment if they were treated in physiotherapy with cervical spine and vestibular rehabilitation compared to a control group [10]. Another study recruited 128 mTBI adults with either PCS or cervicogenic/vestibular symptoms [27], who completed the 22-symptom postconcussion symptoms scale questionnaire. Their results demonstrated that the questionnaire does not reliably discriminate between both types of patients. They concluded that clinicians should consider specific testing of exercise tolerance and perform a physical examination of the cervical spine and the vestibular/ocular systems to determine the etiology of postconcussion symptoms and to consider treating these accordingly [27]. Assessment and treatment of the cervical spine and vestibular system in the presence of persistent dizziness, neck pain, and/or headaches may facilitate functional and symptomatic improvements and shorten recovery in post-mTBI subjects [7, 10].

There is little evidence in clinical trials on the treatment of PTH. A study by Bonk et al. (2000) has shown that physiotherapy treatments decrease pain and increase cervical range of motion compared to a control group in a cervical collar for a period of 6 and 12 weeks after trauma [38]. The physiotherapy programs consisted of active and passive mobilizations, postural strengthening, the application of ice, and exercises that are efficient for PTH.

Regarding the cervical muscular system, several changes are observed following a trauma such as mTBI or whiplash. There is still nonempirical support that stronger neck muscles could reduce the risks of mTBI on the field [11, 39]. In fact, Mihalik et al. (2011) evaluated the effect of cervical strength on head impact in 37 hockey players (average 15 years old) and they concluded that the hypothesis of neck strength decreasing head acceleration was not supported [39]. Recent publications identify the importance of neck musculature in the prevention of concussions. Two hypotheses are presently under debate in the literature. The potentially modifiable risk factors for concussion are neck strength and impact anticipation [40]. Tierney et al. (2005) demonstrated that males have a better head-neck segment dynamic stabilization than females when angular acceleration is sustained by the head in a study including 20 males and 20 females [41]. Furthermore, a descriptive study demonstrated that greater neck strength and anticipatory cervical muscle activation (bracing for impact) can reduce the magnitude of the head's kinematic response in a population of 46 contact sport athletes (male and female) aged between 8 and 30 years [40]. Another study on a group of 49 football players (high school/collegiate) has shown that the odds of sustaining higher magnitude head impacts are reduced with better cervical strength and lower angular displacement following impact [42]. However, their findings did not show that stronger and larger neck muscles in players decreased head impact severity [42]. Meanwhile, Collins et al. (2014) concluded, in their study, which included 6704 high school athletes, that neck strength can be a valuable screening tool to prevent concussion [43]. Further research is needed to clarify these hypotheses and the actual role of neck strength in reducing risk of concussion.

A study by Leddy et al. (2012) for mTBI subjects slow to recover shows that a lightweight level of exercise can be beneficial [44]. Kozlowski et al. (2013) recently published a cross-sectional study about the exercise impact on 34 patients with PCS and a control group of 22 patients [3]. Conclusions showed that patients with PCS had a symptom-limited response to exercise, and the treadmill test was a potentially useful tool to monitor the recovery from PCS [3].

Other physiotherapy treatments, such as vestibular rehabilitation, visual training, cardiovascular training, and the treatment of cervical dysfunctions, have shown some promising avenues, but further studies are needed [4, 10, 14, 17, 20].

7. Conclusion

In conclusion, mTBI is a complex injury and needs to be taken care of by different medical specialists working together toward the same goal, recovery [4]. The evidence of cervical spine involvement in mTBI is becoming apparent, but there is a lack of sound evidence in the literature [25]. Our findings have implications for further research. The hypothesis of cervical spine involvement in post-mTBI symptoms and in PCS is supported by increasing evidence and largely accepted. Health professionals should consider assessing the cervical spine of patients affected by mTBI. Some original data articles support this theory and show that persistent headache and postconcussion syndrome are often related to musculoskeletal pathology of the cervical spine. For the mTBI management and treatment, few articles in the literature are available, but well-defined studies showed interesting results about manual therapy (cervical and vestibular) and exercises as effective tools for health care practitioners. Further studies are needed to establish an adequate evaluation and determine guidelines for treatments. The evaluation and treatment of the cervical region are a major step to improve mTBI rehabilitation.

Appendix

See Figure 1 and Tables 1, 2, 3, and 4, and also see "Summary of the Cervicogenic Headache (CGH) Diagnostic Criteria [33]" in Section 6.2.

Abbreviations

mTBI:	Mild traumatic brain injury
ICL:	Index to Chiropractic Literature
PEDro:	SportDiscus, Physiotherapy Evidence Database
CINAHL:	Cumulative Index to Nursing and Allied Health Literature
CDC:	Centers for Disease Control and Prevention
TBI:	Traumatic brain injury
PCS:	Postconcussion syndrome
MRI:	Magnetic Resonance Imaging
WAD:	Whiplash-Associated Disorder
IHS:	International Headache Society
PTH:	Posttraumatic headache
CGH:	Cervicogenic headache
GCS:	Glasgow Coma Score
SAC:	Standardized Assessment of Concussion
BESS:	Balance Error Scoring System.

Competing Interests

The authors declare that they have no competing interests.

References

[1] C. Tator, G. Bray, and D. Morin, "The CBANCH report—the burden of neurological diseases, disorders, and injuries in Canada," *The Canadian Journal of Neurological Sciences*, vol. 34, no. 3, pp. 268–269, 2007.

[2] M. R. Borich, K. L. Cheung, P. Jones et al., "Concussion: current concepts in diagnosis and management," *Journal of Neurologic Physical Therapy*, vol. 37, no. 3, pp. 133–139, 2013.

[3] K. F. Kozlowski, J. Graham, J. J. Leddy, L. Devinney-Boymel, and B. S. Willer, "Exercise intolerance in individuals with postconcussion syndrome," *Journal of Athletic Training*, vol. 48, no. 5, pp. 627–635, 2013.

[4] P. McCrory, W. H. Meeuwisse, M. Aubry et al., "Consensus statement on concussion in sport: the 4th International Conference on Concussion in Sport held in Zurich, November 2012," *British Journal of Sports Medicine*, vol. 47, pp. 250–258, 2013.

[5] K. G. Harmon, J. A. Drezner, M. Gammons et al., "American Medical Society for Sports Medicine position statement: concussion in sport," *British Journal of Sports Medicine*, vol. 47, no. 1, pp. 15–26, 2013.

[6] E. Hanson, A. Stracciolini, R. Mannix, and W. P. Meehan, "Management and prevention of sport-related concussion," *Clinical Pediatrics*, vol. 53, no. 13, pp. 1221–1230, 2014.

[7] P. G. Brolinson, "Management of sport-related concussion: a review," *Clinical Journal of Sport Medicine*, vol. 24, no. 1, pp. 89–90, 2014.

[8] M. Makdissi, R. C. Cantu, K. M. Johnston, P. McCrory, and W. H. Meeuwisse, "The difficult concussion patient: what is the best approach to investigation and management of persistent (>10 days) postconcussive symptoms?" *British Journal of Sports Medicine*, vol. 47, no. 5, pp. 308–313, 2013.

[9] K. M. Guskiewicz, J. Register-Mihalik, P. McCrory et al., "Evidence-based approach to revising the SCAT2: introducing the SCAT3," *British Journal of Sports Medicine*, vol. 47, no. 5, pp. 289–293, 2013.

[10] K. J. Schneider, W. H. Meeuwisse, A. Nettel-Aguirre et al., "Cervicovestibular rehabilitation in sport-related concussion: a randomised controlled trial," *British journal of sports medicine*, vol. 48, no. 17, pp. 1294–1298, 2014.

[11] C. M. Marshall, "Sports-related concussion: a narrative review of the literature," *The Journal of the Canadian Chiropractic Association*, vol. 56, no. 4, pp. 299–310, 2012.

[12] L. M. Hynes and J. P. Dickey, "Is there a relationship between whiplash-associated disorders and concussion in hockey? A preliminary study," *Brain Injury*, vol. 20, no. 2, pp. 179–188, 2006.

[13] K. A. Scorza, M. F. Raleigh, and F. G. O'Connor, "Current concepts in concussion: evaluation and management," *American Family Physician*, vol. 85, no. 2, pp. 123–132, 2012.

[14] F. Kennedy, *Guideline 2013—Post-Concussion Treatment Guidelines 2013*, 2013.

[15] S. Signoretti, G. Lazzarino, B. Tavazzi, and R. Vagnozzi, "The pathophysiology of concussion," *PM&R*, vol. 3, no. 10, supplement 2, pp. S359–S368, 2011.

[16] J. S. Hecht, "Occipital nerve blocks in postconcussive headaches: a retrospective review and report of ten patients," *Journal of Head Trauma Rehabilitation*, vol. 19, no. 1, pp. 58–71, 2004.

[17] M. M. Weightman, R. Bolgla, K. L. McCulloch, and M. D. Peterson, "Physical therapy recommendations for service members with mild traumatic brain injury," *Journal of Head Trauma Rehabilitation*, vol. 25, no. 3, pp. 206–218, 2010.

[18] J. C. Pelletier, "Sports related concussion and spinal injuries: the need for changing spearing rules at the National Capital Amateur Football Association (NCAFA)," *The Journal of the Canadian Chiropractic Association*, vol. 50, no. 3, pp. 195–208, 2006.

[19] S. Lucas, "Headache management in concussion and mild traumatic brain injury," *PM&R*, vol. 3, no. 10, supplement 2, pp. S406–S412, 2011.

[20] T. K. Watanabe, K. R. Bell, W. C. Walker, and K. Schomer, "Systematic review of interventions for post-traumatic headache," *PM&R*, vol. 4, no. 2, pp. 129–140, 2012.

[21] R. S. Moser, C. Glatts, and P. Schatz, "Efficacy of immediate and delayed cognitive and physical rest for treatment of sports-related concussion," *The Journal of Pediatrics*, vol. 161, no. 5, pp. 922–926, 2012.

[22] T. A. Maugans, C. Farley, M. Altaye, J. Leach, and K. M. Cecil, "Pediatric sports-related concussion produces cerebral blood flow alterations," *Pediatrics*, vol. 129, no. 1, pp. 28–37, 2012.

[23] L. J. Stovner, H. Schrader, D. Mickevičiene, D. Surkiene, and T. Sand, "Headache after concussion," *European Journal of Neurology*, vol. 16, no. 1, pp. 112–120, 2009.

[24] C. Fernández De Las Peñas, L. Palomeque Del Cerro, and J. Fernández Carnero, "Manual treatment of post-whiplash injury," *Journal of Bodywork and Movement Therapies*, vol. 9, no. 2, pp. 109–119, 2005.

[25] O. Leslie and N. Craton, "Concussion: purely a brain injury?" *Clinical Journal of Sport Medicine*, vol. 23, no. 5, pp. 331–332, 2013.

[26] K. J. Schneider, W. H. Meeuwisse, J. Kang, G. M. Schneider, and C. A. Emery, "Preseason reports of neck pain, dizziness, and headache as risk factors for concussion in male youth ice hockey players," *Clinical Journal of Sport Medicine*, vol. 23, no. 4, pp. 267–272, 2013.

[27] J. J. Leddy, J. G. Baker, A. Merchant et al., "Brain or strain? Symptoms alone do not distinguish physiologic concussion from cervical/vestibular injury," *Clinical Journal of Sport Medicine*, vol. 25, no. 3, pp. 237–242, 2015.

[28] W. O. Spitzer, M. L. Skovron, L. R. Salmi et al., "Scientific monograph of the Quebec Task Force on Whiplash-Associated Disorders: redefining 'whiplash' and its management," *Spine*, vol. 20, no. 8, pp. 1S–73S, 1995.

[29] E. Kristjansson and J. Treleaven, "Sensorimotor function and dizziness in neck pain: implications for assessment and management," *Journal of Orthopaedic and Sports Physical Therapy*, vol. 39, no. 5, pp. 364–377, 2009.

[30] N. Bogduk, "On cervical zygapophysial joint pain after whiplash," *Spine*, vol. 36, no. 25, supplement, pp. S194–S199, 2011.

[31] J. Treleaven, G. Jull, and L. Atkinson, "Cervical musculoskeletal dysfunction in post-concussional headache," *Cephalalgia*, vol. 14, no. 4, pp. 273–279, 1994.

[32] A. D. Smith, G. Jull, G. Schneider, B. Frizzell, R. A. Hooper, and M. Sterling, "A comparison of physical and psychological features of responders and non-responders to cervical facet blocks in chronic whiplash," *BMC Musculoskeletal Disorders*, vol. 14, article 313, 2013.

[33] Headache Classification Committee of the International Headache Society, "The International Classification of Headache Disorders, 3rd edition (beta version)," *Cephalalgia*, vol. 33, no. 9, pp. 629–808, 2013.

[34] W. J. Becker, "Cervicogenic headache: evidence that the neck is a pain generator," *Headache*, vol. 50, no. 4, pp. 699–705, 2010.

[35] W. King, P. Lau, R. Lees, and N. Bogduk, "The validity of manual examination in assessing patients with neck pain," *Spine Journal*, vol. 7, no. 1, pp. 22–26, 2007.

[36] J. Gravel, A. D'Angelo, B. Carrière et al., "Interventions provided in the acute phase for mild traumatic brain injury: a systematic review," *Systematic Reviews*, vol. 2, article 63, 2013.

[37] S. A. Reid, D. A. Rivett, M. G. Katekar, and R. Callister, "Sustained natural apophyseal glides (SNAGs) are an effective treatment for cervicogenic dizziness," *Manual Therapy*, vol. 13, no. 4, pp. 357–366, 2008.

[38] A. D. Bonk, R. Ferrari, G. D. Giebel, M. Edelmann, and R. Huser, "Prospective, randomized, controlled study of activity versus collar, and the natural history for whiplash injury, in Germany," *Journal of Musculoskeletal Pain*, vol. 8, no. 1-2, pp. 123–132, 2000.

[39] J. P. Mihalik, K. M. Guskiewicz, S. W. Marshall, R. M. Greenwald, J. T. Blackburn, and R. C. Cantu, "Does cervical muscle strength in youth ice hockey players affect head impact biomechanics?" *Clinical Journal of Sport Medicine*, vol. 21, no. 5, pp. 416–421, 2011.

[40] J. T. Eckner, Y. K. Oh, M. S. Joshi, J. K. Richardson, and J. A. Ashton-Miller, "Effect of neck muscle strength and anticipatory cervical muscle activation on the kinematic response of the head to impulsive loads," *American Journal of Sports Medicine*, vol. 42, no. 3, pp. 566–576, 2014.

[41] R. T. Tierney, M. R. Sitler, C. B. Swanik, K. A. Swanik, M. Higgins, and J. Torg, "Gender differences in head-neck segment dynamic stabilization during head accelaration," *Medicine and Science in Sports and Exercise*, vol. 37, no. 2, pp. 272–279, 2005.

[42] J. D. Schmidt, K. M. Guskiewicz, J. T. Blackburn, J. P. Mihalik, G. P. Siegmund, and S. W. Marshall, "The influence of cervical muscle characteristics on head impact biomechanics in football," *The American Journal of Sports Medicine*, vol. 42, no. 9, pp. 2056–2066, 2014.

[43] C. L. Collins, E. N. Fletcher, S. K. Fields et al., "Neck strength: a protective factor reducing risk for concussion in high school sports," *Journal of Primary Prevention*, vol. 35, no. 5, pp. 309–319, 2014.

[44] J. J. Leddy, H. Sandhu, V. Sodhi, J. G. Baker, and B. Willer, "Rehabilitation of concussion and post-concussion syndrome," *Sports Health*, vol. 4, no. 2, pp. 147–154, 2012.

28

Trajectories of Physical Activity Predict the Onset of Depressive Symptoms but Not Their Progression

Kaisa Kaseva,[1] Tom Rosenström,[1] Taina Hintsa,[1] Laura Pulkki-Råback,[1,2] Tuija Tammelin,[3] Jari Lipsanen,[1] Xiaolin Yang,[3] Mirka Hintsanen,[1,4] Christian Hakulinen,[1] Katja Pahkala,[5,6] Mirja Hirvensalo,[7] Nina Hutri-Kähönen,[8] Olli T. Raitakari,[5,9] and Liisa Keltikangas-Järvinen[1]

[1] *Unit of Personality, Work and Health Psychology, Institute of Behavioral Sciences, P.O. Box 9, University of Helsinki, 00014 Helsinki, Finland*
[2] *Helsinki Collegium for Advanced Studies, Fabianinkatu 24, P.O. Box 4, University of Helsinki, 00014 Helsinki, Finland*
[3] *LIKES, Research Center for Sport and Health Sciences, Rautpohjankatu 8, 40700 Jyväskylä, Finland*
[4] *Unit of Psychology, University of Oulu, P.O. Box 8000, 90014 Oulu, Finland*
[5] *Research Centre of Applied and Preventive Cardiovascular Medicine, Kiinamyllynkatu 10, University of Turku, 20520 Turku, Finland*
[6] *Paavo Nurmi Centre, Sports and Exercise Medicine Unit, Department of Physical Activity and Health, Kiinamyllynkatu 10, University of Turku, 20520 Turku, Finland*
[7] *Department of Sport Sciences, P.O. Box 35 (L), University of Jyväskylä, 40014 Jyväskylä, Finland*
[8] *Department of Pediatrics, P.O. Box 2000, University of Tampere and Tampere University Hospital, 33521 Tampere, Finland*
[9] *Department of Clinical Physiology and Nuclear Medicine, Kiinamyllynkatu 4-8, Turku University Hospital, 20520 Turku, Finland*

Correspondence should be addressed to Liisa Keltikangas-Järvinen; Liisa.Keltikangas-Jarvinen@helsinki.fi

Academic Editor: Ian L. Swaine

This prospective, community-based study examined trajectories of physical activity from childhood to adulthood and whether these trajectories contributed to depressive symptoms in adulthood to a greater degree than adulthood physical activity. Participants ($n = 3596$) were from the ongoing Cardiovascular Risk in Young Finns Study which started in 1980. Depressive symptoms were measured with Beck Depression Inventory (BDI-II) in 2012, and physical activity was assessed from 1980 to 2011 with self-reports. Analyses were adjusted for age, sex, childhood negative emotionality, socioeconomic factors, previous depressive symptoms, social support, body mass index, and smoking status (1980–2007). Highly, moderately, and lightly physically active trajectory groups were identified. Highly active participants reported lower levels of depressive symptoms compared to lightly active ones ($p < 0.001$) and compared to moderately active ones ($p = 0.001$). Moderately active participants had less symptoms than lightly active ones ($p < 0.001$). High levels of adulthood physical activity associated with lower levels of depressive symptoms ($p < 0.001$). The findings did not withstand adjustment for previous depressive symptoms ($p > 0.05$). Lifelong physical activity trajectories or adulthood physical activity was not associated with the progression of depressive symptoms in adulthood. Thus, physical activity history does not contribute to the progression of the depressive symptoms to a greater degree than adulthood physical activity.

1. Introduction

Depressive disorders affect 340 million people (approximately 9%) globally regardless of gender, culture, or ethnicity [1]. From 1990 till present time, depression has been rated one of the leading causes of years lived with disability (YLDs) [2]. Depression associates with a wide range of subsequent health outcomes. For instance, depression predicts future coronary events and cardiac deaths in healthy individuals and in those with established cardiovascular disease (CHD)

[3, 4]. Depression has also been shown to be associated with several other physical diseases, including cancer and osteoporosis [4], as well as with severe psychiatric disorders such as schizophrenia [5]. Furthermore, depression relates to low educational attainment and reduced work productivity [6]. Identifying factors that contribute to depression and developing tools that can be applied in early prevention of depression have been prominently highlighted [7].

Even though some conflicting findings concerning the association between physical activity and depression exist [8, 9], prior evidence provides support for the value of physical activity in reducing depressive symptoms in both healthy and clinical populations [10]. Literature has also indicated that even low doses of physical activity may protect against depression [10]. The relation between physical activity and depression may also be bidirectional, as physical activity may alleviate depressive symptoms, but these symptoms may also decrease the likelihood of initiating physical activity [8, 11]. Physical activity has also been related to neurobiological functioning, which may preempt depressive mood [12]. In addition, physical activity has been shown to be associated with the development of individual qualities such as self-confidence, emotional self-regulation [13], and capacity of social bonding [14], which, in turn, may be protective against depression [13, 14].

Several studies have indicated that regular physical activity associates with reduced risk of depression in all age groups from early childhood to late adulthood [8, 10, 15]. There is also evidence that childhood physical activity may lead to maintenance of lifetime physical activity patterns conducive to well-being (e.g., [16]). These patterns, however, have a tendency to decline towards later adulthood [17]. Many previous findings regarding the association between physical activity and depression derive from cross-sectional designs [10]. Previous longitudinal or intervention designs cover relatively short follow-up phases of physical activity [10, 18]. Prospective studies examining the association between lifelong physical activity and depressive symptoms are very rare [8].

It has been stated that more sophisticated methods are needed when studying the development and etiology of depression [19]. It has also been shown that people's health behaviors may have various developmental tendencies instead of a one growth trajectory [20, 21], and some of these behavioral profiles may be more detrimental to health than others. For instance, it is theoretically possible that physical activity's decline towards later life [17] may start earlier and/or be steeper among specific groups than in others, and thus the different physical activity profiles may associate with distinct health outcomes. The need for examinations assessing the development and decline of physical activity has been acknowledged [17, 22]. It is also essential to study whether long-term physical activity contributes to health over and above the concurrent physical activity. Furthermore, identifying people, whose behavioral tendencies associate with decreased health, might be useful for professionals who aim to adjust lifestyle interventions to targeted groups. It is also important to gain information of the behavioral determinants and contributors of good health [23].

Growth mixture modeling provides an appropriate framework for studying developmental processes [20, 24]. The key advantage of such modeling is that it allows for the estimation of interindividual variability in intraindividual patterns of change over time [20, 24]. Current approaches to growth modeling have also been regarded as flexible for instance in terms of including partially missing data, unequally spaced measurement points, nonnormally distributed or discretely scaled repeated measures, and linearly or nonlinearly shaped trajectories [24]. These issues, or some of these, typically emerge in developmental research. It has been denoted that these issues present challenges for more traditional methods [24].

Extensive adjustment for potential confounders has been lacking in many previous studies regarding physical activity and health outcomes [16, 18]. Development of depression often depends on the interplay of multiple psychological and lifestyle related factors [7] that ideally should be considered when examining associations between health behaviors and depression [25–30]. Child's early emotional experiences (e.g., negative emotionality) may have effects on the development of depression later in life [25]. Childhood family's socioeconomic status has been shown to be associated with the development of health behaviors and well-being [26]. In adulthood, occurrence of depressive episodes has been shown to predict subsequent depression [27]. It has been proven that depression is related to age [28], and women tend to report higher levels of depression than men [28]. Adulthood socioeconomic position, experiences of social support, body mass index, and smoking status are also associated with depression in adulthood [26, 29, 30].

We examined the potential heterogeneity in physical activity trajectories in relation to depressive symptoms over a 30-year period from childhood to adulthood in a population-based sample with six cohorts and including eight study waves. To our knowledge, this is the first study assessing physical activity and depressive symptoms in such design. The analyses were adjusted for several risk factors for depression [25–30]. Physical activity measurements were performed during participants' childhood and adulthood (from the age of 9 to 49), and depressive symptoms were assessed in participants' adulthood (participants aged from 35 to 50). To gain a comprehensive picture of the association between physical activity and depressive symptoms, the association was studied cross-sectionally, with respect to change and with respect to long-term trajectories. The objectives of this study were (1) to explore the potentially distinct trajectories of physical activity from childhood to adulthood, (2) to examine whether physical activity was associated with cross-sectional, short-term, and long-term changes in depressive symptoms in adulthood, and (3) to examine whether the physical activity trajectories contributed to depressive symptoms in adulthood to a greater degree than adulthood physical activity.

2. Methods

2.1. Study Design and Participants. The study participants were from the ongoing prospective Cardiovascular Risk in

Table 1: Descriptive statistics of the original sample (n = 1724–3596)*.

Variables		Measurement year	n	Mean ± SD/%	Range
Covariates	Age	1980	3596	10.44 ± 4.99	3–18
	Childhood negative emotionality	1980	3177	1.06 ± 0.11	1–2
	Parental education†	1980	3540	1.90 ± 0.77	1–3
	Parental income	1980	3453	4.80 ± 1.94	1–8
	Symptoms of depression	1992	2330	2.14 ± 0.60	1–4.57
	Symptoms of depression	1997	2099	2.15 ± 0.67	1–4.57
	Symptoms of depression	2001	2097	2.07 ± 0.67	1–4.62
	Symptoms of depression	2007	2056	2.06 ± 0.68	1–4.67
	Participants' education‡	2007	2022	2.11 ± 0.90	1–3
	Participants' income	2007	2146	3.50 ± 1.56	1–8
	Social support	2007	2055	4.15 ± 0.80	1.08–5.00
	Body mass index	2007	2170	26.00 ± 4.75	16.56–58.82
	Smoking status	2007	2224	3.81 ± 1.53	1–5
Physical activity indices§	Physical activity	1980	2224	9.05 ± 1.83	5–14
	Physical activity	1983	2116	9.03 ± 1.88	5–14
	Physical activity	1986	2320	8.90 ± 2.01	5–14
	Physical activity	1989	2619	8.63 ± 2.10	5–14
	Physical activity	1992	2192	9.08 ± 1.92	5–14
	Physical activity	2001	2442	8.86 ± 1.96	5–15
	Physical activity	2007	2166	8.81 ± 1.81	5–15
	Physical activity	2011	1910	9.02 ± 1.88	5–15
Physical activity trajectory groups§	Lightly physically active	1980–2011	371	10.4%	
	Moderately physically active	1980–2011	3046	85.5%	
	Highly physically active	1980–2011	147	4.1%	
Dependent variable	Symptoms of depression (BDI-II)	2012	1724	5.04 ± 6.60	0–58

*The original sample size was 3596, and 1764 (49.1%) of the participants were males and 1832 (50.9%) were females.
†The frequencies of parents' educational levels were as follows: low, n = 1228 (34.7%), average, n = 1428 (40.3%), high, and n = 884 (25.0%).
‡The frequencies of participants' educational levels were as follows: low, n = 713 (35.3%), average, n = 376 (18.6%), high, and n = 933 (46.1%).
§Physical activity indices ≤ 7 indicate low, >7 to 10 < moderate, and ≥10 high levels of physical activity. Factors scores, which were predicted from physical activity indices (1980–2011) (see Supplementary Table 3), were used in LCGA.

Young Finns Study that began in 1980 [31].The original sample consisted of 3596 children and adolescents (83.2% of those invited, 1832 females and 1764 males) from six birth cohorts (aged 3, 6, 9, 12, 15, and 18). To obtain a representative sample, Finland was divided into five areas based on the locations of universities with medical schools (Helsinki, Kuopio, Oulu, Tampere, and Turku), and the participants were randomly selected based on their social security numbers from nearby urban and rural areas. Informed consent was requested from each participant (or from the parents of small children), and the study was approved by the local ethics committees. The study was conducted according to Declaration of Helsinki and American Psychological Association's ethical principles.

The sample was followed in 8 waves, 1983, 1986, 1989, 1992, 1997, 2001, 2007-2008, and 2012, in which medical, psychological, and physical activity studies were conducted. Physical activity from childhood to middle adulthood was assessed in 1980, 1983, 1986, 1989, 1992, 2001, 2007, and 2011, response rate ranging from 53.1% to 72.8% (n = 1910–2619) of the original study participants (Table 1). Depressive symptoms were measured in 2012 and 47.9% (n = 1724) of the original study subjects participated in the examination (Table 1).

Previous studies of sample attrition have shown that there has not been systematic selection bias regarding study participants' medical profiles or physical activity [31, 32], but some selective attrition with respect to personality and depressive symptoms exists [33, 34]. Participants who were less self-directed and less agreeable and had higher levels of neuroticism as well as depressive symptoms had discontinued the study more often than others [33, 34].

2.2. Measures

2.2.1. Physical Activity. Physical activity was assessed with self-administered questionnaires. Information concerning 3- and 6-year-old children's (born in 1974 and 1977) physical activity levels is missing from this study, because they were not able to self-report their physical activity levels in 1980. Participants, from whom physical activity was assessed, were aged from 9 to 18 in 1980 and from 34 to 49 in 2011.

From 1980 to 1989, physical activity questionnaires consisted of five questions focusing on the intensity and frequency of participants' leisure time physical activity, participation in sports-club training, participation in sports competitions, and participants' usual way of spending leisure time [35]. From 1992 till present time, questionnaires consisted of five questions as well, assessing the intensity and frequency of leisure time physical activity, hours spent on physical activity per week, average duration of a physical activity session, and participation in organized physical activity [32]. From 1980 to 1992, the answers for the questions were coded into 3 categories (ranging from 1 to 3), excluding the items that assessed participation in sports competitions (1980–1989) and participation in organized sports (1992) which had a response range from 1 to 2. From 2001 to 2011, all responses to the questions were coded into 3 categories (response scale ranging from 1 to 3). A sum score (physical activity index) of question responses was created for each participant each year (Table 1), higher scores reflecting higher physical activity level. The index has been found reliable and valid [32].

2.2.2. Depressive Symptoms. Participants' depressive symptoms were assessed with Beck Depression Inventory II (BDI-II) [36]. These symptoms were measured in 2012 when the participants were aged from 35 to 50. BDI-II consists of 21 symptoms with a severity range from 0 (no symptoms) to 3 (severe level of depressive symptoms). A sum score of all items was computed for each participant (Table 1), and no missing items were allowed. The reliability estimate (Cronbach's α) for the depressive symptom scores was >0.90. BDI-II has demonstrated to be a valid instrument [36–38], and it has been regarded as an acknowledged standard in the measurement of depressive mood [36–39]. It is applicable in clinical and nonclinical contexts, including in general populations [36–39]. BDI-II correlates highly with its earlier versions, including modified BDI [36, 38], which has also been considered as a valid measure for assessing depressive symptoms in general populations [34]. Furthermore, BDI-II correlates well with other widely used scales for depression [38]. The instrument has been designed and also demonstrated to be a useful screening tool for potential depressed cases [36, 38].

2.2.3. Covariates. Childhood, adulthood, and general (age, sex, and body mass index) covariates were controlled for in this study (Table 1) [25–30]. Participants' negative emotionality [25] was reported by the primary caretaker via six questions reflecting participants' behavior in childhood (e.g., "The child hits/kicks other children "accidentally""), on a scale from 1 (true) to 2 (not true), and average of the items was calculated for each participant. As some of the participants were adolescents in 1980, their caretakers responded to this question retrospectively. Participants' parents' socioeconomic status was assessed via two indices, educational and income levels [26]. Parents' educational level was determined via educational information collected from participants' mothers' and fathers' (1 = below 9 years/comprehensive school, 2 = 9 to 12 years/secondary school, and 3 = over 12 years/academic education). If parents' educational information differed, we based parental educational status on the information collected from the parent with the higher educational level. If educational information was available for only one parent, family's educational status was determined using his/her educational information. Family's income level was rated in an 8-point scale [1 =< 15 000 marks (~2523 euros) and 8 => 100 000 marks (~16819 euros)].

Symptoms of participants' adulthood depression were determined in 1992, 1997, 2001, and 2007 via a modified version of Beck Depression Inventory, referred to as a modified BDI [34, 40]. Items of the measure were rated in a 5-point scale, and average of the items was computed each year for each participant. Participants' socioeconomic status (2007) was determined via two indices; education was assessed via a 3-category scale (1 = comprehensive school, 2 = secondary school, and 3 = academic level) and income level via an 8-point scale (1 =< 10 000 euros and 8 => 70 000 euros). Additionally, participants' experiences of social support, body mass index, and smoking status measured in 2007 were controlled for [29, 30]. Social support was determined via a 12-question inventory [41] using a 5-point scale, and a mean score of the items was calculated for each participant. Participants' smoking status was examined via a 5-category scale (1 = smokes a cigarette per day or more, 2 = smokes once in a week, 3 = smokes less than once in a week, 4 = has quitted smoking, and 5 = has never smoked).

2.3. Statistical Analyses. Physical activity questionnaires, which were designed for children and adolescents (1980–1989) and adults (1992–2011) differed slightly in their content. To assure that the findings of the present study were based on changes in physical activity and not due to a measurement artifact, a confirmatory factor model was used to examine whether the physical activity indices consisting of five indicator variables had measurement and structural invariance over time [42, 43]. Weighted least squares means and variance adjusted (WLSMV) estimation was used for all analyses [43]. The goodness of fit for scalar invariance was assessed with comparative fit index (CFI), Tucker-Lewis index (TLI), and root-mean square error of approximation index (RMSEA). Factor scores derived from this examination were used in subsequent analyses.

Within the growth mixture modeling framework, Latent Class Growth Analysis (LCGA) was used to explore the trajectories of physical activity from childhood to adulthood. LCGA captures information about developmental processes at inter- and intraindividual levels, detecting subpopulations with distinct growth trajectories [20]. The determination of the number of subgroups for physical activity was based on Akaike's Information Criterion (AIC) [44]. In addition, the determination of the groups was based on the classification quality estimations and practical considerations [20, 45]. Within the LCGA model, the average temporal trajectories in the physical activity groups were modeled by regression equations, in which both the linear and quadratic terms were tested for the independent variable (time).

The associations between physical activity factor scores (assessed from age 9 to 49) and depressive symptoms (participants aged from 35 to 50) were first examined cross-sectionally and longitudinally with linear regression analyses. Due to the potential multiple testing problem, Bonferroni-corrected p values ($p < 0.003$) were used in determining the significant associations. Thereafter, the associations between the physical activity trajectory groups and depressive symptoms measured in 2012 were examined with analyses of variance, and post hoc tests were also performed (Bonferroni's method). Furthermore, we examined the longitudinal associations between physical activity levels assessed in participants' adulthood (2007, including participants aged from 30 to 45) and depressive symptoms (2012) using a linear regression. Due to the number of missing values, the variance analyses and the regression analyses in which the adulthood physical activity (2007) was used as a predictor were performed in another dataset which was imputed using the expectation-maximization (EM) algorithm [46]. Analyses were performed in statistical software programs Mplus (version 7.1 and version 7.2), IBM SPSS (version 21), and Stata (version 13). p values of <0.05 were considered significant.

3. Results

Descriptives of the original sample ($n = 1724$–3596) are shown in Table 1. Supplementary Tables 1 and 2 (see Supplementary Material available online at http://dx.doi.org/10.1155/2016/8947375) provide descriptives of the sample in the complete ($n = 648$) and imputed ($n = 3564$–3596) data, respectively. Although the scalar invariance model for physical activity did not demonstrate strong factorial invariance over time, the fit for partial scalar invariance model was adequate (CFI = 0.90, TLI = 0.90, and RMSEA = 0.047), given partial invariance of the threshold parameters. For RMSEA, values <0.05 indicate a very close model fit, and CFI and TLI values close to 0.90 denote an adequate fit [47]. Since the partial scalar invariance model was considered acceptable, factor scores were predicted for each subject to be used in subsequent analyses (Supplementary Table 3).

The prerequisites of growth mixture modeling (e.g., [24]) were met satisfactorily. LCGA suggested that a three-factor (group) solution was the best fitting model for the data based on AIC indices (AIC = 48915.44, 48915.39, 48901.43, 48902.85, and 48907.08 for 1, 2, 3, 4, and 5 groups, resp.; a lower AIC implies a better model). The classification quality of the three-factor model was also adequate based on the average probability estimates (group 1 = 0.74, group 2 = 0.86, and group 3 = 0.71). Values >0.70 delineate that the group consists of individuals with similar patterns of change [45]. Linear parameter estimates were found for the physical activity groups (Supplementary Table 4). Figure 1 shows the central tendencies of the three groups, lightly ($n = 371$), moderately ($n = 3046$), and highly ($n = 147$) physically active groups by age. Based on the estimated marginal means, participants' physical activity levels remained relatively unchanged from childhood to adulthood in each group, although these levels appeared to diminish minimally towards middle adulthood in all participants (Figure 1).

The regression analyses performed in the original sample ($n = 255$–1467) indicated that low levels of physical activity factor scores were, in most examined ages, associated with higher levels of depressive symptoms in participants' adulthood ($p < 0.05$), although some of the associations attenuated when Bonferroni-corrected p values ($p < 0.003$) were applied (Table 2).

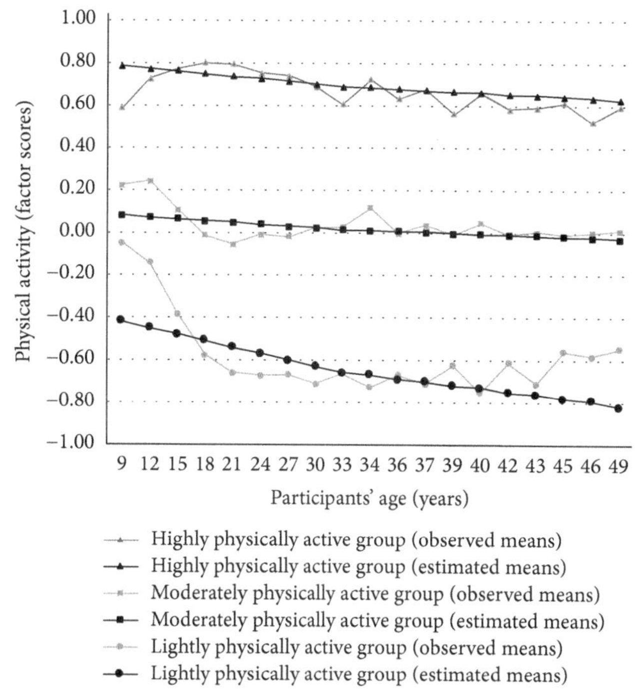

FIGURE 1: Means of the highly physically active ($n = 147$), moderately physically active ($n = 3046$), and lightly physically active ($n = 371$) trajectory groups from childhood to middle adulthood.

The analyses of variance in the original sample ($n = 1722$) indicated that the physical activity trajectory groups predicted symptoms of depression [F (2,1719 = 8.12, $p < 0.001$, adjusted $R^2 = 0.01$)]. Post hoc tests showed that highly physically active group had lower levels of depressive symptoms than lightly active group (mean difference = −3.26; $p < 0.001$, 95%CI: −5.25 to −1.26). Highly physically active participants had lower levels of depression in comparison to moderately active ones (mean difference = −1.92, $p = 0.02$, 95%CI: −3.66 to −0.18). Also moderately active participants had lower levels of depressive symptoms than lightly active participants (mean difference = −1.33, $p = 0.02$, 95%CI: −2.48 to −0.19). Based on the analyses of variance after adjusting for the covariates [25–30], the associations attenuated to nonsignificance [F (2, 631) = 2.13, $p = 0.12$, adjusted $R^2 = 0.25$]. In particular the previous symptoms of depression measured in 1992, 1997, 2001, and 2007 attenuated the associations (for details, see Supplementary Table 5).

We also examined the unadjusted associations in the data with full information on all study variables ($n = 648$), in which case the association between the physical activity trajectory groups and depressive symptoms became only marginally significant [F (2,645) = 2.76, $p = 0.06$, adjusted $R^2 = 0.01$]. As the sample attrition might have affected this association (i.e., by reducing the statistical power), the analyses were also performed in a dataset which was imputed using EM-algorithm ($n = 3564$–3596). This method was applied as the Little's MCAR test [48] confirmed that the data were not missing completely at random ($\chi^2 = 3903.02$, $df = 2923$, $p < 0.001$). In the imputed dataset, physical activity

TABLE 2: Physical activity factor scores (assessed at participants' ages from 9 to 49) as predictors of symptoms of depression (participants aged from 35 to 50) (n = 255–1467).

Participants' age	b	SE	B	p^*	95% CI†
9	−1.06	0.51	−0.07	0.040	−2.06 to −0.05
12	−1.73	0.39	−0.13	<0.001	−2.49 to −0.98
15	−1.72	0.30	−0.15	<0.001	−2.30 to −1.14
18	−1.21	0.29	−0.11	<0.001	−1.78 to −0.63
21	−1.33	0.34	−0.11	<0.001	−1.99 to −0.66
24	−1.53	0.30	−0.15	<0.001	−2.12 to −0.95
27	−1.52	0.35	−0.15	<0.001	−2.21 to −0.84
30	−0.86	0.35	−0.08	0.015	−1.56 to −0.17
33	−1.16	0.47	−0.10	0.014	−2.08 to −0.24
34	−0.51	0.51	−0.06	0.324	−1.52 to 0.50
36	−0.68	0.49	−0.06	0.161	−1.64 to 0.27
37	−0.89	0.60	−0.09	0.140	−2.07 to 0.29
39	−1.59	0.44	−0.15	<0.001	−2.46 to −0.73
40	−0.34	0.72	−0.03	0.643	−1.76 to 1.09
42	−1.96	0.60	−0.18	0.001	−3.14 to −0.79
43	−1.65	0.61	−0.16	0.007	−2.85 to −0.45
45	−1.31	0.57	−0.13	0.022	−2.44 to −0.19
46	−2.22	0.58	−0.21	<0.001	−3.35 to −1.09
49	−1.34	0.54	−0.14	0.014	−2.41 to −0.27

*Bonferroni-corrected p values (α = 0.05/19, p < 0.003) were used in determining significant associations.
†CI: confidence interval.

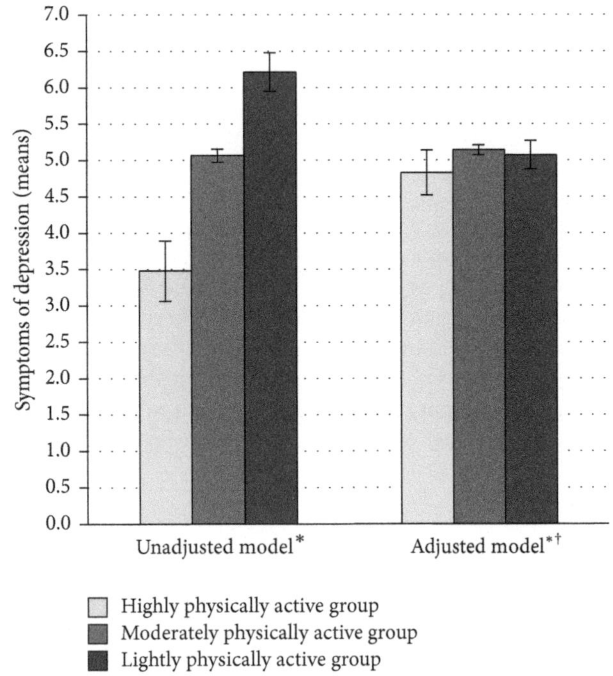

FIGURE 2: Symptoms of depression (2012) in the physical activity trajectory groups in unadjusted* and adjusted models*† (n = 3564). *Standard errors are represented in the figure by the error bars attached to each column. †Participants' age, sex, childhood negative emotionality, parental education, parental income (1980), previous symptoms of depression (1992–2007), participants' education, income, social support, body mass index, and smoking status (2007) were adjusted for in the model.

groups predicted the symptoms of depression [F (2,3561) = 16.74, p < 0.001, adjusted R^2 = 0.01]. Post hoc tests indicated that highly physically active group had lower levels of depressive symptoms than lightly active group (mean difference = −2.74; p < 0.001, 95%CI: −3.91 to −1.56) (Figure 2). Highly physically active participants had lower levels of depressive symptoms in comparison to moderately active ones (mean difference = −1.59, p = 0.001, 95%CI: −2.60 to −0.57) (Figure 2). Also moderately active participants had lower levels of depressive symptoms than lightly active participants (mean difference = −1.15, p < 0.001, 95%CI: −1.81 to −0.49) (Figure 2). When the covariates [25–30] were adjusted for, the results became nonsignificant [F (2,3547) = 0.53, p = 0.59, adjusted R^2 = 0.47]. In particular the previous symptoms of depression measured in 1997 and 2001 attenuated the associations (for details, see Supplementary Table 5).

Thereafter, we examined the longitudinal associations between adulthood physical activity (assessed in 2007, participants' aged from 30 to 45) and symptoms of depression (assessed in 2012). In the original sample, adulthood physical activity was associated with depressive symptoms (b = −1.10, p < 0.001, 95%CI: −1.58 to −0.61, adjusted R^2 = 0.01). When the covariates [25–30] were adjusted for, the association attenuated to nonsignificance (b = −0.17, p = 0.62, 95%CI: −0.85 to 0.51, adjusted R^2 = 0.24). In particular the previous symptoms of depression assessed in 2001 and 2007 attenuated the association (for details, see Supplementary Table 6). Thereafter, the analyses were performed in a sample with full information on all study variables (n = 648), in which case the adulthood physical activity was not associated with depressive symptoms (b = −0.55, p = 0.16, 95%CI: −1.31 to 0.21, adjusted R^2 = 0.002). Due to the sample attrition, the association was studied also in the imputed data (n = 3596), and the results showed that the adulthood physical activity was associated with decreased levels of depressive symptoms (b = −1.07, p < 0.001, 95%CI: −1.36 to −0.78, adjusted R^2 = 0.01). When the covariates [25–30] were adjusted for, the association attenuated to nonsignificance (b = 0.06, p = 0.57, 95%CI: −0.16 to 0.28, adjusted R^2 = 0.47). In particular the symptoms of depression assessed in 2001 and 2007 attenuated the association (for details, see Supplementary Table 6).

4. Discussion

This study examined whether distinct trajectories of lifelong physical activity existed in the data and whether physical activity was related to depressive symptoms in adulthood. We also studied whether the lifelong physical activity trajectories contributed to the outcome to a greater degree than adulthood physical activity. This inspection was important, because the information whether lifelong trajectories contribute to depressive symptoms over and above the concurrent (adulthood) physical activity is lacking. LCGA revealed three distinct groups, the lightly, moderately, and highly physically active groups. Physical activity levels remained relatively similar from childhood to adulthood in each group, although the groups' physical activity levels decreased slightly towards middle adulthood. These results are in line with previous studies demonstrating the decline of physical activity with age [17].

High physical activity associated with lower level of depressive symptoms in adulthood, which is in accord with previous research [10, 18]. The mechanisms behind the observed association can be both physiological and psychological. Physical activity may alleviate depressive symptoms through neurobiological alterations [12]. Physical activity may also relate to enhanced self-confidence, emotion regulation skills, and social capacities that are associated with positive mood [13, 14].

The association between high physical activity and lower levels of depressive symptoms in adulthood, however, disappeared when covariates (age, sex, childhood negative emotionality, parents' socioeconomic status, participants' previous symptoms of depression, participants' socioeconomic status, social support, body mass index, and smoking status) were taken into account. The explanatory power of the fully adjusted models was substantially higher in comparison to the unadjusted ones (46% higher in the imputed data). These same results were found when lifelong physical activity trajectories and adulthood physical activity (assessed in 2007) were used as predictors for depressive symptoms in adulthood. Specifically, physical activity did not predict lower levels of depressive symptoms in adulthood when the experiences of previous depression were taken into account. The bidirectional nature of the association between physical activity and depression has been documented [8, 11]. Hence, it is theoretically possible that the childhood symptoms of depression preceding our first measurement have decreased the likelihood of initiating physical activity [8, 11] or that of maintaining adequate level of physical activity [11].

Summarizing, the study indicated that lifelong physical activity trajectories or adulthood physical activity levels were not associated with the progression of depressive symptoms in adulthood. The study suggests that lifelong physical activity history does not contribute to the progression of the depressive symptoms to a greater degree than adulthood physical activity.

4.1. Limitations and Strengths. Our results need to be interpreted in light of the following limitations. Participants did not provide information regarding each variable across the measurement years, which diminished the complete-sample size considerably. However, we attempted to control the potential attrition bias via an imputation method. The measurements concerning the participants' physical activity focused only on the self-reported leisure time physical activity, not total physical activity or energy expenditure. Also the depressive symptoms were assessed with self-administered questionnaires, and thus the possibility of subjective bias cannot be excluded. However, this is common in epidemiological studies by necessity. To our knowledge, comparably long follow-up studies using diagnostic interviews do not exist. Furthermore, early childhood depression was not assessed in the study, but this deficiency was retrieved to an extent by controlling for the childhood negative emotionality [25].

The strengths of the study were the prospective, population-based study design, relatively large sample size, use of LCGA, and utilization of an extensive set of covariates. In LCGA, the main advantage is that it allows a researcher to model developmental processes at inter- and intraindividual levels [20]. Such modeling has been shown to be especially useful regarding the development of health behaviors [20, 21], and the need for further studies has been recognized [22]. However, in the case of this study, the traditional cross-sectional and longitudinal studies yielded to very similar results. This was not evident *a priori*, and therefore our study adds evidence regarding the etiology of depression [19] by showing that physical activity trajectories appear not to play a special role over and above the adulthood physical activity.

Furthermore, depressive symptoms were studied with a well-validated instrument, BDI-II [36–39].

We were able to study the whole variance of participants' depressive symptoms instead of categorical diagnoses. This is important when attempting to find preventive tools for depression, because functional impairment is much more strongly associated with symptom severity than with diagnostic symptom count [49]. Also the people who have experienced symptoms of depression are at risk of getting a diagnosis [27].

4.2. Conclusions. This study identified three distinct physical activity groups, the lightly, moderately, and highly physically active ones. Each group's physical activity levels remained relatively unchanged from childhood to adulthood, although the levels tended to diminish slightly towards later adulthood. Physical activity was associated with depressive symptoms in adulthood. Highly physically active participants from childhood to adulthood had lower levels of depressive symptoms in adulthood compared to lightly physically active ones. Furthermore, participants' adulthood physical activity assessed in 2007 was associated with decreased levels of depressive symptoms in adulthood. The associations between physical activity and depressive symptoms disappeared when the preexisting symptoms of depression were controlled for, indicating that physical activities did not associate with the progression of depressive symptoms. Thus, the study suggests that lifelong physical activity history does not contribute to the progression of the depressive symptoms to a greater degree than adulthood physical activity. Obtaining information of mental health history might benefit clinicians and other professionals in evaluating the role of physical activity in well-being.

Disclosure

The sponsors had no role in study design, collection, analysis, interpretation of the data, writing the report, and decision to submit the report for publication.

Competing Interests

The authors declare that there is no conflict of interests regarding the publication of this paper.

Acknowledgments

The Young Finns Study has received financial support from the Academy of Finland, Social Insurance Institution of Finland, Kuopio, Tampere and Turku University Hospital Medical Funds, Juho Vainio Foundation, Paavo Nurmi Foundation, Finnish Foundation of Cardiovascular Research and Finnish Cultural Foundation, Sigrid Juselius Foundation, Tampere Tuberculosis Foundation, and Emil Aaltonen Foundation. This study was also supported by Academy of Finland [Grant nos. 258711, 265869, and 258578 (Liisa Keltikangas-Järvinen, Laura Pulkki-Råback, Kaisa Kaseva, Mirka Hintsanen, and Tom Rosenström)], Signe and Ane Gyllenberg Foundation (Liisa Keltikangas-Järvinen, Mirka Hintsanen, and Laura Pulkki-Råback), Emil Aaltonen Foundation (Mirka Hintsanen), Alli Paasikivi Foundation (Mirka Hintsanen), Juho Vainio Foundation (Laura Pulkki-Råback), Finnish Ministry of Education and Culture (Tuija Tammelin, Xiaolin Yang, and Kaisa Kaseva), Finnish Cultural Foundation (Christian Hakulinen), and Urheiluopistosäätiö (Kaisa Kaseva). Irina Lisinen and Mauri Niiniaho are gratefully acknowledged for data management.

References

[1] P. C. Dinas, Y. Koutedakis, and A. D. Flouris, "Effects of exercise and physical activity on depression," *Irish Journal of Medical Science*, vol. 180, no. 2, pp. 319–325, 2011.

[2] T. Vos, A. D. Flaxman, M. Naghavi et al., "Years lived with disability (YLDs) for 1160 sequelae of 289 diseases and injuries 1990–2010: a systematic analysis for the Global Burden of Disease Study 2010," *The Lancet*, vol. 380, no. 9859, pp. 2163–2196, 2010.

[3] R. M. Carney and K. E. Freedland, "Depression, mortality, and medical morbidity in patients with coronary heart disease," *Biological Psychiatry*, vol. 54, no. 3, pp. 241–247, 2003.

[4] D. M. Clarke and K. C. Currie, "Depression, anxiety and their relationship with chronic diseases: a review of the epidemiology, risk and treatment evidence," *Medical Journal of Australia*, vol. 190, no. 7, pp. 54–60, 2009.

[5] K. W. Sax, S. M. Strakowski, P. E. Keck Jr., V. H. Upadhyaya, S. A. West, and S. L. Mcelroy, "Relationships among negative, positive, and depressive symptoms in schizophrenia and psychotic depression," *British Journal of Psychiatry*, vol. 168, no. 1, pp. 68–71, 1996.

[6] J. M. Donohue and H. A. Pincus, "Reducing the societal burden of depression: a review of economic costs, quality of care and effects of treatment," *PharmacoEconomics*, vol. 25, no. 1, pp. 7–24, 2007.

[7] R. F. Muñoz, P. Cuijpers, F. Smit, A. Z. Barrera, and Y. Leykin, "Prevention of major depression," *Annual Review of Clinical Psychology*, vol. 6, pp. 181–212, 2010.

[8] S. M. Pereira, M. Geoffroy, and C. Power, "Investigation of bidirectional associations between depressive symptoms and physical activity from age 11 to 50 years in the 1958 British Birth Cohort," *The Lancet*, vol. 382, supplement 80, 2013.

[9] D. Kritz-Silverstein, E. Barrett-Connor, and C. Corbeau, "Cross-sectional and prospective study of exercise and depressed mood in the elderly: The Rancho Bernardo study," *American Journal of Epidemiology*, vol. 153, no. 6, pp. 596–603, 2001.

[10] M. Teychenne, K. Ball, and J. Salmon, "Physical activity and likelihood of depression in adults: a review," *Preventive Medicine*, vol. 46, no. 5, pp. 397–411, 2008.

[11] M. Azevedo Da Silva, A. Singh-Manoux, E. J. Brunner et al., "Bidirectional association between physical activity and symptoms of anxiety and depression: the Whitehall II study," *European Journal of Epidemiology*, vol. 27, no. 7, pp. 537–546, 2012.

[12] I. Helmich, A. Latini, A. Sigwalt et al., "Neurobiological alterations induced by exercise and their impact on depressive disorders," *Clinical Practice and Epidemiology in Mental Health*, vol. 6, pp. 115–125, 2010.

[13] L. Crust, "A review and conceptual re-examination of mental toughness: implications for future researchers," *Personality and Individual Differences*, vol. 45, no. 7, pp. 576–583, 2008.

[14] E. McAuley, B. Blissmer, D. X. Marquez, G. J. Jerome, A. F. Kramer, and J. Katula, "Social relations, physical activity, and well-being in older adults," *Preventive Medicine*, vol. 31, no. 5, pp. 608–617, 2000.

[15] J. M. Ruuskanen and I. Ruoppila, "Physical activity and psychological well-being among people aged 65 to 84 years," *Age and Ageing*, vol. 24, no. 4, pp. 292–296, 1995.

[16] R. Malina, "Tracking of physical activity across the lifespan," *President's Council on Physical Fitness and Sports Research Digest* , vol. 3, no. 14, pp. 1–8, 2001.

[17] R. Telama and X. Yang, "Decline of physical activity from youth to young adulthood in Finland," *Medicine and Science in Sports and Exercise*, vol. 32, no. 9, pp. 1617–1622, 2000.

[18] X. Yang, M. Hirvensalo, M. Hintsanen et al., "Longitudinal associations between changes in physical activity and depressive symptoms in adulthood: the Young Finns study," *International Journal of Behavioral Medicine*, vol. 21, no. 6, pp. 908–917, 2014.

[19] P. De Jonge and A. M. Roest, "Depression and cardiovascular disease: the end of simple models," *British Journal of Psychiatry*, vol. 201, no. 5, pp. 337–338, 2012.

[20] B. O. Muthén and L. K. Muthén, "Integrating person-centered and variable-centered analyses: growth mixture modeling with latent trajectory classes," *Alcoholism: Clinical and Experimental Research*, vol. 24, no. 6, pp. 882–891, 2000.

[21] N. R. Riggs, C.-P. Chou, C. Li, and M. A. Pentz, "Adolescent to emerging adulthood smoking trajectories: when do smoking trajectories diverge, and do they predict early adulthood nicotine dependence?" *Nicotine & Tobacco Research*, vol. 9, no. 11, pp. 1147–1154, 2007.

[22] S. C. Duncan, T. E. Duncan, L. A. Strycker, and N. R. Chaumeton, "A cohort-sequential latent growth model of physical activity from ages 12 to 17 years," *Annals of Behavioral Medicine*, vol. 33, no. 1, pp. 80–89, 2007.

[23] N. M. Peel, R. J. McClure, and H. P. Bartlett, "Behavioral determinants of healthy aging," *American Journal of Preventive Medicine*, vol. 28, no. 3, pp. 298–304, 2005.

[24] P. J. Curran, K. Obeidat, and D. Losardo, "Twelve frequently asked questions about growth curve modeling," *Journal of Cognition and Development*, vol. 11, no. 2, pp. 121–136, 2010.

[25] K. A. Dodge, "Social-cognitive mechanisms in the development of conduct disorder and depression," *Annual Review of Psychology*, vol. 44, no. 1, pp. 559–584, 1993.

[26] B. Galobardes, M. Shaw, D. A. Lawlor, J. W. Lynch, and G. D. Smith, "Indicators of socioeconomic position (part 1)," *Journal of Epidemiology and Community Health*, vol. 60, no. 1, pp. 7–12, 2006.

[27] J. Karsten, C. A. Hartman, J. H. Smit et al., "Psychiatric history and subthreshold symptoms as predictors of the occurrence of depressive or anxiety disorder within 2 years," *British Journal of Psychiatry*, vol. 198, no. 3, pp. 206–212, 2011.

[28] J. Mirowsky, "Age and the gender gap in depression," *Journal of Health and Social Behavior*, vol. 37, no. 4, pp. 362–380, 1996.

[29] A. Allgöwer, J. Wardle, and A. Steptoe, "Depressive symptoms, social support, and personal health behaviors in young men and women," *Health Psychology*, vol. 20, no. 3, pp. 223–227, 2001.

[30] F. S. Luppino, L. M. de Wit, P. F. Bouvy et al., "Overweight, obesity, and depression: a systematic review and meta-analysis of longitudinal studies," *Archives of General Psychiatry*, vol. 67, no. 3, pp. 220–229, 2010.

[31] O. T. Raitakari, M. Juonala, T. Rönnemaa et al., "Cohort profile: the cardiovascular risk in young Finns study," *International Journal of Epidemiology*, vol. 37, no. 6, pp. 1220–1226, 2008.

[32] X. Yang, R. Telama, M. Hirvensalo et al., "Leadership component of type A behavior predicts physical activity in early midlife," *International Journal of Behavioral Medicine*, vol. 19, no. 1, pp. 48–55, 2012.

[33] T. Rosenström, M. Jokela, C. R. Cloninger et al., "Associations between dimensional personality measures and preclinical atherosclerosis: the cardiovascular risk in Young Finns study," *Journal of Psychosomatic Research*, vol. 72, no. 5, pp. 336–343, 2012.

[34] T. Rosenström, M. Jokela, S. Puttonen et al., "Pairwise measures of causal direction in the epidemiology of sleep problems and depression," *PLoS ONE*, vol. 7, no. 11, Article ID e50841, 2012.

[35] R. Telama, J. Viikari, and I. Välimäki, "Atherosclerosis precursors in Finnish children and adolescents. X. Leisure-time physical activity," *Acta Paediatrica Scandinavica. Supplement*, vol. 74, no. 318, pp. 169–180, 1985.

[36] A. Beck, R. Steer, and G. Brown, *Manual for the Beck Depression Inventory-II*, Psychological Corporation, San Antonio, Tex, USA, 1996.

[37] E. A. Storch, J. W. Roberti, and D. A. Roth, "Factor structure, concurrent validity, and internal consistency of the beck depression inventory—second edition in a sample of college students," *Depression and Anxiety*, vol. 19, no. 3, pp. 187–189, 2004.

[38] Y.-P. Wang and C. Gorenstein, "Psychometric properties of the Beck Depression Inventory-II: a comprehensive review," *Revista Brasileira de Psiquiatria*, vol. 35, no. 4, pp. 416–431, 2013.

[39] A. Beck, R. Steer, and G. Brown, *BDI-II—Beck Depression Inventory®-II: Finnish Standardization*, Psychological Corporation and Psykologien Kustannus Oy, Helsinki, Finland, 2004.

[40] A. T. Beck, C. H. Ward, M. Mendelson, J. Mock, and J. Erbaugh, "An inventory for measuring depression," *Archives of General Psychiatry*, vol. 4, pp. 561–571, 1961.

[41] G. Zimet, N. Dahlem, S. Zimet et al., "The multidimensional scale of perceived social support," *Journal of Personality Assessment*, vol. 52, no. 1, pp. 30–41, 1988.

[42] R. J. Vandenberg and C. E. Lance, "A review and synthesis of the measurement invariance literature: suggestions, practices, and recommendations for organizational research," *Organizational Research Methods*, vol. 3, no. 1, pp. 4–70, 2000.

[43] L. Muthén and B. Muthén, *Mplus User's Guide*, Muthén & Muthén, Los Angeles, Calif, USA, 6th edition, 1998–2010.

[44] S. I. Vrieze, "Model selection and psychological theory: a discussion of the differences between the Akaike information criterion (AIC) and the Bayesian information criterion (BIC)," *Psychological Methods*, vol. 17, no. 2, pp. 228–243, 2012.

[45] H. Andruff, N. Carraro, A. Thompson et al., "Latent class growth modelling: a tutorial," *Tutorials in Quantitative Methods for Psychology*, vol. 5, no. 1, pp. 11–24, 2009.

[46] A. P. Dempster, N. M. Laird, and D. B. Rubin, "Maximum likelihood from incomplete data via the EM algorithm," *Journal of the Royal Statistical Society*, vol. 39, no. 1, pp. 1–38, 1977.

[47] G. W. Cheung and R. B. Rensvold, "Evaluating goodness-of-fit indexes for testing measurement invariance," *Structural Equation Modeling. A Multidisciplinary Journal*, vol. 9, no. 2, pp. 233–255, 2002.

[48] R. J. Little, "A test of missing completely at random for multivariate data with missing values," *Journal of the American Statistical Association*, vol. 83, no. 404, pp. 1198–1202, 1988.

[49] J. Karsten, C. A. Hartman, J. Ormel, W. A. Nolen, and B. W. J. H. Penninx, "Subthreshold depression based on functional impairment better defined by symptom severity than by number of DSM-IV symptoms," *Journal of Affective Disorders*, vol. 123, no. 1–3, pp. 230–237, 2010.

PERMISSIONS

All chapters in this book were first published in JSM, by Hindawi Publishing Corporation; hereby published with permission under the Creative Commons Attribution License or equivalent. Every chapter published in this book has been scrutinized by our experts. Their significance has been extensively debated. The topics covered herein carry significant findings which will fuel the growth of the discipline. They may even be implemented as practical applications or may be referred to as a beginning point for another development.

The contributors of this book come from diverse backgrounds, making this book a truly international effort. This book will bring forth new frontiers with its revolutionizing research information and detailed analysis of the nascent developments around the world.

We would like to thank all the contributing authors for lending their expertise to make the book truly unique. They have played a crucial role in the development of this book. Without their invaluable contributions this book wouldn't have been possible. They have made vital efforts to compile up to date information on the varied aspects of this subject to make this book a valuable addition to the collection of many professionals and students.

This book was conceptualized with the vision of imparting up-to-date information and advanced data in this field. To ensure the same, a matchless editorial board was set up. Every individual on the board went through rigorous rounds of assessment to prove their worth. After which they invested a large part of their time researching and compiling the most relevant data for our readers.

The editorial board has been involved in producing this book since its inception. They have spent rigorous hours researching and exploring the diverse topics which have resulted in the successful publishing of this book. They have passed on their knowledge of decades through this book. To expedite this challenging task, the publisher supported the team at every step. A small team of assistant editors was also appointed to further simplify the editing procedure and attain best results for the readers.

Apart from the editorial board, the designing team has also invested a significant amount of their time in understanding the subject and creating the most relevant covers. They scrutinized every image to scout for the most suitable representation of the subject and create an appropriate cover for the book.

The publishing team has been an ardent support to the editorial, designing and production team. Their endless efforts to recruit the best for this project, has resulted in the accomplishment of this book. They are a veteran in the field of academics and their pool of knowledge is as vast as their experience in printing. Their expertise and guidance has proved useful at every step. Their uncompromising quality standards have made this book an exceptional effort. Their encouragement from time to time has been an inspiration for everyone.

The publisher and the editorial board hope that this book will prove to be a valuable piece of knowledge for researchers, students, practitioners and scholars across the globe.

LIST OF CONTRIBUTORS

Mats Jong
Department of Nursing, Mid Sweden University, Sundsvall, Sweden
Mid Sweden Research & Development Centre, Västernorrland County Council, 851 70 Sundsvall, Sweden

Anton Westman
Department of Physiology and Pharmacology, Karolinska Institutet, 171 77 Stockholm, Sweden

Britt-Inger Saveman
Department of Nursing, Umeå University, 901 87 Umeå, Sweden

Neil D. Clarke
Department of Biomolecular and Sports Sciences, Coventry University, Coventry CV1 5HB, UK

Michael J. Duncan
Human Performance Laboratory, Department of Biomolecular and Sports Sciences, Coventry University, James Starley Building, Priory Street, Coventry CV 5HB, UK

Corey Beals
Department of Surgery,Wexner Medical Center, 395W. 12th Avenue Columbus, OH 43210, USA

David Flanigan
Department of Sports Medicine,Wexner Medical Center, 2050 Kenny Road, Suite 3100 Columbus, OH 43221, USA

Mark R. Lafave and Breda Eubank
Department of Health and Physical Education, Mount Royal University, 4825Mount RoyalGate SW, Calgary, AB,Canada T3E 6K6

Dale Butterwick
Faculty of Kinesiology, University of Calgary, 2400 University DriveNW, Calgary, AB, Canada T2N 1N4

Amitava Halder and Chuansi Gao
Division of Ergonomics and Aerosol Technology, Department of Design Sciences, Faculty of Engineering, Lund University, P.O. Box 118, 221 00 Lund, Sweden

Michael Miller
Division of Physiotherapy, Department of Health Science, Faculty of Medicine, Lund University, P.O. Box 157, 221 00 Lund, Sweden

Yolanda Castellote-Caballero
Hospital Virgen de las Nieves, Servicio Andaluz de Salud, Avenida de las Fuerzas Armadas 2, 18014 Granada, Spain

Maríe C. Valenza
Department of Physical Therapy, Universidad de Granada, Avenida del Hospicio s/n, 18071 Granada, Spain

Emilio J. Puentedura
Department of PhysicalTherapy, School of Allied Health Sciences,University ofNevada Las Vegas, 4505 Maryland Parkway, P.O. Box 453029, Las Vegas, NV 89154-3029, USA

César Fernández-de-las-Peñas
Department of Physical Therapy, OccupationalTherapy, Rehabilitation and Physical Medicine, Universidad Rey Juan Carlos, Avenida de Atenas s/n, Alcorcon, 28922 Madrid, Spain

Francisco Alburquerque-Sendín
Department of Physical Therapy, Universidad de Salamanca, Patio de Escuelas, 137008 Salamanca, Spain

James Fisher and James Steele
Southampton Solent University, East Park Terrace, Southampton SO14 0YN, UK

Pat McKinnon and Stephen McKinnon
Abstract Bodyworks, Precision Exercise, Newbury RG14 5BY, UK

Pedro Silva and Jorge Mota
CIAFEL, Faculty of Sports, University of Porto, 4200-450 Porto, Portugal

Maria Teresa Andrade and Pedro Carvalho
INESC Porto, University of Porto, 4200-450 Porto, Portugal

JohnEric W. Smith, Megan E. Holmes and Matthew J. McAllister
Department of Kinesiology, Mississippi State University, P.O. Box 6186, Mississippi State, MS 39762, USA

Jay H.Williams, Emmanuel Akogyrem and Jeremy R. Williams
Department of Human Nutrition, Foods and Exercise, Virginia Polytechnic Institute and State University, Blacksburg, VA 24060, USA

Matthew Hislop
Brisbane Sports and Exercise Medicine Specialists Clinic, 87 Riding Road, Brisbane, QLD 4171, Australia

Dominic Kennedy, Brendan Cramp and Sanjay Dhupelia
Queensland X-Ray, Greenslopes Private Hospital, Brisbane, QLD 4120, Australia

Mohammad Ali Eshghi
Exercise Physiology Research Center, Baqiyatallah University of Medical Sciences, Tehran, Iran

Ramin Kordi, Amir Hossein Memari and Ahmad Ghaziasgar
Sports Medicine Research Center, Tehran University of Medical Sciences, P.O. Box 14395-578, Tehran, Iran

Mohammad-AliMansournia
Department of Epidemiology and Biostatistics, School of Public Health, Tehran University of Medical Sciences, Tehran, Iran

Seyed Hojjat Zamani Sani
Faculty of Physical Education and Sport Sciences, Shahid Beheshti University, Tehran, Iran

Hamid Arazi and Morteza Purabed
Department of Exercise Physiology, Faculty of Physical Education and Sport Sciences, University of Guilan, Rasht, Iran

Abbas Asadi
Department of Physical Education and Sport Sciences, Payame Noor University, P.O. Box 19395-3697, Tehran, Iran

Alexander M.Wood and Trish Davey
Institute of Naval Medicine, Alverstoke, Hants PO12 2DL, UK

Richard Hales, Michael Chapman and Andrew Nelstrop
Commando Training Centre Royal Marines, Lympstone, Devon EX8 5AR, UK

Andre Keenan and Alexandra Moss
Royal Army Medical Corps, Sandhurst GU15 4PQ, UK

Debbie Palmer-Green
University of Nottingham, Nottingham, UK

Colin Fuller
F-MARC, Zurich, Switzerland

Rod Jaques
English Institute of Sport, Bath, UK

Glenn Hunter
UK Sport, London, UK

Jason Savage
Monash Health, Department of Oral and Maxillofacial Surgery, Melbourne, VIC 3168, Australia

Chloe Hooke
Monash Health, Melbourne, VIC 3168, Australia

John Orchard
School of Public Health, University of Sydney, Sydney, NSW2006, Australia

Richard Parkinson
St Vincent's Hospital, Department of Neurosurgery, Sydney, NSW2010, Australia

Amy Sue Biondich and Jeremy D. Joslin
Department of Emergency Medicine, SUNY Upstate Medical University, Syracuse, NY, USA

Sarah A. Richmond
Child Health Evaluative Sciences, Hospital for Sick Children, 555 University Avenue, Toronto, ON, Canada M5G 1X8
Sport Injury Prevention Research Centre, Faculty of Kinesiology, University of Calgary, 2500 University Drive, Calgary, AB, Canada T2N 1N4
School of Kinesiology and Health Science, York University, 4700 Keele Street, Toronto, ON, Canada M3J 1P3

Patricia K. Doyle-Baker
Sport Injury Prevention Research Centre, Faculty of Kinesiology, University of Calgary, 2500 University Drive, Calgary, AB, Canada T2N 1N4

Alison Macpherson
School of Kinesiology and Health Science, York University, 4700 Keele Street, Toronto, ON, Canada M3J 1P3

Carolyn A. Emery
Sport Injury Prevention Research Centre, Faculty of Kinesiology, University of Calgary, 2500 University Drive, Calgary, AB, Canada T2N 1N4
Alberta Children's Hospital, Institute for Child and Maternal Health, 2888 Shaganappi Trail NW, Calgary, AB, Canada T3B 6A8

Alberto Nettel-Aguirre
Sport Injury Prevention Research Centre, Faculty of Kinesiology, University of Calgary, 2500 University Drive, Calgary, AB, Canada T2N 1N4
Alberta Children's Hospital, Institute for Child and Maternal Health, 2888 Shaganappi Trail NW, Calgary, AB, Canada T3B 6A8

Departments of Pediatrics and Community Health Sciences, Cumming School of Medicine, University of Calgary, 2500 University Drive, Calgary, AB, Canada T2N 1N4

Nicholas M. Beltz, Ann L. Gibson, Len Kravitz and Christine M. Mermier
Health, Exercise & Sports SciencesDepartment, University of New Mexico, Albuquerque, NM, USA

Jeffrey M. Janot
Department of Kinesiology, University ofWisconsin-Eau Claire, Eau Claire,WI, USA

Lance C. Dalleck
Recreation, Exercise & Sports Science Department,Western State Colorado University, Gunnison, CO, USA

Sarah Imhoff and Philippe Fait
Department of Human Kinetics, Universitédu Québec à Trois-Rivières (UQTR), 3351 Boulevard des Forges, Trois-Rivières, QC, Canada G9A 5H7
Research Group on Neuromusculoskeletal Dysfunctions (GRAN), UQTR, 3351 Boulevard des Forges, Trois-Rivières, QC, Canada G9A 5H7
Cortex Médecine et Réadaptation Concussion Clinic, 205-1035 Avenue Wilfrid-Pelletier, Québec City, QC, Canada G1W 0C5
Research Center in Neuropsychology and Cognition (CERNEC), Universit´e de Montr´eal, 90 rue Vincent d'Indy, Montréal, QC, Canada H2V 2S9

Frédérike Carrier-Toutant and Geneviève Boulard
Cortex Médecine et Réadaptation Concussion Clinic, 205-1035 Avenue Wilfrid-Pelletier, Québec City, QC, Canada G1W 0C5
Clinique Neuropsychologique, 206-1379 Chemin Ste-Foy, Québec City, QC, Canada G1S 2N2

Evan Jenkins
Sport and Exercise, the University of Edinburgh, St. Leonard's Land, Edinburgh EH8 8AQ, UK

Andrew Murray
European Tour Performance Institute, Virginia Water GU25 4LX, UK

Roger Hawkes
European Tour Performance Institute, Virginia Water GU25 4LX, UK

Josinaldo Jarbas da Silva and Silvio Luis Pecoraro
Graduate Program in Science of Human Movement, College of Health Science (FACIS), Methodist University of Piracicaba, 13423-070 Piracicaba, SP, Brazil

Priscyla Silva Monteiro Nardi and Julia Maria D'Andréa Greve
Institute of Orthopedics and Traumatology, School of Medicine, University of São Paulo, Laboratory of Kinesiology, 05403-000 São Paulo, SP, Brazil

Paulo Henrique Marchetti
Graduate Program in Science of Human Movement, College of Health Science (FACIS), Methodist University of Piracicaba, 13423-070 Piracicaba, SP, Brazil
Institute of Orthopedics and Traumatology, School of Medicine, University of São Paulo, Laboratory of Kinesiology, 05403-000 São Paulo, SP, Brazil

Brad Jon Schoenfeld
Department of Health Sciences, Program of Exercise Science, CUNY Lehman College, Bronx, NY 10468, USA

Erin Hartigan
Department of PhysicalTherapy, University of New England, Portland, ME 04103, USA

Robert Stanton, Melanie Hayman, Nyree Humphris, Hanna Borgelt, Jordan Fox, Luke Del Vecchio and Brendan Humphries
School of Medical and Applied Sciences, Central Queensland University, Bruce Highway, Rockhampton, QLD 4702, Australia

Hilde G. Nielsen
Division for Society and Health,Department of Health, The Research Council of Norway, P.O. Box 564, 1327 Lysaker,Norway

Olav Øktedalen
Department of Infectious Medicine, Oslo University Hospital, Ullevål, 0407 Oslo, Norway

Per-Kristian Opstad
Norwegian Research Defence Establishment, P.O. Box 25, 2027 Kjeller, Norway
Norwegian Military Academy, 0593 Oslo, Norway

Torstein Lyberg
Department of Medical Biochemistry, Oslo University Hospital, Ullevål, P.O. Box 4956, Nydalen, 0424 Oslo,Norway

Mariè van der Merwe and Richard J. Bloomer
School of Health Studies, The University of Memphis, Memphis, TN, USA

John M. Vasudevan
Department of Physical Medicine & Rehabilitation, University of Pennsylvania, 1800 Lombard Street, Philadelphia, PA 19146, USA

Andrew Logan and Jeffrey J. Koval
Human Performance Lab, Sports Medicine Center, Department of Orthopaedic Surgery, Stanford University, 341 Galvez Street, Lower Level, Stanford, CA 94305, USA

Rebecca Shultz
Human Performance Lab, Sports Medicine Center, Department of Orthopaedic Surgery, Stanford University, 341 Galvez Street, Lower Level, Stanford, CA 94305, USA
Division of Sports Medicine, Department of Orthopaedic Surgery, Stanford University, 450 Broadway Street, Redwood City, CA 94063, USA

Eugene Y. Roh and Michael Fredericson
Division of Sports Medicine, Department of Orthopaedic Surgery, Stanford University, 450 Broadway Street, Redwood City, CA 94063, USA

Michael Morin
Department of Human Kinetics, Université du Québec à Trois-Rivières (UQTR), Trois-Rivières, QC, Canada G9A 5H7
Research Group on Neuromusculoskeletal Dysfunctions (GRAN), UQTR, Trois-Rivi`eres, QC, Canada G9A 5H7

Pierre Langevin
Cortex Médecine et Réadaptation Concussion Clinic, Quebec City, QC, Canada G1W 0C5
Department of Rehabilitation, Faculty of Medicine, Laval University, Quebec City, QC, Canada G1V 0A6

Philippe Fait
Department of Human Kinetics, Université du Québec à Trois-Rivières (UQTR), Trois-Rivières, QC, Canada G9A 5H7
Research Group on Neuromusculoskeletal Dysfunctions (GRAN), UQTR, Trois-Rivières, QC, Canada G9A 5H7
Cortex Médecine et Réadaptation Concussion Clinic, Quebec City, QC, Canada G1W 0C5
Department of Rehabilitation, Faculty of Medicine, Laval University, Quebec City, QC, Canada G1V 0A6
Research Center in Neuropsychology and Cognition (CERNEC), Montreal, QC, Canada H3C 3J7

Kaisa Kaseva, Tom Rosenström, Taina Hintsa, Christian Hakulinen and Liisa Keltikangas-Järvinen and Jari Lipsanen
Unit of Personality,Work and Health Psychology, Institute of Behavioral Sciences, P.O. Box 9, University of Helsinki, 00014 Helsinki, Finland

Laura Pulkki-Råback
Unit of Personality,Work and Health Psychology, Institute of Behavioral Sciences, P.O. Box 9, University of Helsinki, 00014 Helsinki, Finland
Helsinki Collegium for Advanced Studies, Fabianinkatu 24, P.O. Box 4, University of Helsinki, 00014 Helsinki, Finland

Tuija Tammelin and Xiaolin Yang
LIKES, Research Center for Sport and Health Sciences, Rautpohjankatu 8, 40700 Jyväskylä, Finland

Mirka Hintsanen
Unit of Personality,Work and Health Psychology, Institute of Behavioral Sciences, P.O. Box 9, University of Helsinki, 00014 Helsinki, Finland
Unit of Psychology, University of Oulu, P.O. Box 8000, 90014Oulu, Finland

Katja Pahkala
Research Centre of Applied and Preventive CardiovascularMedicine, Kiinamyllynkatu 10, University of Turku, 20520 Turku, Finland
Paavo Nurmi Centre, Sports and Exercise Medicine Unit, Department of Physical Activity and Health, Kiinamyllynkatu 10, University of Turku, 20520 Turku, Finland

Mirja Hirvensalo
Department of Sport Sciences, P.O. Box 35 (L), University of Jyväskylä, 40014 Jyväskylä, Finland

Nina Hutri-Kähönen
Department of Pediatrics, P.O. Box 2000, University of Tampere and TampereUniversityHospital, 33521 Tampere, Finland

Olli T. Raitakari
Research Centre of Applied and Preventive CardiovascularMedicine, Kiinamyllynkatu 10, University of Turku, 20520 Turku, Finland
Department of Clinical Physiology and Nuclear Medicine, Kiinamyllynkatu 4-8, Turku University Hospital, 20520 Turku, Finland

Index

A
Anterior Cruciate Ligament, 76, 79
Artificial Turf, 76-77, 79-81
Athletes, 12, 16, 19-20, 22-23, 25-26, 28, 46, 63-76, 90-97, 99-102, 104-114, 119-125, 131, 137-138, 140, 143, 145, 150, 152-154, 167-170, 176-178, 188-189, 191-195, 202, 206-208, 213-214

B
Ball Wall Throw, 189-194
Biceps Femoris, 161-163
Bone Fractures, 47
Bone Mineral Density, 47, 51-52

C
Caloric Restriction, 65, 134
Carbohydrate, 11-12, 14, 17, 66-68, 70-72, 74, 135
Cardiac Activity, 12
Cardiovascular Disease, 66, 73, 133, 179, 217
Cecs, 84-85
Coronary Heart Disease, 47, 66, 72, 142, 224
Corticosteroid Injection, 20, 23
Cycle Ergometer, 11, 13, 134, 136-137, 140, 173
Cycling Performance, 11

D
Depression, 17, 94, 153, 173, 217-225
Diastolic Blood Pressure, 95-98
Dietary Intake, 13, 66-67, 74
Doppler Ultrasound, 82, 85, 87-88
Dorsiflexion, 32, 35, 40, 43, 85
Dynamometer, 31-33, 36, 38, 165

E
Emergency Medical Services, 25
Endogenous Opioid, 12, 16
Energy Expenditure, 11, 14-16, 18, 56, 64, 67, 71, 73, 80, 223
Ergogenic Aid, 95, 98-99
Exercise Performance, 11-13, 15-17, 64, 67-69, 73-74, 95, 99, 143, 165
Eye Injuries, 155-160

F
Fatigue, 11, 13-14, 16-17, 31-33, 36-39, 45, 51, 67-68, 74, 80-81, 85, 95, 99, 110, 124, 135, 138, 142, 144, 147, 153, 163, 166, 189-190, 206
Femoral Condyle, 20, 22
Femoral Epicondyle, 19-20, 22

G
Gluteus Maximus, 161, 164-165, 190

H
Haemoglobin, 173-174
Hamstring, 39-46, 129, 164, 196
Heart Rate, 11-15, 17, 73, 95-99, 112, 133-134, 137, 140, 142-143, 153, 176
Hip Flexion, 43-44, 165

I
Iliotibial Band Syndrome, 19-20, 22-24
Infectious Diseases, 172, 176
Injury Prevention, 113-114, 127-128, 131, 189, 195
Injury Reporting, 1-2, 5-7, 9
Isometric Force, 31, 35, 37

K
Knee Injury, 19, 27, 29, 127, 129, 131

L
Leg Muscle, 32, 195
Leg Pain, 82, 84, 88
Ligament Injury, 76, 129
Lipopolysaccharide, 173, 178-180, 187

M
Malfunctions, 5-6
Metabolism, 12-13, 16-18, 37, 64, 66-67, 71-74, 125, 141-143
Methylsulfonylmethane, 179, 181, 183, 185, 187
Micronutrients, 64, 69-70, 75
Mood Disorders, 11
Mri Angiography, 85-87
Muscle Contraction, 31, 36, 40, 195
Muscle Cooling, 31-32, 36
Muscle Force, 31, 36
Muscle Strains, 39, 76-77, 79
Muscular Weakness, 19

N
Nerve Conduction, 31, 36, 38
Nervous System, 40-41, 45, 96, 99, 134, 200, 211
Neurodynamic Sliding, 39-41, 43-46
Nonfatal Injury, 2, 7

O
Ocular Injury, 155-156, 158-160
Oxygen Extraction, 31, 141

P
Paes, 82, 84-88
Parachuting, 1, 6, 8-9
Pathophysiology, 19, 22-23, 126, 200, 206, 215
Pediatrics, 63, 69, 72, 74, 94, 127, 141, 152-153, 203, 215, 217
Plantar Flexion, 32-33, 35, 89
Plantarflexion, 43, 84-86, 88
Psychological Stress, 11, 139

R
Recreational Activity, 1
Resistance Training, 47, 50-53, 95, 166
Respiratory Exchange, 13, 18, 68, 135
Rheumatoid Arthritis, 187
Rhodiola Rosea, 11, 13, 15-17
Risk Taking, 8-9

S
Safety Awareness, 4, 8
Semitendinosus, 161-163
Skydiving, 1-2, 4-10
Sports Activity, 12
Sports Nutrition, 64, 71, 73-74, 125, 187
Stomach, 13, 122-123, 125
Straight Leg Raise Test, 40-41, 44
Substrate Oxidation, 14, 16, 18
Supplementation, 11, 16-17, 67, 69-70, 72-73, 100, 179-182, 184, 187
Surface Electromyography, 161-162, 188-189, 192, 194-195

T
Temperature, 31-33, 35-38, 59, 79, 134, 173, 180